Peripheral Arterial Diseases: Medical and Surgical Problems

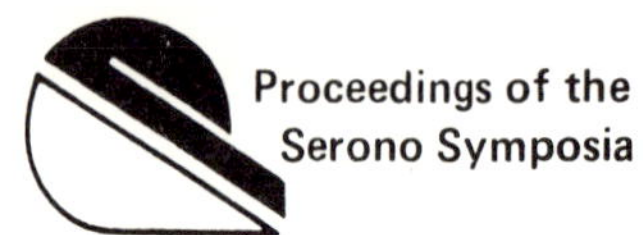

Recent Titles

15. Haemostasis and Thrombosis, *Neri, Serneri and Prentice* 1979
16. Tumor-associated Antigens and their Specific Immune Response, *Spreafico and Arnon* 1979
17. Obesity in Childhood, *Cacciari, Laron and Raiti* 1978
18. The Endocrine Function of the Human Adrenal Cortex, *James, Serio, Giusti and Martini* 1978
19. Neuroendocrinology: Biological and Clinical Aspects, *Polleri and MacLeod* 1979
20A. Emotion and Reproduction, *Carenza and Zichella* 1979
20B. Emotion and Reproduction, *Carenza and Zichella* 1979
21. Research on Steroids Vol. VIII, *Klopper, van der Molen and Sciarra* 1979
22. Clinical Psychoneuroendocrinology in Reproduction, *Carenza, Pancheri and Zichella* 1978
23. Somatomedins and Growth, *Giordana, Van Wyk and Minuto* 1979
24. Immunity and Atherosclerosis, *Constantinides, Pratesi, Cavellero† and Di Perri* 1980
25. Cryptorchidism, *Bierich and Giarola* 1979
26. Medical Complications of Obesity, *Mancini, Lewis and Contaldo* 1979
27. The Immune System: Functions and Therapy of Dysfunctions, *Doris and Eshkol* 1980
28. Obesity: Pathogenesis and Treatment, *Enzi, Crepaldi, Pozza and Renold* 1981
29. Pituitary Microadenomas, *Faglia, Giovanelli and MacLeod* 1980
30. Current Views on Hypoglycemia and Glucagon, *Andreani, Lefebvre and Marks* 1980
31. Fibrinolysis and Urokinase, *Tilsner and Lenau* 1981
32. Problems in Pediatric Endocrinology, *La Cauza and Root* 1980
33. Autoimmune Aspects of Endocrine Disorders, *Pinchera, Doniach, Fenzi and Baschieri* 1981
34. Medical and Surgical Problems of Portal Hypertension, *Orloff, Stipa and Ziparo* 1980
35. The Human Placenta: Proteins and Hormones, *Klopper, Genazzani and Crosignani* 1980
36. Pathophysiology of Puberty, *Cicciari and Prader* 1981
37. Vascular Occlusion: Epidemiological, Pathophysiological and Therapeutic Aspects, *Tesi and Dormandy* 1981
38. Thymus, Thymic Hormones and T Lymphocytes, *Aiuti and Wigzell* 1980
39. The Menopause: Clinical, Endocrinological and Pathophysiological Aspects, *Fioretti, Mattini, Melis and Yen*
40. The "Low T_3 Syndrome", *Hesch* 1981
41. Current Views on Insulin Receptors, *Andreani, De Pirro, Lauro, Olefsky and Roth* 1981
42. The Gonadotropins: Basic Science and Clinical Aspects in Females, *Flamigni and Givens* 1982
43. Medical and Surgical Problems of the Esophagus, *Stipa, Belsey and Moraldi* 1981
44. Peripheral Arterial Diseases: Medical and Surgical Problems, *Stipa and Cavallaro* 1982
45. Immunological Factors in Human Reproduction, *Shulman, Dondero and Nicotra* 1982
46. Markers for Diagnosis and Monitoring of Human Cancer, *Colnaghi, Buraggi and Ghione* 1982
*47. The Genetics of Diabetes Mellitus, *Köbberling and Tattersall*
48. Urokinase: Basic and Clinical Aspects, *Mannucci and D'Angelo* 1982
49. Pituitary Hormones and Related Peptides, *Motta, Zanisi and Piva*
*51. The Endocrines and The Liver, *Langer, Chiandussi, Chopra and Martini*

---

*At the time of going to press these titles were in preparation.

Peripheral Arterial Diseases: Medical and Surgical Problems

Proceedings of the
Serono Symposia, Volume 44

Edited by

S. Stipa and A. Cavallaro

IV Cattedra di Patologia Chirurgica
dell'Università di Roma,
Rome, Italy

1982

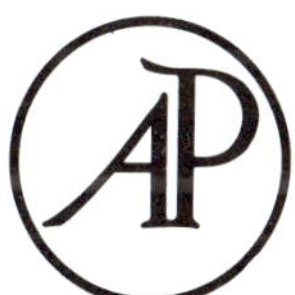

ACADEMIC PRESS

A Subsidiary of Harcourt Brace Jovanovich, Publishers

London New York
Paris San Diego San Francisco São Paulo
Sydney Tokyo Toronto

ACADEMIC PRESS INC. (LONDON) LTD.
24–28 OVAL ROAD
LONDON NW1

U.S. Edition published by
ACADEMIC PRESS INC.
111 FIFTH AVENUE
NEW YORK, NEW YORK 10003

British Library Cataloguing in Publication Data

Peripheral arterial diseases.—(Proceedings of the Serono symposia, ISSN 0308-5503; no. 44)
1. Arteries—Surgery
I. Stipa, Sergio II. Cavallaro, A.
III. Series
617′.413 RD598

ISBN 0-12-671460-6

Typeset by Oxprint Ltd, Oxford
Printed by T. J. Press (Padstow) Ltd., Padstow, Cornwall

CONTRIBUTORS

L.D. ABRAMS Queen Elizabeth Hospital, Birmingham, UK

G. AGRIFOGLIO Institute of Vascular Surgery, University of Milan, Milan, Italy

A. ALESSANDRINI IV Cattedra di Patologia Chirurgica Dell'Università di Roma, Rome, Italy

G. AVELLONE Institute of Clinical Medicine and Medical Therapy of University of Palermo, Palermo, Sicily

A. BASDEVANT Department of Internal Medicine and Nutrition, Hotel Dieu, 1 place du Parvis Notre Dame, F 75004 Paris, France

H.M. BECKER Surgical University Hospital München, Munich, West Germany

S. BHATTACHARYA Department of Cardiovascular Surgery, K.E.M. Hospital and Seth G.S. Medical College, Bombay 400 012, India

S. BONDANINI Cattedra di Chirurgia Vascolare dell'Università di Roma, Rome, Italy

B. BOYCE Research and Development Section, Medical Products Division, W.L. Gore and Associates Inc., Flagstaff, Arizona, USA

D.R. CAMPBELL General and Vascular Surgery, 110 Francis Street, Boston, Mass 02215, USA

J.A. CANNON Research and Development Section, Medical Products Division, W.L. Gore and Associates Inc., Flagstaff, Arizona, USA

A. CARPENTIER Hôpital Broussais, 95 rue Didot, 75014 Paris, France

A. CAVALLARO IV Cattedra di Patologia Chirurgica Dell'Università di Roma, Rome, Italy

S. CISTERNINO IV Cattedra di Patologia Chirurgica dell'Università di Roma, Rome, Italy

P. CORVOL INSERM U 36, 17 rue de Fer à Moulin, 75005 Paris, France

H. DARDIK Vascular Surgical Service, Englewood Hospital, Englewood, New Jersey, USA

G. DAVI' Institute of Clinical Medicine and Medical Therapy of University of Palermo, Palermo, Sicily

A. De GIORGIS VI Cattedra di Patologia Medica dell'Università di Roma, Rome, Italy

D.A. De LAURENTIS University of Pennsylvania School of Medicine, Department of Surgery, Pennsylvania Hospital, 8th and Spruce Streets, Philadelphia, Pennsylvania 19107, USA

L. Di MARZO IV Cattedra di Patologia Chirurgica Dell'Università di Roma, Rome, Italy

J.A. DORMANDY St. James's and St. George's Hospitals, London, UK

L. DROUET Department of Hematology, Hôpital Lariboisiere, 2 rue Ambroise Pare, F 75475 Paris Cedex 10, France

C. DUBOST Clinique Chirurgicale Cardio-Vasculaire, Hôpital Broussais, 96 rue Didot, 75674 Paris Cedex 14, France

E. DUPUY Department of Hematology, Hôpital Lariboisiere, 2 rue Ambroise Pare, F 75475 Paris Cedex 10, France

E.A. EDLINGER Unité de Diagnostic Virologique et Rickettsiales, Institut Pasteur de Paris, Paris, France

V. FARAGLIA Cattedra di Chirurgia Vascolare dell'Università di Roma, Rome, Italy

P. FIORANI Cattedra di Chirurgia Vascolare dell'Università di Roma, Rome, Italy

F. FONTALIRAN Hôpital Boucicaut, Paris, France

L. GABRIELLI Institute of Vascular Surgery, University of Milan, Milan, Italy

M. GAROFALO IV Cattedra di Patologia Chirurgica Dell'Università di Roma, Rome, Italy

J. GAY Hôpital Boucicaut, Paris, France

R. GOTTLOB Abteilung f. Experiment Chirurgie I. Chirurgie University Klinik, Alserstrasse 4, A-1097 Vienna, Austria

C. GUILLAUSSEAU Department of Internal Medicine and Nutrition, Hotel Dieu, 1 place du Parvis Notre Dame, F 75004 Paris, France

P.J. GUILLAUSSEAU Service de Médecine Interne, Hôpital Lariboisière, 2 rue Ambroise Paré, 75475 Paris Cedex 10, France

A. Ter HAAR Division of Transplantation and Vascular Surgery Service, The Johns Hopkins University School of Medicine, 601 North Broadway, Baltimore, Maryland 21205, USA

M. HAIMOV Department of Surgery, Division of Vascular Surgery, Mont Sinai School of Medicine, New York, USA

L.A. HEALEY, The Mason Clinic, Clinical Professor of Medicine, University of Washington, Seattle, Washington, USA

W. HEPP Department of Surgery of the University Ulm, Ulm, West Germany

C.S. HOAR Jr General and Vascular Surgery, 110 Francis Street, Boston, Mass 02215, USA

J.H. JACOBSON II Department of Surgery, Division of Vascular Surgery, Mont Sinai School of Medicine, New York, USA

E. KALOUSTIAN Service de Médecine Interne, Hôpital Lariboisière, 2 rue Ambroise Paré, 75475 Paris Cedex 10, France

A.M. KARMODY Department of Surgery, Vascular Surgery Section, Albany Medical College, Albany, New York, USA

M.D. KELKAR Department of Cardiovascular Surgery, K.E.M. Hospital and Seth G.S. Medical College, Bombay 400 012, India

S.G. KINARE Department of Cardiovascular Surgery, K.E.M. Hospital and Seth G.S. Medical College, Bombay 400 012, India

R.P. LEATHER Department of Surgery, Vascular Surgery Section, Albany Medical College, Albany, New York, USA

R.W. LIGHTFOOT Jr Rheumatology Section, Arthritis Center, Medical College of Wisconsin and Veterans Administration Pilot Rheumatology Project, Wood Veterans Administration Medical Center Milwaukee, Wisconsin, USA

J. LUBETZKI Service de Médecine Interne, Hôpital Lariboisière, 2 rue Ambroise Paré, 75475 Paris Cedex 10, France

E. LUPI-HERRERA Head of Service, National Institute of Cardiology "Ignacio Chavez" Mexico, D.F.

J. MENARD INSERM U 36, 17 rue du Fer à Moulin, 75005 Paris, France

A. MINGOLI IV Cattedra di Patologia Chirurgica Dell'Università di Roma, Rome, Italy

H.D. NAHUM Service de Médecine Interne, Hôpital Lariboisière, 2 rue Ambroise Paré, 75475 Paris Cedex 10, France

S. NOVO Institute of Clinical Medicine and Medical Therapy of University of Palermo, Palermo, Sicily

S.R. PANDAY Department of Cardiovascular Surgery, K.E.M. Hospital and Seth G.S. Medical College, Bombay 400 012, India

G.B. PARULKAR Department of Cardiovascular Surgery, K.E.M. Hospital and Seth G.S. Medical College, Bombay 400 012, India

A.A. PINTO Institute of Clinical Medicine and Medical Therapy of University of Palermo, Palermo, Sicily

H.A. PITT Division of Transplantation and Vascular Surgery Service, The Johns Hopkins University School of Medicine, 601 North Broadway, Baltimore, Maryland 21205, USA

P.F. PLOUIN INSERM U 36, 17 rue du Fer à Moulin, 75005 Paris, France

A.V. POKROVSKY The Bakulev Institute of Cardiovascular Surgery, Moscow, USSR

J.J. RICOTTA Division of Transplantation and Vascular Surgery Service, The Johns Hopkins University School of Medicine, 601 North Broadway, Baltimore, Maryland 21205, USA

R.T. ROLLEY Division of Transplantation and Vascular Surgery Service, The Johns Hopkins University School of Medicine, 601 North Broadway, Baltimore, Maryland 21205, USA

U. RUBERTI Department of Surgery, University of Milan, Milan, Italy

R.B. RUTHERFORD Department of Surgery, University of Colorado Medical Center, 4200 East Ninth Avenue, Denver, Colorado 80220, USA

L.R. SAUVAGE Cardiovascular Reconstruction Division, Bob Hope International Heart Research Institute, The Providence Medical Center, and the Department of Surgery, University of Washington School of Medicine, Seattle, Washington, USA

A. SCIACCA IV Cattedra di Pathologia Medica dell'Università, Policlinico Umberto I 00161, Rome, Italy

V. SCIACCA IV Cattedra di Patologia Chirurgica Dell'Università di Roma, Rome, Italy

S. SEVITT Department of Pathology, Birmingham Accident Hospital, Bath Row, Birmingham 15, UK

D.M. SHAH Department of Surgery, Vascular Surgery Section, Albany Medical College, Albany, New York, USA

S. SHIONOYA Department of Surgery, Nagoya University Branch Hospital, Nagoya, Japan

J.V. SITZMAN Division of Transplantation and Vascular Surgery Service, The Johns Hopkins University School of Medicine, 601 North Broadway, Baltimore, Maryland 21205, USA

R.W. SNYDER USCI C.R. Bard Inc., Box M, Billerica, Massachusetts, 01821, USA

R. SOYER Department of Cardiac Surgery, Hôpital Charles Nicolle, 1 rue Germont, Rouen, France

F. SPEZIALE Cattedra di Chirurgia Vascolare dell'Università di Roma, Rome, Italy

A. STERPETTI IV Cattedra di Patologia Chirurgica Dell'Università di Roma, Rome, Italy

S. STIPA IV Cattedra di Patologia Chirurgica Dell'Università di Roma, Rome, Italy

A. STRANO Institute of Clinical Medicine and Medical Therapy of University of Palermo, Palermo, Sicily

J.P. van der STRICHT Départment de Pathologie Vasculaire à l'Université de Bruxelles, Avenue Henri Jaspar 114, Boite 18, 1060 Brussels, Belgium

D.E. SZILAGYI Department of Surgery, Henry Ford Hospital, 2799 West Grand Boulevard, Detroit, Michigan, 48202, USA

M. TAURINO Cattedra di Chirurgia Vascolare dell'Università di Roma, Rome, Italy

M. THIBONNIER INSERM U 36 17 rue du Fer à Moulin, 75005 Paris, France

R.J.A.M. van DONGEN Department of Surgery, Wilhelminus Gasthuis, University of Amsterdam, The Netherlands

J.F. VOLLMAR Department of Surgery of the University of Ulm, Ulm, West Germany

E.U. VOSS Department of Surgery of the University of Ulm, Ulm, West Germany

A. WARNET Service de Médécine Interne, Hôpital Lariboisière, 2 rue Ambroise Paré, 75475 Paris Cedex 10, France

A.M. WILD Department of Hematology, Hôpital Lariboisière, 2 rue Ambroise Paré, 75475 Paris Cedex 10, France

G.M. WILLIAMS Division of Transplantation and Vascular Surgery Service, The Johns Hopkins University School of Medicine, 601 North Broadway, Baltimore, Maryland 21205, USA

PREFACE

This volume contains the lectures delivered during the International Symposium on Peripheral Arteriopathies held in Rome from May 28th to May 30th 1981.

We welcomed the opportunity of gathering, from several countries, well-known experts who, on the basis of their vast personal experience, are at the top of their chosen fields. In the vast field of vascular pathology, these were selected in relation to their continuing and growing interest as well as to the real or sometimes fictitious — but always exciting — controversies which they tend to create, at meetings and congresses or in discussions in hospital or between practitioners.

The number of vascular patients looking for medical and surgical care is steadily growing; medical practice in this field is, after many years, emerging from the narrow confines of specialized centres and entering the general medical and surgical wards. An increasing number of surgeons and internists, as well as of young residents, need clear data and advice which will enable them to adopt the correct approach to the vascular patient.

Bearing in mind what is said above, we chose the following topics for discussion:

— aneurysms of the abdominal aorta;
— femoro-popliteal and femoro-tibial grafting;
— chronic non-degenerative arteriopathies.

The book was therefore divided into three sections. The first section deals extensively with the problems related to aneurysms of the abdominal aorta, including aetiology, diagnosis, operative indications, surgical techniques and results in elective as well as emergency conditions, operative procedures in high-risk patients and in unusual anatomic situations. A brief survey of aortic traumas and dissections completes this section.

The second section is based on a stimulating survey of the different techniques and materials actually used for femoro-distal grafting. The theoretical advantages and the practical results of each of them are thoroughly described and discussed.

The third section contains the latest developments on chronic non-degenerative arteriopathies, with the clinical standpoint being the predominant one and with special emphasis on Buerger's disease and Takayasu'a arteritis; the controversial role of Rickettsiae is debated. The book comes to a close with a survey on actual views regarding the peculiarities of lower limb arteriopathies in diabetics.

Thanks to the enthusiastic attendance of the lecturers and to the very high quality of their reports, the Symposium was successful; we hope that this book will meet an equally favourable consensus from the wider audience to whom it is, in our intention, aimed.

January 1982

S. STIPA
A. CAVALLARO

CONTENTS

ETIOLOGY OF AORTOILIAC ANEURYSMS

R. B. Rutherford

Department of Surgery, University of Colorado Medical Center, Denver, Colorado, USA

INTRODUCTION

Aneurysms are, in simplest terms, a permanent localized dilatation of an artery or, by extension, an arterial substitute or graft. The aortoiliac segment of the arterial tree is the most commonly affected and, though its predilection for the arteriosclerotic variety of aneurysm is clearly responsible for this, it has also been the site of almost every other type of aneurysm, and therefore provides ample opportunity to discuss the etiology of aneurysms in general.

The factors that contribute to aneurysm formation may be divided into two basic categories, "mural" and "mechanical". The former pertains to the intrinsic strength and structural integrity of the arterial wall, the latter to the mechanical stresses imposed on that wall. The relative contributions of these two factors to the development of the more common types of aneurysms are summarized in Table I. In almost all aneurysms, a mural weakness or defect is primarily to blame. In fact, the only aneurysms which develop in a normal arterial segment, and therefore can be blamed primarily on mechanical factors, are the so-called post-stenotic aneurysms, such as seen in association with coarctation, complete cervical rib, aortic and pulmonary valvular stenoses and popliteal artery entrapment. The fusiform dilatation seen in abdominal coarctation is the only example of this type involving the abdominal aorta. The normal aortic wall, with its interwoven layers of collagen reticulum and elastic fibres is superbly designed to resist the relentless stress placed on it by incessant pulsatile flow at systemic arterial pressures.

Serono Symposium No. 44, "Peripheral Arterial Diseases: Medical and Surgical Problems", edited by S. Stipa and A. Cavallaro, 1982. Academic Press, London and New York.

Table 1. The relative contributions of mural weaknesses or defects and mechanical stresses to the development of common forms of aneurysms.

Type of aneurysm	Presence and type of mural lesion	Abnormal mechanical stresses
Post-stenotic	None	Always
Arteriosclerotic	Diffuse weakness	Often
Anastomotic	Focal defect	Sometimes
Graft, prosthesis	Diffuse weakness or focal defect	Sometimes
Pregnancy related	Diffuse weakness	Usually
Dissecting	Diffuse weakness and focal defect	Often
Congenital	Diffuse weakness	None
Infected	Focal weakness	None
Traumatic	Focal defect	None

This is attested to by the frequency with which aneurysms have developed in every arterial substitute man has used and in every circumstance in which the integrity of the arterial wall has been violated and inadequately repaired. In every type of aneurysm other than post-stenotic, a diffuse or focal weakness or full-thickness defect can be incriminated. Although the normal strains of the systemic circulation are such that no additional abnormal stresses are required for aneurysm formation, these are nevertheless present and contributory in some types of aneurysms, specifically arteriosclerotic and dissecting aneurysms and those related to pregnancy.

That the wear and tear degenerative process called arteriosclerosis does not result more commonly in aneurysm formation is perhaps more remarkable than when it occasionally does. By the same token, the arterial wall's resistance to infection is more remarkable than its being a focus of spirochetal infection or seemingly a favored nesting ground for *Salmonella*. Furthermore, mature saccular aneurysms due to a specific congenital weakness are extremely rare, possibly because such weaknesses allow little chance for chronic arterial dilation, as attested to by the significantly greater risk of spontaneous rupture or acute dissection in such conditions. Finally, it will hopefully be appreciated that, while we understandably must focus on the specific mural lesions that initiate aneurysm development in the vast majority of cases, we should not lose sight of the fact that it may be the mechanical factors that determine the rate of development and the ultimate risk of rupture of these aneurysms.

Classification of Aneurysms

It is not possible to devise a classification of aneurysm based on a single criterion which will completely satisfy the clinician's desire for a scheme in which the groups are distinguishable from each other by their unique origin, special clinical features and predictable natural history and which, therefore, aids in diagnosis and directs treatment. However, those based on form, size, location and structure have less merit in this regard than one based on etiology. The latter also has the advantage of tradition, being the framework upon which most of the factual data in the literature have been reported. It may be noted that the four broad etiologic categories of aneurysms listed in Table II are the same basic categories, with the notable exception of neoplastic (and the expansion of "traumatic" to include other "mechanical" forms), that pathologists apply to all diseases. However, such a broad etiologic classification does not accommodate a unique form like dissecting aneurysms while including several distinct forms under a single etiologic heading. Therefore, to accommodate practical usage, the discussion that follows, though primarily organized along etiological lines, also focuses on those sub-categories of aneurysms whose clinical characteristics hold sufficient meaning and uniqueness to warrant individual consideration, specifically, post-stenotic aneurysms, arteriosclerotic aneurysms, anastomotic and graft aneurysms, "congenital" aneurysms, dissecting aneurysms, aneurysms related to pregnancy, infected or mycotic aneurysms and traumatic aneurysms.

Currently over 90% of all aortoiliac aneurysms are arteriosclerotic in origin, with the other types contributing from less than 1–5% each, the next most common type being anastomotic and graft aneurysms (Table III). A similar distribution is observed for peripheral aneurysms with perhaps a somewhat greater incidence of traumatic and post-stenotic aneurysms. In contrast, thoracic aortic aneurysms include a significantly higher percentage of dissecting, mycotic (luetic) and traumatic aneurysms, although arteriosclerotic aneurysms still predominate. Only in the splanchnic circulation, where pregnancy related, fibrodysplastic and mycotic aneurysms are relatively common, is an overwhelming preponderance of arteriosclerotic aneurysms not the rule.

POST-STENOTIC ANEURYSMS AND THE ROLE OF MECHANICAL FACTORS IN ANEURYSM DEVELOPMENT

Post-stenotic aneurysms are the only type of aneurysm in which no preexisting mural weakness or defect can be implicated, so that aneurysm formation can be attributed solely to mechanical factors. Halstead, in considering the pathogenesis of subclavian artery aneurysms associated with complete cervical rib, was fascinated by this very circumstance and he and Mont Reid conducted a series of experiments, later continued by Emil Holman (1954), to confirm the role of arterial narrowing in aneurysm formation. They succeeded in creating fusiform aneurysms beyond artificially created arterial stenoses in experimental animals and, in correlative clinical studies, described in detail the clinical features of three major examples of this type of aneurysm: thoracic outlet compression, coarctation of the aorta and pulmonary valvular stenosis (Holman, 1954). Post-stenotic aneurysms have sporadically been reported in a wide variety of other circumstances in which the artery has been bound down or impinged upon by some abnormally situated bony, ligamentous, tendinous of fibrous structure. Entrapment of the popliteal artery by an abnormal insertion of the medial head of the gastrocnemius muscle

Table II. Arterial aneurysms: classification schemes.

Etiology	*Degenerative*	*Inflammatory*	*Mechanical*	*Congenital*
	Arteriosclerosis	Syphilitic	Post-stenotic	Cerebral (berry)
	Medial necrosis	Bacterial	Traumatic	Ehlers-Danlos syndrome
	Fibrodysplasia	Viral?	Anastomotic	Marfan's syndrome
	Pregnancy related	Noninfectious?	Prosthetic	Other?
	Graft			

Form	Saccular	Fusiform	Dissecting		
Size	Macroaneurysms	Microaneurysms			
Location	Central	Peripheral	Splanchnic	Renal	Cerebral
Structure	True	False			

Table III. Aortoiliac aneurysms: distribution by type.

200 Consecutive cases		
Arteriosclerotic, infrarenal	89.5%	91%
Arteriosclerotic, suprarenal	1.5%	
Anastomotic (± enteric fistula)	4.0%	5%
Prosthetic deteriorization	1.0%	
Traumatic	1.5%	
Post-stenotic	1.0%	
Infected (no luetic)	1.0%	
Pregnancy related	0.5%	
Congenital	0%	

is one such example. Similarity between this circumstance and popliteal aneurysms developing beyond the sharp tendinous foramen in the abductor magnus muscle known as Hunter's canal, has led to the suggestion that the latter should not be simply dismissed as being arteriosclerotic in origin. The not infrequent location of arteriosclerotic aneurysms in close proximity to arteriosclerotic narrowings has evoked similar speculations (see below). Unfortunately, it is rarely possible to completely dissociate "mural" from "mechanical" factors in most other forms of aneurysms. The only pure post-stenotic aneurysms involving the abdominal aorta occurs in association with abdominal coarctation. When encountered in childhood or early adult life, they are usually simply fusiform dilatations. Later, however, they may become more saccular and have secondary atherosclerotic changes.

Classically, post-stenotic aneurysms have been explained on the basis of a combination of Bernoulli's theorem and LaPlace's law. Acceleration of flow past a point of narrowing creates slower flow lateral to the jet stream beyond the stenosis and increased lateral pressure according to Bernoulli's theorem. This increased pressure, in time, leads to weakening and dilation of a previously normal arterial segment. As critics of this explanation have pointed out, this law of fluid dynamics was developed from the study of steady state flow of Newtonian fluids in rigid walled, cylindrical conduits, and cannot be directly applied to the pulsatile flow of blood through expansile arteries. But, it would seem that similar physical laws must govern the latter situation and explain aneurysmal development (Bruns *et al.*, 1959; Kline *et al.* 1962; Roach, 1979). Certainly, the conversion of normal laminar flow to high velocity turbulent flow must release considerable kinetic energy. With pulsatile flow in expansile arteries, there is a cyclical change in the balance between luminal and mural forces, as the kinetic energy of systole is converted into potential energy by the expanding arterial wall and then the elastic arteries recoil and propel the blood onward during diastole. Should the lateral forces be chronically increased, there will eventually be a fatiguing of the elastic and connective tissue elements in the arterial wall which oppose these forces and a secondary mural weakness will develop and inevitably lead to dilatation. It is likely that the initial fatiguing is due more to vibration than pressure (Stehbens, 1979).

Once dilatation begins, LaPlace's law, "tension (lateral pressure) in the wall of a hollow viscus varies directly with its radius ($T = Pr$)" has been invoked to explain an acceleration of the dilatation process and the increasing risk of rupture with increasing diameter. Again, critics have pointed out that this law should be applied only to very thin-walled structures, i.e. soap bubbles rather than aortas. Since aneurysms rupture when the tangential stress within their walls exceeds the tensile strength of the wall at any point, a formula for tangential stress within the walls of the cylinder might be more appropriate. According to Peterson *et al.* (1960) this is given by $r = Pr_i/\gamma$, where P is the pressure within the cylinder, r_i is the internal radius and γ is the wall thickness. If one uses this formula, an example taken from Sumner (1977), to compare the tangential stress in the walls of a cylinder with the typical dimensions of the abdominal aorta (2-cm diameter, 0.2-cm wall thickness) with that following dilatation to a diameter of 6 cm (and a commensurate thinning of the arterial wall to 0.06 cm), it is apparent that this threefold increase in diameter increases the tangential stress in the wall of the cylinder by a factor of 12.

It would seem clear then that dilatation can occur in a previously normal arterial segment by increased lateral force applied to its wall just beyond a stenosis and that once dilatation begins, other physical laws contribute to perpetuate and accelerate this process. Furthermore, a progressive weakening of the elastic and connective tissue elements and a thinning of the arterial wall add to this vicious cycle. Finally, if dilatation or aneurysm formation occurs for any other cause than stenosis, these same forces come into play for the neck of the aneurysm then acts as a relative stenosis. Thus the mechanical factors identified for the post-stenotic aneurysms ultimately contribute to the development of all aneurysms.

ARTERIOSCLEROTIC ANEURYSMS

As the most common type of aneurysms in almost every location but the splanchnic circulation, arteriosclerotic aneurysms should present the best opportunity for defining responsible pathogenetic mechanisms. However, this does not seem to be the case. There are several reasons for this. Little can be learned from the pathologic study of a thinned out arterial wall and the opportunity for study at earlier stages is limited. Also there seems to have been a relative lack of interest in this aspect of arteriosclerosis in contra-distinction to the atheromatous process. In addition, there is a lack of a good experimental model for arteriosclerotic aneurysms. Many of these limitations now finally seem to be being overcome (*vide infra*).

Many, if not most authors, consider this type of aneurysm simply the result of a wear-and-tear aging process which naturally goes hand in hand with atherosclerosis, with dilatation occurring only in areas not thickened and hardened by the latter process. In contrast to the well-documented evolution of the atheromatous plaque (intimal trauma, platelet aggregation, trans-formation of the myogenic cell, secondary lipid degeneration, cholesterol deposition etc.), discussions of the aneurysmal lesion usually center around histological descriptions of the end-stage lesion. The viewpoint that the elastic fibers of the arterial wall eventually fatigue, fracture and disintegrate under the stresses of the systemic arterial circulation is supported by the histological findings of transverse fracture and relative paucity of elastic lamellae. There is also depletion of the muscular and collagen constituents of the media, but how much of this is primary and how much is secondary to thinning and stretching out of the arterial wall is problematic. The intramural and perivascular collagen formation and calcium deposition, however, are clearly secondary changes.

The unanswered question is still, is there something different about the walls of aneurysmal vessels that determine this end result rather than atheromatous plaque formation? Collagen is the structural fiber principally responsible for the strength of the arterial wall while the elastic fibers absorb and repel the forces of systole. Sumner *et al.* (1970) have studied the stress-strain characteristics and collagen-elastin content of arteriosclerotic aneurysms and the arterial wall proximally and distally, in comparison with the same levels of the aortoiliac segment in atherosclerotic controls. Aneurysms were less compliant, but their elastic moduli did not differ significantly from arteriosclerotic controls. The collagen and elastin percentages were lower and the collagen to elastin ratios were higher in aneurysms suggesting loss of elastin more than collagen. However, these and other changes may represent a dilutional effect by nonfunctional elements (mural thrombus and periadventitial thickening) since total contents were not decreased and the immediately adjacent segments were not significantly different from the same locations in arteriosclerotic controls. These studies suggest these changes were secondary (depletional), not primary or causative. However, the aneurysmal specimens studied were all small and associated with typical arteriosclerotic occlusive disease. None were from large ectatic aneurysms unassociated with arteriosclerotic narrowing.

As expressed in the European literature, there are two distinctly different forms of "arteriosclerotic" aneurysms, one associated with classical arteriosclerotic occlusive lesions and the other in an ectatic tortuous arterial tree with minimal atheromatous change. The British call these "dilating" and "stenosing" aneurysms. Actually the dilating type was described earlier in the French literature by Leriche in 1925 and has subsequently come to be called "Dolicho-Mega-arteries" or "media dystrophies ectasiantes" (Descotes *et al.*, 1976), literally aneurysmal dystrophy of the media. These ectatic or dilating aneurysms differ considerably from the stenotic or sclerosing variety not only in their morphological characteristics but in their natural history, as is expressed in risk of rupture and of thromboembolic and other complications. Martin (1978) has noted statistically significant differences in the frequency of Rh negative blood type (higher) and lipoprotein abnormalities (lower in the "dilating" type). Such observations perpetuate the conviction that there is an inherent difference in the arterial wall of such patients even though definitive studies of the histochemical and/or physical properties of the arterial walls of the two types of aneurysms have not been reported.

Even the pathogenesis of the truly arteriosclerotic or "stenosing" type of aneurysm remains unsettled. Benjamin (quoted by Bergan and Yao, 1974) has theorized that occlusion of the nutritive vessels of the arterial wall causes the degenerative changes which lead to aneurysm formation. He showed that vasovasorum were fewer in number in the abdominal than in the thoracic aorta and speculated that a characteristic finding in abdominal aortic aneurysms, occlusion of the lumbar arteries (which supply the vasovasorum) is primarily responsible.

It has been suggested that the differences between atheromatous and aneurysmal change may be more a matter of degree of depth of the mural involvement, with the atheromatous change focused primarily in the intima and the aneurysmal change focused primarily in the media and its surrounding elastic lamellae. In this regard, Zarins (1980) has performed an interesting experiment in rabbits on an atherogenic diet. By applying three tight ligatures to the aorta for 15 min, a necrosing injury was produced. If the injury was extensive with destruction of the media, an aneurysm resulted with no plaquing, but if there was no significant medial injury, an atheromatous plaque resulted. This suggested to them that the major determinant of aneurysm versus plaque formation was the medial rather than the intimal injury.

The characteristic location of arteriosclerotic aneurysms in the arterial tree has also been a stimulus for conjecture regarding their development. It has been pointed out that aneurysms seem to occur in relatively unfixed segments between branches or bifurcations and it has been proposed (Malcolm, 1957) that abnormal standing waves or resonance is created by these points of fixation. It is assumed that these eventually cause localization of fatigue and degeneration of the structural elements of the artery at their characteristic locations. A significant parallel observation is that the sites of predilection for arteriosclerotic hardening and narrowing occur at the fixation points (bifurcations and branchings) and thus explains the alternating localization of the two processes. In rebuttal, it might be said that aneurysmal degeneration could only occur away from areas thickened and hardened by arteriosclerosis. In a typical arteriosclerotic aneurysm involving the aortoiliac segment, there is a relatively free area between the renal arteries and the first lumbar arteries. At the latter point atherosclerotic thickening and plaque formation begin or increase and involve primarily the posterior aspect of the aorta down to the bifurcation. At the bifurcation of the aorta and again at the bifurcation of the iliac arteries, as well as above at the "neck" of the aneurysm, the artery is thick and strong circumferentially, if not a little narrowed and sclerotic and it is between these three points of relative constriction that the aneurysmal sac balloons out anteriorly and laterally. Another pertinent observation is that aneurysms tend to develop on the inside of curves or lines of flexion in the arterial tree. Aneurysm formation is anterior in the aortoiliac segment and posterior in the popliteal segment, which becomes significant if one considers the fact that most of our lives are spent seated with our thighs and knees flexed. However, this can be viewed in a slightly different perspective by pointing out that the atherosclerotic changes develop on the outside of these same flexion curves allowing aneurysmal development only on the inside of the curves where the walls are not thickened.

Until many of the above speculations are supported by more definitive studies, the least that can be said is that arteriosclerotic aneurysms are an expression of wear-and-tear degenerative changes which may occur with time in response to the relentless stresses of systemic arterial circulation. As such, one should expect these changes to be more common in hypertensive individuals and more extensive in any individuals in whom there is a constitutional weakness of the structural elements of the arterial wall. Furthermore, it is natural that these aneurysmal changes should coexist with, and have a similar general distribution as, arteriosclerotic occlusive disease and that the latter may limit the extent of and determine the points of maximal development of these aneurysms.

ANASTOMOTIC AND GRAFT ANEURYSMS

When grafts are inserted to replace or bypass occluded or aneurysmal segments of the arterial tree, aneurysms can form at the junction between graft and host artery as well as in the body of the graft itself. The former, "anastomotic aneurysm", is essentially a false aneurysm containing no elements of the original arterial wall. It is, in essence, a connective tissue sac protruding through a separation between graft and host artery because the fibrous capsule surrounding the anastomosis lacks the inherent strength to withstand the mechanical stresses of systemic arterial flow. Anything that causes a separation between graft and host artery, therefore, can produce an anastomotic aneurysm (Moore, 1977). The use of silk sutures was once a major cause of this complication because it was not realized that silk was actually biodegradable and would absorb and/or fragment (Moore, 1970). The necrotizing effect of an infection involving the suture line, even if it is eventually controlled, may be responsible for some anastomotic aneurysms, particularly those located in the groin area. Anastomotic leaks with contained hematoma can lead to a false aneurysm in exactly the same manner described in more detail below for traumatic false aneurysms. Anastomotic breakdown is encouraged to occur if inadequate suture purchases are taken in the edge of the artery in constructing the anastomosis. This technical error is now considered one of the major causes of anastomotic aneurysms and is particularly likely to be a factor if the anterior surface of the artery is thinned out (pre-aneurysmal change) or is weakened by concomitant endarterectomy. Finally, even with proper suture technique, anastomotic aneurysms can develop because of abnormal mechanical forces that come to bear on the suture line. With the motion produced by pulsatile blood flow, significant shearing forces can develop at an interface between areas of different compliance. Such differences obviously exist at the junction between any graft and host artery but major "compliance mismatches" are assured if the graft material is particularly rigid, as in the case of a woven graft, or if the artery is particularly weak, as in the case of early aneurysmal degeneration or after endarterectomy (Edwards, 1978). Since most anastomoses are constructed on the side of the artery opposite the arteriosclerotic plaquing, it is also the side most subject to aneurysmal change. Furthermore, the incidence of anastomotic aneurysm is greater when the grafting procedure has been performed for aneurysmal rather than occlusive disease. The shearing forces are made worse by the additional graft motion produced by joint flexion, by hypertension and by the turbulence produced by large anastomotic angles (Berguer and Higgins, 1976). The above etiologic factors are reflected in statistics regarding the incidence of anastomotic aneurysms (Szilagyi *et al.*, 1975). For example, they are much more common in the femoral position, reflecting not only the greater shearing forces produced by joint flexion but also the higher incidence of perigraft hematoma and wound infection and the routine use of end-to-side anastomoses. The incidence of anastomotic aneurysms appears to have been decreased by the abandonment of silk sutures and the woven graft in peripheral arterial reconstructions and possibly also by the routine use of prophylactic antibiotics.

GRAFT ANEURYSMS

Aneurysm formation has developed in the body of almost every arterial substitute used to date. Aneurysmal development was the main stimulus for abandoning arterial homografts. Subsequently, heterografts, or more specifically ficin-digested formaldehyde-treated bovine carotid arteries, also showed a propensity for aneurysm formation (Dale and Lewis, 1976). More recently, the similarly modified human umbilical cord vein graft has had to be reinforced with a circumferential Dacron mesh to avoid aneurysmal development.

Arterial autografts do not become aneurysmal, but vein autografts placed in the systemic arterial tree do. Thinned walled deep veins are not used for arterial substitutes because they essentially all develop aneurysmal dilatation, but the saphenous vein, because it lies unprotected in the superficial tissues and must withstand increased gravitational pressures, is thicker walled and after implantation becomes even thicker by increased connective tissue deposition. Nevertheless, when used in extremity arterial reconstruction, it has a reported incidence of 4% aneurysmal development (Szilagyi *et al.*, 1973). In addition, when placed in the aortorenal position where the flows and pressures are generally higher, the aneurysmal rate is closer to 8%. This has been partly attributed, though without proof, to forceful dilation of the vein graft during its removal and preparation for implantation. This is no longer common practice but there have been no reports as yet reflecting any decrease in aneurysmal development.

Prosthetic grafts have been made of a number of fabrics including Vinyon, Nylon, Orlon, Teflon and Dacron. The first three of these soon developed a number of complications, not the least of which was loss of tensile strength and aneurysm formation. Teflon has been shown to maintain its tensile strength after implantation best of all but has lost its popularity as a "fabric" graft primarily because of its lack of "seating" in the tissues. The overwhelming preference today for prosthetic grafts is Dacron. Woven Dacron grafts achieve hemostasis without pre-clotting and have good patency rates in all aortic locations, but have generally given way to knitted Dacron grafts in the abdominal aorta and more peripheral locations. One reason was that knitted Dacron is more compliant than woven Dacron and thus less likely to contribute to anastomotic aneurysm formation. In addition, the knitted fabric has larger interstices through which capillary ingrowth could reach and nourish and secure the neointima. In an effort to improve this ingrowth, knitted grafts were made progressively more "porous" until reports began to appear of diffuse dilation or fragmentation and aneurysm formation (Ottlinger *et al.*, 1976). Currently the rate of prosthetic aneurysms development is reported to be as high as 4% (Dale, 1979) and has been reported in the following prosthesis: Cooley knitted, Vascolour-D, USCI ultralightweight, Wesolowsky weavenit, DeBakey standard weight knitted, Cooley double velour. Adoption of a velour construction and a "tighter" warp knit may have solved this problem but it takes several years to determine the rate of aneurysmal degeneration. Even the relatively "solid" expanded Polytetrafluoroethylene grafts, as originally constructed, were reported to have a significant incidence of anerysm formation (Campbell *et al.*, 1976). This has since been combated by either adding an outer helical wrap or increasing the graft wall thickness by 50%.

CONGENITAL ANEURYSMS

Is is usually assumed that if an aneurysm appears at an early age, and there is no history of trauma, systemic infection or pregnancy, it must have developed because of some inherent weakness of the arterial wall. The term congenital aneurysm is obviously a misnomer since it is the arterial wall weakness rather than the aneurysm itself which is present at birth. It is often difficult in such aneurysms to identify the responsible congenital factor. Ehlers-Danlos syndrome is often suspected because it is a well-known inherited form of connective tissue weakness. Most reports implicate collagen, probably a defect in cross-linkage, but others suggest that elastin may also be defective (Burnett *et al.*, 1973). Of the six different forms of Ehlers-Danlos syndrome, only the gravis, ecchymotic and mitis types have been associated with aneurysm formation. The gravis type is by far the most common but even in this type there are more dissecting than saccular aneurysms and more thoracic and carotid than abdominal aortic aneurysms (Beighton, 1968). Aneurysms are rare with the ecchymotic type which usually produces spontaneous rupture and hemorrhage. The least common, the mitis type, has been reported to be associated with aneurysms. It is noteworthy because it is the only type that can present in this manner without other obvious stigmata, i.e. hypermobile joints, gaping scars and frequent bruising and bleeding (Burnett *et al.*, 1973). Thus, it would seem that few "congenital" saccular aneurysms are attributable to Ehlers-Danlos syndrome probably because the very nature of the connective tissue defect in the arterial wall makes gradual dilation and saccular aneurysm formation much less likely than spontaneous rupture or acute dissection.

Marfan's syndrome is another inherited form of connective tissue weakness associated with aneurysm formation. The actual basis for this condition is as yet unknown. Afflicted individuals usually have hypermobile joints, lenticular ectopy, aortic and mitral valve insufficiency and dissecting aneurysms of the thoracic aorta. However, not only do almost one-half of the chronic dissecting aneurysms beginning in the thoracic aorta eventually involve the abdominal aorta, but there have been reports of patients with Marfan's syndrome presenting with separate saccular aneurysms of the abdominal aorta as well as of the carotid artery (Killip and Holmquist, 1961). This condition will be discussed further in regard to dissecting aneurysms.

As stated earlier there may be inherent differences between the "dilating" and "stenosing" type of arteriosclerotic aneurysms, but to-date no specific histochemical or physical abnormalities have been demonstrated for the "dilating" type nor do these aneurysms appear at an early age. In the final analysis, most saccular aortic aneurysms occurring in childhood or early adult life cannot be explained on the basis of known defects in connective tissue. Although some as yet unrecognized inherited defect in the connective tissue may be responsible for some, the others are probably due to either unrecognized trauma or inflammatory disease. For example, it has only been recently recognized that Kawasaki's disease (mucocutaneous lymph node syndrome) can not only result in coronary artery aneurysms but aneurysms elsewhere (Takao *et al.*, 1974). This, or some other forms of focal arteritis, could weaken the arterial wall sufficiently to result in aneurysm formation.

ANEURYSMS ASSOCIATED WITH PREGNANCY

Another type of aneurysm that may appear during early adult life and is associated with a connective tissue weakness is the aneurysm which develops in association with pregnancy. Whenever such aneurysms present during pregnancy, it is usually with rupture and exsanguinating hemorrhage, resulting in a high (65%) mortality. One of the most common locations for these aneurysms is the splenic artery. Of 60 splenic artery aneurysms reported by Stanley and Fry (1974) eight were due to fibrodysplasia, six to portal hypertension and three were inflammatory. However, 35, of the 43 in whom no known etiology could be invoked, were women and 40% of these had had six or more pregnancies. The parity of the group was almost twice the national average. Pedowitz and Pertell (1957), in a review of all reports of aneurysms presenting in association with pregnancy, listed 35 splenic, ten renal and five iliac aneurysms. Interestingly, these are all known sites of occurrence of fibrodysplasia, an arteriopathy which has a predilection for females. However, none of these aneurysms were typical of the small aneurysms reported in association with fibrodysplastic stenotic lesions. The same report also included 75 aortic aneurysms, 48 dissecting and 27 saccular. Whereas most of these aortic aneurysms were thoracic in location, some were abdominal and saccular. Thoracic and abdominal saccular aneurysms in childbearing women were, until recently, presumed to be due to unrecognized syphilis, but it is now clear that pregnancy can lead to changes that weaken the arterial wall and, under the increased hemodynamic stresses of pregnancy and/or partuition, lead to spontaneous rupture, dissection and even saccular aneurysm formation. Those aneurysms that do not rupture during pregnancy can present later in life, often with secondary arteriosclerotic changes that causes them to be mislabeled again. Manalo-Estrella and Barker (1967) described decreased acid mucopolysaccarides, fragmentation of reticular fibers and loss of the normal corrugated configuration of elastic fibers in the aortic walls of 16 patients dying during pregnancy of other causes. These changes were not seen in 12 nonpregnant controls of similar age. They also noted that similar changes had previously been described in both pregnant and progesterone-injected experimental animals. While it would seem that such changes, associated with the increased stresses of pregnancy and partuition, can result in either dissecting or saccular aneurysms, its true incidence and the reasons only a certain few develop this complication remain obscure.

DISSECTING ANEURYSMS

Not a distinct etiologic group, dissecting aneurysms deserve separate comment because of their unique form and the unusual etiologic factors which may be involved. It has already been mentioned that aortic changes developing during pregnancy and those observed in association with inherited connective tissue disorders such as Ehlers-Danlos and Marfan's syndromes can result in the development of dissecting aneurysms. In addition, the classic pathologic lesion of dissecting aneurysms, the cystic medial necrosis of Erdheim, is not always demonstrable in the remaining cases. This leaves a significant number of individuals with dissecting aneurysm in whom no specific cause of lesion can be identified. Most of these patients are older and hypertensive and most of such dissections in fact occur during a period of uncontrolled hypertension. The most likely explanation in such cases is that a transverse tear in the inner lining of the aorta occurs during a hypertensive crisis and then dissection is allowed to develop in the same plane in the outer media which vascular surgeons take advantage of in performing an endarterectomy. This view is supported by the lack of differences in histological findings in 83 aortas which had been dissected and 20 hypertensive controls without dissection (Leonard and Hasleton, 1979). An interesting animal model for this type of dissecting aneurysm is found in certain strains of domestic turkey (Collins, 1971) in which there is a significant spontaneous incidence of dissecting aneurysm and probably also periodic hypertension. This incidence can be increased by giving beta aminoproprionitrile and can be decreased by adding reserpine to the feed. In fact, it was this latter observation which led to the current noroperative approach to dissecting aneurysms, i.e. antihypertensive agents and drugs which decrease the cardiac afterload.

TRAUMATIC ANEURYSMS

Traumatic aneurysms are the classic example of a false aneurysm and demonstrate the propensity of a full thickness, focal defect in the arterial wall to lead to a saccular aneurysm even when no abnormal mechanical stresses are involved. In penetrating arterial injuries, when hemorrhage is contained by surrounding tissues, the hematoma may continue to communicate directly through the arterial wall defect with the bloodstream. If this situation persists, the hematoma will be converted into an aneurysm sac by lysis and/or compression of its contents by the pulsatile stream which communicates with it. The risk of rupture is naturally greatest before the restraining surrounding tissues have matured into a definitive sac, but the lack of any true elements of the arterial wall in the aneurysm sac will nevertheless encourage continued enlargement and symptomatic presentation.

Traumatic aneurysms can also occur with nonpenetrating trauma and the best-known example is the traumatic thoracic aortic aneurysm. In this situation a linear tear occurs in the thoracic aorta near the ligamentum arteriosum where the mobile and fixed segments of the thoracic aorta merge and which become the focus of high shearing forces during decelerating injuries (Wilson *et al.*, 1978). It is interesting to note, from an etiologic viewpoint, that although there is a linear tear in the thoracic aorta similar to that occurring with dissecting aneurysms, the aneurysm that results in this instance is a saccular rather than a dissecting aneurysm, ostensibly because of the absence of significant degenerative changes.

INFECTED OR MYCOTIC ANEURYSMS

Though infected aneurysms share an obvious microbial common denominator, they represent a diverse variety of etiologic causes (Wilson *et al.*, 1978). In some the infection is "intravascular" or bloodborne; in others it is "extravascular" (i.e. introduced from the outside). The most common extravascular type of infected aneurysm results from a penetrating wound which introduces contamination at the arterial puncture site and/or into the adjacent hematoma. It is one of the earliest forms of aneurysm encountered by physicians and, during the era in which blood-letting was practised without an understanding of sepsis, this type of aneurysm was almost as common as syphilitic aneurysms. In recent decades we have experienced a resurgence of this type of aneurysm, primarily as a result of the increasingly invasive nature of modern medical practice and, unfortunately, our growing drug culture. Except for penetrating injuries to the abdominal aorta which are contaminated by associated bowel injuries, this form of infected aneurysm does not occur in the aortoiliac segment.

The second form of extravascular infected aneurysm, and one which is commonly represented in this location, is the infected anastomotic aneurysm. Although this is, in other locations, presumed to have originated by contamination at the time of surgery, the aortic location is more commonly the result of erosion of an anastomic aneurysm into the duodenum and less likely the result of a paraprosthetic infection. A third type results from a contiguous extravascular infection. In this situation there is no penetrating wound or anastomotic defect. Its extreme rarity attests to the remarkable ability of the arterial wall to resist extravascular infection in the absence of traumatic or surgical defects.

The least common intravascular type of infected aneurysm is the infection of a pre-existing aneurysm. Even though diseased arteries are more commonly infected during systemic sepsis than normal arteries, this type of aneurysm is still relatively rare. It is often suspected because of inflammatory reaction around an abdominal aortic aneurysm or the suspicious liquifaction of its contents. Routine cultures are positive in as high as 15% but clinical infection occurs in less than 2% of arteriosclerotic aneurysms of the abdominal aorta, a remarkable low incidence considering the frequency of both atheromatous aneurysms and bacteremic infections (Ernst *et al.*, 1977). It appears this complication requires either an infectious agent with a particular affinity for arterial walls or prolonged sepsis with relatively virulent organisms, two circumstances which are a primary cause of the two remaining intravascular types of infected aneurysms.

The incidence of "cryptogenic mycotic" aneurysms secondary to microbial arteritis has greatly decreased since the advent of antibiotics. The classic type, the luetic aortic aneurysm, is now rarely seen in the Western world, whereas it used to be responsible for over 50% of all aneurysms. Some, if not most, of the 10% of abdominal aortic aneurysms formally attributed to syphilis were probably arteriosclerotic aneurysms in patients with positive serologic tests for syphilis. However, syphilitic aneurysms do occur in the abdominal aorta and when they do, they are usually suprarenal. Since they rarely extend up into the thorax, they should not be confused with the ectatic thoraco-abdominal aneurysm of arteriosclerotic origin. Thus, an isolated saccular aneurysm of the suprarenal aorta should be suspected of being syphilitic in origin, particularly if the patient is from a part of the world where this venereal disease has not been well controlled.

The only other microbe that seems to have a particular affinity for arterial walls is *Salmonella* and it is responsible for the majority of infected aortic aneurysms secondary to microbial arteritis. *Salmonella* is considered the prototype of Gram-positive infected aneurysms. The latter predominate four to one and run a much more benign course (25% versus 75% mortality) (Anderson, 1977).

The most difficult infected aneurysms to treat are those encountered in immunosuppressed patients, such as transplant recipients. Not only does one have the problem of continuing immunosuppression, but the nosocomial organisms which cause these aneurysms are often difficult to identify and/or resist to antimicrobial agents. Most instances of aneurysms infected with fungus (i.e. truly "mycotic" aneurysms) are seen in immunosuppressed patients. The final type, secondary, or embolomycotic aneurysms, are the result of infected emboli. The successful treatment of subacute bacterial endocarditis by antibiotics, have made this type of aneurysm fairly rare. The predominant organisms involved are identical with those producing the endocarditis and, therefore, quite different than those seen with other infected aneurysms.

The infectious nature of such aneurysms is frequently not suspected until the time of operation, or worse, after they have been replaced by a prosthesis. They should be suspected in any patient with an intercurrent infection, fever of unknown origin, leucocytosis or elevated sedimentation rate, when aneurysms appear in patients with prolonged illness or immunosuppression or those who have undergone invasive vascular procedures. Finally, a noncalcified aneurysm presenting with rapid growth and signs of compression or erosion of surrounding tissues particularly, in a young or female patient, should arouse suspicion. The classic presentation of regional miliary sepsis (i.e. infected emboli in the legs), is rarely encountered. More will be said of infected and mycotic aneurysms in a later presentation.

Summary

The etiology of aneurysm can be attributed in every case to a combination of congenital or acquired weakness in the arterial wall and mechanical stresses produced by systemic arterial flow. At one end of the spectrum, the mural weakness or defect can lead to aneurysm formation without unusual hemodynamic forces (traumatic, anastomotic, graft and infected aneurysms). At the other end, dilatation can begin in a previously normal artery because of the fatiguing of its elastic and collagen fibers by the lateral forces developed adjacent to the high velocity jet stream of an arterial narrowing. Between these extremes are those aneurysms in which a mural weakness is often combined with unusual hemodynamic forces, most commonly hypertension (dissecting and arteriosclerotic aneurysms and aneurysms associated with pregnancy). The importance of understanding the etiologic background of each of these different forms of aneurysm relates to prevention (post-stenotic, infected, anastomotic and graft aneurysms), prediction of natural history and, therefore, the need for operation, and modifying the operative approach to avoid recurrence (infected, anastomotic and congenital aneurysms).

REFERENCES

Anderson, C.B. (1977). Mycotic aneurysm. *In* "Vascular Surgery" (R. B. Rutherford, Ed.). Saunders, Philadelphia, Pennsylvania.

Beighton, P. (1968). Lethal complications of the Ehlers-Danlos syndrome. *British Medical Journal* **3**(5619), 656.

Benjamin, H. B. and Becker, A. B. (1967). Etiologic incidence of thoracic and abdominal aneurysms. *Surgery Gynecology and Obstetrics* **125**, 1307.

Benjamin, quoted by Bergan, J. J. and Yao, J. S. T. (1974). Modern management of abdominal aortic aneurysms. *Surgical Clinics of North America* **54**, 175.

Berguer, R. and Higgins, R. F. (1976). Deteriorization of grafts and prostheses. *Journal of Cardiovascular Surgery* **17**, 493.

Bruns, D. I., Connolly, J. E., Holman, E. and Stofer, R. C. (1959). Experimental observations of poststenotic dilation. *Journal of Thoracic Surgery* **38**, 662.

Burnett, H. F., Bledsoe, J. H., Char, F. and Williams, G. D. (1973). Abdominal aortic aneurysmectomy in a 17-year-old patient with Ehlers-Danlos syndrome: case report and review of the literature. *Surgery* **74**, 617.

Campbell, C. D., Brooks, D. H., Webster, M. W. and Bahnson, H. T. (1976). Aneurysm formation in expanded Polytetrafluoroethylene prostheses. *Surgery* **79**, 491.

Collins, J. J. (1971). Dissecting aneurysms in turkeys and man. *Archives of Surgery (Chicago)* **102**, 159.

Dale, W. A. (1979). Presented at the International Cardiovascular Society in discussion of Dilation of Synthetic Graft and Junctional Aneurysm by G. E. Kim, A. M. Imparato, I. Nathan and T. S. Riles. Thirty-third Annual Meeting. Opryland Hotel, Nashville, Tennessee, June 28, 1979.

Dale, W. A. and Lewis, M. R. (1976). Further experiences with bovine arterial grafts. *Surgery* **80**, 711.

Descotes, J., Pelissier, P. and Chignier, E. (1976). Dystrophy of the media with aneurysmal tendency in the abdominal aortioliac segment. *Journal of Cardiovascular Surgery* **17**, 413.

Edwards, W. S. (1978). Arterial grafts: past, present and future. *Archives of Surgery (Chicago)* **113**, 1225.

Ernst, C. B., Campbell, H. C., Daugherty, M. E., Sachatello, C. R. and Griffin, W O. (1978). Incidence and significance of intraoperative bacterial cultures during abdominal aortic aneurysmectomy. *Annals of Surgery* **185**, 626.

Halsted, W. S. and Reid, M. R. (1916). An experimental study of circumscribed dilation of an artery immediately distal to a partially occluding band and its bearing on the dilatation of the subclavian artery observed in certain cases of cervical rib. *J. Exper. Med.* **24**, 271.

Holman, E. (1954). The obscure physiology of poststenotic dilation: its relation to the development of aneurysms. *Journal of Thoracic Surgery* **28**, 109.

Killip, T. and Holmquist, N. D. (1961). Aortic surgery in Marfan's syndrome. *Annals of International Medicine* **54**, 431.

Kline, J. L. *et al.* (1962). Poststenotic vascular dilation. *Journal of Thoracic and Cardiovascular Surgery* **44**, 738.

Leonard, J. C. and Hasleton, P. S. (1979). Dissecting aortic aneurysms: a clinicopathological study. *Quarterly Journal of Medicine* **48**, 55.

Malcolm, J. E. (1957). "Blood Pressure Sounds and Their Meanings". Heinemann, London.

Manalo-Estrella, P. and Barker, A. E. (1967). Histopathologic findings in human aortic media associated with pregnancy. *Archives of Pathology* **83**, 336.

Martin, P. (1978). On abdominal aortic aneurysms. *Journal of Cardiovascular Surgery* **19**, 597.

Moore, W. S. (1977). Anastomotic aneurysms. *In* "Vascular Surgery" (R. B. Rutherford, Ed.). Saunders, Philadelphia, Pennsylvania.

Moore, W. S. and Hall, A. D. (1970). Late suture failure in the pathogenesis of anastomotic false aneurysms. *Annals of Surgery* **172**, 1064.

Ottlinger, L. W., Darling, R. C., Wirthlin, L. S. and Linton, R. R. (1976). Failure of ultralightweight knitted Dacron grafts in arterial reconstruction. *Archives of Surgery (Chicago)* **111**, 146.

Pedowitz, P. and Perell, A. (1957). Aneurysms complicated by pregnancy. *American Journal of Obstetrics and Gynecology* **73**, 720.

Peterson, L. H., Jensen, R. E. and Parnell, J. (1960). Mechanical properties of arteries *in vivo*. *Circulation Research* **8**, 622.

Roach, M. R. (1979). Hemodynamic factors in arterial stenosis and poststenotic dilation. *In* "Hemodynamics and the Blood Vessel Wall" (W. E. Stehbens, Ed.). Thomas, Springfield, Illinois.

Stanley, J. C. and Fry, W. T. (1974). Pathogenesis and clinical significance of splenic artery aneurysm, *Surgery* **76**, 898.

Stehbens, W. E. (1979). Arterial aneurysms. *In* "Hemodynamics and the blood vessel wall" (W.E. Stehbens, Ed.), Thomas, Springfield, Illinois.

Sumner, D. S. (1977). The hemodynamics and pathophysiology of arterial disease. *In* "Vascular Surgery" (R. B. Rutherford, Ed.). Saunders, Philadelphia, Pennsylvania.

Sumner, D. S., Hokanson, B. S. and Strandness, D. E. Jr (1970). Stress–strain characteristics and collagen–elastin content of abdominal aortic aneurysms. *Surgery Gynecology and Obstetrics* **30**, 459.

Szilagyi, D. E., Elliot, J. P., Hageman, J. H. *et al.* (1973). Biological fats of autogenous vein implants as arterial substitutes. *Annals of Surgery* **178**, 232.

Szilagyi, D. E., Smith, R. F., Elliot, J. P. *et al.* (1975). Anastomotic aneurysms after vascular reconstruction: problems of incidence, etiology and treatment. *Surgery* **78**, 800.

Takao, A., Kusakawa, S., Hamada, I., Ando, M. and Asai, T. (1974). Cardiovascular

lesion of muco-cutaneous syndrome. *Circulation (Supplement III)* **49** and **50**, 39.
Wilson, S. E., Van Wagenen, P. and Passaro, E. (1978). Arterial infections. *In* "Current Problems in Surgery" (M. M. Ravich, Ed.). Vol XV, No. 9. Yearbook Medical Publishers, Chicago, Illinois.
Zarins, C. (1980). Experimental production of aneurysms by arterial injury in rabbits on an antherogenic diet. *Surgical Forum* **31**, 338.

ANEURYSMS OF ABDOMINAL AORTA: CLINICAL ONSET; DIAGNOSIS

G. Agrifoglio and L. Gabrielli

Institute of Vascular Surgery, University of Milan, Milan, Italy

In the clinical history of abdominal aortic aneurysms we usually distinguish three phases. The first one is asymptomatic or paucisymptomatic, and is characterized by anatomical integrity of the aneurysm wall. It is followed by the fissuration phase and inevitably by the rupture, that is the solution of continuity in the wall that occurs where fissuration determines a huge diminution of superficial resistance. The clinical succession of these three phases in the patient with aortic aneurysm is not constant. The first phase can suddenly be followed by the rupture, which is sometimes the first and only manifestation of the disease.

The asymptomatic aortic aneurysm is usually found during a general examination of the patient. The palpation of the abdomen reveals in fact the presence of an abnormal pulsating mass, which appears to be painless or slightly aching, hard and elastic and is generally roundish with different sizes up to that of the head of a foetus. The mass is commonly located on the mid-line or shifted towards the left; its extension towards the right is blocked by the root of the mesentery and by the inferior vena cava. In the majority of cases (95–96%) the aneurysm develops below the renal arteries. This subrenal origin is testified by the possibility of hooking its upper extremity under the costal arch. It is also possible to delimit its distal extension, unless an aneurysmatic involvement of iliac arteries exists. Often a systolic murmur on the pulsating mass, or distal to it, can be present. Sometimes the patient himself notices the abnormal pulsation in his abdomen. Worried by the

Serono Symposium No. 44, "Peripheral Arterial Diseases: Medical and Surgical Problems", edited by S. Stipa and A. Cavallaro, 1982. Academic Press, London and New York.

discovery, mainly when a slight pain is present, he goes to his family doctor.

The presence of the aneurysm can be revealed by a plain X-ray of the abdomen, an echography or a CAT, made for other reasons. Nowadays this discovery is hardly ever affected during a laparotomy. During the first phase, the symptomatology of the aneurysms has two substrates: the wall of the aneurysms and the compression of the surrounding structures. The stretching of the aortic wall gives rise to a slight pain, also during palpation, with desultory exacerbations which are characterized by continuous, heavy and ill-located pains with dorso-lumbar or inguinal radiation.

The aneurysmatic mass can determine abdominal heaviness, mainly after eating. The compression of the colon, such as the stretching of duodenum, mesentery and mesocolon can lead to a subocclusive condition. The continuous mechanical action exerted on the duodenum can give rise to mucosal erosions (Bernhard and Kleinman, 1979), which manifest themselves mainly with the sudden appearance of haematemesis and melena. The same erosive action can involve vertebral bodies, thus giving rise to a continuous and dull pain which is often attributed to lumbar arthrosis.

The obstructive involvement of ureters in perianeurysmatic fibrosis, typical of inflammatory aneurysms, is peculiar (Goldstone *et al.*, 1978; Lynch and Richie, 1979). However, ureters can be compressed and displaced also by the enlargement of non-inflammatory aneurysms. In any case the typical urological picture is hydronephrosis with progressive uremia.

Above-mentioned inflammatory aneurysms have some peculiar symptomatologic and diagnostic features: generally they do not progress towards the following stages of fissuration and rupture, yet they are noticeably symptomatic (Wylie, 1975). The patient's violent pain leads the surgeon to an emergency operation, fissuration being suspected. It is possible to find some haematologic abnormality, particularly in ESR and inflammatory indices.

Radiographic features will be discussed below: here it is sufficient to say that ureters involved in the perianeurysmatic desmoplastic reaction are displaced medially. On the contrary non-inflammatory aneurysms give, in the majority of cases, the urographic sign of lateral displacement of ureters (Labardini and Ratlife, 1967). Sometimes the first sign of an aneurysm is peripheral ischaemia, due to embolization of endoaneurysmatic thromboatheroma or to aneurysm thrombosis. In the latter case the diagnosis can be particularly difficult since the abdominal mass is not pulsating and sometimes indeed not palpable, if the aneurysm is small or the patient obese. Peripheral ischaemia can also be unrelated to aneurysm and can be mainly due to systemic obliterative atherosclerosis. Sometimes claudicatio abdominis is present, due to superior mesenteric artery involvement by the aneurysm or to atherosclerotic occlusion of mesenteric arteries and celiac artery (Malan and Tiberio, 1967). In such a various symptomatic pattern, the physician has numerous problems of differential diagnosis. In the simplest cases one must differentiate the aneurysm's abnormal pulsation from aortic tortuosity or anterior displacement of the aorta, typical of slender women with marked lumbar lordosis. In these cases it is important to define with precision the lateral margins of the aorta. An evaluated diameter of 3 cm or less does not agree with the diagnosis of aneurysm. In more complex situations the problem is to differentiate an aneurysm from abdominal masses of other nature, transmitting vascular pulsations, especially retroperitoneal ones. However, if an endoaneurysmatic thrombosis occurred, differential diagnosis must consider also non-pulsating masses. Nonetheless, even when the diagnosis of aneurysm is sure, the problem is to ascribe with certainty patient's symptoms to the aneurysm itself, and not to a possible unrelated disease.

The second clinical stage, i.e. fissuration of aneurysms is characterized by continuous intense pain, variously radiated. Sometimes the mass grows rapidly and its palpation gives an excruciating pain. Abdominal defence, paralytic ileum and clinical signs of anaemia can appear. In this stage clinical diagnosis is easy enough. As we said, non-fissurated inflammatory aneurysms show analogous symptoms, but the differential diagnosis is made in the operating room.

Ineluctable progress is towards the rupture, into the retroperitoneum and subsequently the peritoneum or into the inferior vena cava or the duodenum. Retro- and endoperitoneal haemorrhage generally occurs in two stages: at first bleeding is plugged by retroperitoneal structures, but after a period of a few hours of transient improvement, haemoperitoneum ensues and the clinical picture becomes dramatic. Primary rupture into the peritoneum is rare. It happens when the leakage is on the anterior wall or retroperitoneal resistance is strong, "thanks" to perianeurysmal adherences.

Sometimes rupture is the first manifestation of aneurysm. Clinical diagnosis is mainly based on the finding of a mass that "grows under the physician's hand"; the abdomen is contracted, untractable, aching badly, with signs of paralytic ileum. Some hours after the onset of leakage, one can observe haemorrhagic suffusions at lumbar and inguinocrural regions. There is always a very serious state of shock. This classic clinical picture, however, has a great number of variants that raise diagnostic doubts, especially for eventual perforating duodenal ulcers, pancreatitis, cholecystitis, ureteral lithiasis, intervertebral disc rupture and myocardial infarction. Unusual manifestations are those simulating sepsis (Szilagyi *et al.*, 1965) or caval obstruction (Gertner *et al.*, 1978). At the beginning the first manifestation can be an unilateral autosympathectomy due to lumbar sympathetic ganglia destruction (Eastcott and Gardner, 1969). Aorto-caval fistula development is less dramatic (Baker *et al.*). The aneurysm is less painful, less pulsating or not pulsating at all. Auscultation reveals a continuous sisto-diastolic murmur. Lower leg oedema and cyanosis and progressive heart failure at present. Oedema can involve only one leg if rupture develops in the iliac vein. We can distinguish even in the aorto-enteric fistual development (generally in the distal portion of duodenum) an evolution in various phases with progressive increasing episodes of haematemesis and melena which lead the patient to hypovolaemic shock (Bernhard and Kleinman, 1979). Presumptive diagnosis must be made every single time an enteric bleeding is associated with the discovery of abdominal aortic aneurysms.

With few exceptions, fissurated and ruptured aneurysms must be diagnosed only clinically, whereas in the first phase, asymptomatic or paucisymptomatic, instrumental evaluation has a major role. Plain X-ray of the abdomen in search of vascular calcification once was the only non-invasive instrumental diagnostic approach. Evolution of other techniques, more reliable, and some limitations of such a method made it obsolete. Indeed parietal calcifications may be observed only in 55–85% of abdominal aneurysms (therefore error varies between 15% and 45%). In any case, lateral projections are more reliable, for in the anteroposterior ones images top one another and the evaluation of the transverse diameter is difficult. Besides, even intravenous (i.v.) urography has no more space in diagnosis of uncomplicated aneurysms, however, it is still of interest in inflammatory aneurysms: ureters are displaced medially, and not laterally, and are stenosed or obstructed with hydronephrosis. Urography can diagnose correctly about 50% of horseshoe kidneys and helps to make a careful pre-operative planning (Sigler and Geary, 1969). Nowadays, echotomography is the first diagnostic approach. It is a non-invasive greatly reliable method, absolutely harmless and easily repeatable. Therefore echography now cannot be substituted as a means to follow up patients when surgery must be postponed.

Limits of echography are the marked obesity of patients, excessive gas in the bowels, unreliable visualization of visceral vessels especially renal arteries (Gordon *et al.*, 1978), and undetection of complications such as aortocaval fistulas (Karp and Eklof, 1978).

The examination is traditionally made on a patient lying on his back, making xifo-subumbilical longitudinal scans on the mid-line and at bilateral intervals of 1 cm (Fig. 1). Transversal scansions (Fig. 2) on the same extension at intervals of 2 cm are taken (Kristensen *et al.*, 1972). Finally oblique scans can be obtained which measure more accurately the calibre of the aneurysm when it is very tortuous. The vessels are easily recognized as they are

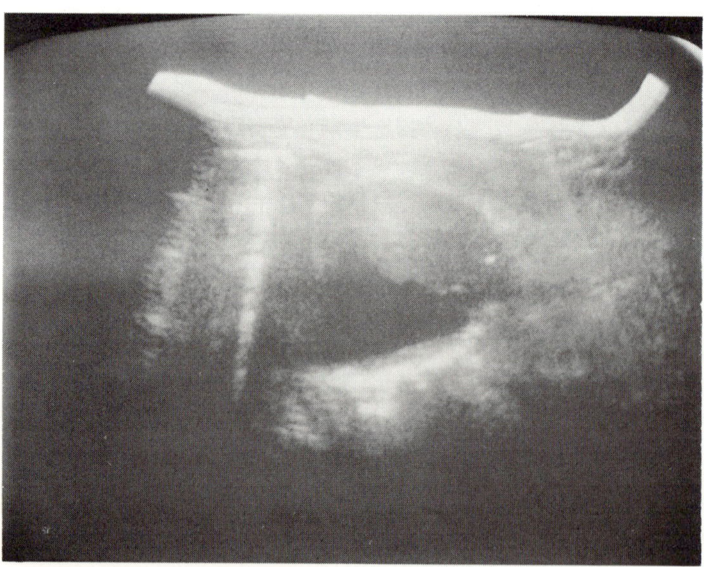

Fig. 1. Echography: longitudinal scan of an aortic aneurysm, showing the true lumen and the thromboatheroma in the lumen.

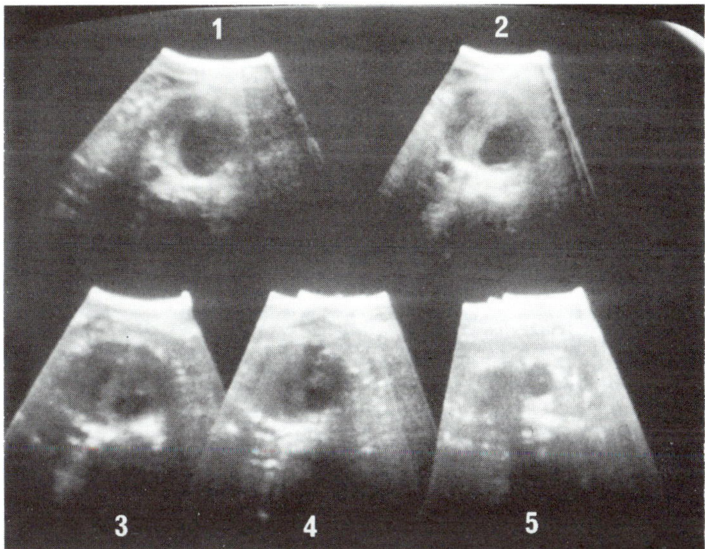

Fig. 2. Ecgography: multiple transverse (scans same case as in Fig. 1).

"sonolucent". In the case of aneurysms it is also rather easy to distinguish the real lumen from the athero-thrombotic material, which is strongly echogenic. Information that is gathered concerns therefore the dimensions (with a margin of error of ± 3 mm), and the thickness of the wall, the form and the contents of the aneurysm and the presence of retroperitoneal haematomas as an index of rupture. In this last case, although there are often technical difficulties, an irregularity of the outer aortic wall becomes evident with disorganized adjacent areas of sonolucency (Fulton *et al.*, 1980). In the case of dissection, sometimes the calcified and dissected intima, which separates the real lumen from the false one and which in transverse scans assumes a crescent-shaped image is visible (Bresnihan and Keates, 1980). In making the echography the diagnostic capacity of the examiner and his specific skill in vascular pathology is very important: in fact, more than the snapshots used to accompany the medical report, it is the observation of the dynamic real-time images which assumes an outstanding importance. From these, informations can be drawn on the aneurysm wall movement, on the presence of a subrenal neck, on its topographical development and on the eventual involvement of iliac arteries. There are therefore precise questions to which the echographist should answer, to give a useful medical report for diagnosis, prognosis and therapeutic indication.

Should there be doubts in interpretation and to have a better surgical planning, it is preferable to take a CAT scan (Axelbaum *et al.*, 1976), which gives clearer images (Fig. 3), but makes the patient undergo quite a large dose of radiations, which however, with the most modern apparatus, are equal to those of a common GI examination (Bernstein *et al.*, 1979). Resolution power is better compared to that of echotomography, especially for the visualization of superior mesenteric artery (Pahira *et al.*, 1979), of renal arteries (Ohlsén

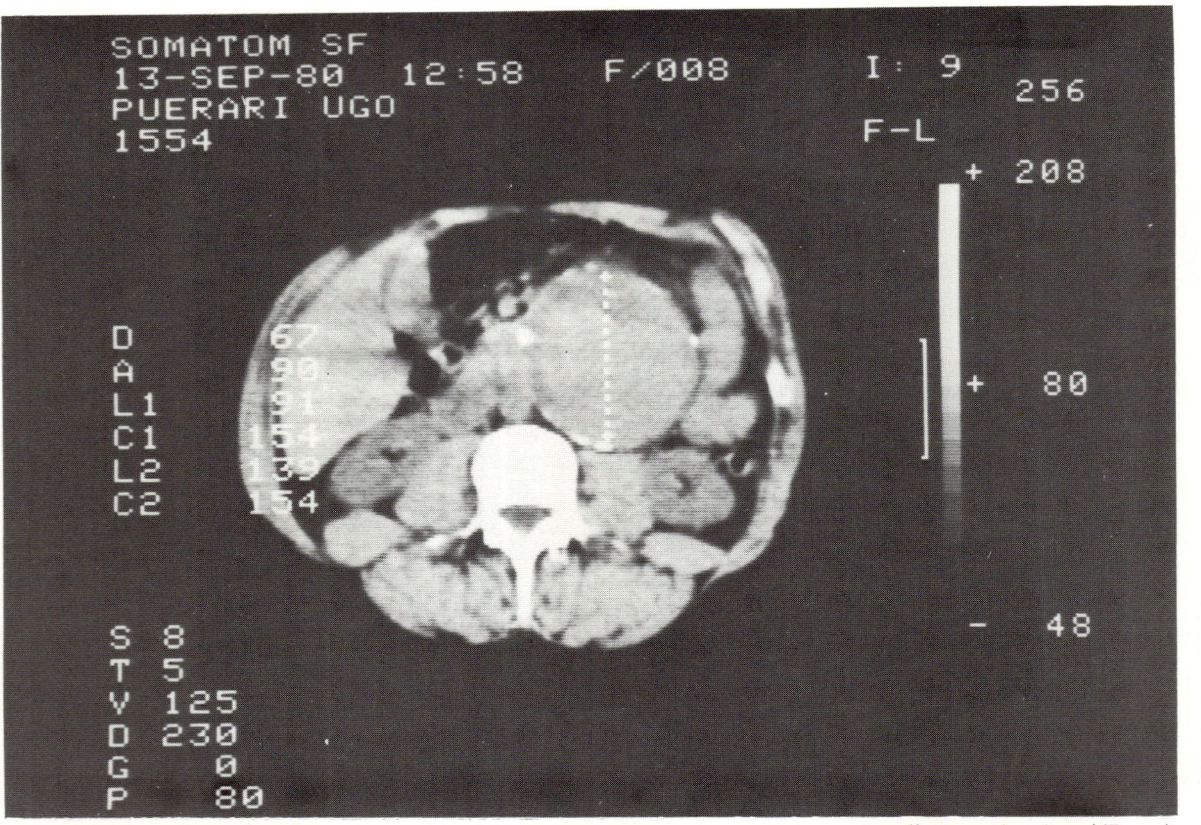

Fig. 3. Computerized assisted tomography of an aortic aneurysm. Anteroposterior diameter is taken (67 mm); calcifications in the outer wall, true lumen and thromboatheroma are visualized.

and Swedenborg, 1980) and for the relations of the aneurysm with the surrounding structures (inferior vena cava, left renal vein, pancreas, eventual horseshoe kidney and other anomalies which may cause problems in surgery).

Aortic lumen is easily evidenced by using a contrast medium, either in bolus or in continuous infusion. In this way the various parietal components are clearly distinguished, especially the calcifications, the intra-luminal clots and the eventual perianeurysmal fibrosis which is typical of inflammatory forms (Young *et al.*, 1980) and which sometimes gives a false image of dissection or rupture (Aiello and Cohen, 1980) or evidences the involvement of the ureters in this periaortic fibrotic sheath (Pahira *et al.*, 1979). In some cases real retroperitoneal haematomas from rupture and real dissections have been demonstrated. In the first case there is a continuity between the aneurysm wall, which is not well outlined, and an isodense formation which becomes continuous and fused in the psoas muscle, whereas in the presence of dissections the formation of a neolumen in the endoaneurysmatic thrombus or in the wall itself can be seen (Fig. 4), in which case calcifications are pushed inside the vessel, giving a crescent-shaped image (Suchato *et al.*, 1980).

Sometimes the CAT scan shows the presence of gas inside the aortic wall, a sure index of mycotic aneurysm (Pripstein *et al.*, 1979). The limits of the method are that even a slight involuntary movement of the patient provokes distortions of the image; besides only the transversal scans are significant. In fact longitudinal reconstructions are coarse and not useful for diagnosis. Artefacts can be caused by the presence of metallic objects (clips etc.).

Angiography is not necessary to confirm the diagnosis of aneurysms. In fact it is known that there is a discrepancy between the external calibre of the aneurysm and its lumen. In a certain percentage of cases, however, it becomes indispensable for a correct surgical planning (Rösch *et al.*, 1978), especially when it is important to know the state of the visceral arteries, particularly of the renal ones, which may be stenotic and may cause nefrovascular hypertension. It is important when the presence of an adequate subrenal neck must be ascertained, as well as the fusiform or saccular morphology and the extension of the aneurysm, with possible involvement of the iliac arteries.

An angiography should be performed also when there is an obliterative peripheral arteriopathy, which must be taken into account during the operation. Angiography is indispensable also in the presence of a horseshoe kidney, to visualize all the ectopic arteries that can come out directly from the aneurysms, and that must be re-implanted. If there is an aortocaval fistula, this is the only examination which can document it adequately (Karp and Eklof, 1978). The aneurysms may be studied either through a suprarenal trans-lumbar aortography or by means of catheterism through the axillary or femoral artery. None of these methods are free of risks but we feel that transfemoral catheterism presents the greater possibility of iatrogenic lesions, unless it is done by expert and careful angiographists, who usually use guides and catheters with a soft and bent tip with multiple lateral holes (Rösch *et al.*, 1978). As the examinations present some risk (rupture, dissection, embolization, allergic reactions etc.) it is wise to do it only in selected cases with an exact indication, since in most patients an echography or a CAT scan is sufficient to formulate correct diagnosis and surgical planning.

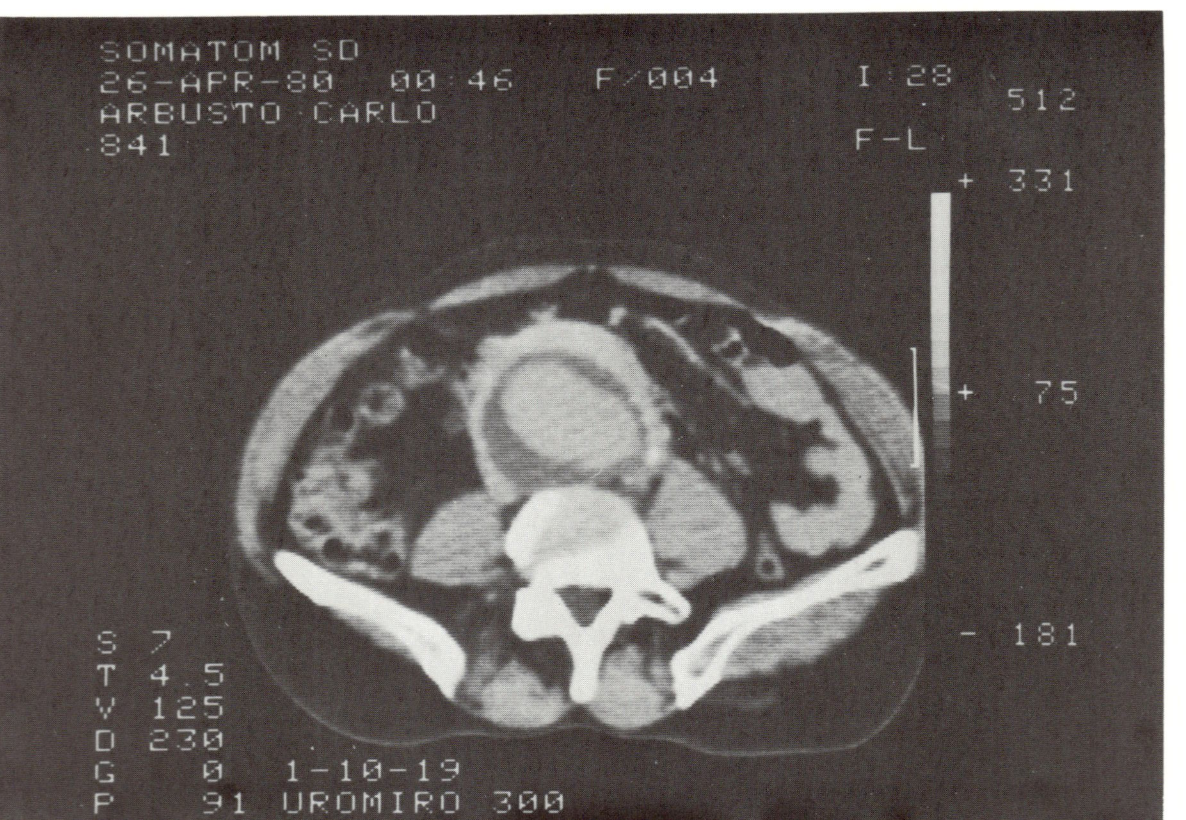

Fig. 4. Contrast enhanced CAT in a case of dissecting aortic aneurysm: double lumen and crescent-shaped image of the intima are observed.

REFERENCES

Aiello, M. R. and Cohen, W. N. (1980). Inflammatory aneurysm of the abdominal aorta. *Journal of Computer Assisted Tomography* **4**, 265.

Axelbaum, S. P., Schellinger, D., Gomes, M. N., Ferris, P. A. and Hakkal, H. G. (1976). Computed tomographic evaluation of aortic aneurysms. *American Journal of Roentgenology* **127**, 75.

Baker, W. H., Sharzer, L. A. and Ehrenhaft, J. C. (1972). Aortocaval fistula as a complication of abdominal aortic aneurysms. *Surgery* **72**, 933.

Bernhard, V. M. and Kleinman, L. M. (1979). Aortoenteric fistulas. *In* "Surgery of the Aorta and Its Body Branches" (J. J. Bergan and J. S. T. Yao, Eds), p. 591. Grune & Stratton, New York.

Bernstein, E. F., Harris, R. D. and Leopold, G. R. (1979). Ultrasound and CT scanning in the non invasive evaluation of abdominal aortic aneurysms. *In* "Surgery of the Aorta and Its Body Branches" (J. J. Bergan and J. S. T. Yao, Eds), p. 43. Grune & Stratton, New York.

Bresnihan, E. R. and Keates, P. G. (1980). Ultrasound and dissection of the abdominal aorta. *Clinical Radiology* **31**, 105.

Eastcott, H. H. G. and Gardner, A. L. (1969). Autosympathectomy in abdominal aortic aneurysms. *Annals of Surgery* **169**, 290.

Fulton, R. E., Stanson, A. W., Forbes, G. S. Miller, W. E., Hattery, P. R. and Williamson, B. (1980). Vascular imaging. *In* "Peripheral Vascular Disease", (Juergens, Spittell and Fairbairn, Eds), p. 193. Saunders, Philadelphia, Pennsylvania.

Gertner, M. H., Hargrove, W. C. and Roberts, B. (1978). A ruptured abdominal aortic aneurysm presenting as inferior vena caval obstruction. *Surgery* **83**, 605.

Goldstone, J., Malone, J. M. and Moore, W. S. (1978). Inflammatory aneurysms of the abdominal aorta. *Surgery* **83**, 425.

Gordon, D. H., Martin, B.L., Schneider, M., Staiano, S. J. and Noyes, M. B. (1978). The complementary role of sonography and arteriography in the evaluation of the atheromatous abdominal aorta. *Cardiovascular Radiology* **1**, 165.

Karp, W. and Eklof, B. (1978). Ultrasonography and angiography in the diagnosis of abdominal aortic aneurysm. *Acta Radiologica Diagnosis* **19**, 955.

Kristensen, J. K., Holm, H. H. and Norby Rasmussen, S. (1972). Ultrasound diagnosis of aortic aneurysm. *Journal of Cardiovascular Surgery* **13**, 168.

Labardini, M. M. and Ratlife, R. K. (1967). Abdominal aortic aneurysm and the ureter. *Journal of Urology* **98**, 590.

Lynch, D. F. Jr and Richie, J. P. (1979). Ureteral obstruction secondary to abdominal aortic aneurysm: a case report. *Vascular Surgery* **13**, 122.

Malan, E. and Tiberio, G. (1967). Clinica degli aneurismi dell'aorta addominale e dei suoi rami. *In* "Atti del XVII Congresso Nazionale della Società Italiana di Gastroenterologia", Genova, Ottobre 1967, p. 1147.

Ohlsén, H., and Swedenborg, J. (1980). Computed tomography in the pre-operative evaluation of abdominal aortic aneurysms. *Vasa* **9**, 4.

Pahira, J. J., Wein, A. J., Barker, C. F., Banner, M. P., Arger, P. M., Mulhern, C. and Pollack, H. (1979). Bilateral complete ureteral obstruction secondary to an abdominal aortic aneurysm with perianeurismal fibrosis: diagnosis by computed tomography. *Journal of Urology* **121**, 103.

Pripstein, S., Cavoto, F. V. and Gerritsen, R. W. (1979). Spontaneous mycotic aneurysm of the abdominal aorta. *Journal of Computer Assisted Tomography* **3**, 681.

Rösch, J., Keller, F. S., Porter, J. M. and Baur, G. M. (1978). Value of angiography in the management of abdominal aortic aneurysm. *Cardiovascular Radiology* **1**, 83.

Sigler, L. and Geary, J. E. (1969). Abdominal aortic aneurysm and unexpected horseshoe kidney. *Journal of Cardiovascular Surgery* **10**, 320.

Suchato, C., Pekenan, P., Singjaroen, T. and Sereerat, P. (1980). Indication of dissecting aortic aneurysm on non contrast computed tomography. *Journal of Computer Assisted Tomography* **4**, 115.

Szilagyi, D. E., Elliott, J. P. and Smith, R. F. (1965). Ruptured abdominal aneurysms simulating sepsis. *Archives of Surgery (Chicago)* **91**, 263.

Wylie, E. J. (1975). Infrarenal Abdominal aneurysms. *In* "Current Surgical Diagnosis and Treatment". (J. E. Dunphy and L. W. Way, Eds), 2nd Edn, p. 703. Lange Medical Publishers, Los Altos, California,

Young, A. E., Lea Thomas, M. and Wright, C. M. (1980). Assessment of abdominal aortic aneurysms by computed tomography. *British Medical Journal* **280**, 765.

ABDOMINAL AORTIC ANEURYSMS: NATURAL HISTORY AND OPERATIVE INDICATIONS

D. E. Szilagyi

Department of Surgery, Henry Ford Hospital, Detroit, Michigan, USA

The natural history of abdominal aortic aneurysms can be best described in three phases: the asymptomatic phase, the phase of symptoms without rupture and the phase with rupture. Without the occurrence of events that change the course of natural evolution of the lesion, every abdominal aortic aneurysm would pass through these phases. Before the advent of surgical treatment, all aneurysms did go through these phases with two exceptions: the aneurysm whose bearer died of an inter-current disease and the aneurysm that skipped the clinical stage of expansion before rupture. One must add that in the latter event, it is very likely that the phase of expansion was indeed present but so briefly as to go clinically unnoticed.

ASYMPTOMATIC ANEURYSM

An abdominal aortic aneurysm is one of the pathological lesions that, though potentially lethal, may be present for long periods of time without giving clinical signs of their existence. The circumstance that makes this characteristic most unusual is that virtually all other commonly seen pathological states that are simultaneously silent and life-threatening are morphologically inconspicuous (for instance, a stenosed coronary or middle cerebral

Serono Symposium No. 44, "Peripheral Arterial Diseases: Medical and Surgical Problems", edited by S. Stipa and A. Cavallaro, 1982. Academic Press, London and New York.

artery), whereas abdominal aortic aneurysms from their inseption are quite bulky.

There are at least three reasons why an aneurysm even though of large dimensions, as long as it has obtained its size gradually, seldom gives rise to symptoms and signs. The mid-abdominal retroperitoneal space is very commodious and hidden, and, unless the patient is thin, a mass of considerable size within it may go unnoticed clinically. Second, there are few organs in this area that would respond by symptoms to pressure by a mass. Very rarely the adjacent vertebrae may be eroded or the ureter compressed and give rise to clinical manifestations but the slow displacement of the duodenum or the pancreas or of the root of the mesentery from behind are symptomless. By contact alone, the slow enlargement of the aneurysm will seldom elicit response from the adjacent organs because of the noninflammatory nonreactive character of the morbid anatomy of its increase in size.

By the laws of physics and in accordance with the rules of morbid anatomy, an aneurysm is destined to increase in size as long as its confines are intact. Given an increase in diameter of a large artery owing to a loss of tensile strength of its walls, the dilatation will be progressive, since with every increment of increase of the diameter there will be, in accordance with the law of Laplace, an increase in the lateral pressure, which, in turn, will further accentuate the dilatation. For every aneurysm there seems to be a critical size at which the wall will yield to the lateral pressure and the rupture will take place. Although the rupture must be caused by identifiable physical factors (such as increase in size, increase in arterial pressure, increase in the intra-abdominal tension, subclinical secondary infection), these factors are usually impossible to identify in an individual case. In this sense the time and circumstances of rupture are unpredictable.

Two factors in the clinical picture, however, have strong predictive values: the size of the aneurysmal sac and the blood pressure. Although small aneurysms (less than 5 cm in diameter), do rupture they do so much less frequently than large ones. If one compares the survival rate of small and large aneurysms — that is the inverse concept of mortality rate — one finds that the small aneurysms have about twice the survival expectancy of large aneurysms. Putting it another way, large aneurysms, greater than 5 cm in diameter, are twice as likely to rupture. In studying the subsequent clinical course of a group of patients in whom surgical treatment for abdominal aortic aneurysms could not be performed for various reasons, we found that a patient bearing an abdominal aortic aneurysm and suffering from hypertension has three times the probability of rupture faced by a normotensive patient.

The natural history of abdominal aortic aneurysms, therefore, can be conceived as one of continuous process of enlargement with an unknown critical size at which rupture will take place. If one represents the life of an abdominal aortic aneurysm as a line made up of a series of points each indicating an increment in size, the farther along this line the aneurysm is, that is, the closer its size is to the critical dimension, the more likely it is to rupture. This fact has an important meaning in establishing reasonable operating indications for abdominal aortic aneurysms.

ANEURYSMS WITH SYMPTOMS AND WITHOUT RUPTURE (EXPANDING ANEURYSMS)

An aneurysm that has not ruptured may lead to symptoms in two ways. It may encroach on a neighboring organ and cause clinical manifestations. We have already seen that this event is extremely rare, constituting less than 1% of the total. In the overwhelmingly large group of patients the aneurysm quite suddenly makes itself known by the appearance of abdominal pain. There is good evidence that this pain is related to and indeed caused by a sudden enlargement of the aneurysmal sac.* Almost without exception the patient is not aware of this increase in size but in many instances the clinician is able to observe it. It is pain that first draws the patient's attention to the change in his clinical course. The pain is almost always severe, constant, unrelated to posture, boring in character and is most commonly located in the lumbar spinal region, in the mid-abdomen or in the pelvis. From any of these primarily near locations the pain may be referred to other points, the most frequent of these being the thigh, testicle or rarely the perineum. The pain may be girdle-like and may be aggravated by raising the intra-abdominal pressure.

On first thought one may assume that the pain is caused by stretching or splitting of the layers of the aortic wall. Indeed, it has been theorized that small hemorrhages into the wall of the aneurysm may be the cause of the pain. Both the pathological findings in the wall of the aneurysm and the type of distribution of the pain contradict this assumption. The essential gross pathological changes consist not of multiple repeated hemorrhages but of extensive edema and inflammatory induration found not in the wall of the sac but in the adventitia and in the periadventitial tissues. Moreover the pain is essentially somatic in type, with only a minor sympathetic component, and this, together with its location and radiation, strongly suggests that its origin is primarily in the retroperitoneal somatic sensory nerve endings and to a lesser extent in the sensory spinal nerve root. The spinal segments affected are usually those from the first to the fifth lumbar and rarely those from the first to the third sacral; the minor visceral component most likely originate in the lumbar sympathetic chain.

It requires no further elaboration that the characteristics of the abdominal pain readily provide opportunity for diagnostic errors.

It appears correct to state, therefore, that this pain is the result of the pressure upon the somatic sensory nerve elements of the retroperitoneal soft tissues in the vicinity of the aneurysmal sac. This mechanism is the same as that seen in ruptured aneurysms, but in the latter case the pathological changes are more extensive, the pressure on the nerve endings more violent and the symptoms more severe.

The outstandingly important characteristic of the expanding abdominal aortic aneurysms is their propensity to progress to rupture. Among 18

---

*This concept justifies the use of the term expanding aneurysm to denote an aneurysm with symptoms and without rupture. The adjectives of "leaking" and "symptomatic" have often been linked with the name of such an aneurysm but the former is inaccurate and the latter is vague.

patients with expanding aneurysms who for a variety of reasons did not have resective treatment, 11 could be followed for at least two years; all were dead at the end of this period, seven having succumbed to rupture (four in less than 12 months) and four to coronary arterial occlusions. The extremely poor prognosis of aneurysm with expansion is even more poignantly illustrated by deaths from rupture of six patients with expanding aneurysms while studies were being carried out preparatory to surgical treatment, the intervals from admission to rupture having ranged from 6 h to four days. Indeed, for the practical purposes of the clinician, expansion of an abdominal aortic aneurysm causing abdominal pain can be regarded as the first stage of an imminent rupture.

ABDOMINAL AORTIC ANEURYSMS WITH RUPTURE

As already described, the first phase of the process that leads to rupture is often an expansion of the aneurysmal sac in terms described in detail above. Judging from the incidence of premonitory signs, a rupture is preceded or accompanied by symptomatic expansion in about 60% of the cases. The event of rupture itself is found on exploration or at autopsy to have taken place in one of three ways.

(1) The tear of an aneurysmal sac may be in the anterior wall and the bleeding may be into the free peritoneal cavity. This type of rupture may be called an *open* rupture.

(2) The rupture site may be retroperitoneal with the formation of a hematoma in the retroperitoneal space. The hematoma varies in size and may be very extensive. Regardless of its size, however, the hematoma ultimately tends to be temporarily self-limited since the retroperitoneal space is relatively confined and favors the development of a compressing or tamponading force. This type may be called *closed* rupture.

(3) Less commonly the rupture may be so small that the escape of blood is effectively walled off by the surrounding tissue reaction in the retroperitoneal space and in the aortic wall. We designate this lesion as a *sealed* aneurysm. Invariably, however, the sealed rupture reopens until eventually it causes massive extravasation of blood. A variant of this rupture is that which breaks into an adjacent hollow viscus or into a vein.

With the exception of small sealed lesions, in which the picture may remain stationary for days or weeks, once rupture has taken place the clinical events progress in one of two characteristic fashions, and at usually considerable speed. In an unconfined rupture the blood loss may be so massive and rapid that the patient loses consciousness from the sudden fall of blood pressure; except in wide anterior rupture, in which the patient may bleed to death in a matter of a few minutes, but which fortunately are very rare, the natural course of events tends to tamponade the site of rupture; the accumulation of a firm clot and the lowering of blood pressure are circumstances that result in effective albeit transient control of bleeding. At this stage the patient continues to complain of severe abdominal pain, and, in addition presents the picture of hemorrhagic shock to varying degrees.

SEALED RUPTURE

Although sealed ruptures are uncommon, constituting only 5% of the total, they deserve special emphasis because of the diagnostic difficulties they often present. Since these lesions are usually of small or moderate dimensions, they are difficult to palpate and since they may be accompanied by repeated extravasation of blood, they may readily mimic retroperitoneal infection with respect to distention, anorexia, vomiting, leucocytosis and fever. These circumstances open the way for serious diagnostic mistakes. The pathological characteristics of sealed rupture readily explain its clinical evolution. Since the aneurysm that may manifest this complication is usually a small one and still has a structurally fairly strong wall, the original tear is limited in extent. Since the perforation is always posterior, the adjacent tissues tend to respond to extravasation of blood with fibroblastic reaction. The patients are usually normotensive, which is an important factor in limiting the extent of hemorrhage. Thus, the first hemorrhage is encapsulated and may remain so for relatively long intervals, but in most instances the tear does not heal and the hemorrhage soon recurs. On the clinical level the pain will recur or continue, the escaped blood will provoke systemic reaction such as fever, leucocytosis and hypohemoglobinemia. As the blood loss is protracted, the pulse and blood pressure do not change appreciably, but with each episode of escape of blood the connective tissue barrier weakens and eventually a wide rupture takes place. By this time the hematoma–aneurysm complex may have grown sufficiently in size to become palpable.

Since the clinical course of sealed rupture is so reminiscent of retroperitoneal septic process, questions have been raised regarding the part that infection may play in its causation. The occurrence of secondary infection in an existing abdominal aortic aneurysm has been mentioned by some authors and the claim has even been made that the secondary involvement by infection, resulting from bacteremia of septicemia may be the cause of some cases of expansion or rupture. Similarly one may raise the question whether the lesion under discussion might not actually be a mycotic aneurysm, that is an aneurysm originating in a metastatic supportive infection of the vascular wall. Actual observations disproved this possibility. In the case of mycotic aneurysms the clinical picture is dominated by manifestations of septicemia, and pain is an unimportant feature. The gross morphologic characteristics of mycotic aneurysms are likewise dissimilar. Finally, whenever blood cultures and cultures of tissues removed at the time of aneurysmectomy are obtained, they are invariably negative.

It should be mentioned in this connection, however, that occasionally in abdominal aortic aneurysms positive cultures have been obtained and there have been very rare instances of rupture of abdominal aortic aneurysms which can be traced to the localization of systemic infection in the wall of the aneurysm.

A specific variant of sealed rupture is the fistulization between the abdominal aortic aneurysm and an adjacent large vein, usually the vena cava or a hollow viscus. In the former case the clinical picture is dominated by the hemodynamic changes due to the arteriovenous communication. The extent of these changes, of course, is directly related to the size of the communication. When the aneurysm has perforated into a hollow viscus (almost invariably the small intestine), the dominant change, indeed usually the only clinical manifestation, is gastrointestinal bleeding.

OPERATIVE INDICATIONS

In general, the surgeon's decision to operate for a given case of disease can be represented by a cost–benefit equation; if the benefit in terms of prolongation of life or improvement in function or quality of life exceeds the rate of operative mortality and morbidity, the surgical intervention is justified. Needless to say in case of symptomatic or ruptured aneurysms there is no room for the consideration of such formulas: operative treatment is mandatory regardless of risk. In the case of asymptomatic abdominal aortic aneurysms, however, the formula is valid but its calculation must take into account a complex set of factors.

(1) There is a probability of dying from rupture, the magnitude of which depends to an important degree on (a) the size of aneurysm, (b) the degree of coronary and other organ atherosclerosis that seriously influences not only the operative mortality but also longevity irrespective of the type of treatment.

(2) Advanced age, which virtually always is a part of a clinical picture, brings in its train associated degenerative diseases and primarily determines the life expectancy.

(3) Life expectancy, while important to all cases, is a consideration of particular importance in the evaluation of the operability of small aneurysms, which require a substantial length of time before they can evolve to the stage at which they rupture.

(4) Operative mortality, determined by many factors in addition to the degree of advancement of atherosclerosis, notably by a variety of degenerative diseases common to advanced age.

(5) The expected technical difficulties in a given case are also of importance, and their consideration may become decisive when the physiological risk factors are marginal.

Soon after the inception of our experience with surgical treatment of these lesions we adopted an aggressive approach to the treatment of asymptomatic abdominal aortic aneurysms. We felt that this aggressive approach was justified since, once established, abdominal aortic aneurysms increase in size continually, silently and capriciously; since they may rupture while still small; since in most of the cases rupture is completely unheralded; since when symptoms appear they are often misleading and, most importantly, since, untreated, all the lesions rupture unless the patient succumbs to some other disease earlier. Based on these considerations, and even in the absence of strong statistical evidence to support it, we felt that all abdominal aortic aneurysms called for surgical treatment unless one or more of the following set of contraindications were present.

(1) Myocardial infarction of less than three months standing.

(2) Intractable congestive cardiac failure.
(3) Intractable angina pectoris.
(4) Severe pulmonary insufficiency (dyspnea at rest).
(5) Disabling residuals of cerebrovascular accident.
(6) Severe decrease in renal function (blood creatinine greater than 3 mg%).
(7) Associated lethal disease with less than three years' survival expectancy.
(8) Small size of aneurysm (less than 6 cm in diameter) in patients over 75 years.
(9) Advanced age (greater than 80 years).

This liberal policy of case selection appeared well justified by surgical results but, as mentioned before, statistical evidence was lacking for its support. This objective proof was gathered from a rather large retrospective case study, which I would now like to summarize.

The principal goal of the study was the comparison of the survival experience, that is the length of life in years after diagnosis, in two groups of patients: one group comprising patients with aneurysms who had had nonsurgical treatment (which in essence means no treatment) and the other made up of patients who had had their aneurysms removed. In addition, certain factors that have an important effect on survival were evaluated in each group. There were 233 patients in the nonsurgical and 480 patients in the surgical group. In the detailed statistical analysis these numbers were reduced since only those patients were retained in the two groups to be compared that fulfilled a set of criteria of uniformity with respect to the same essential clinical features. By this method of standardization the surgical and nonsurgical groups were rendered similar, that is, to some degree they were caused to resemble two randomly selected samples of population.

The study revealed that in the surgical group the leading cause of loss of life after operation was the immediate operative mortality which averaged 13.6% for the total group. Next in importance in the surgical cases was death from coronary atherosclerosis which had an incidence of 9.4%. In the nonsurgical group by far the most common cause for loss of life was rupture of the aneurysm which was calculated at 35%. The second leading cause of death in this group was likewise coronary atherosclerosis, which had an incidence of 17%.

The survival experience in each group was calculated according to the life-table method and showed that the survival rate for surgical patients was far superior at every chronological interval from one to 12 years postoperatively. As examples one may quote the survival rates in percentages respectively for the surgical and nonsurgical cases as 80 against 44 at two years, 62 against 22 at four years, 48 against 18 at six years and 20 against four at ten years. The total survival experience of all the surgical cases in comparison with the nonsurgical cases was approximately doubled.

It has been a subject of debate whether or not the operability of small aneurysms should be judged by radically different criteria than are large aneurysms. The question is particularly important since during the past 20 years the incidence of small aneurysms seen by the clinician has increased from about 30% to 52% of all aneurysms encountered.

The study showed that the rupture rate in small aneurysms was considerably lower than in large aneurysms, 19.5% compared with 43.3%, but it still was a significant cause of death. It was also true that the average survival of small aneurysms was roughly twice that of large aneurysms.

Nevertheless, the post-operative survival rate of small aneurysms that had been subjected to operation was found to be about 50% better than the total survival experience of the aneurysms of small size that had been treated by observation.

These findings firmly supported the aggressive attitude of management we had adopted and appeared to confirm the validity of our liberal case selection policy. Very recently we conducted another study which looked at the problem of the validity of our operative criteria from a different vantage point. In this study, we surveyed the clinical course of 156 patients with asymptomatic abdominal aortic aneurysms that between 1950 and 1971 had been deemed unfit for surgical treatment because of coexistant risk factors. Subsequently 29 patients eventually came to have surgical treatment. Thus in the group that we analysed statistically there were 127 patients who received no surgical treatment at any time. Among these, 90 died during the subsequent 20-year follow-up period.

We found that the rate of rupture in the series we studied earlier composed of patients who failed to receive surgical treatment not because of medical contraindications but because of the unavailability of surgical methods was twice as large as in the recent series in which the surgical treatment was not recommended owing to medical reasons. In the recent group the incidence of atherosclerosis as cause of death was twice as high as in the earlier group. It appears that the gain of life expectancy due to the lower incidence of rupture in recent series was almost exactly counter-balanced by a higher incidence of atherosclerosis. This would suggest that our set of surgical indications in the past up to and including the time of the study was a correct one.

An incidental but very important finding of this study was that the incidence of rupture in patients with arterial hypertension was seven times that in the group that did not have rupture. Putting it another way, the presence of hypertension was a very important factor in leading to rupture as a cause of death.

One can make a theoretical calculation of the value of the salvage of life under the operative indications described. The operative mortality during the time the recent group of cases was observed was 7%. If one relates the rate of loss of life from rupture to the rate of loss of life from surgical treatment, assuming a rate of rupture in unselected patients of 35% with a salvage rate by surgical intervention of 50%, one finds that the surgical treatment reduced the expected loss of life by the ratio of 2.3 to 1, that is, by a factor of more than two.

Since this study, the operative mortality of abdominal aortic aneurysmectomy in our experience has been further reduced, and currently is 3.5% in all asymptomatic cases. With this improved mortality rate and with the newer available methods for treating certain manifestations of coronary atherosclerosis, it would seem reasonable to enlarge our operative indications. At the present time people with intractable angina pectoris, who otherwise fulfilled the operative criteria, are studied for coronary artery disease and subjected to corrective surgery on the coronary arteries whenever feasible. Subsequently, the aneurysmectomy can be carried out with very acceptable risk of surgical mortality. In cases of large aneurysms, that is aneurysms larger than 6 cm in diameter, we have further liberalized indications for surgical treatment in elderly patients. In fact we do not recognize a chronological age limit, and a patient with a large aneurysm will be recommended surgical treatment regardless of age as long as the physiological state of the patient does not violate the operative indications other than age. We also look with a more liberal attitude at pulmonary insufficiency, residuals of cerebrovascular accident and deficiency of renal function.

ELECTIVE SURGERY OF ABDOMINAL AORTIC ANEURYSMS: TECHNIQUES AND RESULTS

J. F. Vollmar and W. Hepp

Department of Surgery of the University of Ulm, Ulm, West Germany

The infrarenal segment of the abdominal aorta is the most frequent location of aortic aneurysms. Only in 5% of cases is the suprarenal segment affected mostly under the pattern of a thoraco-abdominal aneurysm. Concerning aetiology, arteriosclerosis is the predominant lesion (95%) (Heberer *et al.*, 1972; Baird *et al.*, 1978). Dissecting aneurysms or those from syphilitic, mycotic or traumatic origin are very rare conditions. More frequently anastomotic false aneurysms may be seen. But these will not be discussed in this paper. In the last ten years there has been a remarkable increase in elective surgery for the treatment of abdominal aortic aneurysms (Hepp *et al.*, 1980; Scobie *et al.*, 1977). This evolution is mainly caused by improvements in the diagnostic and operative approach.

The broad application of computerized tomography (CT) and ultrasound investigations offer today excellent non-invasive–diagnostic tools for early diagnosis. Most vascular centres are using now routinely these techniques in all suspected cases.

For elective surgery a pre-operative aortogram should be performed regularly. The arteriogram may give additional informations on concomitant stenotic lesions of the visceral branches and/or of the run-off vessels but also on the involvement of the suprarenal aorta.

Serono Symposium No. 44, "Peripheral Arterial Diseases: Medical and Surgical Problems", edited by S. Stipa and A. Cavallaro, 1982. Academic Press, London and New York.

INDICATION FOR SURGERY

In principle every diagnosed abdominal aortic aneurysm should be considered for surgical repair. Neither its size nor the presence of calcification are reliable parameters in respect to the risk of rupture. There are two main arguments for early elective surgery.

(1) The significant improvement of life expectancy in the group of operated patients.

(2) The reduced operative mortality, especially in patients with intact aortic aneurysms. There are still some contraindications such as cardiac or pulmonary insufficiency, incurable cancer or other consuming diseases. Age beyond 80 years should not contradict surgery in good-risk patients.

Concomitant carotid artery stenosis should be repaired before aortic surgery.

SURGICAL TECHNIQUES

The technique of aneurysm resection has changed remarkably in the last ten years following the 3-S principle, i.e. make the procedure simpler, safer and shorter. Some important technical details may be mentioned and emphasized.

(1) The patient should be placed on the operating table in a right-tilted position. Using a long mid-line incision complete eventration of the bowels is very easily accomplished (Fig. 1).

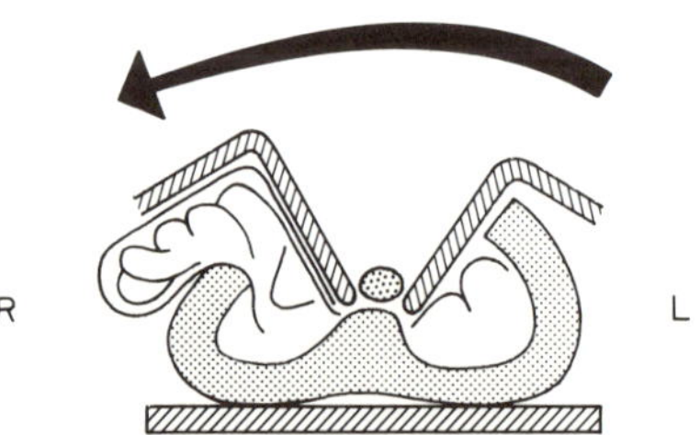

Fig. 1. "V" principle for the exposure of the infrarenal aorta.

(2) Covering of the whole bowel in a plastic sheet is easier to realize than the use of a plastic bag which includes the danger of strangulation of bowel loops. Two retractors should be inserted in a V-shaped fashion with the abdominal aorta at the deepest point of the "V", which allows free access for the surgeon.

(3) After reflection of the duodenum to the right the most important landmark, i.e. the left renal vein is exposed. It crosses usually anteriorly to the neck of most infrarenal aneurysms. For bleeding control it is sufficient to put clamps on the neck of the aneurysm and the common iliac arteries. Without further dissection aortic aneurysm is incised longitudinally between the three vascular clamps (Fig. 2). After taking out the clots from the

aneurysmatic sac the inner atheromatous layer of the aneurysm is removed, the orifices of some back bleeding lumbar arteries are suture ligated. Usually the take off of the inferior mesenteric artery must be transsected and ligated closely to the aorta.

(4) The inlay technique of prosthetic substitution offers a time-saving arterial reconstruction using a continuous suture leaving the posterior wall of the aneurysm *in situ* (Fig. 2d); 4.0 prolene–suture, double-armed, is our preferred suture material. For all elective reconstructions a high-porous knitted velour prosthesis is the substitute of choice. Woven grafts are preferred for emergency interventions in patients with ruptured aneurysms in shock. The level of the distal anastomoses depends on the extension of the vascular lesions. In our hands in over 90% of patients a bifurcated graft is necessary. Due to concomitant stenotic iliac lesions in 40% the distal anastomoses are done to the common femoral arteries. If there is a block in the superficial femoral artery a long end-to-side anastomosis to the deep femoral artery is performed following the principle of a profundaplasty in combination with a lumbar sympathectomy (L4–L5).

The most frequent technical faults are kinking of the limbs. The best way of preventing this is to use a short mainstem of the bifurcated prosthesis at a high level resulting in a nearly vertical course of the prosthetic limbs. The prosthesis may be covered by suturing the outer layer of the aneurysm over the prosthesis or covering the graft by an omentum flap.

The post-operative care includes drainage of the retroperitoneal space. In all high-risk cases a controlled pulmonary ventilation is sustained for 24 h with continuous control of pO_2 and electrolyte balance. A post-operative heparin medication is contraindicated. In all vascular cases the risk of bleeding is higher than the advantage of thromboembolic protection.

SURGICAL RESULTS

These are based on a retrospective evaluation of 162 patients operated between 1970 and 1979. Four clinical groups were differentiated (Table I). Asymptomatic aortic aneurysms were most frequently diagnosed in patients investigated for claudication (59%). Symptomatic aneurysm are those causing abdominal pain, disturbing pulsating sensations in the abdominal cavity or signs of embolic events in the distal arterial tree. Seventy-six per cent of patients were admitted with "staged rupture", every second in shock condition. Twenty-four per cent of patients with ruptured aneurysms suffered from a free rupture in the abdominal cavity. All of them were in severe shock with oliguria or anuria since several hours.

Two time periods were differentiated. The second one (1975–1979) was characterized by the use of a standardized and simplified dissection technique, by an increased number of operations performed by the same group of four–five surgeons and by an intensive pre- and post-operative care, i.e. controlled respiration support in an intensive care unit during the first 24 h after surgery.

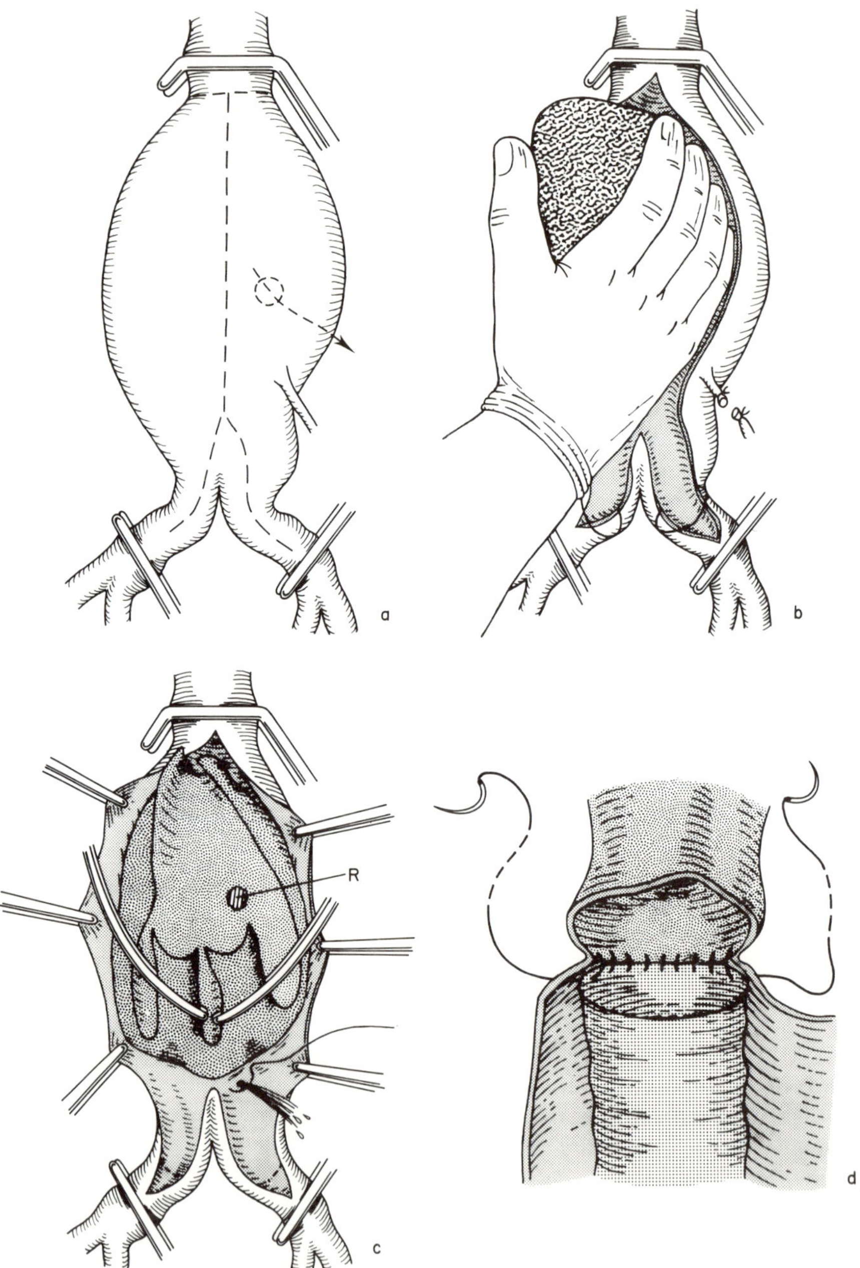

Fig. 2. Dissection technique for abdominal aortic aneurysms: (a) exclusion of the aneurysm by putting on a central aortic clamp and two distal clamps on the common iliac arteries. The aneurysm is now opened longitudinally; (b) manual evacuation of the clots; (c) the atheromatous inner layer is pulled off similarly to the technique used

Table I. Operative mortality in aneurysms of the infrarenal abdominal aorta ($n = 162$) 1970–1979 (Reg. No.: 63 - 4293).

	No. of patients		Operative mortality	
	1970–1974	1975–1979	1970–1974	1975–1979
Closed aneurysms	28	72	4 (14.3%)	2 (2.8%)
Asymptomatic	14	41	0 (0.0%)	0 (0.0%)
Symptomatic	14	31	4 (28.6%)	2 (6.5%)
Ruptured aneurysms	18	44	11 (61.1%)	23 (52.3%)
Covered rupture	14	33	7 (50.0%)	17 (51.5%)
Free rupture	4	11	4 (100.0%)	6 (54.5%)

Comparing the results of both time periods, the post-operative mortality in the group of closed aneurysms drops down from 14.3% to 2.8%, and in the group of ruptured aneurysms from 61.6% to 52.3% (Table I). There was no death in patients operated on asymptomatic closed aortic aneurysms. In the first period all four patients with a free rupture died. In the second period five from 11 patients survived. The most important risk factors in relation to operative mortality and survival rate were the age of person, concomitant hypertension and pulmonary insufficiency. Patients with ruptured aneurysms were on average nine years older than those with closed aneurysms. Coronary heart diseases was not a statistical significant factor for the post-operative outcome. The same is true for patients with concomitant distal arterial occlusive lesions. After surgery the patients life expectancy approaches that of the average population. (Fig. 3). The survival curves run parallel but operative mortality reduces the course of the line to a lower level. These results are

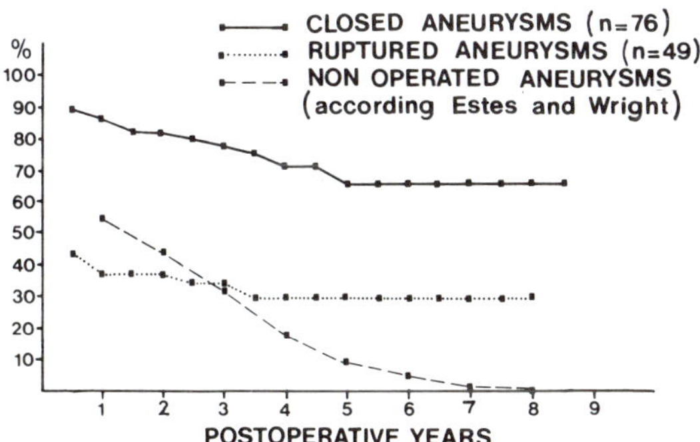

Fig. 3. Cumulative survival rate in patients with infrarenal abdominal aortic aneurysms.

---

for TEA. The remaining posterior wall of the aneurysm frequently adherent to the inferior vena cava is left *in situ*. The orifices of lumbar arteries are suture ligated transluminally (R: area of rupture). (d) Inlay technique of graft insertion. Continuous suture of the posterior wall of the prosthesis with the central aortic stump.

similar to those published by others (Crawford *et al.*, 1966; Szilagyi *et al.*, 1966; Thompson *et al.*, 1975; Vollmar and Noble, 1975).

The remarkable improvement concerning the surgical outcome of patients operated on in the last five-year period is mainly caused by the following factors.

(1) Simplification and standardization of the surgical techniques, i.e. doing the vascular repair safer and quicker. The operating time could be reduced to 2–3 h.

(2) An improved pre-, intra- and post-operative care of high-risk patients specially in the presence of arterial hypertension and pulmonary insufficiency. The intra-operative monitoring of pressure and flow in the pulmonary artery helps much to keep the patients in a steady state of their cardiovascular condition.

There is only little doubt that in Europe many of aortic aneurysms get diagnosed not at all or too late. Some figures may illustrate these facts. The ratio between closed and ruptured aortic aneurysms in the United States is approximately 10 to 2 and in most European countries, also in our series, it is only 1.5 to 1.0. These figures represent a surgical challenge to all European surgeons for the need of earlier diagnosis. On the other hand, our Anglo-American colleagues are more familiar with the dilating form of arteriosclerosis specially under the pattern of abdominal aortic aneurysm. Several autopsy studies gave evidence that the morbidity of aortic aneurysm in the European population is different to the population of the United States. In our countries the obliterative type of arteriosclerosis is approximately three times more frequent as in the United States.

SUMMARY

(1) Surgery for closed abdominal aortic aneurysms offers a remarkable chance of long-term survival escaping the danger of rupture. Surgical repair of asymptomatic closed aneurysms can be done with a very low risk, i.e. a mortality rate below 1.0%. A main prerequisite for such a protective surgery is an early diagnosis, best done by a routine examination of all elderly people suffering from arterial hypertension, peripheral arterial occlusive disease or other signs of arteriosclerosis. Computerized tomography and ultrasound–doppler technique gained a predominant position for such a protective screening programme.

(2) Standardization and simplification of the operative techniques, i.e. make surgical repair simpler, safer and shorter, has recently remarkably reduced the operative risk for patients with intact aneurysms. But the surgical progress is very limited in emergency surgery for ruptured aneurysms. As a further consequence, this type of vascular surgery should be restricted to special units with a highly trained surgical team. Repair of aortic aneurysms, closed or ruptured, should no longer be a case for occasional surgery.

REFERENCES

Baer, U., Häring, R. and Kunkel, M. (1978). Zur klinik und therapie des abdominalen aortenaneurysmas. *Zëntrablatt für Chirurgie* **103**, 1194.

Baird, R. J., Gurry, J. F., Kellam, J. F. and Wilson, D. R. (1978). Abdominal aortic aneurysms: recent experience with 210 patients. *Canadian Medical Association Journal* **118**, 1229.

Bremner, D. N., Shand, J. E. G. and Kenyon, G. S. (1977). Ruptured abdominal aortic aneurysms. *Journal of the Royal College of Surgeons Edinburgh* **22**, 400.

Crawford, E. S., De Bakey, M. E., Morris, G. C., Garrett, H. E. and Howell, J. F. (1966). Aneurysm of the abdominal aorta. *Surgical Clinics of North America* **46**, 963.

Estes, E. J. (1950). Abdominal aortic aneurysm: A study of 102 cases. *Circulation* **2**, 258.

Heberer, G., Sachweh, D. and Giessler, R. (1972). Zur chirurgischen Behandlung des infrarenalen arteriosklerotischen Bauchaortenaneurysmas. *Chirurg* **43**, 162.

van Heeckeren, D. W. (1970). Ruptured abdominal aortic aneurysms. *American Journal of Surgery* **119**, 402.

Hepp, W., Vollmar, J. and Krier, S. (1980). Das aneurysma der infrarenalen aorta abdominalis. *Chirurg* **51**, 330.

Key, J. A. and Sokol, D. M. (1973). The symptomless abdominal aneurysm: A 15-year review. *Canadian Journal of Surgery* **16**, 297.

Scobie, K., McPhael, N. and Hubbard, C. (1977). Early and late results of resection of abdominal aortic aneurysms. *Canadian Medical Association Journal* **117**, 147.

Szilagyi, D. E., Smith, R. F., Derusso, F. J., Elliott, J. P. and Sherrin, F. W. (1966). Contribution of abdominal aortic aneurysmectomy to prolongation of life. *Annals of Surgery* **164**, 678.

Thompson, J. E., Hollier, L. H., Patman, R. D. and Persson, A. V. (1975). Surgical management of abdominal aortic aneurysms: factors influencing mortality and morbidity — a 20-year experience. *Annals of Surgery* **181**, 654.

Vollmar, J. (1980). "Reconstructive Surgery of the Arteries". Thieme, Stuttgart.

Vollmar, J. and Nobbe, F. (1975). "Arteriovenöse Fisteln — Dilatierende Arteriopathien (Aneurysmen)", p. 161. Thieme, Stuttgart.

Wright, I. S., Urdaneta, E. and Wright, B. (1956). Reopening the case of the abdominal aortic aneurysm. *Circulation* **13**, 754.

SURGICAL TREATMENT OF RUPTURED ABDOMINAL AORTIC ANEURYSMS: SPECIAL PROBLEMS

R Soyer[1] and Ch. Dubost[2]

Department of Cardiac Surgery, Hôpital Charles Nicolle, Rouen[1] and Department of Cardiac Surgery, Hôpital Broussais, Paris,[2] France

Since Charles Dubost's report of the first resection and homograft replacement of an abdominal aortic aneurysm in 1951 (Dubost *et al.*, 1952) great strides have been made in the control of this disease. Its surgical treatment has been well standardized and the indications for operation have been more clearly defined (Alpert *et al.*, 1970; De Bakey *et al.*, 1964; Dubost *et al.*, 1970; Szilagyi *et al.*, 1966).

There has been a consistent decrease in the mortality and morbidity associated with surgical treatment of non-ruptured abdominal aortic aneurysm. On the other hand, only a moderate decrease has been observed in the published series of ruptured abdominal aneurysm; the surgical management of this disease thus continues to present a challenge to the vascular surgeon.

The results of operation for ruptured abdominal aortic aneurysm vary considerably in the literature and many of them fail to give sufficient details on the condition of the patient at the time of operation. This study will consider only patients with frank rupture of the aneurysm wall, with retroperitoneal or intraperitoneal bleeding or both, who underwent emergency aortic surgery. Those with impending or imminent rupture are excluded.

Serono Symposium No. 44, "Peripheral Arterial Diseases: Medical and Surgical Problems", edited by S. Stipa and A. Cavallaro, 1982. Academic Press, London and New York.

MATERIAL AND METHODS

Between 1951 and 1980, 534 patients underwent resection for abdominal aortic aneurysms in the Department of Cardiovascular Surgery at the Broussais Hospital in Paris and at Charles Nicolle Hospital in Rouen with a peri-operative mortality of 3.1%. Seventy-six (14.2%) of these required emergency operation for ruptured abdominal aortic aneurysm. The mean age was 76.5 in a range of 50 to 87 years. There were 52 males and 24 females. Coronary artery disease was diagnosed in 26 patients of whom 20 had electrocardiographic evidence of myocardial ischaemia or previous infarct (Lagaaij *et al.*, 1970). Ten patients had clinical diabetes and 26 had hypertension (Table I). It is, however, most important to note that 24 patients had previously been aware of their aneurysms and that 14 were transferred from other surgical units where the rupture had been diagnosed during operation for another cause (acute pancreatitis). For these, the delay was highly dangerous, and indeed fatal in six cases.

Table I. Ruptured abdominal aortic aneurysms (76 operated cases).

Age 50–87 years (76.5)	
Associated medical lesions	
Coronary disease	26
Previous infarct	13
Diabetes	10
Hypertension	26
Chronic renal disease	8

At time of operation, 34 patients had had symptoms for 24 h or less and 42 for more than 48 h. On arrival, six patients had unrecordable blood pressure and three were in a state of cardiac arrest; they were rushed to the operating room. Forty-one patients were in profound shock with systolic blood pressure less than 70 mmHg, whereas 26 patients had no significant pre-operative hypotension on arrival but this developed later. In these cases, operation was performed at a mean interval of 3 h after admission Table II).

Table II. Ruptured abdominal aortic aneurysms (76 operated cases).

Duration of symptoms prior to operation	
1–24 h	34
≥ 48 h	42
Condition of the patient	
Unrecordable blood pressure	6
Cardiac arrest	3
Profound shock (≤ 70 mmHg)	41
No shock	26

Any delay due to preoperative tests should obviously be minimal. In patients whose blood pressure is relatively stable, at least two large intravenous cannulae should be inserted for infusion. A central venous cannula is then placed in the internal jugular vein and transfusion starts. The patient is prepared and draped before anaesthesia and intubation. A vertical incision is made from xyphoïd to pubis. Rapid control of the aorta is achieved, first manually by direct approach through the haematoma to the neck of the aneurysm, and then by placing an aneurysm clamp below the renal arteries, or on the aorta below the diaphragm through the gastro-hepatic omentum, if the aorta is palpable. Care must be taken not to damage the oesophagus, which is close to the antero left lateral aspect of the aorta at this level (two cases). This technique of abdominal aortic control was used in 56 cases (Table III).

Table III. Ruptured abdominal aortic aneurysms (76 operated cases).

Surgical technique	
Abdominal control	56
Left thoracotomy	20
Intra-operative findings	
Retroperitoneal haematoma	76
Free blood	40
Seat of the rupture	
Posterior	13
Left lateral	52
Right lateral	11

Digital compression of the proximal part of the abdominal aorta is a method that is commonly used but which we have found to be somewhat less than satisfactory. It obscures the field, is often cumbersome to maintain and makes the application of the aortic clamp difficult.

The transthoracic approach of the aorta was used in 20 cases, and we believe this method of control continues to offer a number of unique advantages: the incision is made in the fifth intercostal space and can usually be accomplished in a matter of seconds, with minimal bleeding. Furthermore, the aorta is readily accessible for control and the proximal compression diverts needed blood to the coronary and cerebral circulation for vital tissue perfusion. Cardiac resuscitation can be performed if necessary.

Injuries to such structures as renal vessels and/or vena cava can be avoided by a more clearly visualized operative field. This approach lends itself well to a concomitant approach by laparotomy by a second member of the team, so that supradiaphragmatic clamping time may be reduced to a minimum. It also reduces the risk of abdominal decompression following caeliotomy in patients presenting retro and intraperitoneal haematoma.

It is usually easy to obtain distal control by opening the aneurysm, where Foley catheters may be directly inserted in the iliac arteries and inflated to achieve temporary control. When the patient is relatively stable and vascular clamps are secure below the renal arteries and on the common iliac arteries, the laminar clot is evacuated and the orifices of the inferior mesenteric and lumbar vessels are suture ligated from within the sac.

Graft replacement is performed using a tightly woven Dacron tube or bifurcation graft. Limited dissection is considered essential to minimize blood loss. The graft may be pre-clotted and flushed in an autoclave for 3 min. No attempt is made to resect the aneurysm.

Prior to completion of the distal suture line, appropriate flushing is carried out; on completion of the suture line, the proximal clamp is slowly removed to avoid hypotension. If satisfactory backflow is not obtained during the flushing procedure, Fogarty catheters may be introduced to retrieve any embolus present.

The wall of the aneurysm is sutured over the proximal suture line and the graft. It is very important to separate the small bowel from the aortic suture line with a layer of viable periaortic tissue. If this presents any difficulty, a cuff of Dacron graft may be placed around the proximal suture line (Fig. 1).

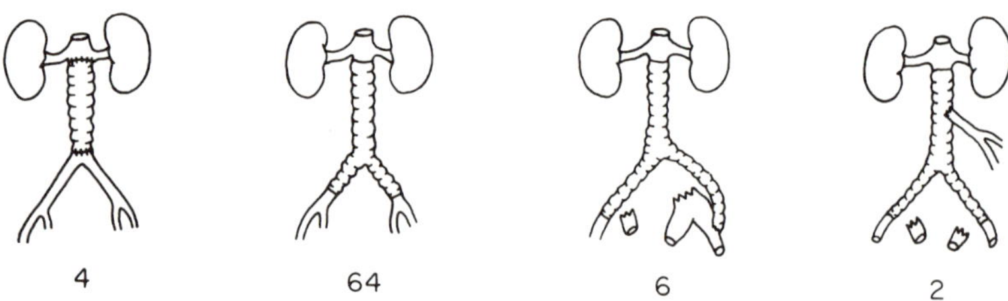

Fig. 1. Ruptured abdominal aortic aneurysms, 76 operated cases. Tube graft: 4; bifurcation graft: 72.

Although clamp control of the ruptured abdominal aortic aneurysm is essential, there are other important considerations if the patient is to make a full recovery. The aims of preventing cerebral and renal ischaemia and clotting abnormalities must be emphasized. The resanguination of the patient is top priority in order to restore blood volume and blood pressure and to give adequate tissue perfusion. We insist on the fact that the best replacement therapy for haemorrhagic shock is blood. A Swan Ganz catheter may be inserted for monitoring the left atrial pressure if the patient is not entirely stable upon transfer to the intensive care unit.

Post-operatively, in addition to routine management, the endotracheal tube is left in place to assist ventilation for 24 h. It is removed when the patient is able to maintain satisfactory blood-gas levels.

RESULTS

We considered the successfully treated patient to be one who survived the operation for 30 days and left the hospital. In our series, out of the 76 patients with a ruptured aneurysm, 23 (30%) died (Table IV). Eleven patients died in

Table IV. Ruptured abdominal aortic aneurysms (76 operated cases — causes of death).

Peri-operative deaths 11	Cardiac arrest	6
	Uncontrolled bleeding	1
	Myocardial infarction	4
Post-operative deaths 12	Cerebral and renal failure	8
	Myocardial infarction	2
	Pulmonary embolism	1
	Colonic ischaemia	1

the operating room: volume depletion and unresponsive intra-operative cardiac arrest accounted for six of the immediate deaths (two patients at intubation, four at mid-line incision). One patient died from uncontrolled bleeding of a retroaortic vena cava when the clamp was placed on the aorta, and four from confirmed immediate post-operative infarction and ventricular fibrillation. Twelve patients died 1–12 days after operation: eight from irreversible damage of the brain and kidneys, two from myocardial infarction, one from a massive pulmonary embolism and one from colonic ischaemia.

Post-operative complications in the survivors included one patient with acute renal failure requiring temporary haemodialysis (Table V), one with significant acute respiratory insufficiency, two with a peripheral embolus requiring embolectomy, one with gastro-intestinal bleeding. No patient required re-exploration for post-operative bleeding and of the nine with no recordable blood pressure or cardiac arrest prior to induction of anaesthesia, five survived aortic resection. One patient developed a recurrence of the aneurysm at the level of the superior aortic suture line two years later. Five patients died from causes having no connexion with their aneurysms two, three, five and seven years after operation. We have received to date satisfactory news of 35 patients for a maximum period of 16 years after operation.

Table V. Ruptured abdominal aortic aneurysms (76 operated cases).

Post-operative complications in survivors	
Renal failure	1
Acute respiratory insufficiency	1
Peripheral embolus	2
Gastro-intestinal bleeding	1

COMMENTS

Based on autopsy statistics, the rate of aneurysm rupture is approximately 28% (ranging from 15% to 50%) rising to 31 % in five clinical series

(Blondeau and Sautot, 1967; De Bakey *et al.*, 1964; Lawrie *et al.*, 1979; Szilagyi *et al.*, 1966; Van Heeckeren, 1970). In our series, however, the rate was only 14%

Without operation the mortality rate of ruptured aneurysms is essentially 100%, and, for this reason, we considered that practically no patient should be refused operation. Advanced age is not a contraindication, nor is the severity of shock an absolute guide to prognosis, since, of the patients admitted to the operating room with cardiac arrest or with no recordable blood pressure prior to the induction, five survived operation and were subsequently discharged from hospital (Table VI). Three patients were considered inoperable: two of these were in coma, the third for medical reasons.

Table VI. Mortality statistics related to profound shock prior to surgery.

Year	Author	Patients	Deaths
1969	Van Heeckeren	57	34 (60%)
1970	Darling	39	22 (56%)
1975	Sink	12	10 (83%)
1979	Dubost	41	21 (51%)
1979	Lawrie	14	4 (28%)

Once a ruptured aortic aneurysm has been diagnosed, we feel it is crucial that the patient be taken to the operating room as soon as possible. Irreversible damage to the heart, brain, kidneys or lungs from pre-operative hypotension was the most common cause of death in our patients.

The clinical picture of rupture was similar to that described in other reported series. The importance of early diagnosis is emphasized by the fact that, in our experience, almost one-third of our patients were aware of their aneurysm and that one-quarter of our initially normotensive patients became hypotensive prior to induction.

The seat of the rupture was posterior in 13 cases, left lateral in 53 cases and right lateral in 11 cases. Rupture was always accompanied by extensive retroperitoneal haematoma, with intraperitoneal bleeding in 40 cases.

A description of the operative technique for emergency aortic aneurysmectomy is now fairly well standardized: our conception and method evolved with time and experience (Soyer *et al.*, 1974, 1979).

Anaesthesia should not be induced until the operating suite and surgeons are in total readiness.

The primary objective is arrest of the aorta proximal to the aneurysm. Two techniques may be used: abdominal or transthoracic approach. We feel strongly that left thoracotomy for proximal control of the aorta prior to laparotomy provides advantages over the abdominal route in patients entering the operating room with a very low or unrecordable blood pressure or in cardiac arrest. (Four patients in our series died from the effect of decompression following laparotomy.) Not only is it a more rapid and direct approach to the aorta but also iatrogenic tears or injuries can be avoided by a clearly visualized operative field. The segment below the renal arteries may then be better exposed after which an occluding clamp may be applied and the upper occluding clamp released (Alpert *et al.*, 1970; Soyer *et al.*, 1974, 1979; Stephenson and Lockhart, 1977).

In the other cases, the techniques of intra-abdominal proximal control may be used. Dissection through the haematoma should be by a blunt technique and should be directed towards the left side of the neck of the aneurysm to avoid entering the left renal vein or vena cava. Sometimes, in large aneurysms, control above the left renal vein will be easier than attempting control below it.

If the aneurysm involves the bifurcation and common iliac arteries up to but not beyond their bifurcation, a bifurcation graft is anastomosed end-to-end. If atherosclerosis affects the common iliac arteries, the limbs of the Dacron bifurcation graft may be anastomosed end-to-side to the external iliac or common femoral arteries. Care must be taken to preserve blood flow at least into the left or right internal iliac artery to ensure adequate supply of the rectosigmoid.

The results of operation for ruptured abdominal aortic aneurysms vary considerably in the literature. In our series, factors that influence mortality include age of the patient, associated diseases, condition of the patient at time of operation and intra-operative findings:
retroperitoneal haematomas alone were found in 36 patients of whom nine died, combined intraperitoneal and retroperitoneal haemorrhage occurred in 40 patients of whom 14 died. Factors influencing survival, as can be expected, appear to be related to the previous experience of the physician with the problem. Lethal complications are directly related to the degree and persistence of hypovolaemia, hypoperfusion of the tissues and the ability of the surgeon to cope with intra-operative complications.

Post-operative deaths and complications are primarily due to the ravages of the haemorrhage, specifically myocardial, cerebrovascular and renal ischaemia or infarction (Alpert *et al.*, 1970;, Blondeau and Sautot, 1967; Kouchoukos *et al.*, 1967; Lawrie *et al.*, 1979; Lagaaij *et al.*, 1970; Shumaker *et al.*, 1973; Sink *et al.*, 1976; Soyer *et al.*, 1979; Stephenson and Lockhart, 1977).

Although there has been some improvement in operative mortality in recent years, elective resection of the unruptured aneurysm still appears to offer the best chance of preventing deaths from ruptured lesions.

It has been widely advocated and we support this concept on the basis of our experience. Many studies found that elective resection doubled the patient's life expectancy, whereas 30% of unoperated patients with known aneurysms died of rupture (Blondeau and Sautot, 1967; Darling, 1970; Szilagyi *et al.*, 1966; Van Heeckeren, 1970).

All ruptured abdominal aortic aneurysms occur below the renal arteries. However, on rare occasions, a ruptured aneurysm of the upper abdominal aorta will occur, requiring replacement of the visceral branches. In addition, some anatomical variations which complicate the operative management, such as retroaortic left renal vein, persistent left vena cava (one case), horseshoe kidney or visceral branches arising from the aneurysm may be present.

Primary aorto-duodenal fistula is rare and occurs when an abdominal aortic aneurysms ruptures into the terminal portion of the duodenum. Although primary repair of the bowel and graft replacement of the aneurysm have been successful, the possibility of delayed graft infection is increased. Two techniques may be used: closure of the duodenum and the aorta, with axillo-femoral bypass or anastomosing a Dacron bifurcation graft end-to-side from the descending thoracic aorta to both common iliac arteries (Beall *et al.*, 1963; Brewster *et al.*, 197; Dubost *et al.*, 1970; Garret *et al.*, 1963).

Aortocaval fistula is rare. Operative treatment consists of control of the aneurysm with vascular clamps. The aneurysm is opened and the fistula controlled manually or with a Foley catheter. This is inserted uninflated through the fistula and the balloon is filled. The catheter is then gently pulled until the balloon occludes the fistula (Beall *et al.*, 1963; De Bakey *et al.*, 1958; Dubost *et al.*, 1970; Yashar *et al.*, 1969).

CONCLUSION

It is obvious that further improvement in results will be achieved only by earlier operation, preferably prior to rupture.

Control of bleeding at the earliest possible moment is essential. Alternative technical approaches in controlling exsanguination of aortic blood flow are available. The advantages of the trans-thoracic approach have been presented and should be resorted to in selected patients. Unfavourable prognostic factors in our series are the condition of the patient before and during operation, age, intra-operative findings, free blood in the peritoneal cavity.

The high mortality of ruptured aneurysms (30%) may best be avoided by elective resection of the unruptured aneurysm.

SUMMARY

Of 534 consecutive patients operated for aneurysm of the abdominal aorta between 1953 and 1980, 76 (52 men and 24 women) underwent emergency operation for ruptured abdominal aortic aneurysm, giving an incidence of 7.2%. Their mean age was 76.5 with a range of 50 to 87 years. Hypotension ($\leq$ 70 mmHg stystolic) was present in 47 patients (61%) on admission to hospital. Operation was begun in nine patients with an initially unrecorded blood pressure or in cardiac arrest. Twenty-three patients died. The two most important factors were age and the condition of the patient prior to operation (shock, magnitude of blood loss). The results of our experience suggest the need for avoiding technical problems during operation and also, as emphasized, earlier referral of patients with known abdominal aortic aneurysms, and early diagnosis with immediate operation for ruptured aortic aneurysms.

REFERENCES

Alpert, J., Donald, K., Brief and Victor Parsonnet (1970). Surgery for the ruptured abdominal aortic aneurysm. *Journal of the American Medical Association* **212**, 1359.

Beall, A. C., Cooley, D. A., Morris, G. C. *et al.* (1963). Perforation of arteriosclerotic aneurysm into inferior vena cava. *Archives of Surgery (Chicago)* **86**, 136.

Blondeau, P.. and Sautot, J. (1967). Les résultats éloignés de la chirurgie artérielle restauratrice de l'aorte sous rénale. Rapport au 69e congrès français de chirurgie, Paris, 1967.

Brewster, D. C., Ottinger, L. M. and Darling, R. C. (1977). Hematuria as a sign of aorta-caval fistula. *Annals of Surgery* **186**, 766.

Darling, R. C. (1970). Ruptured arteriosclerotic abdominal aortic aneurysms. A pathologic and clinical study. *American Journal of Surgery* **119**, 397.

De Bakey, M. E., Cooley, D. A., Morris, G. C. and Collins, H. (1958). Arterio-venous fistula involving abdominal aorta: report of four cases with successful repair. *American Surgeon* **147**, 646.

De Bakey, M. D., Crawford, E. S., Cooley, D. A. *et al.* (1964). Aneurysm of abdominal aorta. Analysis of results of graft replacement therapy one to eleven years after operation. *Annals of Surgery* **160**, 622.

Dubost, Ch., Allary, M. and Oeconomos, N. (1952). Resection of an aneurysm of the abdominal aorta: re-establishment of the continuity by a preserved human arterial graft, with result after five months. *AMA Archives of Surgery* **64**, 405.

Dubost, Ch., Guilmet, D. and Soyer, R. (1970). La Chirurgie des Anévrysmes de l'Aorte, Vol. 1. Masson, Paris.

Garret, H. E., Beall, A. C., Jordan, G. L. *et al.* (1963). Surgical consideration of massive gastro-intestinal tract hemorrhage caused by aortoduodenal fistula. *American Journal of Surgery* **105**, 6.

Kouchoukos, N. T., Levy, J. F. and Butcher, H. R. Jr. (1967). Mortality from ruptured abdominal aortic aneurysm. *American Journal of Surgery* **113**, 232.

Lawrie, G. M., Morris, G. L. Jr., Crawford, E. S. *et al.* (1979). Improved results of operation for ruptured abdominal aortic aneurysms. *Surgery* **85**, 483.

Lagaaij, M. B., Terpstra, J. L. and Vink, M. (1970). Ruptured aneurysms of the abdominal aorta. *Journal of Cardiovascular Surgery* **11**, 440.

Shumacker, H. F. Jr., Barnes, D. L. and King, H. (1973). Ruptured abdominal aortic aneurysms. *American Surgeon* **177**, 772.

Sink, J. D., Myers, R. T. and James, P. M. Jr. (1976). Ruptured abdominal aortic aneurysms: review of 33 cases treated surgically and discussion of prognostic indicators. *American Surgeon* **42**, 303.

Soyer, R., Deloche, A., Brunet, A., Lessana, A., Deliere, T. and Dubost, Ch. (1979). Rupture des anévrysmes de l'aorte abdominale sous rénale. Réflexions à propos de 66 cas. *Annales de Chirurgie Thoracique et cardio-vasculaire* **33**, 211.

Soyer, R., Eisenman, B., Deloche, A., Diamant-Berger, F., Haas, Cl. and Dubost, Ch. (1974). Traitement des anévrysmes rompus de l'aorte sous rénale. *NPM* **3**, 81.

Stephenson, H. E. Jr. and Lockhart, C. G. (1977). Treatment of the ruptured abdominal aorta. *Surgery Gynecology and Obstetrics* **144**, 855.

Szilagyi, D. E., Smith, R. F., De Russo, F. J. *et al.* (1966). Contribution of abdominal aortic aneurysmectomy to prolongation of life. *Annals of Surgery* **164**, 678.

Van Heeckeren, D. W. (1970). Ruptured abdominal aortic aneurysms. *American Journal of Surgery* **119**, 402.

Yashar, J. J., Hallman, G. L. and Cooley, D. A. (1969). Fistula between aneurysm of aorta and renal vein. *Archives of Surgery (Chicago)* **99**, 546.

MANAGEMENT OF ABDOMINAL AORTIC ANEURYSMS IN HIGH-RISK PATIENTS WITHOUT DIRECT-GRAFT REPLACEMENT

A. M. Karmody, D. M. Shah and R. P. Leather

Department of Surgery, Vascular Surgery Section, Albany Medical College, Albany, New York, U.S.A.

Although the natural history of the abdominal aortic aneurysm has been recognized for over 400 years, it is only in the recent past that satisfactory methods of treatment have been developed for this type of arterial pathology. The propensity of these aneurysms to rupture before their presence is known or suspected by either the patient or physician is well recognized. The mortality attendant on this event still generally hovers around 50% (Upstate New York Registry Report, 1980) except in a few reports. In addition, apart from the threat of rupture, limb loss because of microembolization from the aneurysm is a more recently recognized problem (Karmody *et al.*, 1976) although it is less frequent than that of rupture. The modern treatment of replacement of the aneurysm by prosthetic grafts dates back to the pioneer efforts of Voorhees *et al.*, which was first reported in 1951. As a result of this work, prosthetic grafts of many types have been developed and are now an essential part of the vascular surgical discipline. Direct-graft interposition serves both the purpose of eliminating the risk of rupture as well as restoration of blood supply to the lower limbs. This method of treatment remains the procedure of choice and has been shown by long-term studies to restore normal life expectancy in all such patients (Szilagyi *et al.*, 1966). The operative mortality for such graft replacement of aneurysms over a wide

---

Serono Symposium No. 44, "Peripheral Arterial Diseases: Medical and Surgical Problems", edited by S. Stipa and A. Cavallaro, 1982. Academic Press, London and New York.

spectrum of surgical practice patterns remains at 5% or less (Upstate New York Registry Report, 1980; Stokes and Butcher, 1973).

However, certain categories of patients cannot be so fortunately dealt with. In patients with certain serious medical conditions, the peri-operative mortality (30-day period) will reach 20% and has been reported to be as high as 60% (Gardner *et al.*, 1978). In addition, some patients may also have specific intra-abdominal pathology which clearly contraindicates attempted graft replacement (Berguer *et al.*, 1978). In such patients, therefore, the surgeon is confronted with a decision that balances the risks of graft replacement of the aneurysm against those of the known complications. We have managed these patients by means of an alternative to direct-graft replacement which offers a much smaller surgical morbidity. This procedure has as its end-point the removal of the aneurysmal sac from continuous exposure to aortic pressure by the induction of aneurysmal sac thrombosis distal to the origin of the renal arteries. This surgical procedure is referred to as nonresective treatment of abdominal aortic aneurysm (Leather *et al.*, 1979).

SURGICAL TREATMENT

The principle of the method is that of producing acute thrombosis of the aneurysm while maintaining blood flow to the lower limbs via axillo-bilateral femoral grafts (Fig. 1). When the relevant investigations for the associated medical and surgical conditions determine that this approach should be used, each patient underwent pre-operative ultrasound examination of the aneurysm and angiographic visualization of the aorta, iliac and infrainguinal femoral arteries. The method of ensuring blood flow to the limbs is the use of the well-known axillo-bifemoral bypass grafts. The first part of the procedure consists of the placement of these grafts using the right axillary artery as the inflow source in every case (Blaisdell and Hall, 1963). In 36 patients, uncrimped external velour Dacron grafts (special order — USCI) were used. In nine patients Polytetrafluoroethylene (PTFE) (WT Gore) grafts were used. These grafts (8-mm main stem and 6-mm limbs) are individually constructed by ourselves using a geometric pattern (Table I).

The method of producing aneurysmal sac thrombosis was accomplished by means of complete acute obstructions of its immediate outflow tracts by surgical and/or radiological means. When the internal iliac arteries were patent in 18 instances, the common iliac arteries were interrupted surgically to preserve perfusion of the internal iliac territory (Fig. 2). However, when the common iliac arteries were not anatomically suitable for surgical interruption because of aneurysmal change or extensive calcification, the internal iliac and external iliac arteries were separately interrupted surgically at their origins (Fig. 3). This was done in 35 instances. In the last two patients in whom patent internal iliac arteries were demonstrated at the time of angiography, a trans-axillary aortic catheter was used to deposit Dacron-tufted metal coils within the internal iliac arteries to initiate thrombosis of these arteries. This obviated the necessity for any surgical procedure in the region of the abdomen (Fig. 4). External iliac interruption was then surgically carried out through the femoral

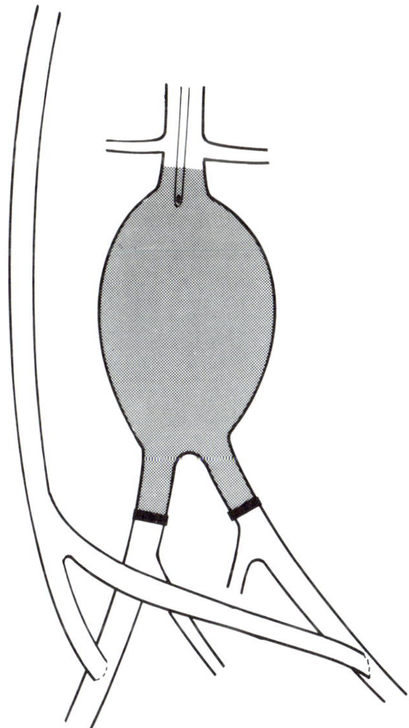

Fig. 1. General schema of the procedure of axillo-femoral bypass followed by outflow interruption and aneurysmal sac thrombosis. The common iliac arteries are ideally ligated to allow internal iliac retroperfusion (see also Figs 2 and 6). The proximal catheter is depicted to indicate the mechanism of completion of aneurysmal thrombosis post-operatively.

Table I. Special materials.

Special materials
Uncrimped external velour Dacron (special order USCI)
"Hemoclips" (large) with right angled applicator (Weck, Inc.)
No. 2 Ethicon (Ethilon, Inc.)
Occluding spring embolus (Cook, Inc.)

incision beneath the inguinal ligament, proximal to the origin of the deep circumflex and inferior epigastric branches. During this procedure it was found best to divide the anterior crossing deep circumflex vein to prevent unpleasant accidental tears which may extend into the external iliac vein. When the internal iliac arteries were not patent the external iliac artery was interrupted as described above through the femoral incision (Fig. 5). This was done in 23 instances. In 12 instances in which revascularization of a severely ischemic limb was a specific therapeutic goal, the common iliac artery was

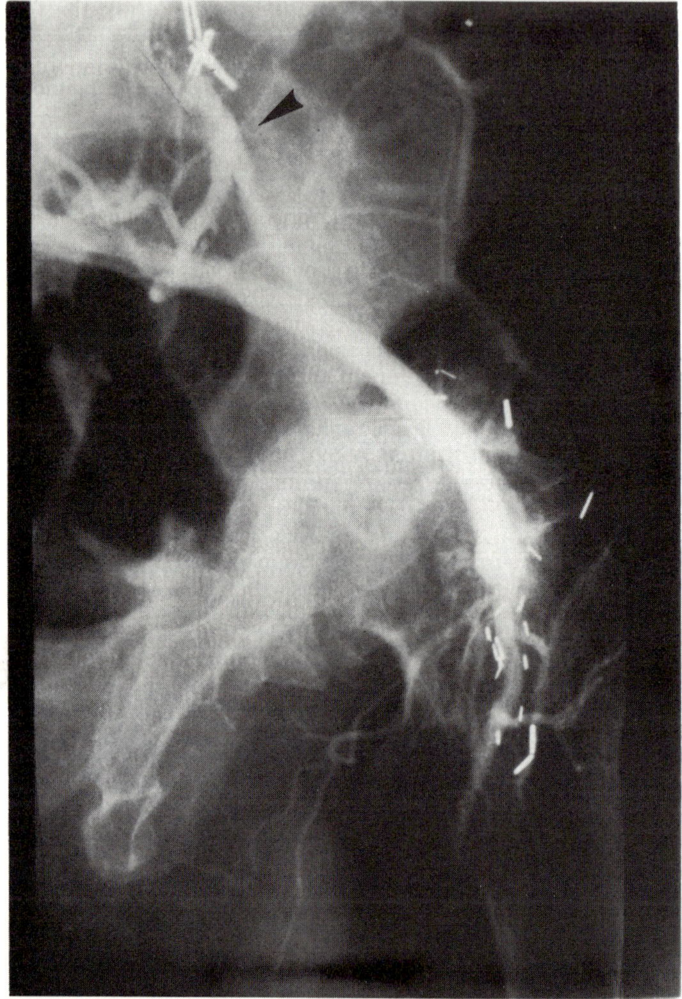

Fig. 2. Left limb of axillo-femoral bypass placed into the profunda-femoris artery. The common iliac artery has been interrupted with metal clips and the internal iliac (arrow) is being retroperfused.

pathologically occluded and no interruptive procedure was required. In one patient, because of severe stenosis of the common and internal iliac arteries on both sides, only the external iliac arteries were ligated as described and no attempt was made to completely interrupt the immediate aneurysmal outflow tract. This instructive case will be discussed later. Surgical interruption of these arteries was accomplished by the use of heavy metal Weck "hemoclips" or No. 2 Ethicon monofilament sutures (Table I). In patients of small build it was possible to use a single (usually left) retroperitoneal incision to reach both

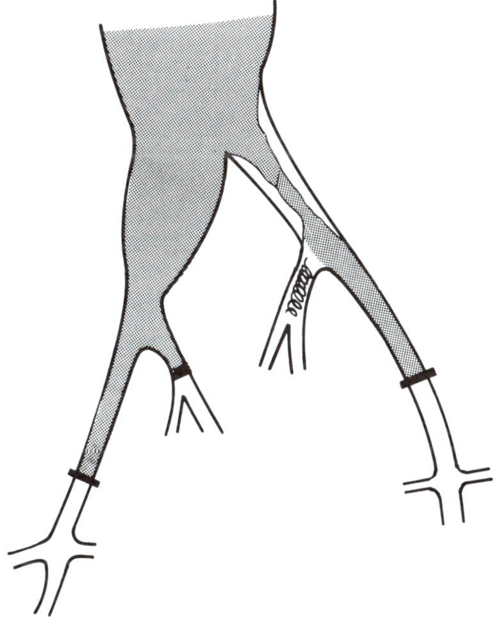

Fig. 3. Alternatives if the common iliac artery is aneurysmal or too rigid for ligation. On the right side both external and internal iliacs have been surgically interrupted (see also Fig. 7). On the left side a thrombogenic coil has been introduced into the internal iliac by angiographic catheter (see Fig. 4) and the external iliac is interrupted below the inguinal ligament.

common iliac arteries and their bifurcations. In patients of larger girth it was sometimes necessary to use bilateral retroperitoneal exposures to expose these vessels. However, in the last five patients who required common or internal iliac interruptions a lower mid-line incision was used to gain entry to the retroperitoneal space on both sides for accomplishing these goals.

Flow in the aneurysm was monitored post-operatively by the disappearance of expansile pulsations and Doppler ultrasound and was confirmed by radionucleide aortic flow studies (Fig. 6) three days later. In those patients in whom aortic thrombosis did not occur within 72 h transaxillary aortography was used to identify the outflow vessels responsible for continued patency of the aneurysm. In three patients, Bucrylate, a tissue adhesive, was then introduced by coaxial catheter into these vessels. Because of the unique property of this compound to solidify immediately on contact with charged ions, permanent segmental vascular occlusion was obtained by these means (Fig. 7) (Goldman *et al.*, 1978). In the last such case tufted coils have been successfully used for this purpose (Fig. 8, Table I). In 12 patients 1 ml of 1% thrombin solution was injected proximal to the points of interruption to initiate thrombosis of the obstructed artery more rapidly. This is no longer done (see Medical Complications).

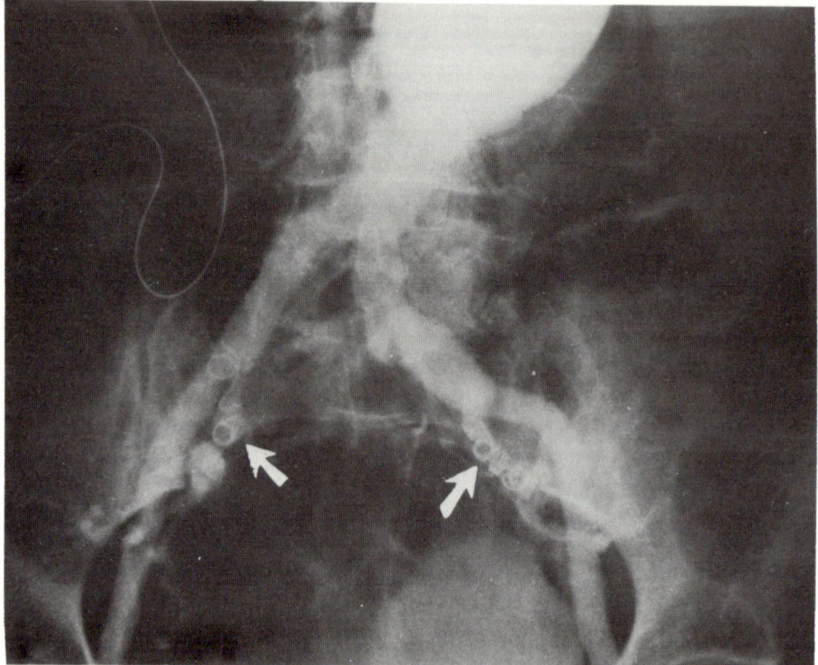

Fig. 4. Pre-operative placement of coils in both internal iliac arteries (arrow). This allows external iliac ligation through the femoral incision, thus avoiding abdominal wounds.

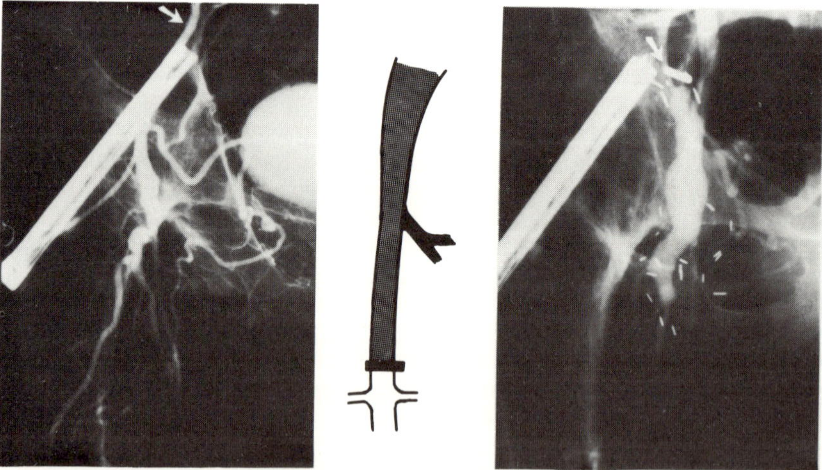

Fig. 5. When the common and external iliacs are patent (left) (arrow) but the internal is pathologically occluded (right) the external iliac is interrupted under the inguinal ligament *proximal* to the deep circumflex and inferior epigastric arteries (arrow). Note in left part the stenotic lesions of the common femoral and lateral circumflex arteries and the absence of the profunda main stem. These arteries were reconstructed for limb salvage.

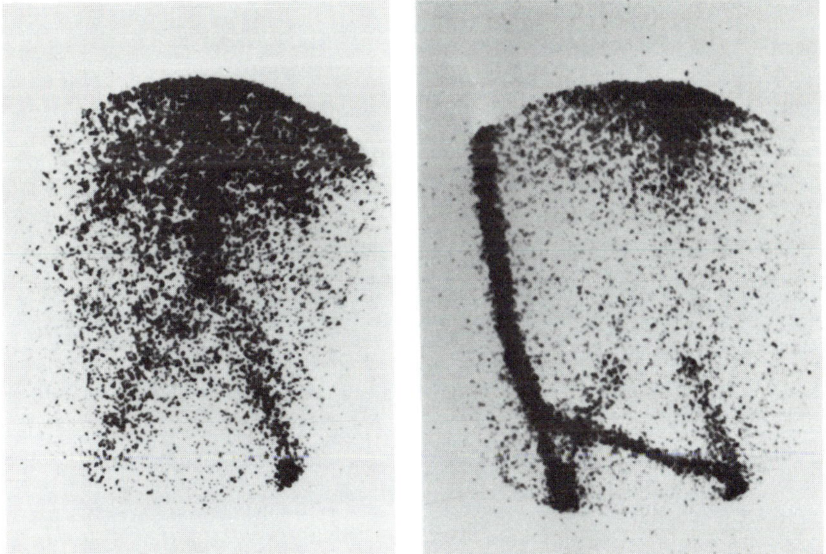

Fig. 6. Pre- and post-operative radionucleide aortic flow studies. In the post-operative study, the aortic stump is shown above together with the axillo-femoral bypasses supplying the lower limbs and the pelvis by retroperfusion of the internal iliac arteries.

CLINICAL MATERIALS

Forty-five patients have undergone the general procedure of non-resective treatment of abdominal aortic aneurysm with the details already described. Specific indications for treatment of the aneurysm apart from its presence are shown in Table II. Of particular interest are the seven patients who had severe chronic occlusive arterial disease which itself necessitated a surgical procedure for limb salvage irrespective of the presence of the aneurysm. In one patient with severe retroperitoneal fibrosis, scarring was of such intensity that clamps could not be placed to allow graft interposition. In another patient who had undergone eight intra-abdominal surgical procedures, the intra-peritoneal and retroperitoneal spaces were so disturbed by fibrous adhesions that direct graft replacement of the aneurysm seemed to be unnecessarily risky. The vast majority of patients were, however, treated by this method because of severe cardiac, renal and respiratory insufficiency and associated morbid obesity. These factors are defined in Table III. The cardiac risk is based on the New York Heart Association classification of functional capacity and therapeutic end point (New York Heart Association, 1973). All patients with cardiac problems were either graded as class III or IV. Respiratory risk was based on the findings that patients with a forced expiratory volume (FEV) of less than 1 liter in 1 s carry a high risk of respiratory failure after major intra-abdominal surgery (Auchinloss, 1974). Severe renal insufficiency is

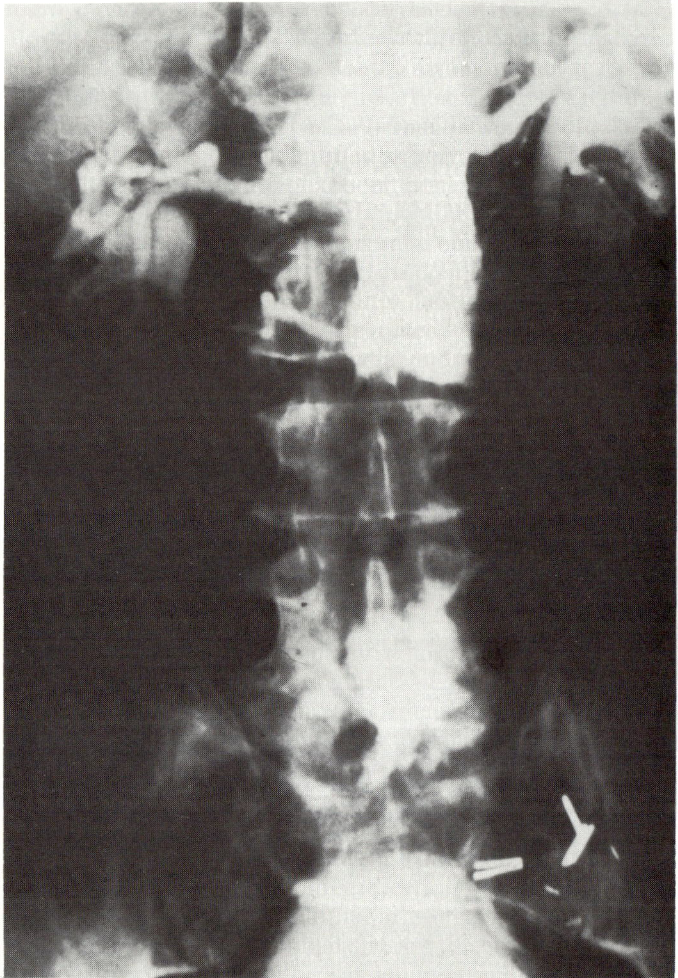

Fig. 7. Aneurysmal thrombosis induced by Bucrylate (arrow). On the left side the external and internal iliacs have been separately clipped.

defined as a 24-h creatinine clearance of less than 40 ml/min^{-1}. It has previously been shown that patients with this degree of renal functional disturbances carry a high mortality rate after surgical procedure because of permanent deterioration in renal performance (Powers *et al.*, 1964). The risk factor for morbid obesity is defined as a body weight that is 45 kg and/or 100% more than the ideal weight–height correlation for a given patient (Consensus Conference on Surgical Management of Obesity, 1978). The frequency with which specific medical problems were encountered in these patients is shown in Table IV. It will be noted from Table IV that, in most cases, each patient had two or more risk factors operating simultaneously.

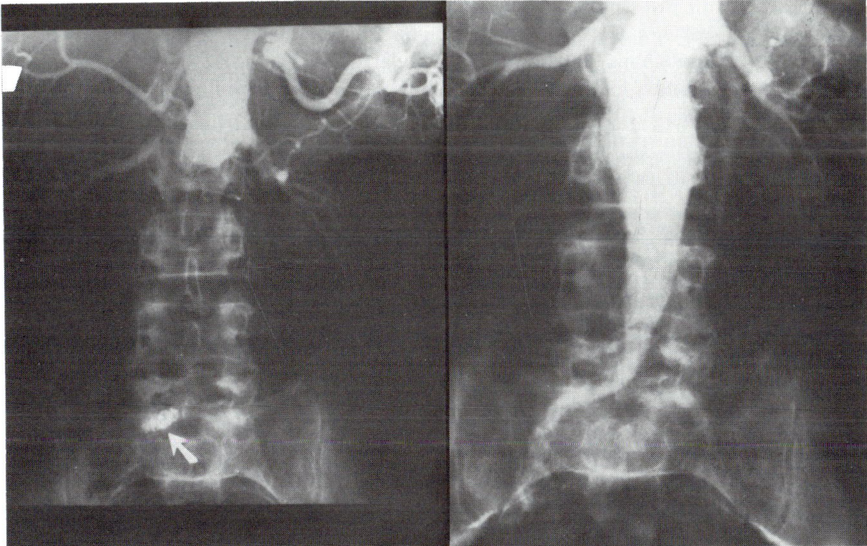

Fig. 8. Similar case to that in Fig. 7. Aneurysmal flow was maintained by a patent branch of the internal iliac. Introduction of a thrombogenic coil by catheter (arrow) has resulted in immediate infrarenal aortic thrombosis.

Table II. Surgical indications.

Symptomatic	6
Rapid expansion	12
Associated with limb salvage	7
Greater than 8 cm	10

Table III. Definition of medical risk factors.

Cardiac
NYHA — classes III and IV
Renal
24-h creatinine clearance < 40 ml min^{-1}
Respiratory
FEV_1 less than 1 liter or 50% predicted value
Obesity
45 kg or 100% more than ideal H/W ratio

Table IV. Medical indications.

Type	Absolute	Relative
Cardiac	15	26
Respiratory	11	5
Renal	23	5
Obesity	10	5

RESULTS

There was no intra-operative mortality. All of the patients felt and showed minimal physiological disturbances from the surgical procedure in the immediate post-operative period. Only one required bank blood transfusion because of the development of disseminated intravascular coagulation (see Medical Complications). In 41 patients thrombosis of the aneurysm occurred within 72 h. In the symptomatic patient pain and tenderness abated as aortic thrombosis occurred. In four patients patent though diseased internal iliac arteries were sufficient for continued aortic patency. These were treated by transaxillary catheter deposition of either Bucrylate or thrombogenic coils into the relevant vessels within seven days of the surgical procedure. Two patients died in the peri-operative (30-day) period, both from myocardial infarctions. One of these patients who had had a previous stroke suffered from unremitting hypotension in the post-infarct period and had a further profound stroke. The other had severe cardioelectric disturbances which were uncontrolled by all known forms of therapy. Six patients died in the post-operative period (Table V). Three died from cardiac failure two, two and six months after operation. One patient with chronic renal failure died after a concomitant severe hemorrhage from diverticular disease of the colon. In this series of cases the second patient treated by this procedure died four months later because of rupture of the abdominal aneurysm. The influence of this case on our subsequent approach is considered more fully in this paper. The 37 surviving patients (follow-up period was one month to three years) are alive and have continued to function within the limits of their medical restrictions. There has yet been no evidence of proximal progression of aortic thrombosis into the renal or other visceral arteries in these patients.

Table V. Post-operative deaths (6).

Type	Number	Time interval (months)
Cardiac	3	2, 2 and 6
Renal failure	1	4
Ruptured aneurysm	1	4
CA colon	1	10

The surgical complications are shown in Table VI. Four patients have had axillary graft thrombosis necessitating graft thrombectomies. Three of these patients were those in whom the operation was carried out for limb salvage as well as for aneurysmal obliteration. There was a false aneurysm at one femoral anastomosis in one patient which required surgical correction. There was one inguinal wound infection in an obese woman which required treatment by radical excision and a musculocutaneous flap. Two male patients are now experiencing buttock claudication and impotence eight months after operation. In one of these patients both internal iliac arteries were ligated at their origins but in the other the common iliac arteries were ligated on each side but thrombosis has nevertheless progressed to involve the internal iliac arteries as well (Fig. 9). Lack of internal iliac perfusion is presumably the cause of both buttock claudication and impotence in these two patients.

Table VI. Surgical complications.

Axillary graft thrombosis	4
Buttock claudication and impotence	2
Wound infection	1
False aneurysm	1

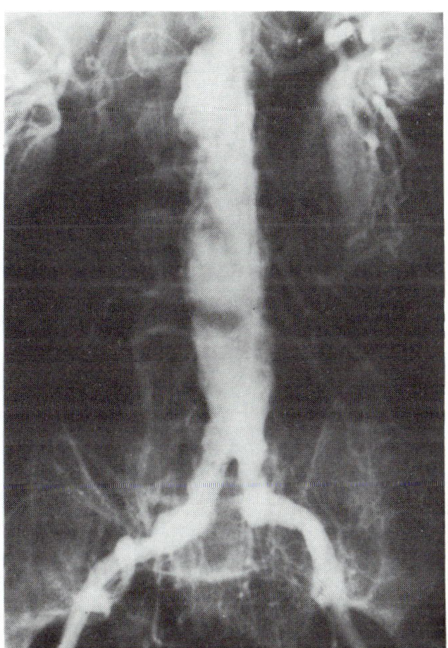

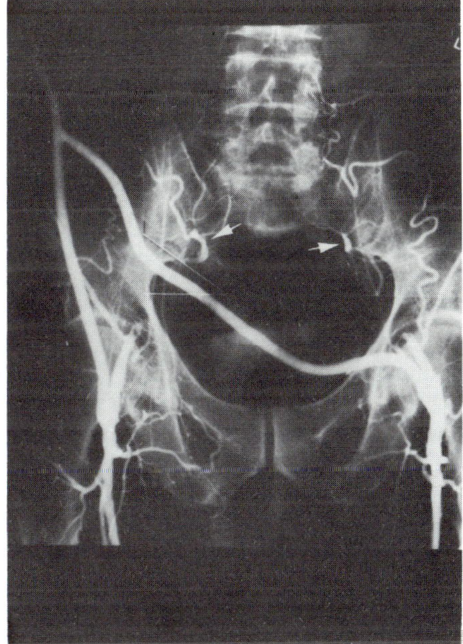

Fig. 9. One of two patients with buttock claudication and impotence. The common iliac arteries were ligated in this patient well proximal to their bifurcation but thrombosis of the external iliac has nevertheless occurred. The remnants of the internal iliac are shown by arrows.

The medical complications are listed in Table VII. Apart from the deaths already described there have been two non-fatal myocardial infarcts and one patient in whom the serum creatinine has risen from 2.8 to 4.2 mg % and remained at this level for the past year. However, as far as we can judge by isotope imaging and clearance studies the renal arteries themselves are not involved by proximal thrombotic progression. In one patient in whom thrombin was introduced into the proximal common iliac artery after its ligation in order to hasten the initiation of thrombosis, a florid state of disseminated intravascular coagulation took place which required consider-

Table VII. Medical complications.

Myocardial infarcts	2
Thrombin DIC	1
Renal dysfunction	1

able intra-operative hematological correction. The peri-operative (30-day) mortality in this series has been 4.4% and the subsequent mortality from the medical conditions which dictated this approach has been 11% over a period of three years.

DISCUSSION

It has long been recognised that intrasaccular thrombosis of aneurysms would alleviate symptoms and prevent their rupture (Dale, 1974). A variety of methods have been used to promote this event. The principle of inflow ligation as a mode of treatment of aneurysms dates back to the second century when it was frequently used as a treatment for traumatic aneurysms of the limbs. As a point of surgical history this type of ligation is referred to as Hunterian ligation because of its use by John Hunter in the management of syphilitic popliteal aneurysms. Within the body cavities aneurysms were first treated in 1817 when Sir Astley Cooper attempted ligation of the neck of an abdominal aortic aneurysm but nearly 150 years would elapse before the first successful ligation of such an aneurysm was reported (Blaisdell *et al.*, 1965). Wire coils introduced into the aneurysmal sac both at operation and percutaneously have also been used with and without electric current augmentation to induce rapid thrombosis (Hicks and Rob, 1978). However, devascularization and death of the lower limbs after induced thrombosis of abdominal aortic aneurysms have remained a serious problem. In addition to intrasaccular thrombosis various methods have been used to induce fibrosis of the aneurysm wall in order to strengthen it and arrest its enlargement. These include cellophane wraps, mesh wraps, fascia lata and metal bands as well as sprays such as diacetic phosphate. These treatments are rarely used nowadays since they involve a degree of surgical trauma that differs but little from the formal procedure of graft replacement of the aneurysm.

Although the mortality for elective aneurysmectomy is consistently at or below 5% (McCombs and Roberts, 1979; Bergan and Yao, 1974) many investigators (Szilagyi *et al.*, 1966; Thompson *et al.*, 1975; De Bakey *et al.*, 1964) have demonstrated that in those patients treated by graft replacement the coexistence of pre-existing cardiorespiratory disease will cause an increase of significant proportions in the mortality rates. This increase in peri-operative mortality is causally related to the complications of atherosclerotic heart disease probably because its incidence is greater in the elderly who provide the bulk of these patients. It has also been shown that patients with creatinine clearances of less than 40 ml/min^{-1} have a tremendously increased mortality when undergoing major abdominal surgery (Gardner *et al.*, 1978; Powers *et al.*, 1964).

One of the known effects of aortic cross-clamping in the standard operation of graft replacement of an aneurysm is a sudden increase in the cardiac afterload. The potential risk of this physiological readjustment is myocardial ischemia, cardiac arrhythmias or intra-operative myocardiac infarction. The technique described here eliminates this risk not only because the aorta is not cross-clamped but also because the axillo-femoral bypass provides a safety valve for decompression of this afterload while thrombotic occlusion of the aorta is occurring. The relatively slow rate of this occlusive process compared with the sudden application of a clamp is also beneficial in this respect. These factors may be particularly important in patients with severe myocardial disease.

It is, therefore, clear that although graft replacement remains the ideal treatment for abdominal aortic aneurysm this particular operation may result in an unacceptably high mortality in certain medically compromised patients. The fact that four of the six late deaths were caused by the conditions that dictated this particular choice of treatment serves to emphasize the extent of medical risks in this group. The high incidence of patients with both abdominal aortic aneurysms and threatened limb survival is also worthy of note (Fig. 10). This appears to be indicative of a greater deterioration of the

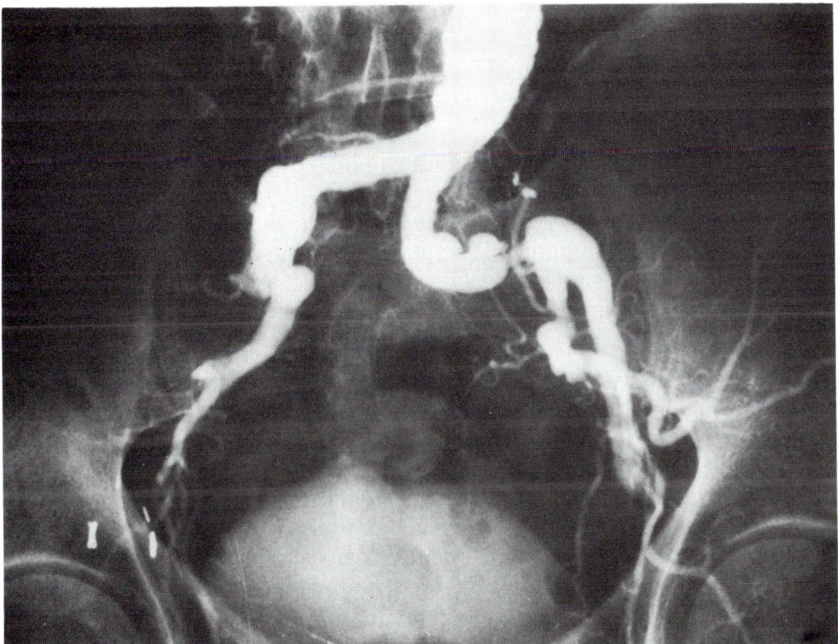

Fig. 10. Severe stenosis of right internal and left common iliac arteries were sufficient to allow aneurysm patency and subsequent rupture. The internal iliac artery or its branches are the most common offenders in this respect.

arterial tree in these patients when compared with patients with abdominal aortic aneurysms who have no apparent compromise of the arterial circulation to the lower limbs. It is, therefore, not surprising that these patients also exhibit marked evidence of cardiopulmonary and renal impairment. In addition, the consistent problems experienced with the axillo-femoral grafts in this group of patients are a well-recognized fact of life and will probably represent the inability of severely compromised outflow arterial tract to allow high enough flow rates to keep these grafts patent.

Although the role of angiography in the management of abdominal aortic aneurysm is not fully agreed on this is a mandatory pre-operative investigation in these patients. It identifies three potential problems.

(1) It determines the position and importance of the renal and inferior mesenteric arteries. A low-lying main or accessory renal artery may undergo thrombosis with resulting loss of renal parenchyma or it may serve as an outflow tract of sufficient size to allow continued flow through the aneurysm. An enlarged inferior mesenteric artery may also contribute to aneurysmal patency in similar fashion but, worse yet, if it is a major intestinal arterial source acute thrombosis may result in a fatal gastro-intestinal insult (Karmody *et al.*, 1976).

(2) The patency of the hypogastric arteries must be determined so that their interruption can be accomplished.

(3) Outflow problems of the infrainguinal femoral arteries (common, superficial and profunda) must be identified to ensure that there are no hemodynamically critical lesions of the predominant outflow tract distal to the proposed site of anastomosis that would compromise the achievement of the highest possible graft flow rates and thus short-term function and long-term patency.

Probably the most important aspect of this procedure is the minimizing of tissue trauma, blood loss and respiratory difficulties that attend intra-abdominal replacement. Blood loss has been minimal and only one patient has required a post-operative transfusion. All regained unimpaired gastro-intestinal function within 24 h. Of 45 patients 40 were discharged after an uneventful convalescence which did not include any extraordinary means of cardiopulmonary or renal support.

The first case report of the use of this method was published by Berguer *et al.* (1978). In this patient massive retroperitoneal lymphomatous involvement prevented direct-graft replacement. After axillo-femoral bypass the common iliac arteries were occluded by balloon catheters passed retrogradely through exteriorized external iliac arteries. Occlusion of the aneurysm was accomplished by the installation of thrombin, Gelfoam and crushed muscle into the aortic bifurcation via a transaxillary aortic catheter. These materials were infused into the aneurysmal sac under radiological control until thrombosis was achieved within 12 h. Both Berguer and ourselves have since treated other patients in whom balloon occlusions of the common iliac arteries were attempted unsuccessfully with the Hunter-Session or Fogarty occlusion balloons. Attempts are now underway to achieve common iliac occlusion without their direct surgical exposure at the time of axillo-femoral bypass by using detachable balloons (Berguer *et al.*, 1981). The results of these efforts may well further simplify the performance of this procedure.

In our second patient, referred to previously (Fig. 10) the right internal iliac artery was stenosed at its origin and there was severe stenosis of the left common iliac artery as well. We believed that flow through these internal iliac arteries was so compromized that it would be insufficient to support patency of the aneurysm and that thrombosis would slowly but definitely occur. This patient was discharged in this state and was lost sight of until four months later when he was readmitted with obvious signs of rupture of the aneurysm. This was treated by intraperitoneal occlusion of the neck of the aneurysm with interrupted sutures but these efforts did not prevent his death. This experience has indicated that even severely diseased iliac arteries could maintain aortic flow. Subsequently, strenuous attempts have been made to obliterate all iliac outflow tracts whenever these were seen to be patent on angiography.

In our experience, aneurysmal thrombosis will generally occur (92%) within 72 h if the iliac outflow tracts are completely obstructed. Although we have not had any instance in which there was immediate post-operative rupture of the aneurysm after interruption of the major iliac outflow vessels, our observation of intrasaccular thrombosis within 72 h has been so pronounced that in our opinion, when aortic flow persists beyond this interval, transaxillary aortography should be undertaken to identify the outflow tract responsible for continued aortic patency. Under radiological control this vessel can be obliterated by the deposition of a number of materials including thrombin, Gelfoam, crushed muscle, Bucrylate or thrombogenic coils, or even by surgical interruption if the surgeon prefers. Usually, aneurysmal thrombosis will then take place immediately and can be angiographically documented. In four patients when Doppler ultrasound and radionuclear examinations showed continued patency of the aneurysm, these patients had aortic thrombosis induced by these means. Although Bucrylate was originally used as a thrombogenic agent, the availability of this material is now restricted by the FDA and indeed it has showed a somewhat alarming propensity to be swept distally before solidification has occurred. Our experience with thrombogenic metal coils has been more benign and is the present method of election. Savarese *et al.* (1981) have also used coils very successfully to accomplish these ends in six patients of this type.

The operation itself is greatly facilitated by two teams of surgeons. Although speed is not of great consequence some procedures have been completed within 75 min and none have exceeded 150 min. The choice of available graft material is obviously wide. In the interest of saving time and blood, nine procedures have been done with PTFE grafts. However, the authors' preference is for external velour Dacron grafts and these have been used in the remainder (Yates *et al.*, 1978). It is possible that when unobstructed lower limb vessels are present either material will be equally satisfactory. In our hands, however, uncrimped external velour Dacron seems to be the material of choice for outflow tracts of poorer quality. Recent work reported by Moore (1981) appears to support this choice.

One of the most important and difficult surgical aspects of this procedure has been the complete interruption of the iliac vessels. The common iliac vessels are frequently both aneurysmal and heavily calcified and may be firmly adherent to the adjacent veins. As we have experienced, ligatures may sever such soft vessels or may incompletely occlude the lumen because of its atherosclerotic rigidity. Although it is ideal to interrupt the aneurysms outflow at the common iliac level to permit retrograde internal iliac perfusion this maneuver may prove to be unrewarding and/or dangerous. In this event it is preferable to interrupt the external and internal iliac arteries separately. When carefully applied, large metal clips have been useful because of their broader area of contact but if ligatures are preferred, a sizable monofilament suture is the best choice. Successful though sporadic use of braided umbilical tape has also been reported by others who have carried out this procedure.

We have deliberately ligated the internal arteries separately in over one-half of our patients without incident and have seen no complications related to ischemia of the pelvic organs or sigmoid colon. However, in the two male patients who now complain of buttock claudication and impotence, thrombosis of the internal iliac arteries may clearly have had these undesirable side effects. Whether this will prove to be a statistically important complication remains to be seen. However, when comparing high-risk graft replacement of the abdominal aneurysm and the lower morbidity of this method with these potential complications, surgical judgement after frank consultation with each patient will have to be exercised in each decision. It should also be pointed out that in most of these patients (females, elderly males) the potential problem of impotence is largely academic and that in the relatively young potent male the risk of impotence after direct-graft replacement is also considerable.

CONCLUSION

We wish to stress again that the good-risk patient with an abdominal aortic aneurysm deserves the tried and tested operation of direct-graft replacement. Although the patency rates of axillo-femoral and aorto-iliofemoral bypasses are comparable (LoGerfo *et al.*, 1977) the axillary bypasses are, at least, subject to mechanical misadventure because of their subcutaneous positions. However, their use together with iliac outflow occlusion represents a simple and potentially effective alternative to the standard surgical treatment of abdominal aortic aneurysms. In this well-defined group of patients this procedure has resulted in a decrease in morbidity and mortality when prohibitive problems may have been anticipated after extensive intra-abdominal surgery.

REFERENCES

Auchinloss, J. H. (1974). Preoperative evaluation of pulmonary function. *Surgical Clinics of North America* **54**, 1015.

Bergan, J. J. and Yao, J. S. T. (1974). Modern management of abdominal aortic aneurysms. *Surgical Clinics of North America* **54**, 175.

Berguer, R., Schneider, J. and Wilner, H. I. (1978). Induced thrombosis of inoperable

abdominal aortic aneurysm. *Surgery* **83**, 425.
Berguer, R., Feldman, A. J. and Karmody, A. M. (1981). Intravascular thrombosis of abdominal aortic aneurysm in high-risk patients. *Vascular Diagnosis and Therapy* **1**, 24.
Blaisdell, F. W. and Hall, A. D. (1963). Axillo-femoral bypass for lower extremity ischemia. *Surgery* **54**, 563.
Blaisdell, F. W., Hall, A. D. and Thomas, A. N. (1965). Ligation treatment of abdominal aortic aneurysms. *American Journal of Surgery* **109**, 560.
Consensus Conference on Surgical Management of Obesity (1978). National Institute of Health, December 1978.
Dale, W. A. (1974). The beginnings of vascular surgery. *Surgery* **76**, 849.
DeBakey, M. E., Crawford, E. S., Cooley, D.A. *et al.* (1964). Aneurysm of the abdominal aorta: analysis of results of graft replacement therapy one to 11 years after operation. *Annals of Surgery* **160**, 622.
Gardner, R. J., Gardner, H. L., Tarnay, T. J. *et al.* (1978). The surgical experience and one- to 16-year follow-up of 277 abdominal aortic aneurysms. *American Journal of Surgery* **135**, 226.
Goldman, M. L., Freeny, C., Tallman, M. *et al.* (1978). Transcatheter vascular occlusion therapy with isobutyl 2-cyanoacrylate (Bucrylate) for control of massive upper gastrointestinal bleeding. *Radiology* **129**, 41.
Hicks, G. L. and Rob, C. (1978). Abdominal aortic aneurysm wiring: an alternative method. *American Journal of Surgery* **131**, 664.
Karmody, A. M., Jordan, F. R. and Zaman, S. N. (1976a). Left colon gangrene after acute inferior mesenteric artery occlusion. *Archives of Surgery (Chicago)* **111**, 972.
Karmody, A. M., Powers, S. R. Jr., Monaco, V. J. and Leather, R. P. (1976b). Blue toe syndrome: an indication for limb salvage surgery. *Archives of Surgery (Chicago)* **111**, 1263.
Leather, R. P., Shah, D. M., Goldman, M., Rosenberg, M. and Karmody, A. M. (1979). Nonresective treatment of abdominal aortic aneurysms: use of acute thrombosis and axillo-femoral bypass. *Archives of Surgery (Chicago)* **114**, 1402.
LoGerfo, F. W., Johnson, W. C., Corson, J. D. *et al.* (1977). Comparison of late patency rates of axillo-bilateral and unilateral femoral grafts. *Surgery* **81**, 33.
McCombs, P. R. and Roberts, B. (1979). Acute renal failure after resection of abdominal aortic aneurysm. *Surgery Gynecology and Obstetrics* **148**, 175.
Moore, W. S. (1981). The influence of graft porosity and design on healing characteristics. *American Journal of Surgery* (In press).
New York Heart Association (1973). "Nonenclature and Criteria for Diagnosis of Disease of the Heart and Gross Vessels". Little, Brown, Boston, Massachusetts.
Powers, S. R., Kiley, J. E. and Boba, A. (1974). Renal failure in surgical patients. *Current Problems in Surgery* 10–18, November, 1964.
Savarese, R. P., Rocenfeld, J. C. and DeLaurentis, D. A. (1981). Alternatives in the treatment of abdominal aortic aneurysm. *American Journal of Surgery* (In press).
Stokes, J. and Butcher, H. R. (1973). Abdominal aortic aneurysm: factors influencing operative mortality and criteria of operability. *Archives of Surgery (Chicago)* **107**, 297.
Szilagyi, D. E., Smith, R. F., DeRusso, F. J. *et al.* (1966). Contribution of abdominal aortic aneurysmectomy to prolongation of life. *Annals of Surgery* **164**, 678.
Thompson, J. E., Hollier, L. H., Patman, R. D. *et al.* (1975). Surgical management of abdominal aortic aneurysm. *Annals of Surgery* **181**, 654.
Upstate New York Registry Report (1980). Authors data.
Voorhees, A. B., Jaretzki, A. and Blakemore, A. H. (1952). The use of tubes constructed from Vinyon "N" cloth in bridging arterial defects. *Annals of Surgery* **135**, 332.

Yates, S. G., Aires, A. B., Knute, B. O. *et al.* (1978). The preclotting of porous arterial prostheses. *Annals of Surgery* **188**, 611.

SURGERY OF ABDOMINAL AORTIC ANEURYSMS IN PECULIAR ANATOMIC SITUATIONS

D. A. DeLaurentis

Department of Surgery, University of Pennsylvania School of Medicine, Pennsylvania Hospital, Philadelphia, Pennsylvania, USA

INTRODUCTION

There has been a progressive decrease in the mortality and morbidity rate for surgery of abdominal aortic aneurysm since the original report by Dubost (1952). The reasons for this improvement are related primarily to better respiratory support, a more detailed understanding of associated athero-sclerotic lesions, sophisticated hemodynamic monitoring, improved arterial prostheses and sutures, the nonresectional technique introduced by Creech in 1966 and lastly, a more comprehensive knowledge of the surgical anatomy of this aneurysm. For a surgeon to obtain a good result, knowledge of normal anatomy is necessary. To obtain superior results, however, it is essential that he understands and recognizes anatomical variations and peculiarities. The possible anatomical variants in surgery for abdominal aortic aneurysm involve mainly the following systems or areas.

(1) Venous.*
(2) Arterial.*
(3) Urological.*
(4) Retroperitoneal.*
(5) Gastro-intestinal.
(6) Neurological.

Serono Symposium No. 44, "Peripheral Arterial Diseases: Medical and Surgical Problems", edited by S. Stipa and A. Cavallaro, 1982. Academic Press, London and New York.

(7) Lymphatic.
(8) Pelvic viscera.

The purpose of this paper is to describe the more common anatomical peculiarities encountered in surgery for abdominal aortic aneurysms (*) and methods used to deal with these variants. Between January 1967 and December 1980, the author and his group have operated upon 273 patients with abdominal aortic aneurysms. Two hundred and eight of these procedures were carried out on an elective basis with 15 deaths giving a mortality rate of 7%. There were 65 patients with ruptured abdominal aortic aneurysms of which 28 died giving a mortality rate of 43%. Nineteen patients with ruptured abdominal aneurysms traveled more than 100 miles to our institution for definitive therapy. Of these 19 patients, 13 survived and six died providing a mortality rate of 32%. In the elective group, there were 164 males (79%) and 44 females (21%). In the ruptured group, there were 53 males (82%) and 12 females (18%). The ages of these patients varied between 48 and 88 years in the elective group (average of 66 years) and 53–94 years in the ruptured group (average of 69 years). It is from this group of 273 patients that our experience with some of the anatomical variants encountered in this type of surgery is derived.

MAJOR VENOUS ANOMALIES

Abdominal aortic aneurysms are "framed" with adherent large veins. There is little question that the major source of uncontrolled and massive hemorrhage in surgery of abdominal aneurysms is related to venous injuries. Consequently, it is imperative that the surgical anatomy and anomalies of these veins be thoroughly understood. These anomalies are primarily related to the *inferior vena cava* and the *left renal vein*. The aortic "frame of veins" can better be understood if we consider the embryology of this area. The caval system is derived from the modification of three parallel sets of veins: the postcardinal, the subcardinal and the supracardinal. The postcardinal, a primitive system develops in association with the mesonephros, anastomoses with the developing subcardinal system and persists only as the iliac bifurcation. The right and left subcardinal veins are in a plane ventral to the aorta, anastomose together and divert blood to the right subcardinal system that forms the suprarenal portion of the inferior vena cava. Finally, the supracardinal system appears in a plane dorsal to the aorta and anastomoses with the subcardinal system and itself. This group of anastomoses (intersubcardinal, subcardinal–supracardinal and the intersupracardinal) join to form a collar of veins that surrounds the aorta. The right supracardinal vein persists as the normal infrarenal right inferior vena cava, and the ventral part of the circumaortic ring persists as the normal left renal vein (Fig. 1). The left supracardinal vein may persist, resulting in either a doubled inferior vena cava or a single left-sided inferior vena cava. The entire circumaortic ring may persist or the ventral portion may disappear, leaving only a retroaortic left renal vein (Milloy *et al.*, 1962). This simplified description accounts for the four major venous anomalies.

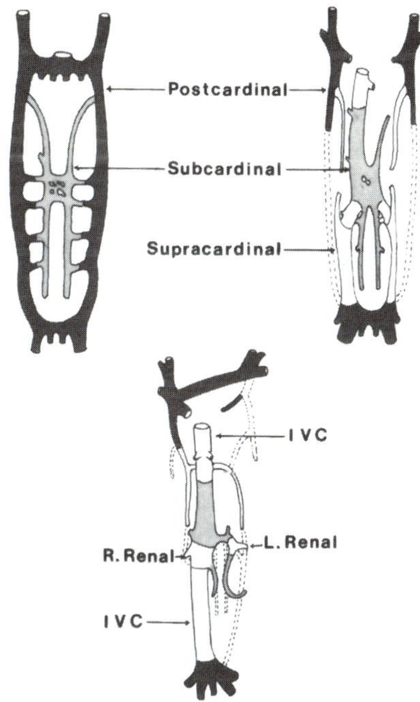

Fig. 1. Embryological derivations of the inferior vena cava and renal veins.

(1) Left-sided inferior vena cava.
(2) Duplicated inferior vena cava.
(3) Retroaortic left renal vein.
(4) Circumaortic renal collar.

Although anomalies of the lumbar, azygos, prevertebral and ascending lumbar veins are common, these veins are covered by the psoas muscle and are not usually of any consequence to the vascular surgeon except for anomalous left lumbar veins. These lumbar veins can drain into a retroaortic left renal vein and form large plexuses behind an abdominal aortic aneurysm. If injured during surgery, massive and, at times, uncontrollable hemorrhage ensues. During elective surgery, many of these peculiar venous patterns can be recognized if one is careful and looks for them. In patients with ruptured abdominal aortic aneurysms, however, the retroperitoneal hematoma camouflages the anomalies and this circumstance is undoubtedly another reason why the mortality rate for patients with ruptured abdominal aortic aneurysms is still high.

MANAGEMENT OF LEFT-SIDED VENA CAVA

If this anomaly is retroaortic, we can leave it alone, being extremely careful not to injure it during mobilization of the neck of the aneurysm and the common iliac arteries. If the left-sided inferior vena cava is preaortic, however, one may have to handle this by gentle retraction to the left along with retraction of the renal veins. If this does not allow sufficient exposure, the inferior vena cava can be transected below the renal veins, or the right renal vein can be transected close to the confluence with the inferior vena cava (Fig. 2). However, the right renal vein in this anomaly does not always have the collateral venous drainage found in the normal left renal venous system. Therefore, this latter procedure would be the least desirable choice and should not be done unless the function of the left kidney is known to be normal. As pointed out by DuPont (1971), the isolated left inferior vena cava is very rare and only one-tenth as common as the double inferior vena cava.

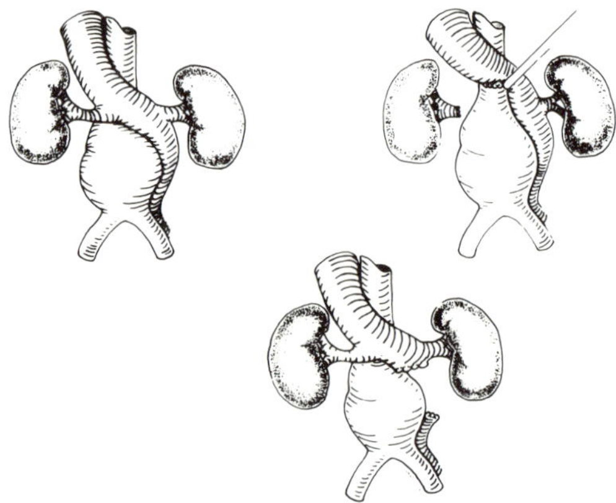

Fig. 2. Anatomy of the left-sided vena cava and techniques used to approach the aneurysm neck.

MANAGEMENT OF THE DOUBLE INFERIOR VENA CAVA

If the left side of a double inferior vena cava is small and posterior, nothing but careful dissection is necessary. If the left side is small and crosses the abdominal aortic aneurysm anteriorly, we may divide it. If the left-sided inferior vena cava is large and anteriorly placed, the left inferior vena cava can be transected below the confluence with the left renal vein or the left renal vein can be transected at the inferior vena cava (Fig. 3). In the report by Brener *et al.* (1974), major caval anomalies were found in nine patients. They were all handled successfully with no significant problems related to hemorrhage or renal function. In our series, we encountered a double caval system in two patients. In the first patient, this was recognized as the left portion of this system passed anterior to the abdominal aortic aneurysm to join the left renal vein. This situation was managed by ligation below the left renal vein. The second patient had a very large abdominal aortic aneurysm with a tight, short, kinked neck. Because control of the neck of the aneurysm could not be

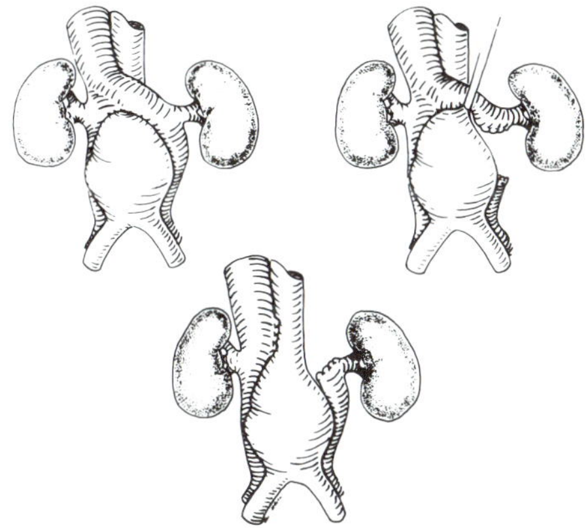

Fig. 3. The double inferior vena cava and methods used to approach the aneurysm neck.

achieved, it was elected to transect the iliac arteries and mobilize the aorta enough posteriorly to allow unkinking of the neck. During this maneuver, a large, posteriorly located, left inferior vena cava was recognized and injured. The laceration was controlled and the abdominal aortic aneurysm was resected without incident.

MANAGEMENT OF RENAL VEIN ANOMALIES

It must be emphasized that during the early mobilization of the neck of an abdominal aortic aneurysm, one must always carry out the dissection cephalad until the left renal vein can be identified crossing the aorta anteriorly. This normal anatomy occurs in about 90% of patients (Fig. 4). If the left renal vein cannot be identified anteriorly, one must identify the

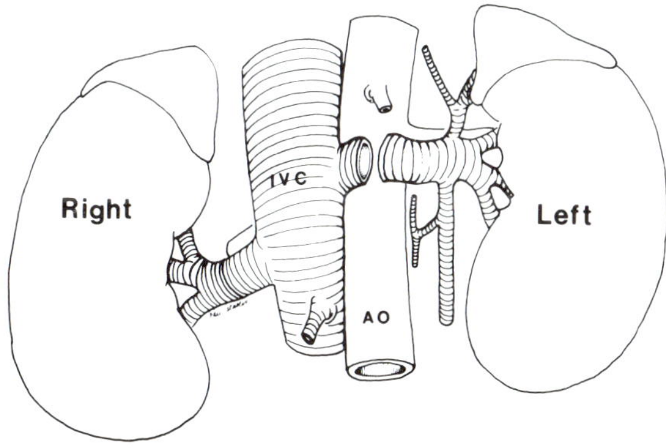

Fig. 4. Normal anatomy of left renal vein showing anterior or ventral position to the aorta.

inferior vena cava and, if present normally, one must assume that the left renal vein lies behind the aorta and dissection should proceed carefully, deliberately and under direct vision. When the left renal vein is located posterior to the aorta, it usually has an oblique course caudally as it joins the inferior vena cava behind the abdominal aortic aneurysm (Fig. 5). Also, this

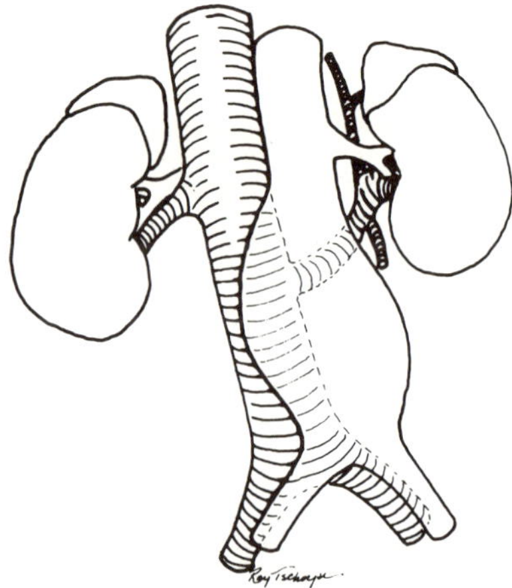

Fig. 5. The retroaortic left renal vein. Note caudal course of left renal vein.

retroaortic left renal vein is often joined by a plexus of large lumbar and retroperitoneal veins. This arrangement makes it particularly vulnerable to injury and resultant massive bleeding. This anomaly was encountered 20 times in the Brener and Darling series (Brener *et al.*, 1974) and there were nine major injuries with two deaths directly related to the injury and hemorrhage. Even when the normal occurring anterior left renal vein is identified, one must still be ever on the alert for a circumaortic collar, the other important left renal vein anomaly (Fig. 6). One of the clues to this anomaly is that the circumaortic collar is very adherent and intimate to the neck of the abdominal aortic aneurysm. When this occurs, one must suspect a collar and

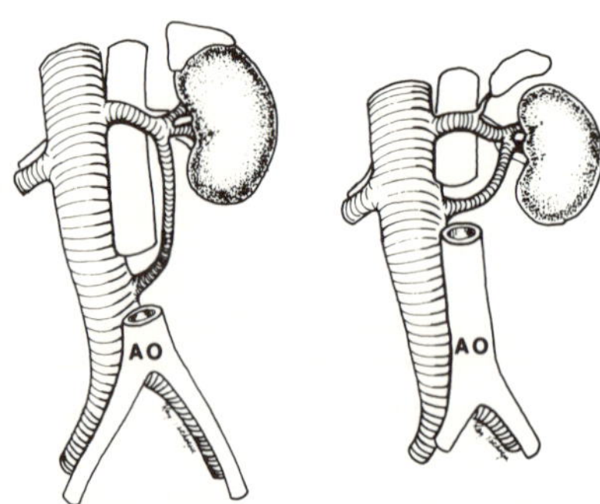

Fig. 6. Circumaortic left renal venous collar.

proceed carefully. If the collar is too tight and does not allow dissection and mobilization of the neck of the aneurysm, one may divide the anterior portion of the collar at the confluence with the inferior vena cava. Again, one must be very careful not to injure the posterior portion of the collar during mobilization of the neck. We have encountered a retroaortic left renal vein on five occasions. In four patients, the resection of the abdominal aortic aneurysm was elective, the vein was identified and not injured. In one patient with a ruptured abdominal aortic aneurysm, this retroaortic renal vein was not recognized, it was injured and led to additional massive hemorrhage and death of the patient. A circumaortic collar was encountered in one patient and successfully managed by dividing the anterior portion of the collar.

In summary, although venous anomalies are rare, they can be treacherous and the venous variant leading to most mortality and morbidity is the retroaortic left renal vein.

LIGATION AND DIVISION OF NORMAL OCCURRING PREAORTIC LEFT RENAL VEIN

Although not a peculiarity or anomaly, it seems appropriate to discuss this subject at this time since it is an adjunct to the surgical treatment of abdominal aortic aneurysms. Although in most patients the left renal vein can be retracted out of the way while the neck of the aneurysm is being mobilized and sutured, in some situations, division of this vein increases the exposure considerably and allows for better control of the neck of the aneurysm. Since the report by Neal and Shearburn in 1967, we have ligated and divided the normal occurring left renal vein in 26 patients undergoing abdominal aortic surgery. This maneuver was done most frequently (21 patients) during resection of an abdominal aortic aneurysm (8%). The left renal vein can usually be divided with impunity if the division is at the inferior vena cava and preserves collaterals to the left renal vein; i.e. the adrenal, phrenic, spermatic and ascending lumbar veins (Fig. 7). One must be certain that right renal

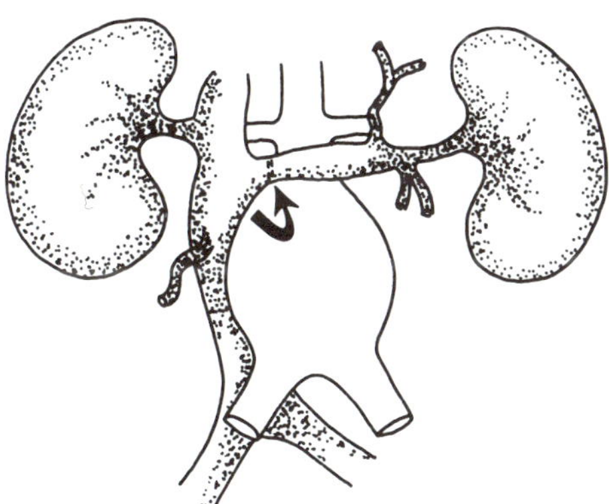

Fig. 7. Proper site to divide left renal vein when more exposure of this area is necessary.

function is present prior to ligation and division of the left renal vein. Our studies with left spermatic vein venography in 14 patients has demonstrated that the drainage of the left kidney is primarily by way of the ascending lumbar, hemiazygos and azygos system (DeLaurentis and Iyengar, 1970) (Fig. 8). In certain patients a very rapid and high degree of venous hypertension occurs when this vein is ligated, consequently, we have been measuring routinely the left renal vein stump pressure. If this pressure is much higher than 60 mmHg, we do not feel it is safe to ligate and divide the left renal vein (McCombs and DeLaurentis, 1979). Although this was a clinical impression, we have recently completed an experimental evaluation of left renal vein pressure in dogs and found that with pressures below 60 mmHg, very little parenchymal damage is done to the kidney. However, pressures above this level produce definite and sometimes irreversible renal changes. Consequently, if very high pressures are observed and the left renal vein is divided, one must be prepared to accept possible injury or loss of function of the left kidney. We do not recommend that the left renal vein be ligated and divided if there is a possibility of having to occlude the right renal artery for any length of time. This was done in one of our patients with a ruptured abdominal aortic aneurysm and he developed acute renal failure which did fortunately respond to repeated dialysis.

ARTERIAL ANOMALIES

The value of pre-operative arteriography in patients with abdominal aortic aneurysms can no longer be disputed (Rosch *et al.*, 1978). If this is done carefully, much information concerning arterial peculiarities can be obtained and the vascular surgeon has a good "road map". One must emphasize, however, that the diagnosis of an abdominal aortic aneurysm is not made by aortography but by physical examination, plane X-rays of the abdomen, ultrasonography and computerized automated tomography (CAT scan). Although arterial anomalies are more frequent than venous, they are usually easier to recognize and manage. If we postpone the discussion of anomalous arteries associated with horseshoe kidney, we can approach this subject by considering three common arterial variants.

(1) Accessory renal arteries.
(2) Low-lying renal arteries arising from the abdominal aortic aneurysm.
(3) The dominant inferior mesenteric artery (meandering artery).

Accessory renal arteries are present in approximately 15–20% of patients with abdominal aortic aneurysms (Fig. 9). They are managed by re-implantation in the prosthetic graft if they arise from the abdominal aortic aneurysm (Hardy and Timmis, 1971). The same holds true for low-lying renal arteries arising from the abdominal aortic aneurysm (Fig. 10). The technique involves making a "button" about the orifice of the artery (1–1.5 cm in diameter) and then re-implanting this button in the prosthetic graft (Fig. 11). If the orifice is stenotic, endarterectomy should be done prior to re-implantation. We infuse chilled heparinized Ringer's lactate solution in the renal artery and external

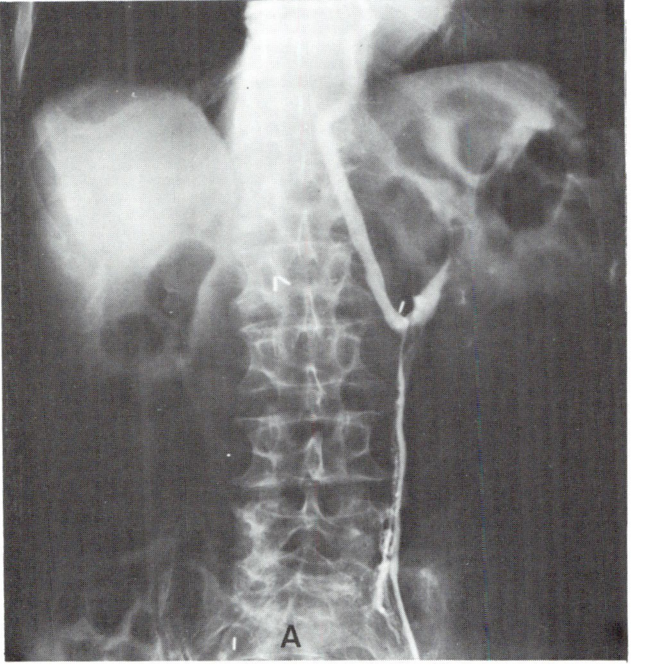

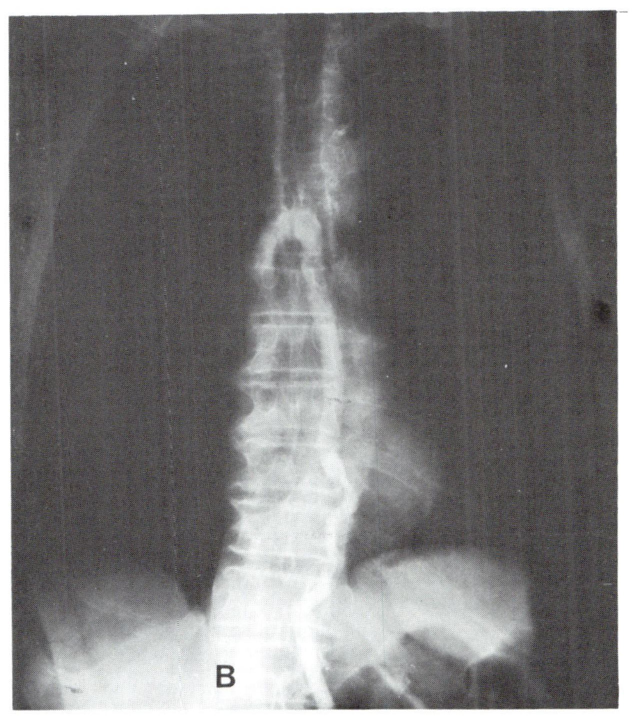

Fig. 8. Left spermatic vein venogram in a post-operative patient in which the left renal vein was divided. (A) Spermatic vein, ascending lumbar and hemiazygos venous channels. (B) Final drainage into the azygos vein.

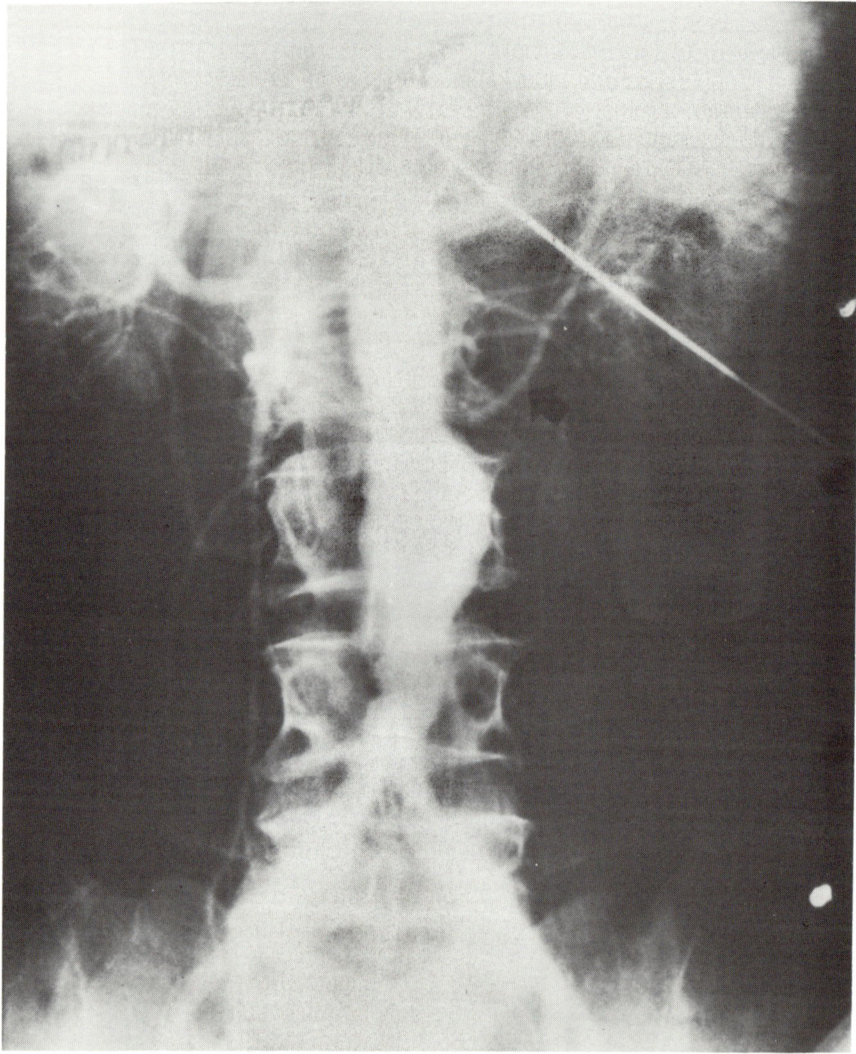

Fig. 9. Left accessory renal artery arising from the neck of an abdominal aortic aneurysm.

saline slush on the kidney to help reduce ischemia when renal arteries are re-implanted. The re-implantation should be done immediately after the proximal aortic anastomosis and then the proximal clamp is applied distal to the re-implanted artery (again to decrease the ischemia). If there is any question as to the success of the repair, the kidney should be carefully inspected to determine areas of ischemia. If areas of necrosis are present or if repair cannot be done, resection of the ischemic portion of the kidney should be carried out.

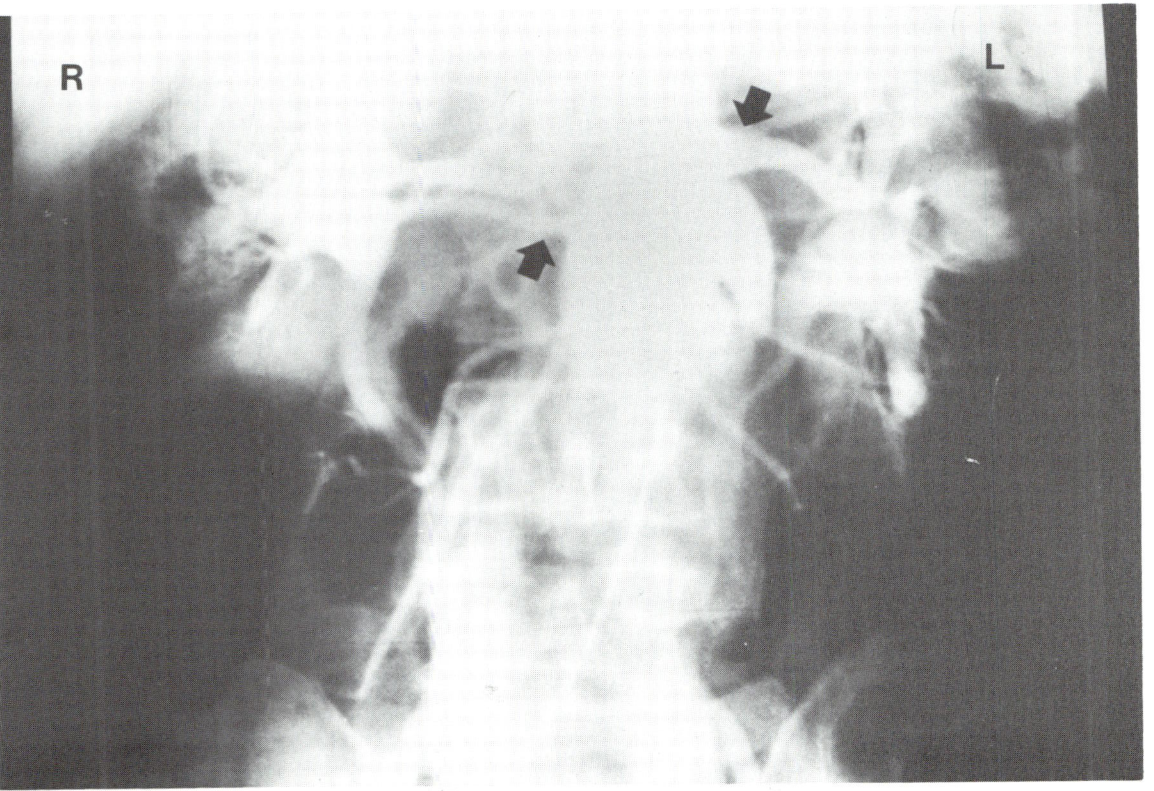

Fig. 10. Patient with a large abdominal aortic aneurysm demonstrating accessory renal artery on right and low-lying renal artery on left.

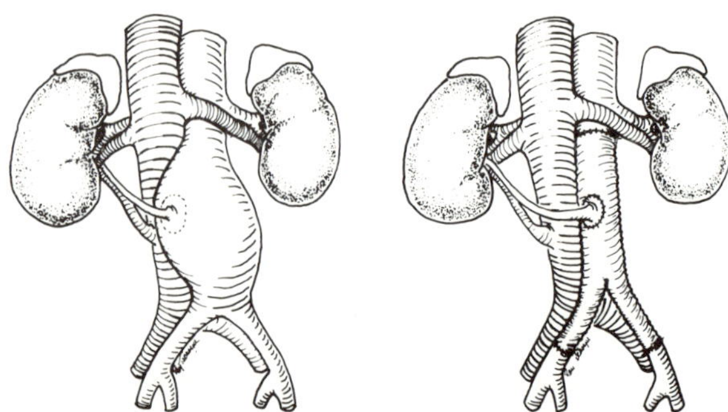

Fig. 11. Technique for reimplanting renal arteries arising from wall of abdominal aortic aneurysm.

The dominant inferior mesenteric artery is usually identified on pre-operative arteriograms (Figs 12a and 12b), however, if a pre-operative arteriogram was not done, one must be on the alert for this anatomical peculiarity. It occurs when there is occlusion of the superior mesenteric artery and flow to the area covered by the superior mesenteric artery is supplied by the inferior mesenteric artery. This "meandering" artery is large and prominent and must be preserved in order to prevent ischemia and necrosis of the small and large bowel. Again, the technique is that of re-implanting a button consisting of the orifice of the artery and portion of the aneurysm (Fig. 13). Following re-implantation, bowel color and mesenteric arterial pulsations must be evaluated to make sure perfusion is occurring. If for some reason the re-implantation cannot be done, a bypass to the superior mesenteric artery from the prosthetic graft should be carried out. If there is any doubt about the re-implantation or if the patient has had prior signs and symptoms of intestinal angina, both procedures should be carried out. Although the inferior mesenteric artery in most abdominal aortic aneurysms is occluded at its orifice, we make a point of *not* dividing the inferior mesenteric artery until the aneurysm is entered and either occlusion or back bleeding at the orifice is demonstrated. In this manner, if there is a large patent orifice with no back bleeding, a collar can be made and the artery can be re-implanted.

UROLOGICAL ANOMALIES

The most common urological anomaly associated with abdominal aortic aneurysm is the horseshoe kidney, although there have been reports of pelvic kidney (Fuller *et al.*, 1974) and also crossed renal ectopia (Bigley *et al.*, 1977). (Figs 14a,b,c,d). Horseshoe kidney associated with abdominal aortic aneurysm is an uncommon anatomical variant which has been reported in at least 56 patients as of December 1980 (Connelly *et al.*, 1980). This anatomical peculiarity is probably more common than reported since many centers have treated but not reported this anomaly when associated with an abdominal aortic aneurysm. For instance, we have had experience with two patients that had abdominal aortic aneurysms and horseshoe kidneys but have not previously reported them in the surgical literature. In this congenital anomaly, the kidneys remain lower and anterior since their ascent has been aborted due to fusion of the lower poles. This fused area usually crosses the mid-line at the level of the fourth lumbar vertebra. The fusion is brought about by the abnormal connection of the two renal blastemas and occurs between the fourth and eighth week of embryonic life (Fig. 15). The fused portion of the kidney is called the isthmus and usually lies anterior to the aorta. The ureters characteristically arise from the upper anteromedial aspect of each side of the kidney and pass down anterior to the isthmus. The reported incidence of horseshoe kidney is 1:600–800 and is present mostly in males (80%) (Starr *et al.*, 1981). When associated with an abdominal aortic aneurysm, the presence of a horseshoe kidney adds significant technical problems. Two factors largely determine the ease of aneurysm resection in this situation: (1) whether the renal isthmus is thin and fibrous and consequently can be divided (Fig. 16) and (2) the presence of anomalous renal arteries that may supply an isthmus consisting mainly of functioning renal parenchyma. Usually, a thick functioning isthmus has an anomalous blood supply arising from the abdominal aortic aneurysm wall and, therefore, cannot be divided (Fig. 17).

Abdominal aortic aneurysm associated with horseshoe kidney presents not only problems of vascular compromise but can lead to complications such as urinary leakage and urinary obstruction. The key to managing this problem is to recognize it *prior* to surgery. This should be possible in all elective cases since no abdominal aortic aneurysm should be resected without either intravenous urography or arteriography. If the intravenous pyelogram is suggestive of an abnormality, it must *always* be followed by comprehensive arteriography.

A recent review of this problem by Connelly *et al.*, (1980) shows that many patients had a previous history of urinary tract infection, hydronephrosis and stone formation. However, in 30% of patients there was no antecedent history. In their collective review of 70 patients with horseshoe kidney associated with aortic disease, there was an operative mortality rate of only 4.3%. Vascular anomalies associated with horseshoe kidney and abdominal aortic aneurysms are present in at least 60% of patients. Although the renal veins in these patients are also often anomalous, they are infrequently a problem. Careful dissection is necessary, and all aberrant renal vessels of any size should be preserved. If the arteries are small, and one contemplates ligation, they should be gently occluded first to see whether any ischemic changes occur in the kidney. If an artery is ligated, it may be necessary to remove the ischemic tissue. Re-implantation of these arteries is done by using the button technique previously described. In his report, Connelly notes that division of the isthmus (symphysiotomy) was performed in 34% of the cases reviewed. Despite their possibility, complications such as renal leakage and graft infection did not occur in these patients. In summary, horseshoe kidney in the presence of an abdominal aortic aneurysm presents additional, but not overwhelming, complexities. In elective cases, careful pre-operative evaluation of

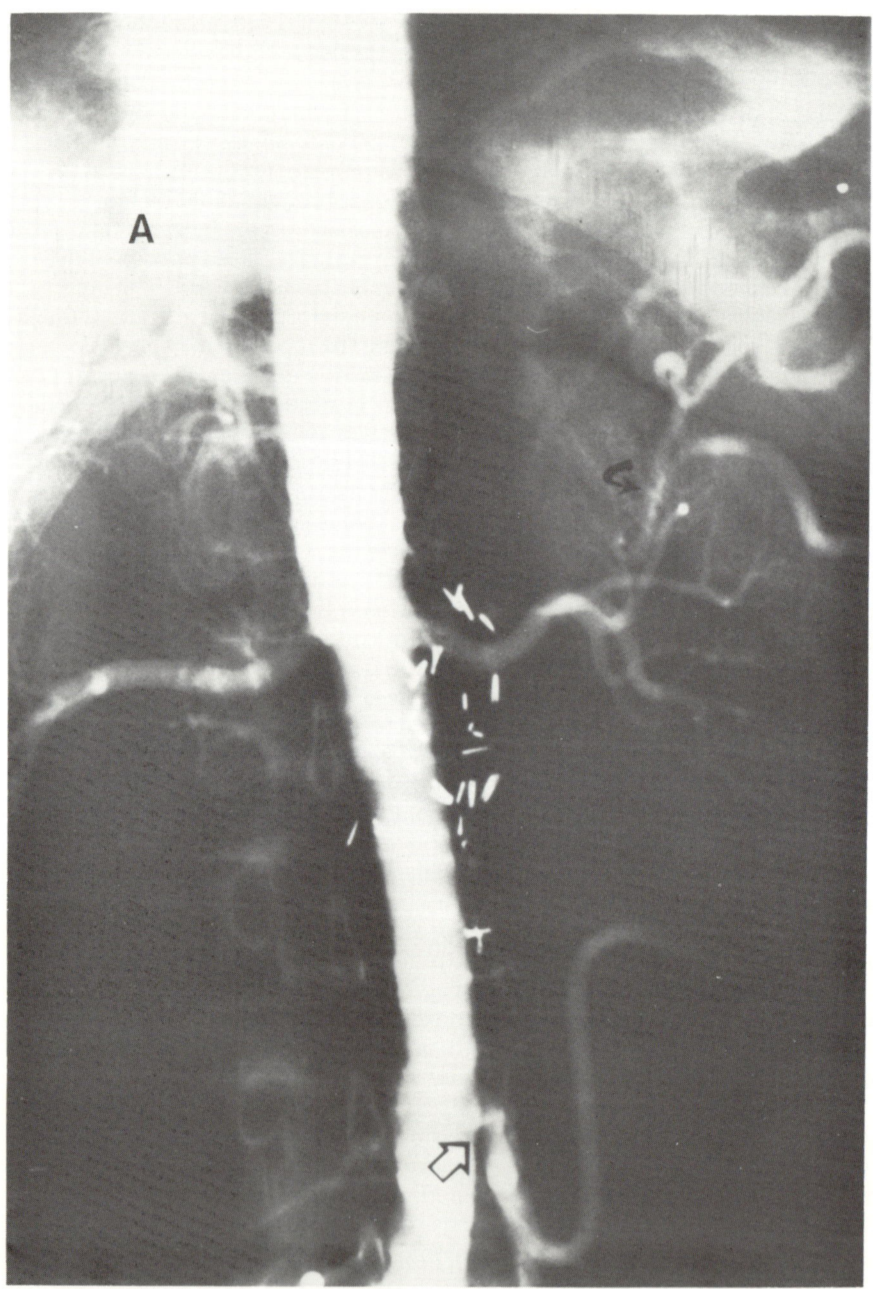

Fig. 12A. Dominant inferior mesenteric artery, i.e. "Meandering" artery.

Fig. 12B. Lateral view showing occlusion of orifice of celiac axis and superior mesenteric artery.

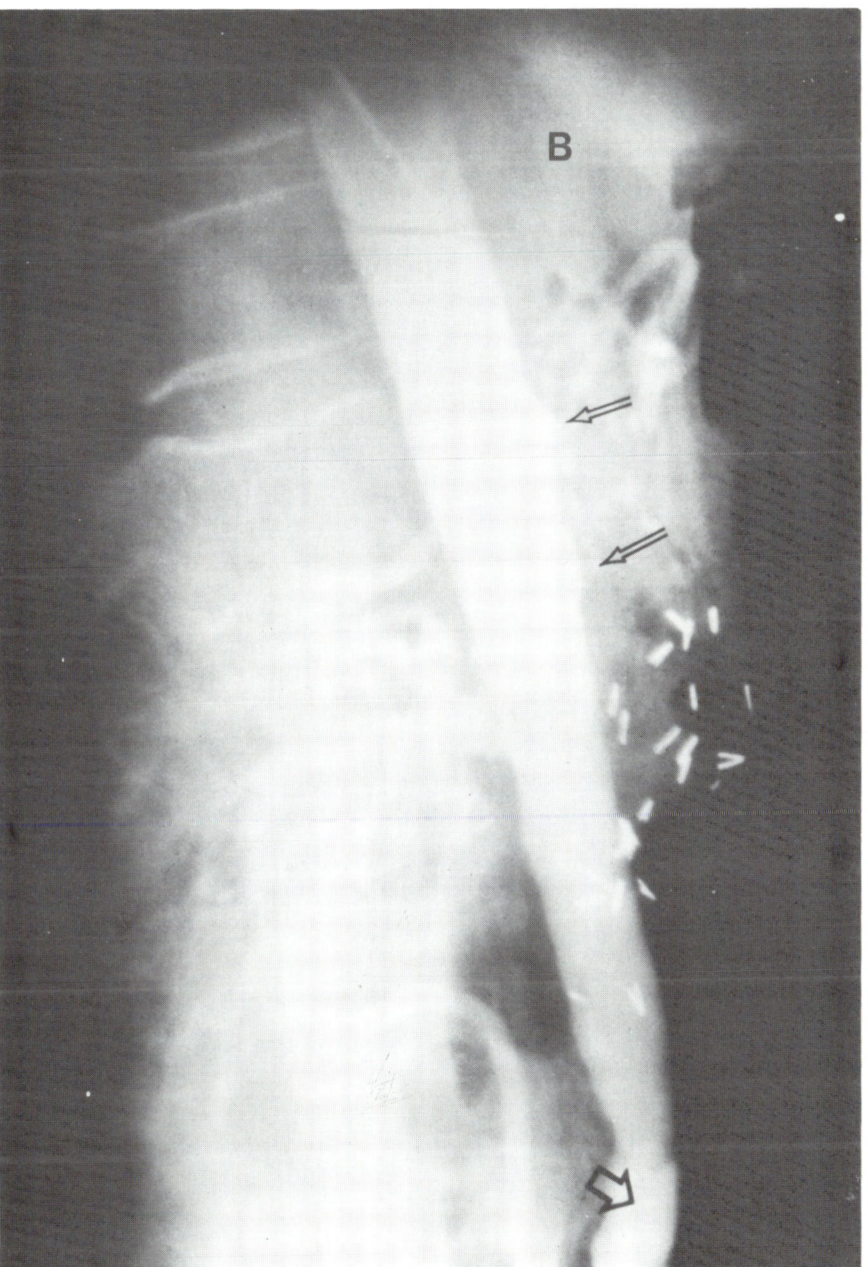
B

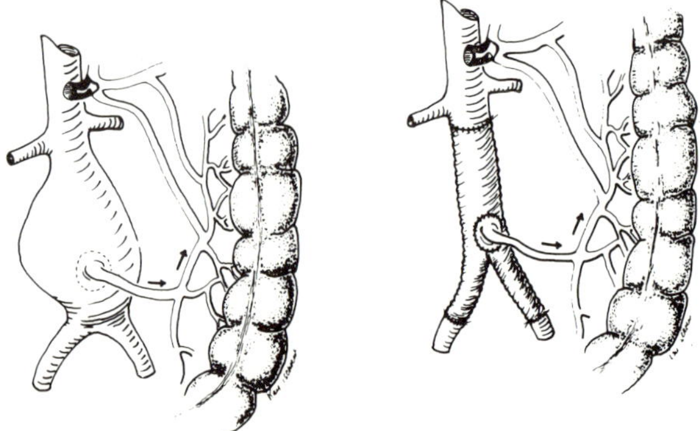

Fig. 13. Method of reimplanting dominant inferior mesenteric artery.

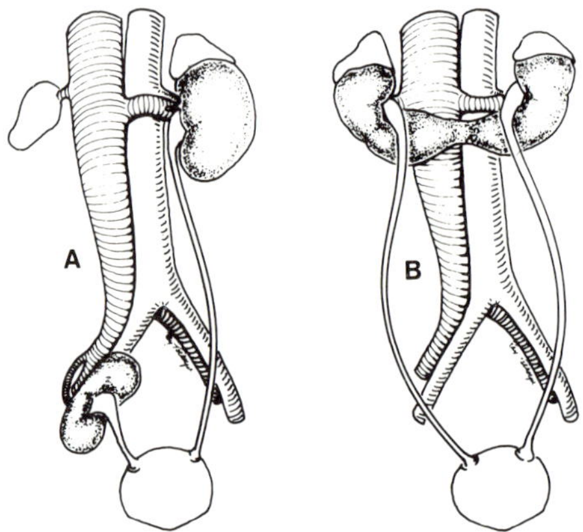

Fig. 14. (a) Pelvic kidney. (b) Horseshoe kidney.

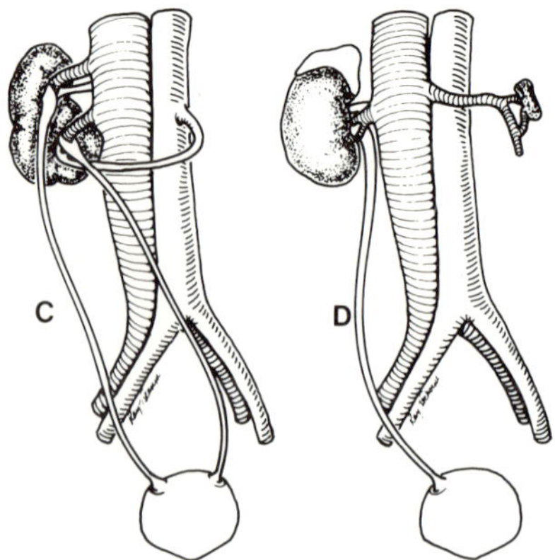

Fig. 14. (c) Crossed renal ectopia. (d) Renal agensis.

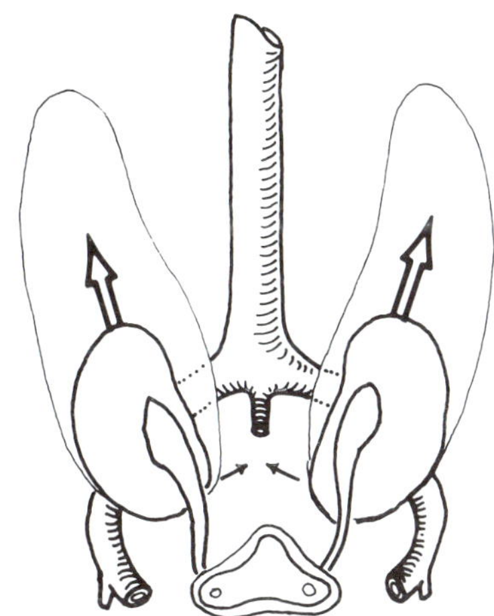

Fig. 15. Embryology of horseshoe kidney includes the abnormal fusion of the two renal blastemas between the fourth and eighth week of embryonic life.

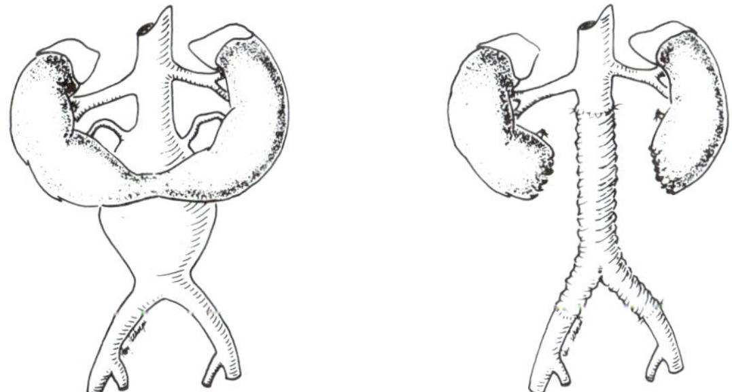

Fig. 16. Renal isthmus is thin and can be divided, however, the small renal arteries should be re-implanted if possible and not automatically ligated as demonstrated.

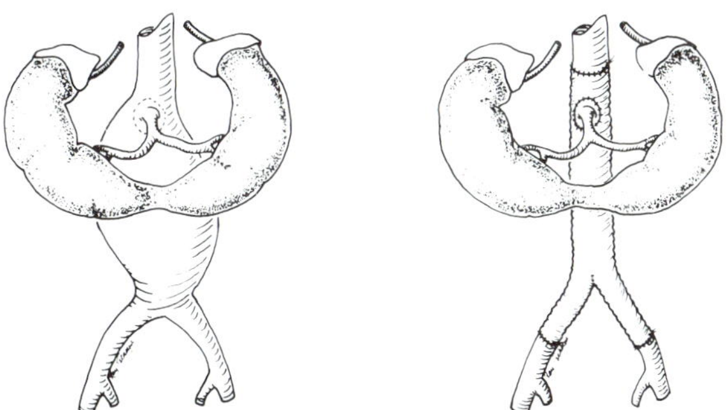

Fig. 17. Thick isthmus with a large supplying artery must be preserved and the isthmus not transected.

arterial supply, treatment of urinary tract infection and obstruction are most important. In patients with ruptured abdominal aortic aneurysms, a horseshoe kidney again can be bothersome (Cayten *et al.*, 1972). However, the reported literature seems to indicate that the survival of patients with ruptured abdominal aortic aneurysms associated with horseshoe kidney is the same as that without horseshoe kidney. The many variations of this anomaly have been carefully recorded by Bietz and Merendino (1975), Connelly *et al.* (1980) and Sidell *et al.* (1979). These references should be referred to in order to appreciate the many variations that can occur with this urological anomaly. We have had experience with two patients with nonruptured abdominal aortic aneurysm and a horseshoe kidney.

Case 1

J.F. is a 67-year-old man, previously in good health except for mild hypertension, he was found to have an abdominal aortic aneurysm when he became conscious of his heart beat in the abdomen and consulted his physician. A large, pulsating, nontender mass was found and ultrasonography demonstrated a large abdominal aortic aneurysm. Repeat ultrasonography a month later demonstrated an increase in size and he was referred to us. Arteriography was carried out and a horseshoe kidney in addition to an abdominal aortic aneurysm was demonstrated. On surgery, the major blood supply was from two normally placed renal arteries supplying the kidney from the superior poles (Fig. 18). The abdominal aortic aneurysm was resected without transection of the kidney and without ligation of any major vessels. His post-operative course was uneventful.

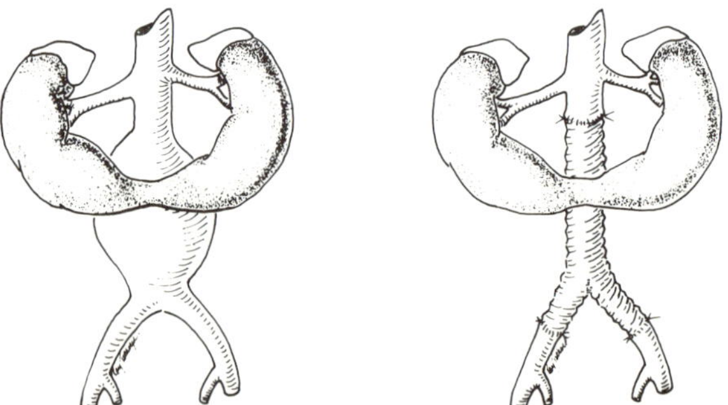

Fig. 18. Patient J.F. aneurysm resected without ligation of any major vessel and without division of the isthmus.

Case 2

J.U., a 68-year-old male, was diagnosed as having carcinoma of the bladder in June of 1979. It was also discovered at that time that he had a horseshoe kidney. He underwent a diverting ureterostomy and ileal loop and then subsequently had radiation therapy to his bladder. He developed radiation enteritis with peritonitis but eventually recovered. He was re-hospitalized in October of 1979 and underwent a total cystectomy. It was noted at that operation that he had a large abdominal aortic aneurysm. He was referred to us for evaluation of his abdominal aortic aneurysm in April 1980. We favored an axillo-bifemoral bypass and thrombosis of the aneurysm, rather than a classical aneurysm resection because of the previous irradiation, the ileostomy and the presence of the horseshoe kidney (Savarese *et al.*, 1981). On April 22, 1980, we performed a left axillo-bifemoral bypass and bilateral external iliac artery ligation. We intended to ligate each internal iliac artery as well, but because of the presence of the ileal loop, previous irradiation and horseshoe kidney, this was not feasible. Eight days after the axillo-bifemoral bypass, the aneurysm was thrombosed by inserting Gianturco-Wallace coils and gelfoam into each internal iliac artery and the abdominal aortic aneurysm (through a catheter inserted into the right axillary artery) (Fig. 19). For several days after this procedure, the patient experienced fever and diarrhea. All blood cultures were negative, and sigmoidoscopy failed to reveal any evidence of ischemic colitis. The diarrhea and fever eventually subsided. A translumbar arteriogram, performed prior to discharge, confirmed that the aneurysm was completely thrombosed up to the proximal row of coils, but not up to the renal arteries (Fig. 20). This suggested that there might be small lumbar arteries at this level. He continued in good health when examined one year later in April 1981.

RETROPERITONEAL PECULIARITIES

The inflammatory abdominal aortic aneurysm (perianeurysmal retroperitoneal fibrosis syndrome) is a pathological and anatomical variant that deserves discussion. Like retroperitoneal fibrosis without abdominal aortic aneurysm, the etiology is unknown. This lesion is probably a variant of atherosclerosis, since many times the retroperitoneal process recedes following excision of the abdominal aortic aneurysm. Although chronic use of ergot alkaloids can produce retroperitoneal fibrosis, our patients with fibrosis and abdominal aortic aneurysm and those that have been reported in the literature, have not had this as an etiological agent. That the etiology may be due to small repeated aneurysm leaks seems unlikely since studies of this tissue fail to show evidence of hemosiderin. This lesion can produce ureteral obstruction and patients are often first seen by urologists presenting with bilateral ureteral obstruction, hydronephrosis, infection or even anuria (Fridel *et al.*, 1973). Goldstone noted that in their ten patients with inflammatory abdominal aortic aneurysms, eight had symptoms (80%) (Goldstone *et al.*, 1978). This incidence of symptoms was much higher than in noninflammatory aneurysms where symptoms were present in only 31% of unruptured aneurysms. Inflammatory aneurysms are usually larger and they occur predominantly in males. Rupture can occur in spite of the very thickened anterolateral aneurysmal wall. At operation, the characteristic findings are a large abdominal aortic aneurysm which is encased in dense, thick, shiny, white fibrotic reaction which often involves the adjacent retroperitoneum and

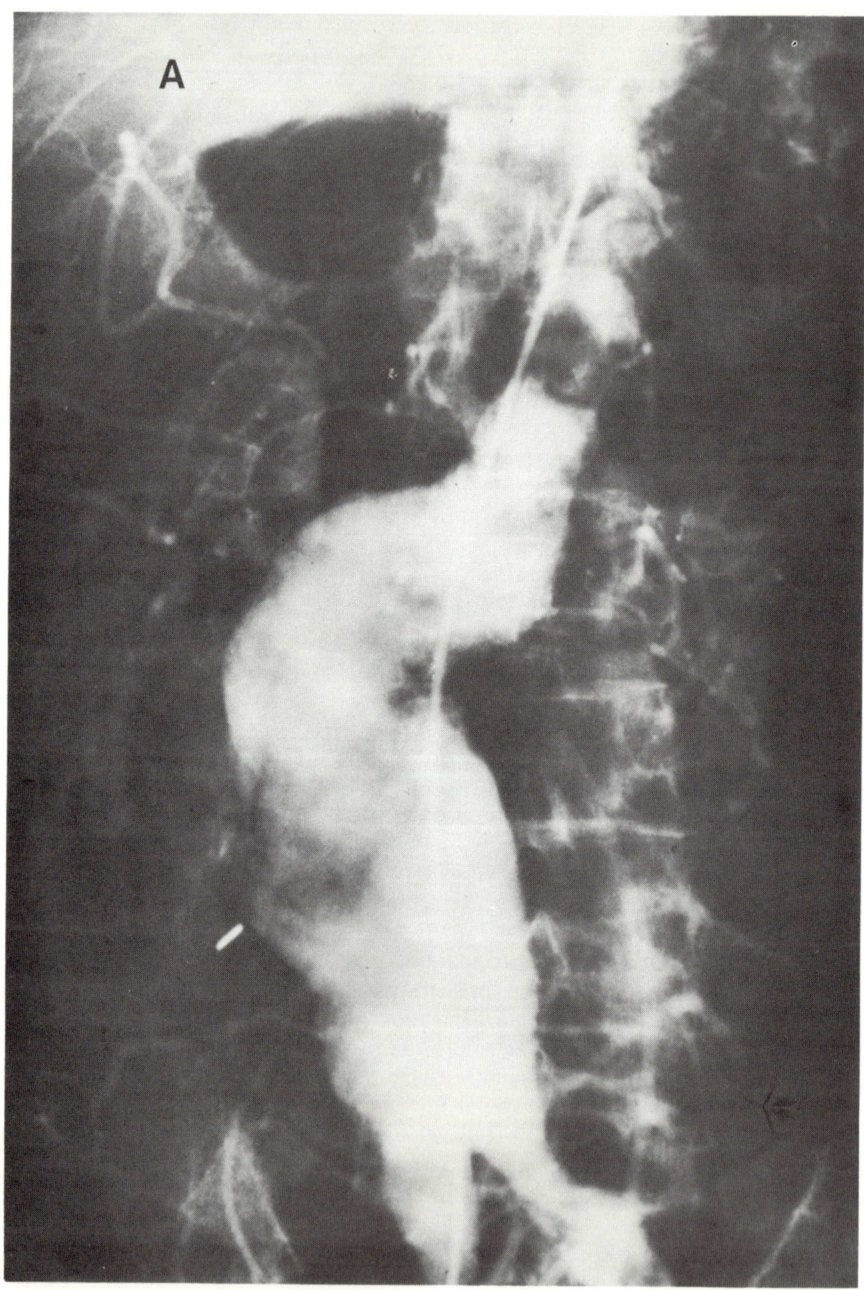

Fig. 19. Patient J.U. (A) abdominal aortic aneurysm before thrombosis. (B) and (C) Various stages during the thrombosis process.

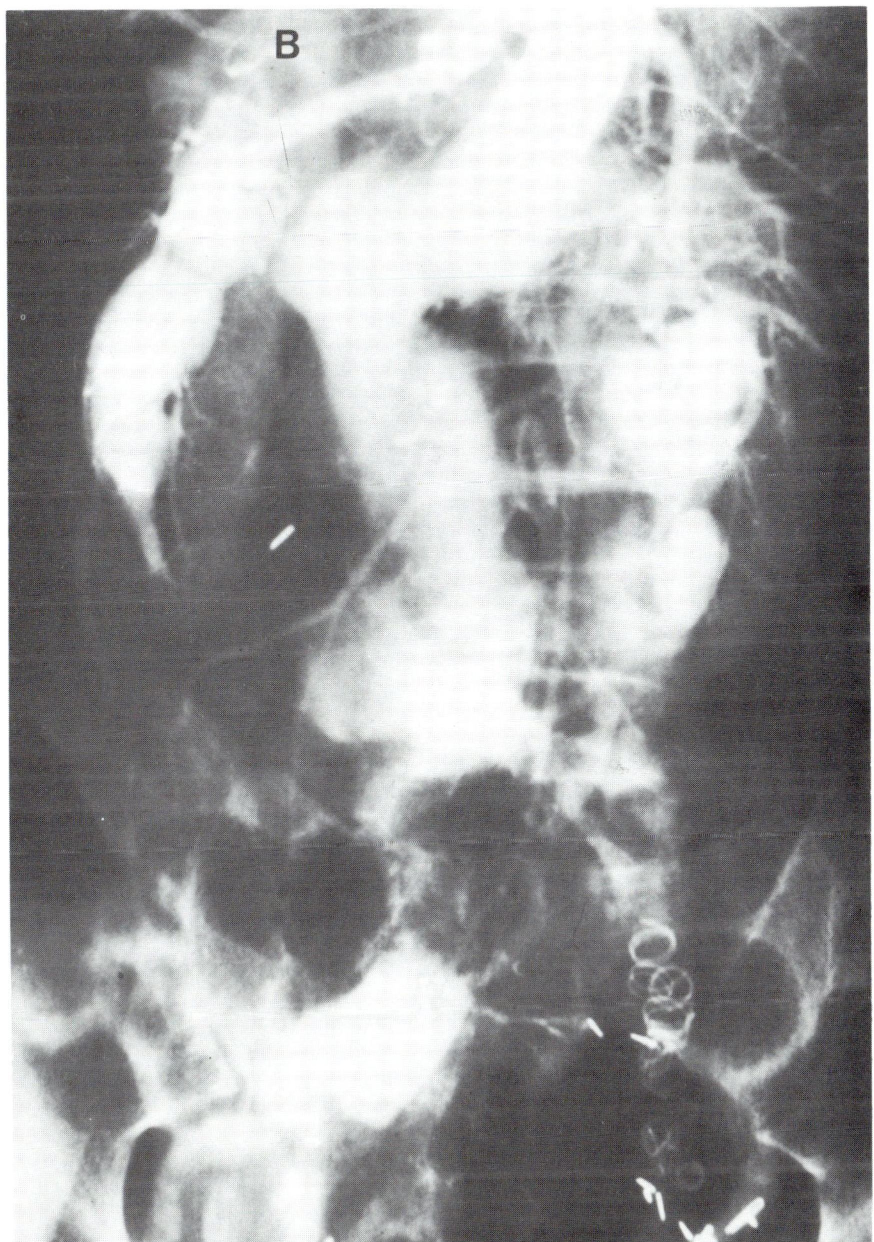
B

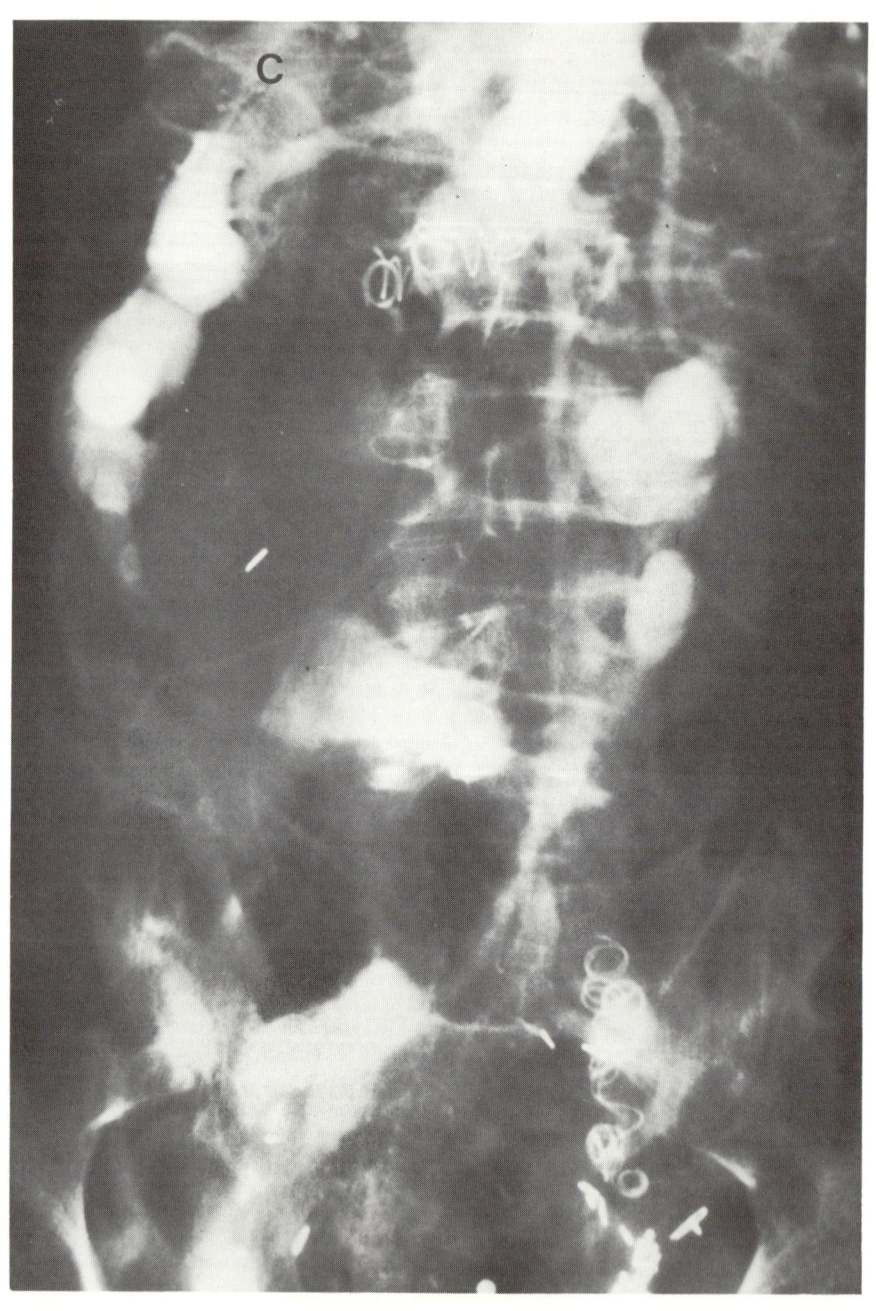
C

almost always involves to a great extent the fourth portion of the duodenum (Olcott *et al.*, 1978). The ureters, small bowel and large bowel can also be involved. These inflammatory abdominal aortic aneurysms are easily identified at surgery but the approach must differ from the routine abdominal aortic aneurysm resection. With the inflammatory variant, minimal mobilization is done especially of the duodenum which should be left in place since leakage can be catastrophic. After proximal and distal control, the inflammatory aneurysm is opened, and the operation is completed in the usual way. If ureters are involved and obstructed, a complete ureterolysis should be carefully done (Darke *et al.*, 1977). The histopathology of this lesion shows a nonspecific thick desmoplastic adventitial layer with no hemosiderin. No bacteria have been found, and the layer is relatively acellular with aggregates of lymphocytes.

Ureteral displacement is usually lateral in large noninflammatory abdominal aortic aneurysms. However, with inflammatory abdominal aortic aneurysms the ureters tend to be pulled medially by the contracting fibrotic reaction (Peters and Cowie, 1978) (Fig. 21). Until recently it was difficult to diagnose inflammatory abdominal aortic aneurysms except at the time of surgery. Now, it is possible to make a pre-operative diagnosis with the use of ultrasound (Fig. 22) and CAT scan. The use of these techniques have been aptly described by Henry *et al.* (1978) and Pahira *et al.* (1979).

We have treated five patients with retroperitoneal fibrosis and abdominal aortic aneurysms, i.e. inflammatory abdominal aortic aneurysms. All were males and all were symptomatic. One of these patients had a ruptured abdominal aortic aneurysm. Resection and successful grafting was carried out in all but one patient. This latter patient (F.C.) had a very large, 12 cm, inflammatory abdominal aortic aneurysm in which mobilization and resection was impossible because of the severe desmoplastic reaction (Fig. 21). We treated this patient successfully with axillo-bifemoral bypass and several days later with percutaneous transarterial thrombosis of the abdominal aortic aneurysm (Fig. 23). If ureteric obstruction becomes a problem, we may have to resort to steroids as reported by Clyne and Abercrombie (1977).

SUMMARY

The common anatomical variants associated with surgery of abdominal aortic aneurysms have been reviewed and various modes of management have been considered. The most dangerous anomalies are those related to the venous system and especially the retroaortic left renal vein. The arterial anomalies are best managed by preservation of a button of aortic wall and re-implantation into the prosthetic graft. Renal anomalies are most often due to a horseshoe kidney and the results with this anomaly as reported in the literature are quite good. The management of this variant involves control and reconstruction of the veins and arteries associated with the horseshoe kidney. The key to successful management of abdominal aortic aneurysm and horseshoe kidney is comprehensive pre-operative arteriography. The inflammatory abdominal aortic aneurysm is best handled by minimal dis-

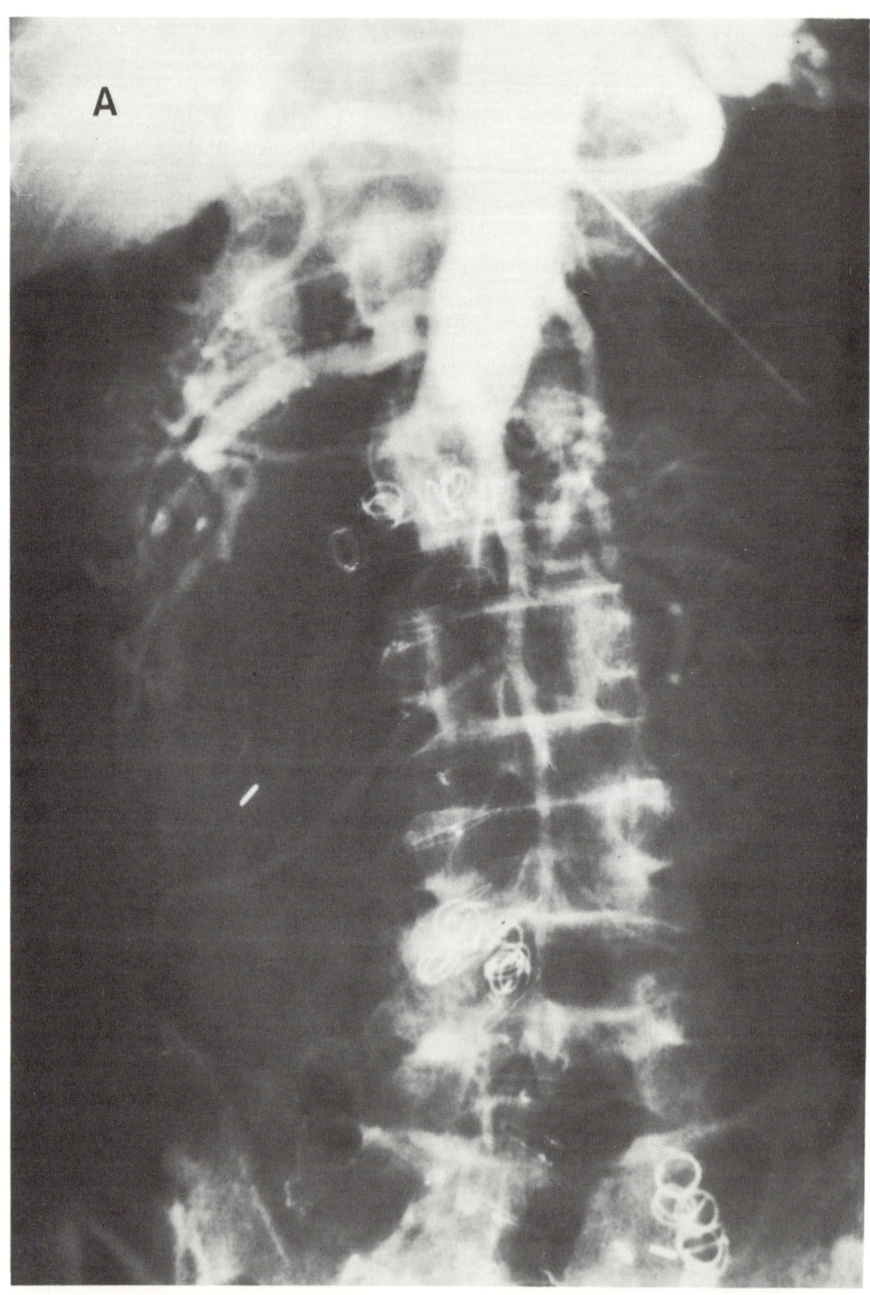

Fig. 20. Patient J.U. (A) aortogram just prior to discharge showing thrombosis of abdominal aortic aneurysm. (B) Nephrogram of large horseshoe kidney.

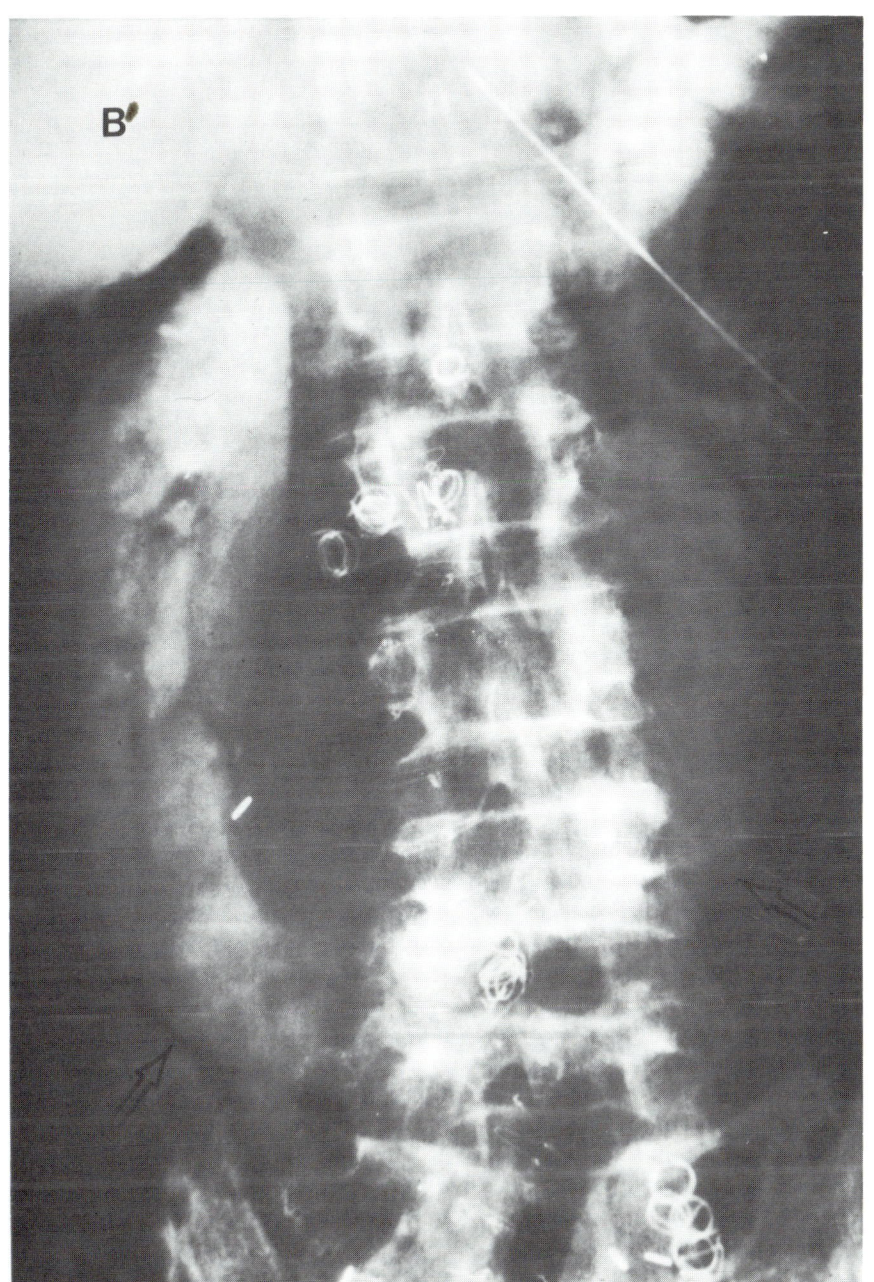
B′

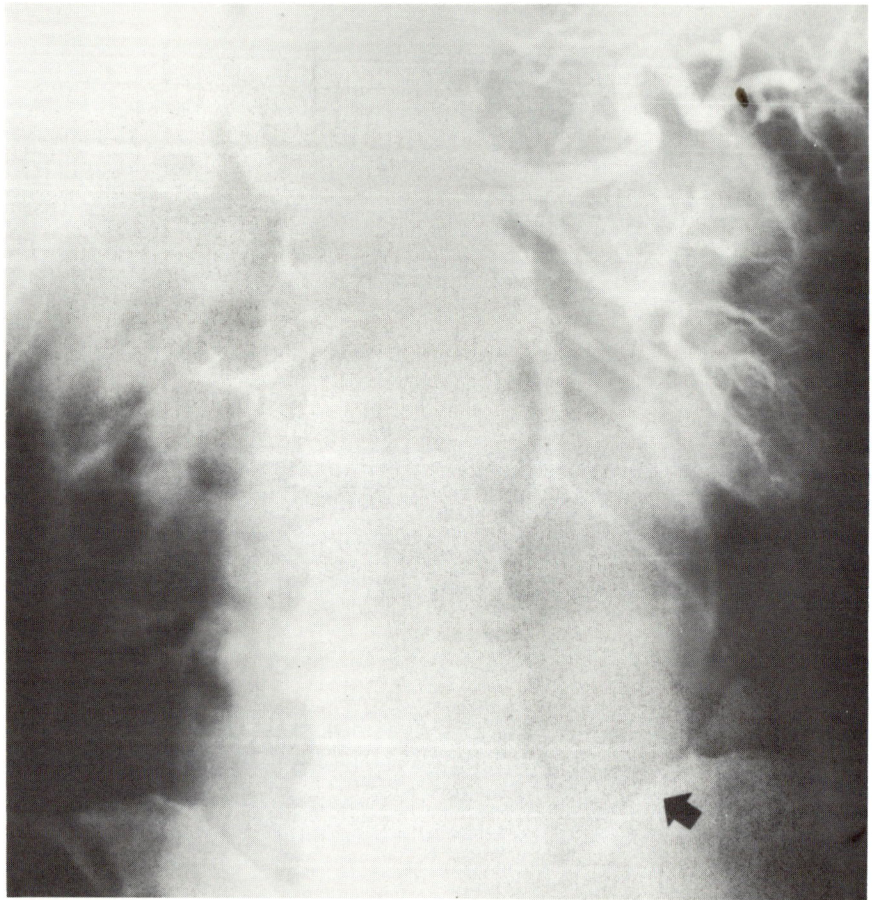

Fig. 21. Large inflammatory aneurysm in patient F.C. in which the ureter is displaced laterally and not medially as usually described in this syndrome.

section (especially the duodenum) and intra-aneurysmal repair and grafting. Although this type of abdominal aortic aneurysm shows a very desmoplastic thickened wall, they do rupture and indications for resection should be the same as all other abdominal aortic aneurysms. Although the variants that have been considered in this paper are not common, they must be appreciated and adequately handled if one expects to obtain excellent results in the surgical treatment of abdominal aortic aneurysms.

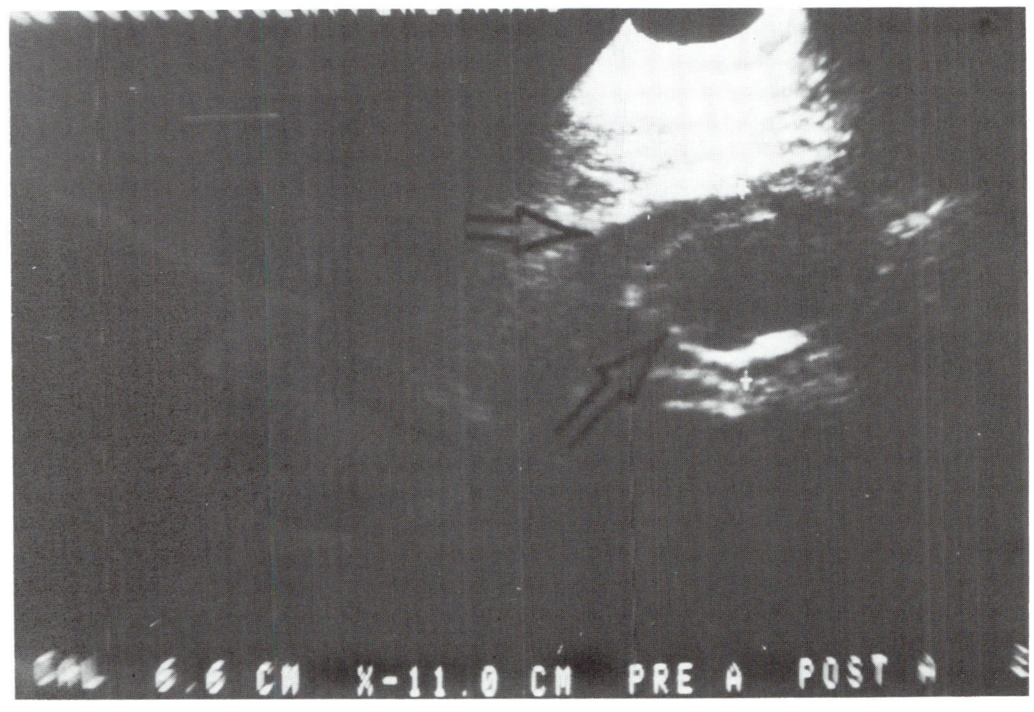

Fig. 22. Ultrasonography to demonstrate inflammatory abdominal aortic. Arrows demonstrate extent of thickened aortic wall.

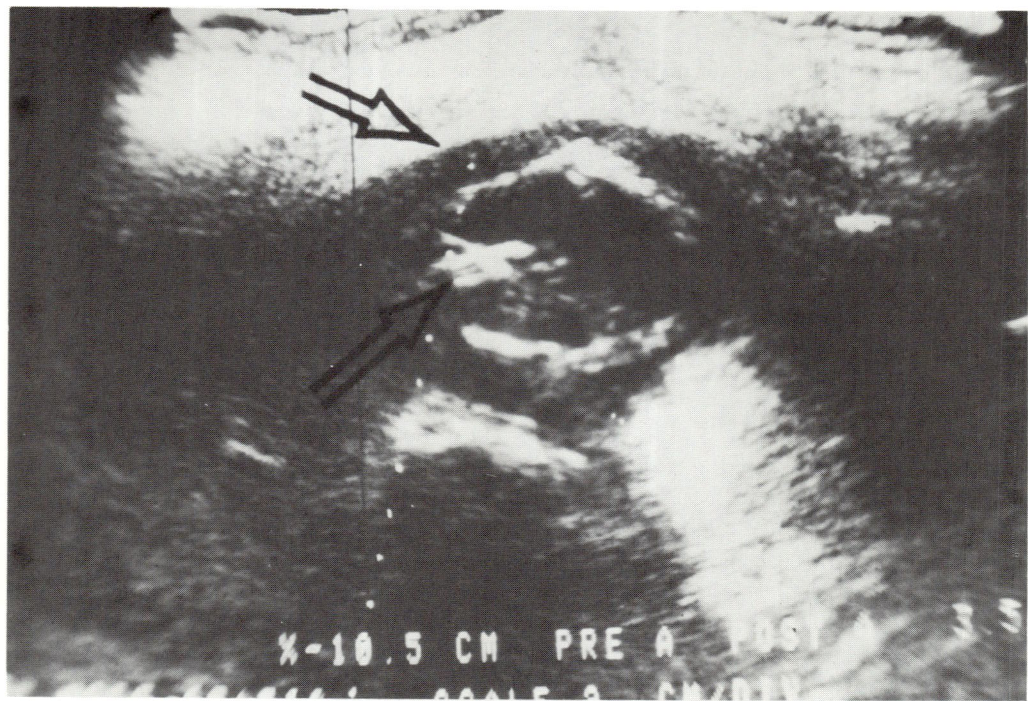

Fig. 23. Patient F.C., post thrombosis ultrasound showing steel wire coils in aneurysm (lower arrow). The upper arrow demonstrates thick "inflammatory" type aortic wall.

REFERENCES

Bietz, D. S. and Merendino, K. A. (1975). Abdominal aneurysm and horseshoe kidney: a review. *Annals of Surgery* **181**, 333.

Bigley, H. A., Barreca, J. P. and Chenault, O. W. (1977). Crossed renal ectopia and abdominal aortic aneurysm. *Urology* **10**, 573.

Brener, B. J., Darling, R. C., Frederick, P. L. and Linton, R. R. (1974). Major venous anomalies complicating abdominal aortic surgery. *Archives of Surgery (Chicago)* **108**, 159.

Cayten, C. G., Davis, A. V., Berkowitz, H. D. and Roberts, B. (1972). Ruptured abdominal aortic aneurysms in the presence of horseshoe kidneys. *SGO* **135**, 945.

Clyne, C. A. C. and Abercrombie, G. F. (1977). Perianeurysmal retroperitoneal fibrosis: two cases responding to steroids. *British Journal of Urology* **49**, 463.

Connelly, T. L., McKinnon, W., Smith, R. B. and Perdue, G. D. (1980). Abdominal aortic surgery and the horseshoe kidney. *Archives of Surgery (Chicago)* **115**, 1459.

Creech, O. Jr. (1966). Endo-aneurysmorrhaphy and treatment of aortic aneurysm. *Annals of Surgery* **164**, 935.

Darke, S. G., Glass, R. E. and Eadie, D. G. A. (1977). Abdominal aortic aneurysm: perianeurysmal fibrosis and ureteric obstruction and deviation. *British Journal of Surgery* **64**, 649.

DeLaurentis, D. A. and Lyengar, S. R. K. (1970). Renal function and a technique for venography after left renal vein ligation. *American Journal of Surgery* **120**, 41.

Dubost, C., Allary, M. and Oeconomos, N. (1952). Resection of an aneurysm of the abdominal aorta: re-establishment of the continuity by a preserved human arterial graft with the results after five months. *Archives of Surgery (Chicago)* **64**, 405.

Dupont, J. R. (1971). Isolated left sided vena cava and abdominal aortic aneurysm. *Archives of Surgery (Chicago)* **102**, 211.

Friedel, W. E., Smith, T. R. and Herman, J. R. (1973). Anuria caused by peri-aneurysmal retroperitoneal fibrosis. *Journal of Urology* **110**, 516.

Fuller, C. H., Spence, H. M. and Willbanks, O. L. (1974). Management of horseshoe kidney and pelvic kidney during operations. *Southern Medical Journal* **67**, 492.

Goldstone, J., Malone, J. M. and Moore, W. S. (1978). Inflammatory aneurysms of the abdominal aorta. *Surgery* **83**, 425.

Hardy, J. D. and Timmis, H. H. (1971). Abdominal aortic aneurysms: special problems. *Annals of Surgery* **173**, 945.

Henry, L. G., Doust, B., Korns, M. E. and Bernhard, V. M. (1978). Abdominal aortic aneurysm and retroperitoneal fibrosis. *Archives of Surgery (Chicago)* **113**, 1456.

McCombs, P. R. and DeLaurentis, D. A. (1979). Division of the left renal vein, guidelines and consequences. *American Journal of Surgery* **138**, 257.

Milloy, F. S., Anson, B. J. and Cauldwell, E. W. (1962). Variations in the inferior caval veins and in their renal and lumbar communications. *SGO* **115**, 131.

Neal, H. S. and Shearburn, E. W. (1967). Division of the left renal vein as an adjunct to resection of abdominal aortic aneurysm. *American Journal of Surgery* **113**, 763.

Olcott, C., Holcroft, J. W., Stoney, R. J. and Wylie, E. J. (1978). Unusual problems of abdominal aortic aneurysms. *American Journal of Surgery* **135**, 426.

Pahira, J. J., Wein, A. J., Barker, C. F., Banner, M. P., Arger, P. H., Mulhern, C. and Pollack, H. (1979). Bilateral complete ureteral obstruction secondary to an abdominal aortic aneurysm with perianeurysmal fibrosis: diagnosis by computed tomography. *Journal of Urology* **121**, 103.

Peters, J. L. and Cowie, A. G. A. (1978). Ureteric involvement with abdominal aortic aneurysm. *British Journal of Urology* **50**, 313.

Rosch, J., Keller, F. S., Porter, J. M. and Baur, G. M. (1978). Value of angiography in the management of abdominal aortic aneurysm. *Cardiovascular Radiology* **1**, 83.

Savarese, R. P., Rosenfeld, J. C. and DeLaurentis, D. A. (1981). Alternatives in the treatment of abdominal aortic aneurysms. *American Journal of Surgery* (In press).
Sidell, P. M., Pairolero, P. C., Payne, W. S., Bernatz, P. E. and Spittell, J. A. (1979). Horseshoe kidney associated with surgery of the abdominal aorta. *Mayo Clinic Proceedings* **54**, 97.
Starr, D. S., Foster, W. J. and Morris G. C. (1981). Resection of abdominal aortic aneurysm in the presence of horseshoe kidney. *Surgery* **89**, 387.

ANEURYSMS OF ABDOMINAL AORTA WITH INVOLVEMENT OF VISCERAL BRANCHES

R. J. A. M. van Dongen

Department of Surgery, Wilhelmina Gasthuis, University of Amsterdam, The Netherlands

AORTIC ANEURYSM ASSOCIATED WITH UNILATERAL OR BILATERAL RENAL ARTERY STENOSIS

Aneurysms of the abdominal aorta are frequently associated with unilateral or bilateral renal artery stenosis since arteriosclerosis is the underlying pathogenic factor in both aneurysm and occlusive arterial disease. Such patients may have hypertension, or the discovery of the renal artery lesions may be a casual finding during aortography.

During the last 12 years 450 patients have been submitted to surgery for non-bleeding aneurysm of the abdominal aorta. Eighty-eight of these patients had an associated lesion of one or both renal arteries, that is 20%. This large number of cases can be explained by our practice of performing aortograms as a routine pre-operative study in patients with abdominal aortic aneurysms, except in emergency cases.

Many such renal artery lesions are unimportant and need not be corrected because the patients are normotensive and have normal renal function. Whether or not to perform combined renal artery reconstruction in such patients should be based on several factors.

(1) The presence and severity of hypertension.
(2) Renal function.

Serono Symposium No. 44, "Peripheral Arterial Diseases: Medical and Surgical Problems", edited by S. Stipa and A. Cavallaro, 1982. Academic Press, London and New York.

(3) The severity of the renal lesions on arteriography and on surgery.
(4) Intrarenal vascular disease.
(5) The condition of the contralateral kidney.
(6) The patient's age and general medical condition.

That few such patients with associated renal artery lesions require renal revascularization is emphasized by our own work: only 40 patients (that is 9%) underwent aortic and renal artery surgery. Twenty-six patients had an associated stenosis or occlusion of one renal artery; in 14 cases both renal arteries were affected.

About one-half of these 40 patients were hypertensive but this was seldom the reason for reconstruction of the renal artery. In most patients reconstruction of the renal artery was carried out because they had a greater than 90% renal artery stenosis. Repair of such severely affected renal arteries is required because of the danger of total occlusion from progressive arteriosclerotic disease.

In all patients simultaneous treatment of both the aneurysm and the renal artery lesion was carried out at the same time for two reasons. Firstly, additional post-operative complications, such as renal insufficiency or other sequelae of renovascular hypertension, are prevented by the repair of the renal artery; second, reconstruction of the renal artery lesion later on is technically more difficult and increases the danger of failure.

In patients with associated unilateral renal artery stenosis three different techniques were used for the revascularization of the kidney.

Five patients with left-sided renal artery stenosis had an arterial splenorenal anastomosis performed. All patients had a large-sized splenic artery, as demonstrated by angiography. Moreover, flow and pressure measurements during the operation demonstrated good patency of this artery and good flow.

In all cases the splenic artery was dissected free after elevation of the lower border of the pancreas, mobilized over its entire length, transected in the hilum of the spleen and anastomosed end-to-end to the post-stenotic segment. The renal artery being repaired, the aortic aneurysm was resected and replaced by a prosthesis.

In 11 patients with stenosis in the proximal part of long left or right renal arteries, the transected post-stenotic renal artery was re-implanted into the infrarenal aorta or into the aortic part of the prosthesis without graft interposition.

Sometimes the infrarenal part of the aorta is of normal size over a sufficient length to be used for re-implantation of the renal artery.

If the infrarenal part of the aorta is involved in the aneurysm, a short proximal part of the aneurysmal sac can be preserved. By excising a wedge-shaped part of the anterior wall and joining the edges of the opening by a continuous suture a sufficiently long infrarenal aortic stump of normal size is obtained, which can be used for the re-implantation of the post-stenotic renal artery. Finally, the post-stenotic renal artery can be re-implanted into the aortic part of the prosthesis.

In ten patients with stenosis of short renal arteries, re-implantation was carried out using an interposition graft. This interposition graft was anastomosed, either to the infrarenal aortic stump or to the aortic part of the prosthesis. In all these cases only autogenous venous interposition grafts were used.

Fourteen patients had associated bilateral renal artery stenosis. In all cases, revascularization of both kidneys was achieved with an aortorenal bridge angioplasty, using a single venous graft. After resection of the valves the venous graft is anastomosed side-to-side to either the anterior wall of the infrarenal part of the aorta (Fig. 1A–C) or to the aortic part of the prosthesis. The ends of the graft are anastomosed to the post-stenotic renal arteries.

In some patients an aortic aneurysm is associated with stenosis of one renal artery and total occlusion of the other. In most cases the branches beyond the occlusion are patent and then the artery can be reconstructed. Revascularization of both kidneys can be achieved using the aortorenal venous bridge angioplasty.

Two early post-operative deaths occurred in this group of 40 patients. The mortality (5%) was not higher than after isolated aortic or renal procedures.

AORTIC ANEURYSM ASSOCIATED WITH OCCLUSION OF THE UPPER INTESTINAL ARTERIES

In patients with aneurysm of the abdominal aorta associated with occlusion of the superior mesenteric artery and coeliac trunk, there is a great risk of ischaemia of the left colon, particularly if blood flow through the inferior mesenteric and hypogastric arteries is insufficient. In such cases at least one of the upper intestinal arteries has to be reconstructed. In one patient only the coeliac trunk has been revascularized, using a venous bypass transplant between the infrarenal aorta and the hepatic artery.

The venous bridge angioplasty allows the possibility of revascularizing both the superior mesenteric artery and the coeliac artery using a single venous graft, which is anastomosed side-to-side to the infrarenal aorta. One end of the venous bridge is attached to the hepatic artery, the other end to the superior mesenteric artery beyond the occlusion. We used this method in five patients with these combined lesions, without mortality.

AORTIC ANEURYSM ASSOCIATED WITH STENOSIS OF RENAL AND INTESTINAL ARTERIES

In six of our patients the aneurysm of the abdominal aorta was associated with occlusive disease of renal as well as intestinal arteries. Resection of the aneurysm and reconstruction of all arteries during the same operation were carried out in all cases. Various reconstructive procedures can be used. One of the methods is shown in Fig. 2A–C. In this case there was, apart from the aneurysm, stenosis of the right renal artery and occlusion of the superior mesenteric artery. After resection of the aneurysm and replacement by a bifurcation prosthesis, endarterectomy with aorterenal patch graft angioplasty was performed on the narrowed right renal artery. The post-occlusive

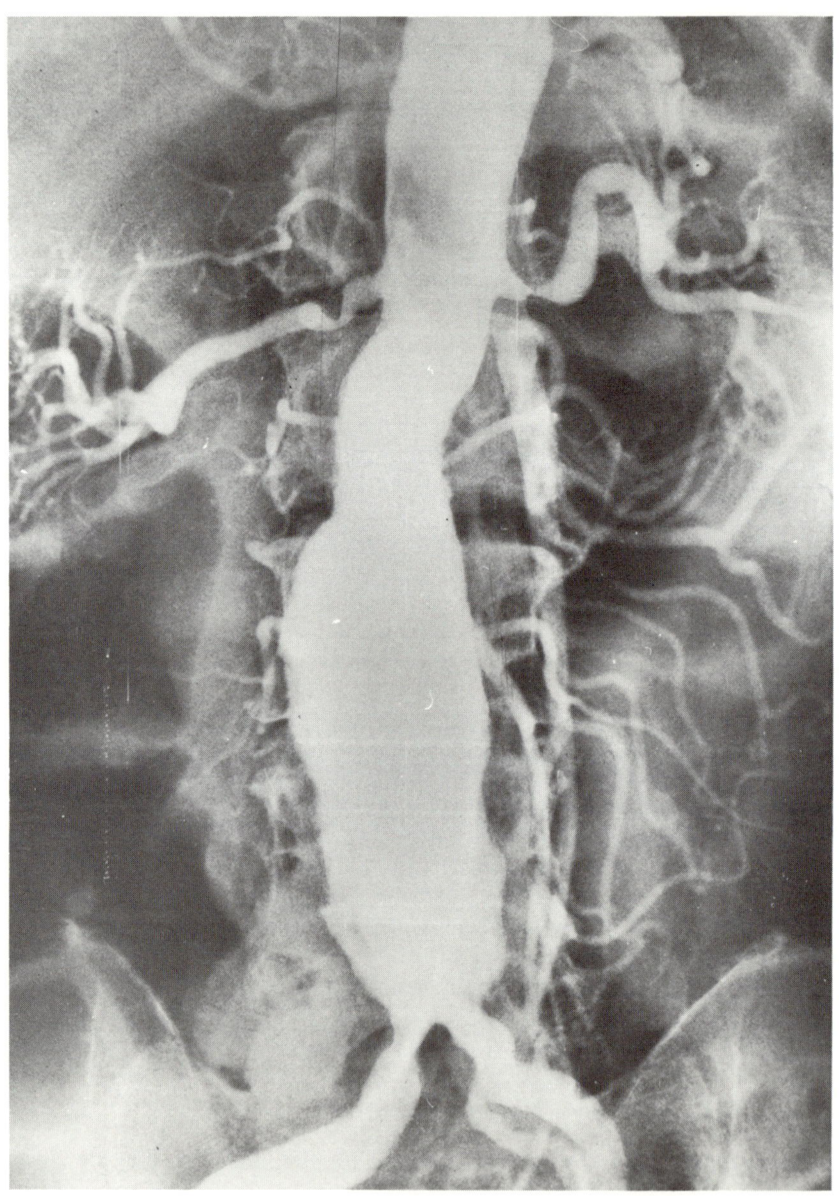

Fig. 1A. Aortic aneurysm with associated bilateral renal artery stenosis.

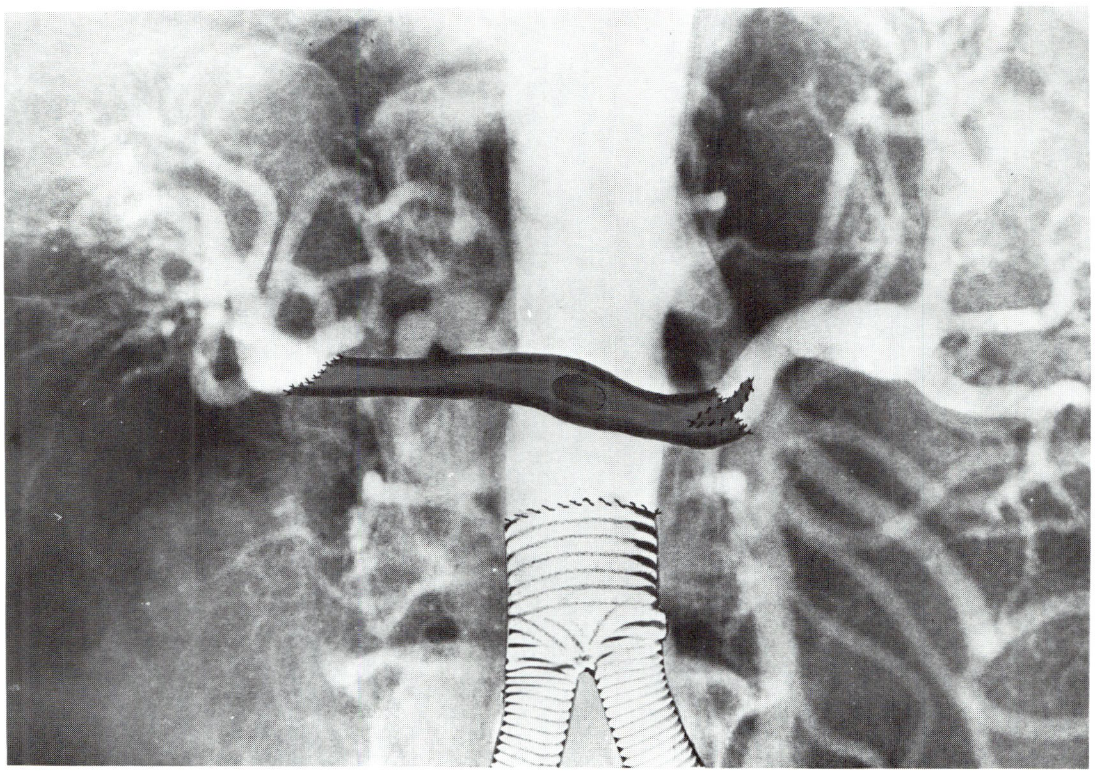

Fig. 1B. Resection of the aneurysm and replacement by bifurcation graft. Revasculariztion of the kidneys by aortobirenal bridge angioplasty using a single venous graft.

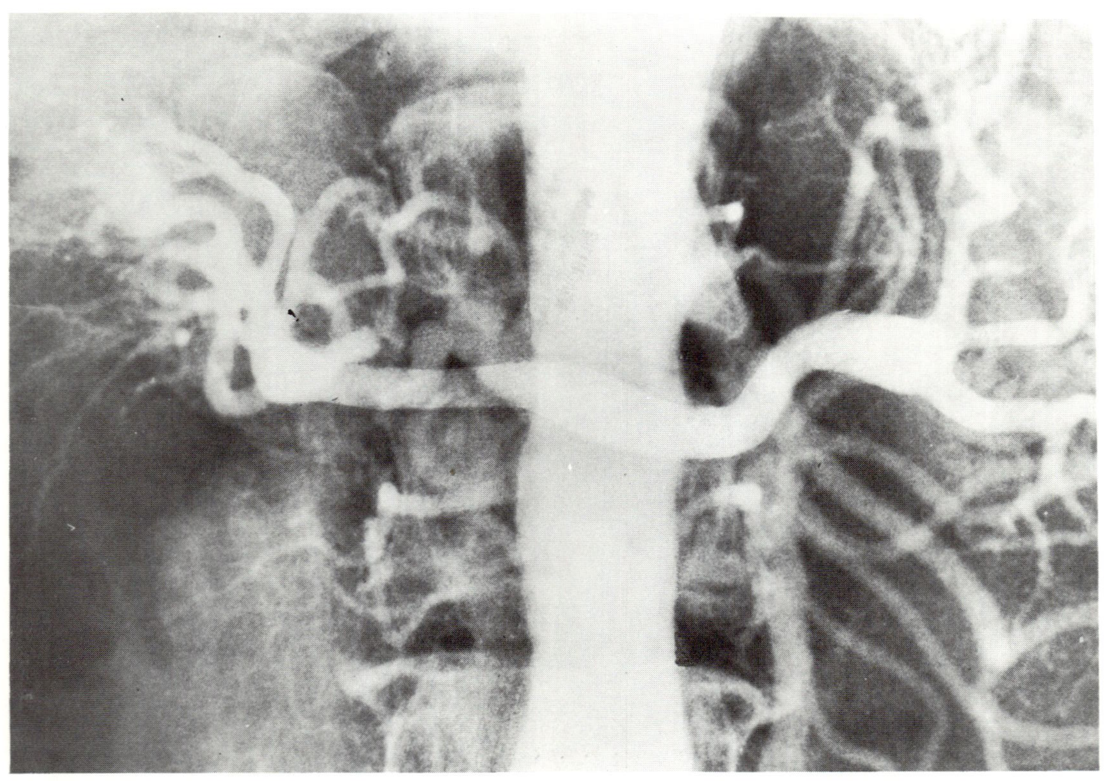

Fig. 1C. Post-operative angiogram.

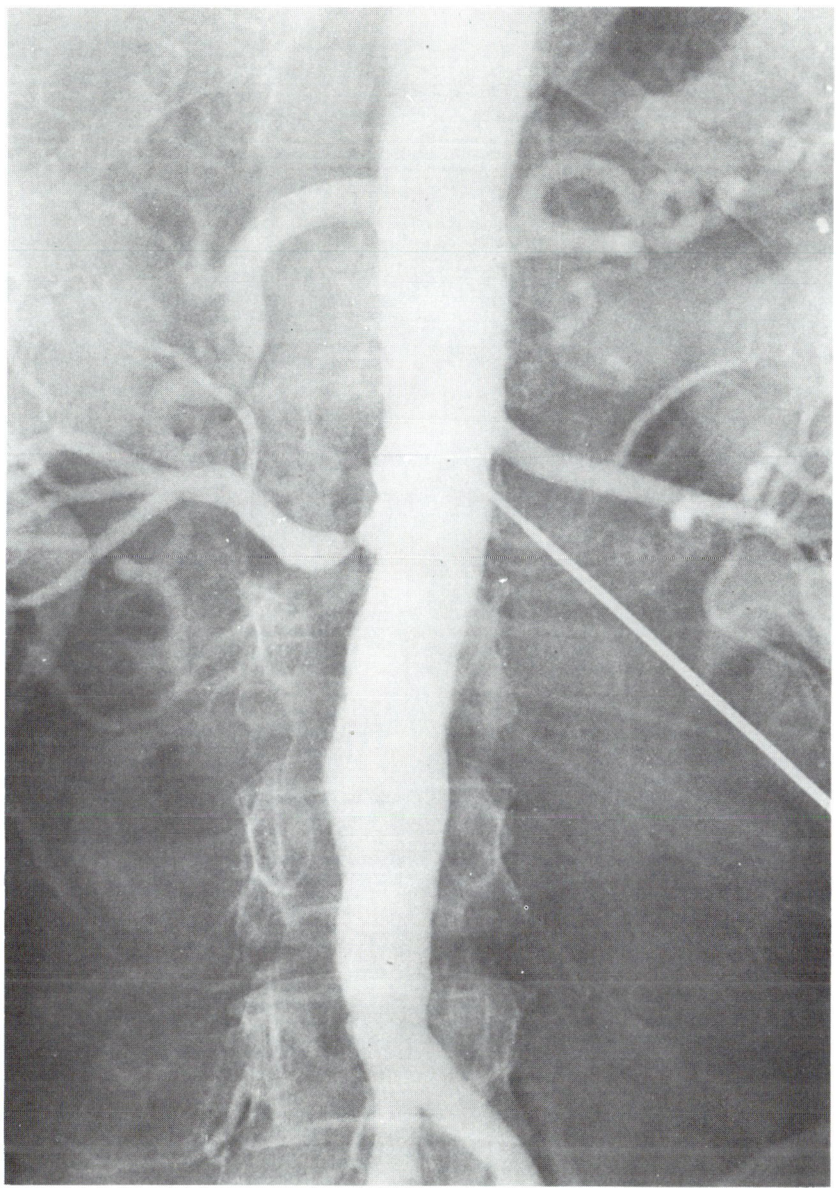

Fig. 2A. Aortic aneurysm associated with stenosis of the right renal artery and occlusion of the superior mesenteric artery.

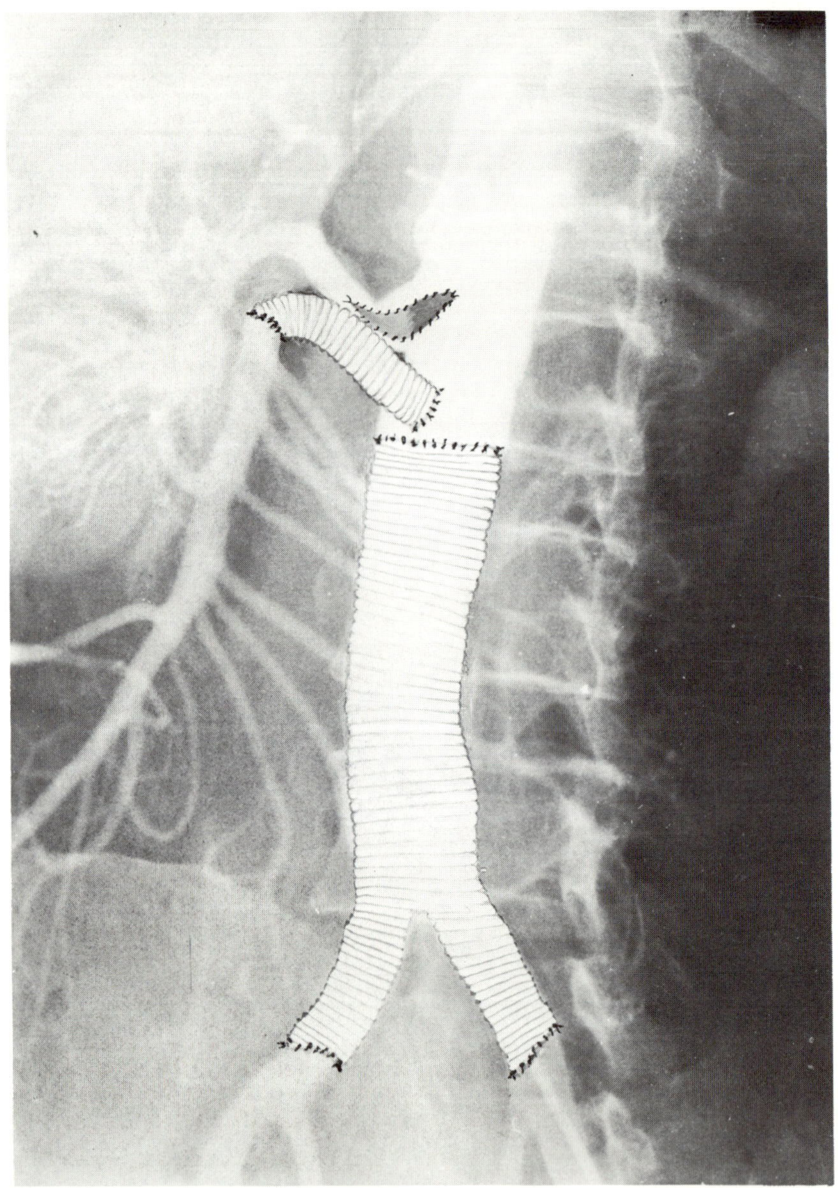

Fig. 2B. Resection of the aneurysm and replacement of bifurcation graft. Repair of the right renal artery by endarterectomy and venous aortorenal patch graft angioplasty.

Re-implantation of the post-occlusive superior mesenteric artery with interposition of a prosthetic graft.

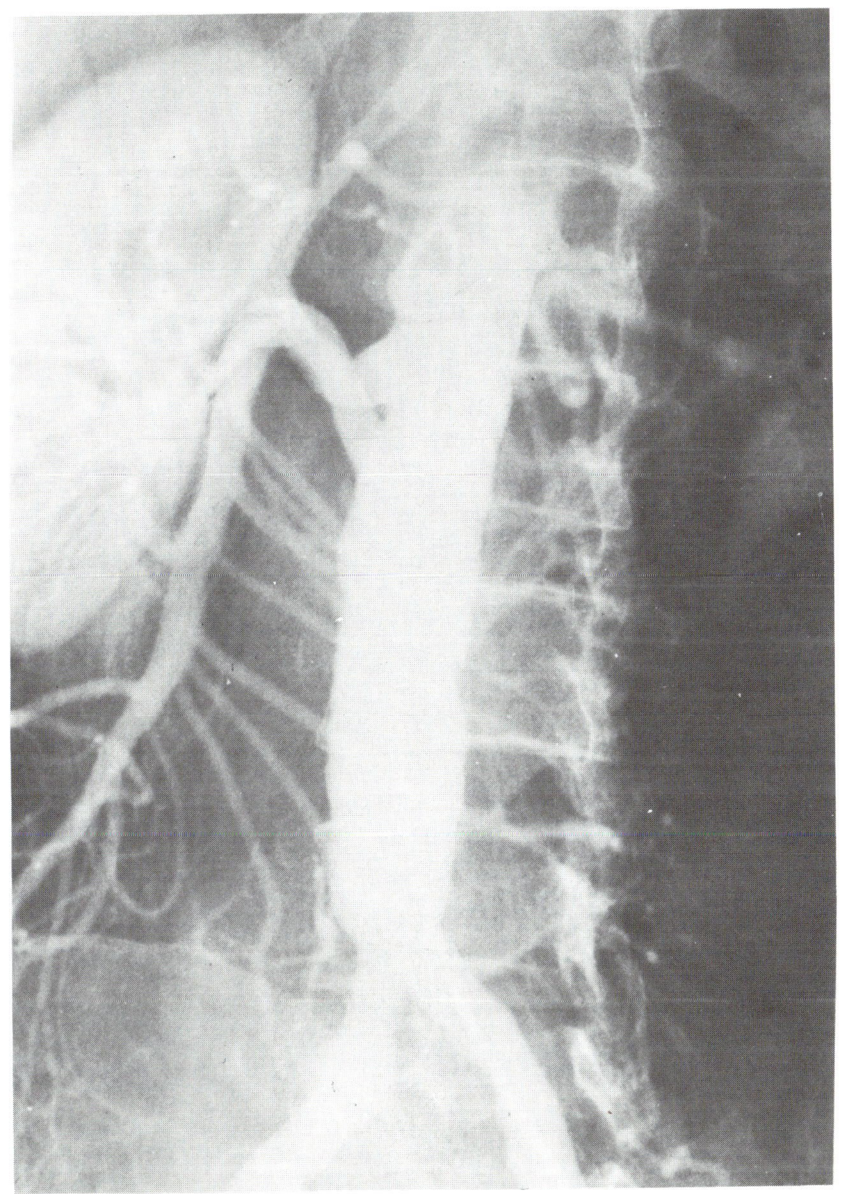

Fig. 2C. Post-operative angiogram.

portion of the superior mesenteric artery was re-implanted into the infrarenal part of the aorta with interposition of a Dacron graft.

Another possibility is to reconstruct both arteries with the bridge angioplasty using a single venous graft, which is anastomosed side-to-side to the anterior wall of the infrarenal aorta. One end of the graft is connected end-to-end to the post-occlusive part of the superior mesenteric artery, and the other end of the graft is anastomosed end-to-end to the post-stenotic renal artery.

AORTIC ANEURYSM AND ARTERIAL CONGENITAL ABNORMALITIES

In as many as 5% of our patients with aortic aneurysm an arterial congenital abnormality was demonstrated by pre-operative diagnostic procedures.

The most frequently seen abnormalities are supernumerary renal arteries. An accessory renal artery is an end artery, without intercommunications with the main renal artery. When such an accessory renal artery arises from the aneurysmal part of the aorta, it must be re-implanted into the wall of the prosthesis.

Since such accessory arteries are usually small sized, special measures must be taken to guarantee an adequate and reliable anastomosis. There are many possibilities. Sometimes we widen the ostium of the accessory renal artery with a wedge-shaped venous patch. This result in a funnel-shaped enlargement of the mouth of the small-sized artery (Fig. 3A). In other cases a so-called Carrel patch is used (Fig. 3B).

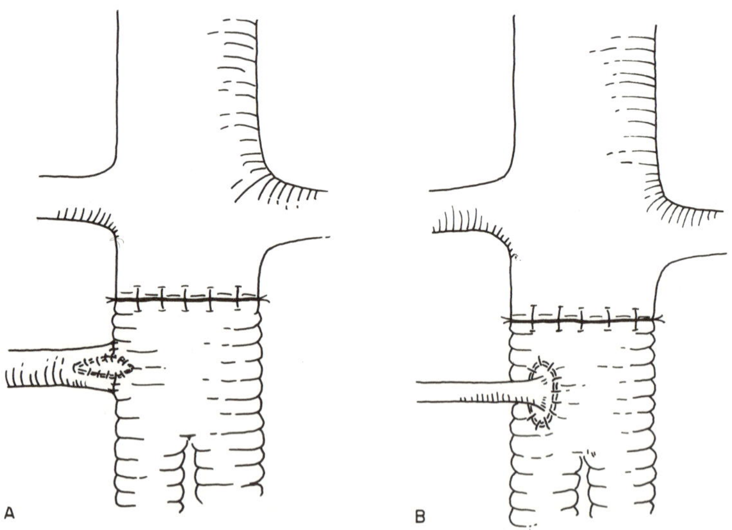

Fig. 3(A). Widening of the re-implanted accessory renal artery with a venous patch sutured into the anastomosis. (B) Re-implantation of the accessory renal artery using a Carrel patch.

An aortic aneurysm is rarely associated with a horseshoe kidney, only 60 cases being reported up to 1979. In most cases the presence of a horseshoe kidney is a casual finding, established by pre-operative aortography. The diagnosis can be missed unless pre-operative aortography is performed. This is one of the reasons why pre-operative diagnosis includes angiographic examination. Without knowledge of the vascularization of such abnormalities adequate treatment is impossible. Review of our own experience and that reported in the literature reveals that the arterial anatomic variations may be classified into five groups. Pre-operative studies of the arterial supply makes it possible to select the site of transection of the isthmus of the kidney and to decide which arteries can be sacrificed and which must be preserved or re-implanted into the prosthesis. The most serious problem faced by the surgeon in such cases is that of deciding the functional importance of the small aberrant vessels. Trial occlusion is then necessary and if a large part of the renal mass appears compromised, preservation or re-implantation of the involved artery may be required.

Unusual technical problems are encountered in patients with aortic aneurysm associated with crossed renal ectopia. Figures 4A–C shows an example. Both kidneys on the left are supplied with blood by four arteries. The uppermost artery could be preserved. Preservation of the other three arteries consisted of excising them with a patch of aortic wall, and sewing this to the side of the prosthesis.

As a guide to operative management we classify the different possibilities of arterial supply in all these cases of aneurysms associated with congenital abnormalities into four groups.

In type A the aberrant arteries arise from the neck of the aneurysm. In such cases the aberrant artery can be preserved by either oblique transection of the aorta or excising a wedge-shaped part of the anterior wall of the proximal part of the aneurysmal sac and joining the edges of the opening.

In type B part of the kidney is supplied with blood by arteries originating distal to the aneurysm. Preservation of these arteries is possible by performing distally an end-to-side or a bevelled end-to-end anastomosis.

In type C the kidney is completely supplied by an artery originating from the aneurysmal wall of the aorta. In such cases this renal artery must be re-implanted into the prosthesis. To perform this anastomosis a so-called Carrel patch can be used. If this is impossible and the connexion must be made directly, a safe wide anastomosis can be established by suturing an aortorenal dilating patch in it.

Finally in type D, of multiple arteries originating from the aneurysmal sac, it will be necessary to excise two or more groups of arteries with elliptical segments of aortic wall and sew them to corresponding windows made in the wall of the prosthesis.

SUPRARENAL AORTIC ANEURYSM

Sometimes only a single renal artery originates from the upper part of the aneurysm. This artery must then be re-implanted into the prosthesis, either

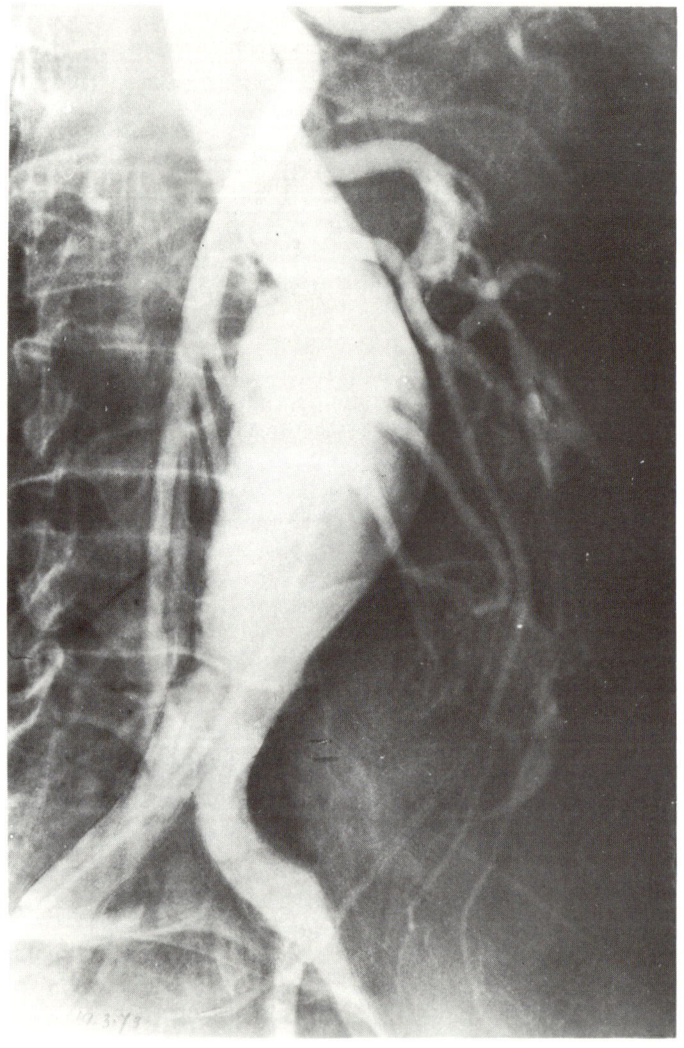

Fig. 4A. Aortic aneurysm associated with crossed renal ectopia. Both kidneys on the left are supplied by four arteries.

directly or with interposition of a graft.

In 2% of our patients the aneurysm extended proximally involving both renal arteries. If the origin of the superior mesenteric artery is free of the aneurysmal sac, the aortic part of the prosthesis can be connected to the aorta at a level just distal to the superior mesenteric artery and revascularization of the kidney can be achieved by re-implanting the renal arteries with Carrel patches into windows in the prosthetic wall. However, when using this technique there is a great risk of renal damage because of prolonged ischaemia time. It is impossible to perform a triple anastomosis in less than 30 min.

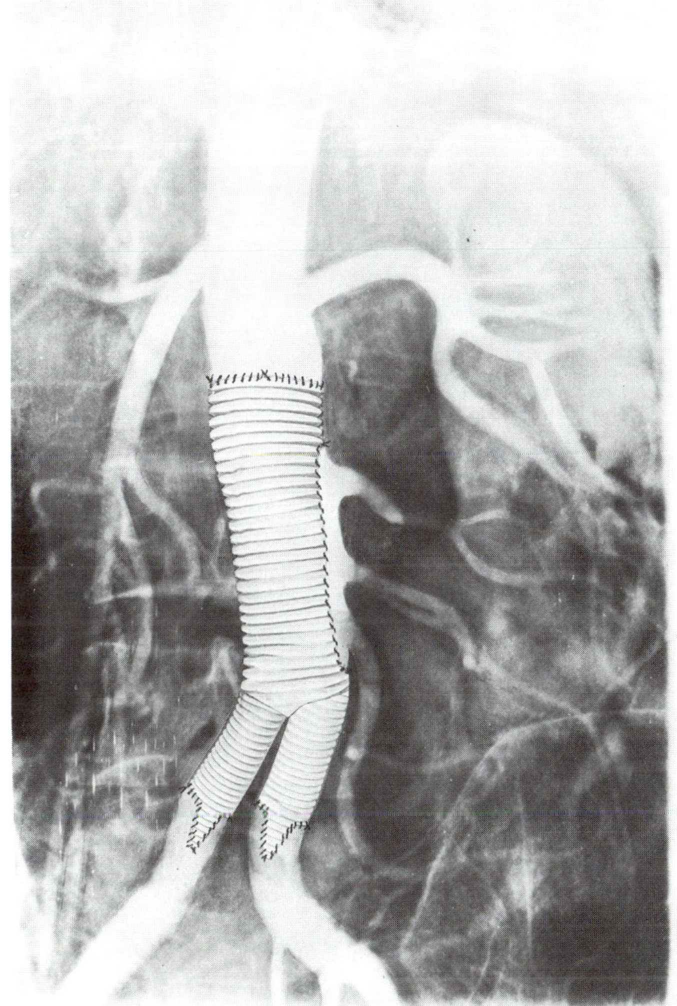

Fig. 4B. Resection of the aneurysm and replacement by prosthetic bifurcation. Re-implantation of the three distal renal arteries into a window made in the prosthesis using a patch of aortic wall.

When revascularizing both kidneys in such cases there is less risk using the venous bridge angioplasty. Before the aorta is transected between the origins of the superior mesenteric and renal arteries and before the proximal anastomosis is performed, a venous transplant is attached to a window made in the anterior aortic wall proximal to the origin of the coeliac trunk using a partial tangential occlusion clamp. The renal arteries are transected subsequently and connected to the ends of the venous bridge. If no suitable venous graft is available a Dacron graft can be used for this bridge angioplasty.

Aneurysmal involvement of the upper abdominal aorta and its major

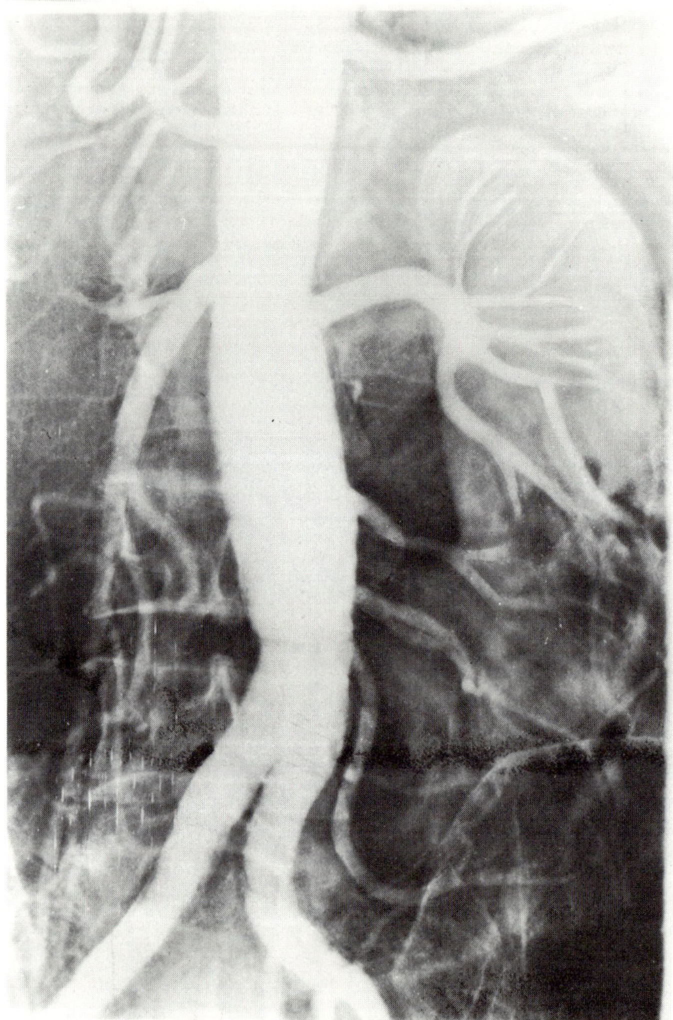

Fig. 4C. Post-operative aortogram.

visceral branches occurred in ten of our patients. In five the lower descending thoracic aorta was also involved. These aneurysms present a very serious challenge to the surgeon, but they may be resected successfully, with graft replacement in most cases. In all patients we used a modification of an old technique, the double deviation procedure without the use of prosthetic material for the visceral branches. Using this double deviation procedure, a Dacron bypass is inserted between the thoracic aorta and the aortic bifurcation behind the left renal vein. This is the first deviation. Then the neck of the aneurysm is transected and the proximal stump closed with interrupted sutures. Blood flow to the aneurysm and visceral branches is maintained through the graft. The splenic artery is then dissected free, transected close to the spleen and attached to a window in the graft. This is the second deviation.

After dividing the celiac trunk and oversewing the stumps, blood flow to the hepatic artery is maintained by retrograde flow through the splenic artery and to the superior mesenteric artery via the pancreatic duodenal arteries. The next step is transection of the left renal artery, which is directly attached to a window in the graft, using a tangential occluding clamp. The left renal occlusion time is never more than 15 min. The superior mesenteric artery is detached from the aneurysm and occluded. To prevent clot formation in the proximal segment of this artery a drip influsion with heparin solution is introduced. Because the entire gastro-intestinal tract is provided with blood through the splenic artery, re-implantation of the superior mesenteric artery can wait.

The next step is excision of the right renal artery out of the aneurysmal wall and resection of the anterior wall of the aneurysm. The graft is moved to the right after which the right renal artery is sutured to a window in the graft. The occlusion of the right renal artery is limited to about 20 min. Finally the superior mesenteric artery is sutured to a window made in the anterior wall of the graft. This procedure has two advantages. Firstly, the period of temporary circulatory arrest to each branch is kept to an absolute minimum; it is about 15–20 min. Second, no synthetic material is used for the reconstruction of the renal and intestinal arteries. This technique was used in all patients. One patient died because of haemorrhage due to coagulopathy. There were no ischaemic gastro-intestinal complications, no renal damage and no ischaemic lesions of the spinal cord.

Associated stenosis or occlusion and involvement of the visceral arteries in patients with aortic aneurysm is often seen more frequently than is generally assumed. The treatment of these lesions poses special problems. Simultaneous treatment of both the aneurysm and the lesions of the visceral branches during the same operation may protect the patient from post-operative renal and intestinal complications.

COMPLICATIONS OF ABDOMINAL AORTIC ANEURYSM SURGERY

U. Ruberti

Department of Surgery, University of Milan, Milan, Italy

Many complications of the surgery of "aneurysms of the abdominal aorta" (AAA) have been described. Some of these are not specific to this kind of surgery and can occur following any major surgical procedure and, therefore, will not be treated in this paper; these are mainly involvement of the respiratory system, urinary infections, phlebitis etc. More specifically, the surgical treatment of AAA may aggravate a pre-existing involvement of the coronary, carotid, renal or peripheral arteries already compromised by the same primary atherosclerotic disease that caused the aneurysm itself (Fig. 1). Aortic cross-clamping or declamping can also bring very peculiar disturbances to the coronary or cerebral circulation. The involvement of the coronary system during aortic manipulation has been widely demonstrated (Longo *et al.*, 1971) (Fig. 2). Similar consequences may also occur to the supraaortic trunks as well specially during declamping with a consequent fall in the carotid pressure and flow; for these reasons an accurate evaluation of the cerebral circulation in those patients affected also by lesions to the supraaortic trunks is mandatory prior to surgery.

Finally, the renal arteries may be intra-operatively damaged due to their proximity to the aneurysm itself. In conclusion, the factors that can possibly induce specific post-operative complications are as follows.

Serono Symposium No. 44, "Peripheral Arterial Diseases: Medical and Surgical Problems", edited by S. Stipa and A. Cavallaro, 1982. Academic Press, London and New York.

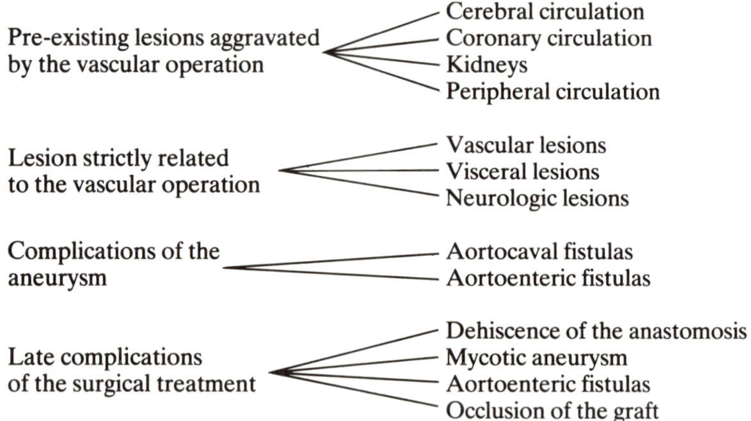

Fig. 1. Complications of abdominal aortic aneurysms surgery.

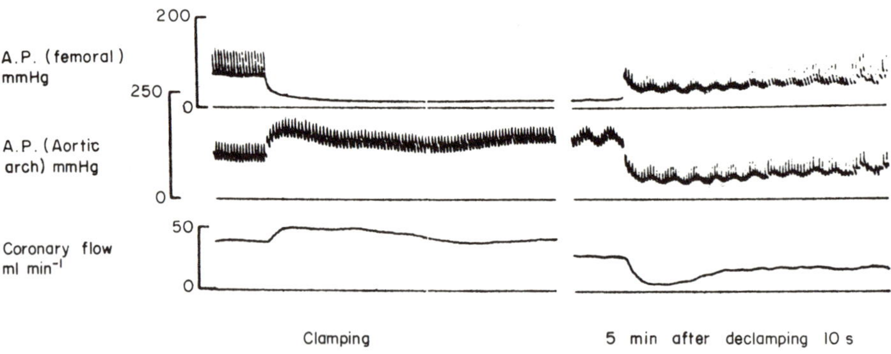

Fig. 2. Graphic shows disturbances of coronary flows in dog during and after aortic cross-clamping (5 min) above renal arteries. (After Longo *et al.*, 1971).

(1) Temporary renal ischaemia.
(2) Embolization.
(3) Aortic declamping.
(4) Reabsorption of the haematoma.

The temporary renal ischaemia after below-renal aortic cross-clamping, according to many authors (AAA), is believed to be induced by the hypertension and the consequent secondary arteriolar vasoconstriction. In our experience this kind of complication did not frequently occur. On the other hand, very severe involvement of the renal vascular bed in case of aortic cross-clamping above the renal arteries has been widely experienced by our group as well as by many other authors. Embolization in the renal arteries from thrombi or atherosclerotic debris during manipulation and preparation of the aneurysm is also possible but not very frequent in our experience. Porter *et al*. (1966) has reported this kind of complication in 17% of the cases.

The involvement of the renal arterial bed is markedly more severe during clamping and declamping procedures with a fall of the renal flow (Fig. 3). Renal involvement induced by aortic declamping during surgery for AAA is usually more severe than the one that occurs during surgery for aortic or peripheral arterial occlusion since in this case the distal arterial bed is widely patent. Finally, most relevant is the renal damage induced by reabsorption of the haematoma in case of ruptured aneurysms.

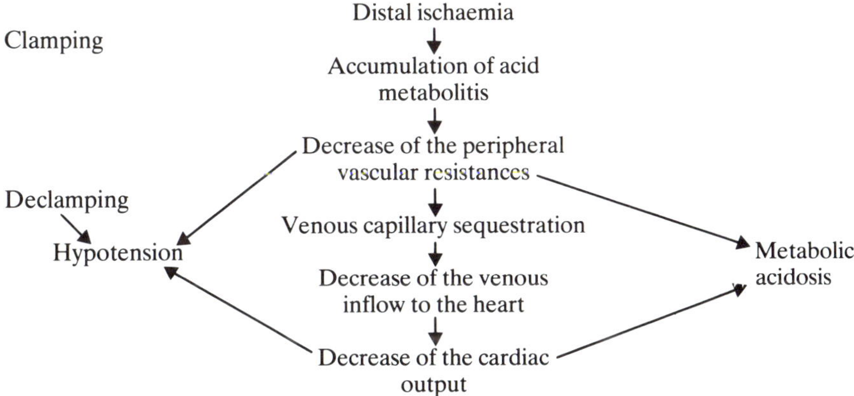

Fig. 3. Effects of aortic clamping and declamping.

In emergency surgery for ruptured aneurysms, the renal involvement is of course much more severe for the shock, the technical difficulties in isolating and clamping the aorta, the massive blood transfusion, the possible long-time ischaemia and, most important, the retroperitoneal haematoma that can often induce an acute renal failure (Fig. 4).

Surgical treatment for AAA may complicate with a peripheral ischaemia to the lower limbs due to distal embolization or thrombosis or to the aortic cross-clamping; 32% of our patients operated on for AAA were also affected by peripheral arteriopathies at various stages. Nevertheless, in many cases the arteries of the lower limbs are mostly patent, there is a very poor collateral circulation and the ischaemia time due to aortic clamping is very badly tolerated. For those reasons surgery for AAA requires delicate manipulation of the aneurysm, accurate application and release of the clamps, short operative times, heparinization of the distal and sometimes of the renal vascular bed, moderate blood losses. Ruptured aneurysms are often complicated in the post-operative course by the reabsorption of the retroperitoneal haematoma.

In our experience, the peritoneal dialysis that we routinely start in the immediate post-operative course with the aim at reducing the acute renal failure consequent to the blood reabsorption, should be highly recommended

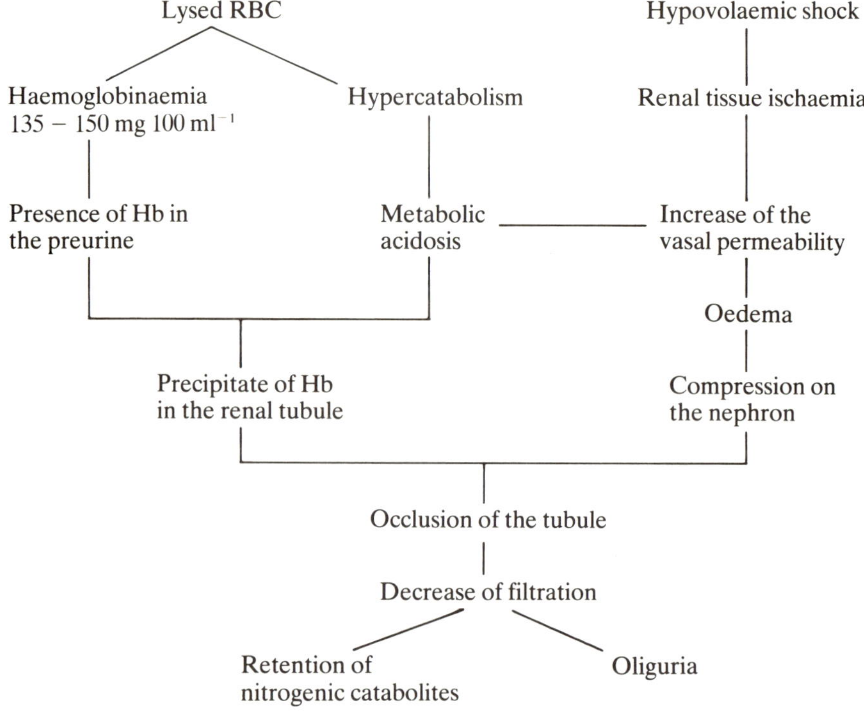

Fig. 4. Mechanism of renal damage in ruptured aneurysms.

in the post-operative treatment of ruptured aortic aneurysms. Some other complications are strictly related to the surgical procedures such as venous disruptions of the vena cava or iliacs. The careful isolation of the right side of the AAA does not need to be very extensive and accurate as long as the place for a safe aortic and iliac clamping is obtained. Disrupture of the main abdominal veins gives in most of the cases very severe and troublesome haemorrhages.

Episodes of paraplegia due to occlusion or ligation of a medullar artery emerging from the aorta at the level of the aneurysm have been reported. Most of the times these medullary lesions are irreversible and have a very severe prognosis (Szilagyi, 1978). Complications such as aorto-enteric (most often involved is the duodenum) or aortocaval fistulas pre-existing the operation, necessitate an emergency surgical repair and in many cases may complicate the post-operative course. In such circumstances, specially when the fistula involves the alimentary tract, the implant of an artificial graft in the retroperitoneum might raise many infective sequelae and therefore should be avoided. In these cases, the aortic ligation and the construction of an extra-anatomic bypass graft (axillo-femoral or from the thoracic aorta to distal arteries) could represent the treatment of choice. Better tolerated are the aortovenous fistulas; there are no infective implications and, in case of aortocaval fistula, the venous rupture can be easily repaired from the intra-aneurysmatic aspect. Aortic fisutlas, specially aortoenteric, may occur in the post-operative course as consequence of a dehiscence of the graft and mycotic aneurysm. Also in these cases the aortic reconstruction should be avoided and the application of an extra-anatomic bypass graft is recommended.

Our experience is based on the surgical treatment of 603 AAA; 409 patients underwent elective surgery and 194 emergency surgery for ruptured AAA. The overall mortality rate has been 7.3% for the elective cases and 53% for the emergency cases. It is worthwhile to note that in the last two years the corresponding mortality rates have dropped to 2.2% and 30% respectively. In Table 1 are summarized the complications occurred in 76 patients who underwent elective surgery (18.5%).

Table I. Complications in patients operated upon electively for AAA.

Total number of cases: 409	Times	(%)
Worsening of a pre-existing cardiopathy	19	4.64
Pneumonia	18	4.40
Renal insufficiency	10	2.40
Jaundice	5	1.22
Urinary tract infections	43	10.51
CIA	2	0.48
TIA	3	0.73
Haemorrhagic enteritis	8	1.94
Stress ulcer	2	0.48
Phlebitis of the lower limbs	9	2.20
Nevritis	3	0.73
Gangrene of the lower limbs	3	0.73
Occlusion of one leg of the graft	3	0.73
Intestinal occlusion	3	0.73

The events that complicated the emergency operations for ruptured AAA are more difficult to define being rupture itself a very severe complication of the aneurysmatic pathology (Table II).

Table II. Cause of death in 61 patients operated on for ruptured AAA.

Acute renal insufficiency	34 times
Respiratory insufficiency	12 times
Myocardial infarct	5 times
Ischaemia of the pelvis and limbs	3 times
Acute ischaemic colitis	3 times
DIC	2 times
Peritonitis	2 times

To conclude it is worthwhile to remind that surgical therapy represent the only reliable treatment of AAA; it prevents the future rupture which is the unavoidable consequence of untreated aneurysms. Qualified centres with well-trained experience in this kind of pathology can achieve very good and promising results for intact AAA as well as for ruptured AAA. Possible complications that can render the post-operative course very eventful and sometimes fatal can be prevented and avoided.

REFERENCES

Longo, T., Marchetti, G. and Vercellio, G. (1971). Coronary hemodynamic changes induced by aortic cross clamping. *Journal of Cardiovascular Surgery* **12**, 52.

Porter, J. M., McGregor, F., Acinapura, A. J. and Silver, D. (1966). Renal function following abdominal aortic aneurysmectomy. *Surgery, Gynecology and Obstetrics* **123**, 89.

Szilagyi, D. E. (1978). Paraplegia following abdominal aortic surgery. *Surgery* **1**, 123.

MYCOTIC AND INFECTED ANEURYSMS OF THE ABDOMINAL AORTA

R. B. Rutherford

Department of Surgery, University of Colorado Medical Center, Denver, Colorado, USA

The term mycotic was applied by Osler in 1885 to infected aneurysms resulting from septic emboli originating from bacterial endocarditis. Properly, it should be reserved for such aneurysms, but unfortunately it is now used interchangeably with "infected aneurysms" rather than to indicate a special type of the latter. Infected aneurysms are one of the most treacherous challenges a surgeon can face, one which infected penetrating wounds and venereal disease have presented us with since early civilization. Briefly, during the 1800s, in the era before antisepsis, the practice of blood-letting briefly challenged wars and syphilis as the major contributor of infected aneurysms. More recently, with the increasing application of invasive diagnostic and therapeutic vascular procedures, iatrogenic causes again threaten to dominate the other sources of infected aneurysms. With this and with his control, by the use of antibiotics, of most of the bloodborne forms of infected aneurysms, the physician truly "giveth" and "taketh away".

Although they share a microbial common denominator, infected aneurysms represent a very diverse group in regard to origin of infection, responsible organisms, location and natural courses; all of which ultimately affect surgical management. Close to 20% of all infected aneurysms occur in the abdominal aorta, yet less than 2% of abdominal aortic aneurysms are clinically infected. Infected aneurysms in this location are not as easily detected as when they occur in the extremities, neck or thorax. They are also

Serono Symposium No. 44, "Peripheral Arterial Diseases: Medical and Surgical Problems", edited by S. Stipa and A. Cavallaro, 1982. Academic Press, London and New York.

more prone to rupture freely, with exsanguinating hemorrhage, than all but infected thoracic aneurysms, and, by their very location, they present special problems in operative management. Their similarities and dissimilarities with infected aneurysms in other locations will be emphasized in the discussion that follows.

MECHANISM OF INFECTION AND ETIOLOGIC CLASSIFICATION

Like all other infected aneurysms, those located in the abdominal aorta may be infected via the bloodstream or by contamination introduced from the outside. Furthermore, these intravascular and extravascular forms can each be subdivided into three subtypes as outlined in Table I. Although infected aneurysms themselves are uncommon, comprising less than 2% of all aneurysms, primary or cryptogenic mycotic aneurysms, i.e. those due to microbial arteritis, are a relatively common type in the abdominal aorta being three times more common than peripheral locations (Mundth *et al.*, 1969). Diseased arteries are more prone to infection during bacteremia so it is understandable why the infrarenal aorta would be a site of predilection. In a review of the literature of salmonellosis and aneurysm of the distal abdominal aorta, Reichle *et al.* (1970) collected 20 cases from the literature and added one of their own. All the cases were in their sixth to eighth decade and all but *three* had atherosclerosis of the abdominal aorta. Sixty-five percent of *Salmonella*-infected aneurysms occur in the abdominal aorta (Wilson *et al.*, 1978).

Table I. Types of mycotic or infected aneurysms.

Source	Etiology	Nomenclature
Intravascular	1. Emboli of endocardial origin	Mycotic, embolomycotic, secondary mycotic
	2. Arteritis secondary to bacteremia	Primary or cryptogenic mycotic, microbial arteritis
	3. Infection of pre-existing aneurysm	Intramural infected aneurysm
Extravascular	4. Vascular trauma with secondary infection	Traumatic infected pseudoaneurysm
	5. Infected graft or suture line	Infected anastomotic aneurysm
	6. Contiguous infection	Nontraumatic (extramural) infected pseudoaneurysm

Syphilitic arteritis can affect the abdominal aorta and cause a saccular aneurysm in this location. In fact, as late as the 1950s, syphilis was thought to contribute up to 10% of all abdominal aortic aneurysms. In retrospect, many of these were probably arteriosclerotic aneurysms in patients with a positive serologic test for syphilis but, when they do occur, syphilitic aneurysms are usually saccular in form, suprarenal in location and rarely extend above the diaphragm (Crisler and Bahnson, 1972). This should be kept in mind whenever such an aneurysm is encountered, particularly in a patient from a region in which this venereal disease has not been well controlled.

Secondary or embolomycotic aneurysms, the condition for which Osler originally applied the term mycotic, are becoming as rare as their cause, subacute bacterial endocarditis (SBE). However, in 1923 at a time that this type contributed close to 80% of all infected aneurysms, Stengel and Wolferth (1923), reported that approximately 25% of infected aneurysms secondary to SBE were aortic in location. This possibility should be considered in any patient with a history of heart disease or cardiac surgery.

In the remaining intravascular form of infected aneurysm, a pre-existing aneurysm becomes secondarily infected. In view of the relative frequency of systemic bacteria infections and abdominal aortic aneurysms, this type of infected aneurysm is not seen as commonly as one would expect. Often, infection of an aortic aneurysm is suspected at the time of surgery because of inflammatory reaction surrounding the aneurysm or the suspicious appearance of its contents. Usually cultures of the aneurysm wall or its contents in such cases are sterile, although in one report by Ernst *et al.* (1977), 15% of 80 cultured aneurysms grew bacteria. However only two of the 80 cases developed graft sepsis and most of the cultures grew *Staphylococcus epidermidis*. Therefore, it was concluded that either such infections were not clinically significant or resection and antibiotic therapy had modified the end result. Nevertheless, Gram smears and cultures of suspicious aortic aneurysms are still recommended because of the consequences of not making this discovery.

Currently, extravascular causes of infected aneurysms are far more common than intravascular. The increasing frequency of invasive vascular diagnostic and therapeutic procedures are mainly responsible for this. Infected grafts and anastomoses contribute significantly, combining as they do, a violation of the integrity of the arterial tree with risk of intra-operative bacterial contamination. This complication has been significantly reduced but not eliminated by prophylactic antibiotics in elective cases (Kaiser *et al.*, 1978). A special variant of this type of infected aortic aneurysm is one presenting as an aortoenteric fistula. On the one hand, a primary or secondary, anastomotic aneurysm may erode into adjacent bowel, usually duodenum, with secondary infection and eventually, serious gastro-intestinal hemorrhage. On the other hand, paraprosthetic infection can lead to aneurysm formation with enteric fistulization occurring later. The former mechanism has been generally thought to predominate, although experiments by Busuttil *et al.* (1979) suggest that infection may play a more primary role. Other invasive procedures (cardiac catheterization, arterial sampling for blood gas analysis, angioaccess for renal dialysis etc.) all contribute to the frequency of this type of aneurysm. However, they produce peripheral rather than aortic infected aneurysms. The same can be said for mycotic aneurysms resulting from unsterile drug abuse practices. Abdominal wounds which penetrate the aorta are a potential but infrequently reported source of this type of mycotic aneurysm because of associated contamination from concomitant bowel injuries. A final form of extravascular infected aneurysm that, due to contiguous (extramural) suppuration, is rare, attesting to the ability of the normal (undiseased, uninjured) aortic wall to resist infection. In fact, even in the days when psoas abscesses were relatively common, tuberculous pseudoaneurysms were exceedingly rare. Thus by far the most common extravascular form of infected aortic aneurysm involves an infected graft of anastomotic aneurysm and commonly presents as an aorto-duodenal fistula.

BACTERIOLOGY

The lower incidence of bacterial endocarditis, the predominance of peripherally located infected aneurysms and improvements in culturing techniques have all contributed to a change in the frequency spectrum of bacteria involved in infected aneurysms because the type of organism recovered depends on etiologic type, location and ease of culture (Anderson, 1977). Aneurysms secondary to bacterial endocarditis are usually due to hemolytic *Streptococcus*, and *Staphylococcus* which composed 44–32% of the total in one series (Wilson *et al.*, 1978). Other types of infected aneurysms are more likely to be caused by *Salmonella* or *Staphylococcus* but enterobacteria, *Klebsiella*, *Proteus*, *Escherichia coli*, *Pseudomonas*, *Bacteroides* and *Peptostreptococcus* have all been reported (Anderson, 1977). Infected aneurysms of the abdominal aorta due to bacteremias other than SBE demonstrate growth in only about one-half of the cultures but in almost one-half of these *Salmonella* is implicated (Mundth, 1969). There appears to be a predilection of *Salmonella* for diseased arterial walls, particularly the abdominal aorta and the superior mesenteric artery. Other bacteria found in infected aortic aneurysms include *Staphylococcus*, *Gonococcus*, *Pneumococcus*, *Streptococcus*, *E. coli* and *Proteus*. In a number of infected aortic aneurysms with negative cultures, Gram-positive cocci can be identified histologically and these have been presumed to be *Staphylococcus epidermidis* (Anderson, 1977), so *Staphylococcus* is also a relatively frequent cause of infected aortic aneurysms, but it does not dominate to the extent it does in peripheral sites.

Identification of the responsible bacteria is extremely important, for appropriate antibiotic therapy should be based on culture and antibiotic sensitivity testing. It may also be of prognostic significance. Generally infected aneurysms caused by Gram-negative organisms have a much higher mortality than when Gram-positive bacteria are responsible (Anderson, 1977; Jarrett *et al.*, 1975). However, this striking difference may be partly because peripheral aneurysms are more likely to be due to Gram-positive and central aneurysms to Gram-negative organisms, i.e. the location, as much as the cultured organisim, is affecting the prognosis. Despite this, it would appear that Gram-negative aortic infections, primarily those due to *Salmonella*, run a more fulminant course (Wilson *et al.*, 1978).

DIAGNOSIS

Pre-operative diagnosis of infected aortic aneurysm correlates well with successful treatment. This is not only because infected aneurysms can present unexpectedly with exsanguinating hemorrhage but because prosthetic reconstruction of the aortoiliac segment without realizing the infected nature of the aneurysm can also result in catastrophic outcome. Though there is no characteristic size or shape for mycotic aneurysms, this diagnosis obviously should be suspected in any patient presenting with aneurysm and with fever of unknown etiology, leucocytosis or elevated sedimentation rate. Similarly, patients with known intercurrent infections, prolonged illnesses, immunosuppression, or who have undergone invasive vascular procedures, should be suspected of harboring an infected aneurysm. This suspicion is strengthened by lack of calcification of an aneurysm and evidence of rapid growth or signs of compression or erosion, particularly in a young or female patient. The classic presentation of regional miliary sepsis is rarely seen. Repeated positive cultures are strongly supportive of the diagnosis, particularly if taken from an artery in the same distribution as the aneurysm. Arteriography is not generally helpful; CAT scans may demonstrate satellite gas formation in certain bacterial infections (Haaga *et al.*, 1978); both CAT and ultrasound scans may identify abnormal fluid collections around the abdominal aorta or a prosthesis.

TREATMENT OF INFECTED AORTIC ANEURYSMS

The proper management of infected aneurysms of the abdominal aorta adheres to very similar principles of those governing the treatment of the more frequent problem, graft sepsis. Together, these two conditions constitute one of the most challenging situations confronting vascular surgeons today. Unfortunately, the two major therapeutic goals, eradicating the infection and maintaining adequate circulation to the distal tissues, conflict directly with each other. Spontaneous or antibiotic-treated cures are unusual enough to warrant single case reports but should not be considered a reasonably achievable result. Experience dictates that the surgical management of infected aneurysms (and grafts) adheres to several principles which are enumerated and discussed below (Anderson, 1977; Moore, 1977; Liekweg and Greenfield, 1977; Willwerth and Waldhausen, 1974).

Remote Proximal and Distal Control of Hemostasis

Even under circumstances less urgent than rupture or fistulization of an infected aortic aneurysm, the problem of obtaining proximal and distal control is often complicated by the presence of an intervening inflammatory mass and/or reaction in the surrounding tissues. This is particularly true of paraprosthetic infections and aortoenteric fistulas. In addition, infected aneurysms are friable and more liable to rupture if manipulated. Other approaches than the usual method of gaining proximal control are worth considering. One may position an aortic occlusion balloon catheter (Fogarty 8-22F) just above the aneurysm through a left upper brachial artery cut-down. Then, if exsanguinating hemorrhage develops during the dissection, the balloon catheter can be quickly inflated. Another alternative is to employ the left posterior lateral approach to the upper abdominal aorta recommended by Crawford (1974) for suprarenal aneurysms. To gain exposure of the aorta through clean tissue planes above the involved segment, all the left-sided abdominal viscera except the kidney and adrenals are mobilized forward and to the right, providing safe access to the upper abdominal aorta.

Remove All Infected Tissues and Foreign Bodies Including the Entire Length of Any Involved Vascular Graft

Even if the infection seems localized, one should resist the temptation of leaving part of a prosthesis in place. In this regard, it should be realized that sepsis can induce graft thrombosis but this does not arrest at the intra-luminal spread of infection. Therefore, all clotted segments, even though they do not appear grossly infected, should be removed. On the other hand, if one is dealing with one of the intravascular forms of infected aneurysms and there is no evidence of transmural penetration of the infection, one may elect to simply excise the aneurysm *en bloc* with cuffs of normal artery proximally and distally.

Obtain Multiple Aerobic, Anaerobic, and Fungal Cultures of Removed Infected Material

Unless the offending organisms have already been identified with certainty.

Ligate or Oversew the Proximal and Distal Arteries

The closure of the proximal artery may be extremely treacherous, particularly in the extravascular types, and this is the most common cause of failure in cases in which the graft is removed. Monofilament suture should be used (e.g. horizontal mattress sutures of 00 Polypropylene) and, if there is room, an additional proximal occluding row of sutures, a heavy ligature or a row of staples should be placed. The suture line should be further isolated from the rest of the wound by a peritoneal flap or pedicle of greater omentum (Goldsmith *et al.*, 1968).

Provide Adequate Drainage

This principle is easy to follow when dealing with peripheral mycotic aneurysms but presents special problems when applied to infected aortic aneurysms. If there is suppuration or gross contamination, multiple soft latex rubber (Penrose) drains should be placed and led out through a left flank wound. Additional catheters, for infusion and aspiration of topical antibiotics or antimicrobial solutions might be employed (Diethrich *et al.*, 1970), though they probably are of little benefit beyond 24–48 h.

Restore Distal Flow Only if Limb Viability is Threatened and Perform an Extra-anatomic Rather than Direct Bypass

Except in the case of infection of a prosthesis placed for peripheral arterial occlusive disease, flow to the legs will often be inadequate after removal of the abdominal aorta or an infected aortic prosthesis. In such cases, a bypass must be performed or inevitable amputation accepted. Occasionally, however, the extremities will be viable as indicated by good capillary return, venous filling, lack of ischemic pain or ischemic neuropathy. This impression can be confirmed by demonstrating audible flow in pedal arteries by a Doppler velocity detector. In such cases, no arterial reconstructive procedure should be performed. Otherwise flow should be restored by extra-anatomic bypass. Although reports of successful direct reconstruction are in the literature, many of these have short follow-up periods and, even if one could occasionally "get away with" repair or reconstruction *in situ*, this does not justify employing it in other than very selected instances. The major categorical exception to this would be intravascular forms of infected aneurysms in which there was no evidence of transmural spread of the infection. These may be reconstructed *in situ*. If the aortic bifurcation has been preserved after removing the infected aneurysm, a unilateral axillary femoral bypass will suffice. If not, an axillobifemoral graft (a combination of an axillary femoral and femoro-femoral graft) will be required. Under less urgent circumstances, extra-anatomic bypass should be performed before dealing with the infected aneurysm itself. This avoids most of the penalties of prolonged aortic cross-clamping required while the infected aneurysm is removed and before the axillobifemoral bypass can be completed. Circumstances in which one would not perform the extra-anatomic bypass first include (1) the diagnosis of infected aortic aneurysm is not certain, (2) reasonable possibility that immediate revascularization may not be necessary, (3) bleeding or other complication does not allow time and (4) systemic sepsis is poorly controlled and may infect the new graft if the infected aneurysm is not first excised.

Rarely, infected abdominal aortic aneurysms will involve visceral or renal branches and create additional reconstructive problems. Usually at least the superior mesenteric artery can be grafted to a more proximal site in the aorta and at least one kidney can be preserved by similar anastomosis, or if an extra-anatomic bypass has already been performed, by re-implantation to the iliac vessels.

Administer Appropriate Antibiotics for a Minimum of Six Weeks

In the case of *Salmonella* infection, Chloramphenicol is often given for extended periods of time similar to those employed in the treatment of SBE. For six months to two years, the patient should have his temperature monitored every evening and have leucocyte counts and sedimentation rates performed every two to four weeks.

RESULTS

As recently as 1967 Bennett and Cherry reported that infected abdominal aortic aneurysms were invariably fatal. In 1954 Barker reported that barely 20% were salvagable because they were beyond the scope of surgical extirpation. However, with intensive surgical care, better antibiotics and improved surgical techniques, particularly the use of extra-anatomic bypass, this 4:1 mortality to survival ratio should soon be reversed with survival to be expected if diagnosed early before threatening complications have developed (Smith *et al.*, 1962). The main causes of failure are recurrent sepsis, bleeding from the aortic closure and renal failure, all potentially avoidable if one adheres to the approach recommended above.

REFERENCES

Anderson C. B. (1977). Mycotic aneurysms. *In* "Vascular Surgery" (R. B. Rutherford, Ed.). Saunders, Philadelphia, Pennsylvania.

Barker, W. (1954). Mycotic aneurysms. *Annals of Surgery* **139**, 85.

Bennett, D. and Cherry, J. (1967). Bacterial infection of aortic aneurysms. *American Journal of Surgery* **113**, 321.

Busuttil, R. W., Rees, W., Baker, J. D. and Wilson, S. E. (1979). Pathogenesis of aorto-duodenal fistula: experimental and clinical correlates. *Surgery* **85**, 1.

Crawford, E. S. (1974). Thoracoabdominal and abdominal aortic aneurysms involving renal, superior mesenteric, and coeliac arteries. *Surgery* **179**, 763.

Crisler, C. and Bahnson, H. T. (1972). Aneurysms of the aorta. *In* "Current Problems in Surgery" (M. M. Ravitch, Ed.), Vol. 9. Yearbook Medical Publishers, Chicago, Illinois.

Diethrich, E. B., Noon, G. P., Liddicoat, J. E. and DeBakey, M. E. (1970). Treatment of infected aortofemoral arterial prosthesis. *Surgery* **68**, 1044.

Ernst, C. *et al.* (1977). Incidence and significance of intraoperative bacterial cultures during abdominal aortic aneurysmectomy. *Annals of Surgery* **185**, 626.

Goldsmith, H. S., De Los Santos, R., Vanamee, P. and Beattie, E. Jr. (1968). Experimental protection of vascular prosthesis by omentum. *Archives of Surgery* **97**, 872.

Haaga, J. R., Baldwin, G. N., Reich, N. E. *et al.* (1978). CT detection of infected synthetic grafts: preliminary report of a new sign. *American Journal of Radiology* **131**, 317.

Jarrett, F. *et al.* (1975). Experience with infected aneurysms of the abdominal aorta. *Archives of Surgery (Chicago)* **110**, 1281.

Kaiser, A. B., Clayson, K. R., Mulherin, J. L. *et al.* (1978). Antibiotic prophylaxis. *In* "Vascular Surgery". Presented at the Annual Meeting of the American Surgical Association April 26–28, 1978, Dallas, Texas.

Liekweg, W. G. and Greenfield, L. J. (1977). Vascular prosthetic infections: collected experience and results of treatment. *Surgery* **81**, 335.

Moore, W. S. (1977). Infection in prosthetic grafts. *In* "Vascular Surgery" (R. B. Rutherford, Ed.). Saunders, Philadelphia, Pennsylvania.

Mundth, E. *et al.* (1969). Surgical management of mycotic aneurysms and the complications of infection in vascular reconstructive surgery. *American Journal of Surgery* **117**, 460.

Reichle, F. *et al.* (1970). Salmonellosis and aneurysm of the distal abdominal aorta. *Annals of Surgery (Chicago)* **171**, 219.
Smith, R., Szilagyi, E. and Colville, J. (1962). Surgical treatment of mycotic aneurysms. *Archives of Surgery (Chicago)* **85**, 663.
Stengel, A. and Wolferth, C. (1923). Mycotic (bacterial) aneurysms of intravascular origin. *Archives of International Medicine* **31**, 527.
Willwerth, B. M. and Waldhausen, J. A. (1974). Infection of arterial prostheses. *Surgery, Gynecology and Obstetrics* **139**, 446.
Wilson, S. E., Van Wagenen, P. and Passaro, E. Jr. (1978). Arterial infection. *In* "Current Problems in Surgery" (M. M. Ravitch, Ed.). Vol. XV, No. 9. Yearbook Medical Publishers, Chicago, Illinois.

MEDICAL TREATMENT OF AORTIC DISSECTION

J. Menard, P. F. Plouin, M. Thibonnier and P. Corvol

Inserm U 36, Paris France

In the past 15 years, the role of medical therapy in aortic dissection has been carefully examined. After the first report by Wheat and Palmer (1968), application of medical therapy was extended to many cases of aortic dissections (Slater and Desanctis, 1979). Even though a randomized trial between medical and surgical therapy is not available at the present time, and, probably, it is not feasible, a majority of authors reported excellent results of the medical treatment for distal or descending dissections (type III), whereas a surgical treatment was preferred for dissections originating in the ascending aorta (MacFarland *et al.*, 1972). MacFarland *et al.* reported a 12% mortality during the initial hospital admission of 26 patients, and 61% of these patients survived for at least a mean of 36 months.

As suggested by Wheat and Palmer (1968), there are two major objectives of medical therapy. The first is to lower blood pressure, and the second is to reduce the velocity with which the contracting left ventricle ejects blood. Reducing arterial blood pressure diminishes the force exerted against the damaged aortic wall, whereas decreasing cardiac ejection velocity attenuates the shearing force that tends to initiate and propagate dissection. A third objective is to maintain sodium balance and renal function by counteracting the reactions of the kidney to the pharmacological decrease in renal perfusion pressure.

The clinical corollary of these observations is that drugs or combination of drugs should be used that both reduce the arterial pressure and diminish ejection velocity. Patients should be admitted to an intensive care unit where

Serono Symposium No. 44, "Peripheral Arterial Diseases: Medical and Surgical Problems", edited by S. Stipa and A. Cavallaro, 1982. Academic Press, London and New York.

blood pressure, pulse rate, electrocardiogram and also urine output can be continuously monitored. A sudden decrease in urinary output can reflect the fall in renal perfusion pressure but can also be the consequence of an extension of the dissection to one or both renal arteries.

Since new antihypertensive drugs are now available, it is worth while to review their main characteristics, in order to know if the medical treatment of aortic dissections can be improved from two points of view: efficacy and tolerance. Many drugs are available and their choice must be performed according to precise criteria.

The haemodynamic characteristics of the different antihypertensive drugs constitute the first criteria (Bhatia and Frohlich, 1973). The second is their ease of administration and the time course of their hypotensive effect (Koch-Weser, 1974). For the first few hours of treatment, the need for hypotension is often urgent and drug administration should be parenteral. Moreover, gastro-intestinal absorption is frequently unreliable and surgery may be imminent for some patients. Another criteria is the duration of action of the drug to avoid a rebound or an excessive hypotension.

Three antihypertensive drugs have the same haemodynamic profile and must be avoided: diazoxide, hydralazine and minoxidil. Moreover, this last drug cannot be used parenterally. The fall in blood pressure induced by these three antihypertensive drugs is due to a direct dilatation of peripheral resistance vessels, with little effect on capacitance vessels, and no interference with sympathetic reflexes. Their hypotensive action is accompanied by tachycardia, increased cardiac output, and increased oxygen myocardial consumption. These cardiac effects are undesirable since they increase the shearing forces that propagate dissection and also the cardiac work in patients who have frequently a patent or latent coronary heart disease (Bhatia and Frohlich, 1973).

Nifedine has been recently used in the treatment of hypertension. Its myocardial effects minimize the risk of myocardial ischaemia. However, since it increases both pulse rate and cardiac output, it cannot be considered as a drug useful for the treatment of aortic dissection (Olivari *et al.*, 1979; Soto *et al.*, 1981).

Many other antihypertensive drugs are able to decrease blood pressure without increasing cardiac output, or, even more, are able to decrease cardiac output and heart rate.

The ganglionic blocking agent, Trimetaphan, lowers arterial pressure by arteriolar vasodilatation and by decreasing cardiac output. It is no longer indicated since it has all the side effects of ganglionic blockade: urinary retention, constipation and tachyphylaxis (Koch-Weser, 1974).

Whereas the cardiac effects of beta blockers (decrease in heart rate and cardiac output) are constant and immediate after intravenous injection, their hypotensive effect is unpredictable in hypertension (Menard *et al.*, 1980). For this reason, propranolol (0.15 mg kg^{-1}, intravenously) cannot be used as a unique treatment of medical dissection. It is also contraindicated if heart failure is suspected or if asthma is present in the patient's medical history. The main advantage of propranolol is to allow the use of a vasodilator, such as intravenous hydralazine. This combination reduces arterial pressure in less than 10 min. The vasodilator action of hydralazine persists, whereas its cardiac effects are neutralized by propranolol.

Labetalol is a new beta blocker which has also alpha-blocking properties. Its intravenous administration, either by a 50 mg injection or by the continuous infusion of 10–160 mg h^{-1} induces a fall in blood pressure, with a decrease in pulse rate and no change in cardiac output at least in recumbent posture (Pearson and Havard, 1978; Koch, 1977). It fulfils the two haemodynamic criteria for medical treatment of aortic dissections. Moreover, oral administration of the drug is possible after initiation of the treatment by parenteral administration. A chronic treatment by labetalol 1200–1600 mg daily has the same potency as the combination of a beta blocker (acebutolol 400–800 mg daily) and dihydralazine (50–100 mg daily) (Thibonnier *et al.*, 1980).

Theoretically, clonidine, a centrally active alpha-sympathomimetic agent has many advantages. It is effective in less than 15 min when administered intramuscularly or by continuous infusion and it decreases peripheral resistances, cardiac output and heart rate. Its rapid intravenous injection is prohibited, since a rapid and short rise in blood pressure occurs before hypotension. It acts in less than 30 min when 300 μg are administered orally. This oral administration of clonidine, in case of emergency far from a hospital, is able to facilitate patient's transportation to a specialized centre, without cardiac risk. Sedation is, under these circumstances, a useful side effect of clonidine. Unfortunately, the major disadvantage of clonidine is the possibility of a rebound in blood pressure and heart rate, when the drug will be withdrawn (Rosei *et al.*, 1976).

The converting enzyme inhibitor captopril has an haemodynamic profile which seems quite favourable: fall in blood pressure without increase in heart rate or cardiac output (Tarazi *et al.*, 1980). It cannot be administered intravenously, but an oral administration of 1 mg kg^{-1} captopril is effective between 15 and 30 min, and a 17% decrease in mean arterial blood pressure is obtained around the 90th minute (Soto *et al.*, 1981). The efficacy of captopril is certainly dependent on the initial status of the patient's renin–angiotensin system. It is more effective in high renin than in low renin patients. For this reason, its use during aortic dissection has too high a risk of ineffectiveness, especially in the absence of a previous negative sodium balance. We have successfully used captopril in a patient whose right renal artery was injured during the extension of his aortic dissection, with the appearance of a renovascular hypertension well documented on the intravenous pyelography.

This review of the advantages and disadvantages of several new antihypertensive agents explain why a drug which is rather difficult to use, sodium nitroprusside, is still considered as the most effective agent for immediate reduction of blood pressure.

A solution of 50–100 mg in 500 ml of dextrose 5% is injected at an initial rate of 25–50 μg min^{-1}. Not more than 1 mg kg^{-1} should be given during the first 3 h and a maximum of 0.2–0.3 mg kg^{-1} h^{-1} thereafter. The hypotensive effect is immediate, and disappears immediately when infusion is stopped.

Monitoring this treatment is not easy: photosensitivity of the nitroprusside sodium solution, rapidity of onset and cessation of the drug's action, thiocyanate toxicity after 48 h of treatment, first indicated by confusion, hyper-reflexia and convulsions. Blood thiocyanate levels can be monitored and levels below 10 mg % are well tolerated. Associated with the hypotension is a fall in cardiac output, total peripheral resistances and also left ventricular ejection rate (Bhatia and Frohlich, 1973). Heart rate increases (Fig. 1). The

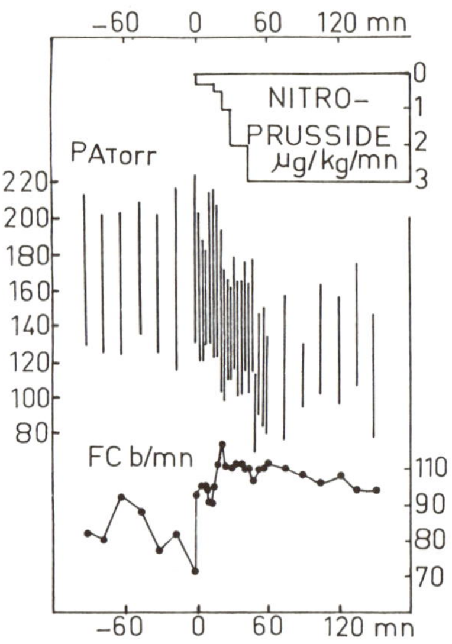

Fig. 1. Rapid hypotensive effect of sodium nitroprusside administered to a 72-year-old man with a dissection of his descending aorta. The fall in blood pressure is accompanied by a reflex tachycardia (from Lechevoir, 1977).

diminished left ventricular ejection rate results from the reduced cardiac filling and stroke volume. Reflex tachycardia can be blocked by adequate simultaneous beta adrenergic blockade. Later on, the decrease in perfusion pressure is accompanied by a fall in urinary volume and sodium output. Fluid retention is avoided by concomitant administration of diuretics such as furosemide. Orally active drugs will be administered after the first hour of parenteral therapy, for instance hydralazine in beta blocker treated patients, clonidine, methyl dopa or labetalol. A careful blood pressure monitoring is necessary when sodium nitroprusside is stopped and the antihypertensive effect becomes exclusively dependent on orally active drugs (Fig. 2).

If long-term medical therapy is selected, systolic blood pressure should be maintained at 140 mmHg or less. Beta adrenergic blockade is a requisite part of definitive medical therapy. Regular follow-up studies are required by all patients with routine X-rays every three to six months, ultrasonic measurements of the abdominal aorta and repeat angiography if there is any suspicion of redissection.

In conclusion, a complete knowledge of the time course of action, dosage and mechanism of action of all the available antihypertensive drugs is neces-

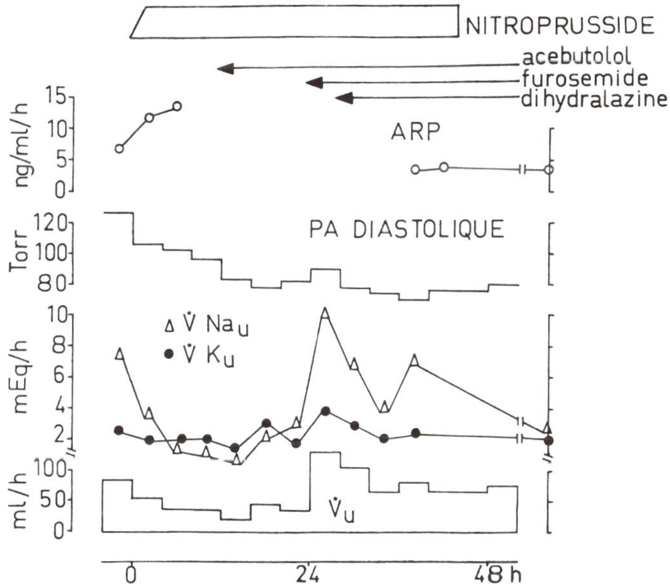

Fig. 2. Oral acebutolol treatment suppresses the reflex tachycardia induced by sodium nitroprusside and the rise in plasma renin activity. Oral dihydralazine, given after beta blockade, is substituted to sodium nitroprusside, whereas furosemide treatment counteracts the fall in urinary volume and natriuresis secondary to hypotension (from Lechevoir, 1977).

sary to determine the optimum therapy for each individual patient. Therapy should be started as soon as acute dissection is suspected and chronic oral therapy is the treatment of choice for uncomplicated dissections of the distal aorta, and for patients with proximal dissections and contraindications to surgery.

REFERENCES

Bhatia, S. K. and Frohlich, E. D. (1973). Hemodynamic comparison of agents useful in hypertensive emergencies. *American Heart Journal* **85**, 367.

Koch, G. (1977). Acute hemodynamic effects of an alpha and beta-receptor blocking agent (AH 5 158) on the systemic and pulmonary circulation at rest and during exercise in hypertensive patients. *American Heart Journal* **93**, 585.

Koch-Weser, J. (1974). Hypertensive emergencies. *New England Journal of Medicine* **290**, 211.

Lechevoir, X. X. (1977). MD Thesis, Paris.

MacFarland, J., Willerson, J. T., Dinsmore, R. E., Austen, W G., Buckley, M. J., Sanders, C. A. and Desanctis, R. W. (1972). The medical treatment of dissecting aortic aneurysms. *New England Journal of Medicine* **286**, 115.

Menard, J., Bautier, P., Plouin, R. F., Thibonnier, M. and Corvol, P. (1980). Beta-adrenoceptor blocking drugs and the renin-angiotensin system. *In* "Clinical

Pharmacology Therapy Proceedings of the First World Conference (P. Turner, Ed.), p. 264. Macmillan, London.

Olivari, M. T., Bartorelli, V., Polese, A., Fiorentini, C., Moruzzi, P. and Guazzi, M. D. (1979). Treatment of hypertension with nifedipine, a calcium antagonistic agent. *Circulation* **59**, 1056.

Pearson, R. M. and Havard, C. W. H. (1978). Intravenous labetalol in hypertensive patients given by fast and slow injection. *British Journal of Clinical Pharmacology* **5**, 401.

Rosei, E. A., Brown, J. J., Lever, A. F., Robertson, A. S., Robertson, J. I. S. and Trust, P. M. (1976). Treatment of phaeochromocytoma and of clonidine withdrawal hypertension with labetalol. *British Journal of Clinical Pharmacology* **3**, (4) (Suppl. 3), 809.

Slater, E. E. and Desanctis, R. W. (1979). Dissection of the aorta. *Medical Clinics of North America* **63**, 141.

Soto, M. E., Thibonnier, M. Sire, O., Menard, J., Corvol, P. and Milliez, P. (1981). Antihypertensive and hormonal effects of a single oral dose of Captopril or nifedipine in essential hypertension. *British Journal of Clinical Pharmacology* (In press).

Tarazi, R. C., Bravo, E. L., Fouad, F. M., Omvik, P, and Cody, R. J. Jr. (1980). Hemodynamic and volume changes associated with Captopril. *Hypertension* **2**, 576.

Thibonnier, M., Lardoux, M. D. and Corvil, P. (1980). Comparative trial of labetalol and acebutolol, alone or associated with dihydralazine in treatment of essential hypertension. *British Journal of Clinical Pharmacology* **9**, 561.

Wheat, M. W. Jr. and Palmer, R. F. (1968). Dissecting aneurysms of the aorta. Present status of drug versus surgical therapy. *Progress in Cardiovascular Diseases* **11**, 198.

TREATMENT OF ACUTE DISSECTIONS OF THE AORTA

Ch. Dubost and A. Carpentier

Clinique Chirurgicale, Cardio-Vasculaire, Hôpital Broussais, Paris, France

The current treatment of aortic dissections is based on the following principles.

(1) The goal is not to treat the dissection but to prevent the worst complications.
(2) The method of treatment depends on the inclusion or not of the ascending aorta (De Bakey *et al.*, 1965; Dubost *et al.*, 1971; Anagnostopoulos, 1975).

This approach which is essentially palliative has greatly improved the prognosis of surgical cures and has discredited the radical attempts at complete cure which included an extremely high mortality rate. The two techniques which we describe herein are those we use at Broussais Hospital in Paris; they are derived from those of De Bakey and have been improved upon over the years with increasing experience.

DISSECTING ANEURYSMS INVOLVING THE ASCENDING AORTA

This type of aortic dissection requires urgent surgical treatment. This approach might seem simplistic and brusque to those who remember the medical hypotensive treatment of Wheat, but the statistics of Daily *et al.* (1970) and Wolfe and Moran (1977) have shown the medical treatment to be ineffective. We use hypotensive treatment only in patients older than 70

Serono Symposium No. 44, "Peripheral Arterial Diseases: Medical and Surgical Problems", edited by S. Stipa and A. Cavallaro, 1982. Academic Press, London and New York.

years. The emergency is all the more important in the presence of certain signs of gravity: major aortic insufficiency, cardiac tamponade, oligoanuria, ischaemia of the lower limbs, visceral ischaemia.

In Principle

The intervention is limited to the correction of the aortic insufficiency by resection and replacement with a Dacron graft of the ascending aorta. This palliative approach advocated by De Bakey proposes to remove the most fragile part of the aorta.

Preparation

The surgery on dissecting aortic aneurysms is difficult, one of the most difficult in all of cardiovascular surgery. Failures are dominated by one cause — excessive bleeding from sutures placed with difficulty in friable tissues. Success often depends on correct preparation before surgery including typed and matched blood in sufficient quantities, Teflon pledgets, surgical glue and Cooley type Dacron prosthesis, an extracorporeal circulation with a membrane oxygenator to conserve platelets, three branches off the main arterial lines for possible carotid artery perfusion and cardioplegic solution at 4°. Two central venous catheters should be inserted before the operation. Continuous EEG and cervical arteries blood pressure (BP) monitoring are more than a precaution, for us they are a necessity. The patient is placed in the dorsal decubitus position with the two femoral arteries and the left axillary artery included in the operative field, the carotid arteries and the pedal arteries should be accessible to the anaesthesiologist.

The operation

It begins with the placement of two arterial cannulae for the extracorporeal circulation; one in the left axillary artery, the other in the healthiest of the femoral arteries. These two arterial lines are connected in a "Y" to the extracorporeal circulation.

The next step is a pre-sternal incision followed by mid-line sternotomie. The aorta and the roots of the cervico-cephalic blood vessels are exposed which sometimes involves cutting the left brachio-cephalic vein.

The pericardium is not opened until an open precautionary clamp is placed on the aorta at the base of the brachio-cephalic artery. This clamp can be immediately closed if the ascending aorta ruptures from decompression when the haemopericardium incises. Two cannulae are placed in the venae cavae and a vent is prepared for the left ventricle.

The extracorporeal circulation is started through the two arterial cannulae already in place. The EEG should be verified as should the BP in the brachio-cephalic and left carotid arteries. The diuresis should also be monitored.

Body temperature is brought down to 28°. At 32° the left ventricular vent is put in place and the aorta is test clamped at the base of the brachio-cephalic artery while verifying the EEG and cerebral arterial BP in order to determine the best combination of the arterial lines to insure a normal perfusion of the cerebral and visceral arteries. Often all the cannulae are needed. The brachiocephalic trunk should also be test clamped with EEG and BP monitoring to determine if the trunk can be clamped later if necessary. At 28° the heart should fibrillate and the aorta is definitively clamped. The outside cylinder of the dissecting aneurysm is opened transversally (Fig. 1). The dissection often extends proximally to the aortic ring while generally leaving the part of the aorta in relationship with the pulmonary artery intact. The intimal tear of the internal cylinders found, it is generally transversal and above the aortic leaflets, but it can be helicoidial and descend to the right aortic sinus, generally the coronary arteries themselves are untouched. The aorta is then widely opened while the heart is protected by cardioplegia injected through the coronary sinus in a retrograde way.

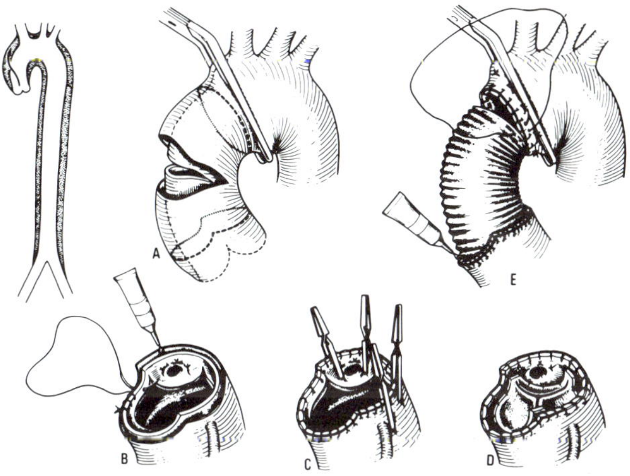

Fig. 1. Surgical treatment of type I A dissection. (A) After incision of the external cylinder, representation of the intimal tear. Dashes show where the aorta is to be resected distally and proximally. (B–C) Preparation of the proximal segment: approximation of the two cylinders with surgical glue and continuous sutures. (D) Placement of an aortic valve bioprosthesis. (E) Sutures of the aortic graft proximally and distally by continuous sutures. The sutures are placed in the Dacron graft then the aortic tissues.

Aortic insufficiency is corrected by valvuloplasty or prosthetic replacement. Valvuloplasty is possible if the valve tissue is healthy and the insufficiency is due to prolapse of a leaflet following detachment by the dissection. Valve replacement is necessary if the valves are the slightest bit altered, which is usually the case.

Suturing of the proximal end of the Dacron graft requires careful preparation of the aorta where the sutures will be placed. The two cylinders are excised just above the aortic leaflets and can even be incised proximally in the posterior sinus down to the aortic annulus. The space between the two concentric cylinders is then cleaned, carefully dried and covered with surgical glue as proposed by Guilmet *et al.* (1977). The two cylinders are approximated before the glue and held together by a bulldog clamp and a large continuous suture over the cut end. The Dacron graft is sewn in place with continuous sutures of 20- to 100-mm monofilaments. The sutures are first placed in the prosthesis from outside in, then in the aorta from the inside out. This method holds the grafts firmly against the aortic tissues and reduces the risks of later tears. The finished sutures are then covered with glue. The utility of Teflon pledgets to reinforce the aortic wall remains debatable. We personally avoid their use for two reasons: first of all they are no longer necessary when surgical glue is used and second they hinder the localization of bleeding sutures. To help find bleeding from suture points the following method might help: once the anastomosis is completed, clamp the graft 5 cm from the suture line and fill it with blood (introduced with a coronary cannula through a hole cut in the graft) or iced saline mixed with blood (50 cc syringe); any bleeding points are then stanched with additional sutures placed in Teflon pledgets. This method has the advantage of checking the impermeability of the sutures under controlled pressure, of allowing the prosthesis to be pulled forward to expose the posterior sutures, and of allowing sufficient time while the heart is still protected from necrosis.

The sutures in the distal end of the graft are no less difficult and require the same careful preparation and the same organization of the various steps (preparation and gluing of the two cylinders, suturing the Dacron and aorta and control of bleeding points).

There is, however, one problem which is different from the proximal end, namely the difference in size (often quite large) between the internal and external cylinders and their functional role. This is particularly true in dissections which are days or even weeks old. Thus it is necessary to unclamp the aorta to verify the reflux through the internal cylinder. In order to adapt the Dacron graft to the diameter of the internal cylinder it is better to remove a long triangular piece, then stitch the graft, then to try and fold the cylinder and thus create many potential bleeding points.

After the sutures are completed and verified for bleeding points, the patient is brough back to normal body temperature, the aorta is unclamped and the coronary arteries are naturally perfused, and the heart cavities are checked for air bubbles. The progressive take over of the circulation by the heart is a critical movement and pressures should be checked in the cerebral vessels, the renal arteries and the femoral arteries.

Particular Situations and Their Treatment

(1) Aortic rupture on pericardial incision. The aorta should be clamped and the extracorporeal circulation started by aspirating the blood in the pericardium and the right atrium using two aspirating cannulae. The venae cavae cannulae should be inserted later.

(2) EEG abnormalities, insufficient carotid pressures or insufficient diuresis after start-up of the extracorporeal circulation or aortic clamping: verify by sequential clamping of the femoral and axillary lines which has the most efficient flow.

(3) Intimal tear involving a coronary artery: perform coronary bypass anastomosed to the Dacron grafts.

(4) Intimal tear continuing distal to the aortic clamp (type 1B). (a) If pressures verified by the test clamping of the brachio-cephalic trunk allow it, clamp this trunk and move the aortic clamp between the left carotid artery and the brachio-cephalic trunk. If the dissected aneurysm can then be excised, do so and re-implant the brachio-cephalic trunk on the prosthesis. (b) If the brachio-cephalic trunk cannot be clamped, use one of the prepared arterial line branches to perfuse the right carotid artery. (c) If the intimal tear extends distal to the left carotid, both carotid arteries should be perfused and the dissected aneurysms excised beyond the intimal tear. The brachio-cephalic trunk and the left carotid artery are then re-implanted in the prostheses.

(5) Insufficient perfusion pressures after removal from the extra-corporeal circulation: reconnect the extracorporeal circulation at maximum flow rate and perform a bypass between the brachio-cephalic trunk and the carotid artery and the aortic graft using a bifurcating graft of Dacron anastomosed to the graft.

DISSECTING ANEURYSM BEYOND ASCENDING AORTA

Dissections of this type have a short-term prognosis, which is better than if the ascending aorta is involved. The acute phase can be controlled with hypotensive treatment. This should be done in an intensive care unit since there is a danger of anuria, ventricular arrythmias and hypotensive shock.

Medical Treatment

Standard treatment includes Trimetaphan (Arfonad) which decreases myocardial contractility and peripheral resistance. This is given intravenously 1–2 mg in dextrose 5% in water. The perfusion rate should be adapted to obtain a systolic blood pressure of 100–120 mmHg. The ECG, the central venous pressure and the urinary debit should be monitored. If after 24 h the results are not satisfactory, other drugs can be used. Reserpine 1–2 mg i.m. q. 4 h; Guanethedine 50 mg p.o.; Propranolol 10 mg day^{-1} i.m. or 80–120 mg day^{-1}; Phentolamine 10–30 mg h^{-1}; or Nitroprusside 25–100 mg h^{-1}.

The ineffectiveness of the medical treatment, an increase in the size of the aneurysm, a repetition of painful crises, ischaemia of the limbs, oligoanuria or visceral ischaemia should prompt a surgical cure, which in any case would be indicated six weeks after the initial dissection. This type of dissecting aneurysm when it is extensive has a long-term prognosis barely better than those of the ascending aorta.

Principles and Preparation for Surgery

Here again the goal is not to cure the lesions but to prevent the complications. Complete excision is impossible because of the spinal blood supply and it is recommended to stop at T-9. Preparation is the same as for the previous type: we prefer an extracorporeal circulation as added security, whereas others prefer a moderate hypothermia of 30° or a Gott aortoaortic bypass. Extra-corporeal circulation can be total but is usually partial and insures abdominal vascularization by femoro-femoral or femoral–atrial shunt. The patient is operated on in the right lateral decubitus and the posterior tibial and pedal arteries are accessible to the anaesthesiologist.

Controlled Intervention (Type III C)

Access is through a lateral thoracotomy in the 4th intercostal space with disinsertion of the chondral extremity of the 5th rib. The extracorporeal circulation is placed between the femoral artery and the iliac vein on the same side. Into this venous line is branched an accessory aspirator to be used if the iliac drainage is insufficient; this line can be placed in the pulmonary infundibulum. The aorta is clamped at the base of the subclavian artery proximally and the T-10 distally. Two precautions are necessary to avoid a dissection progressing proximally from the subclavian clamp: maintain a systolic pressure of no more than 100 mmHg in the territory proximal to the clamp and clamp the aorta progressively with a large non-traumatizing clamp which is closed with the minimum pressure closing the aorta.

The excision of the proximal part of the descending aorta should be performed in healthy tissue proximal to the intimal tear. Suturing is done with 20- to 100-monofilaments. The distal excision is at the level of T-9. The two cylinders are glued and approximated with a continuous suture and then the Dacron graft is sewn to the two cylinders already joined together. Unclamping requires several precautions: evacuation of any air bubbles and progressive unclamping to avoid surges in the pressures.

Particular Situations and Their Treatment

The intimal tear extends proximal to the proximal clamp (type III B): the rule requiring that the proximal anastomis be made before the intimal tear is hard and fast, otherwise there is a risk of retrograde dissection. Thus it is necessary to clamp the aorta before the left subclavian artery or the left carotid artery after EEG monitoring of the effects of this clamping.

Insufficient perfusion pressure in the femoral or renal arteries after unclamping means perform an aortic bi-iliac bypass anastomosed to the graft.

The technique of partial resection and grafting of the aorta has had good results with an operative mortality of 20–40% and a long-term mortality of 5–10% per year, acceptable figures for such a disease; however, criticism can be made.

(1) A part of the damaged aorta is left in place which exposes the patient to eventual extension of the dissection, rupture of the aneurysm and visceral ischaemia.

(2) Suturing the graft to the aorta which is friable due to the dissection is difficult at best no matter what precautions are taken.

Two new techniques have tried to solve these problems. One is deliberately palliative and tries to reduce the bleeding problems by changing the suture techniques and the methods of joining the aortic graft. The other is more curative and tries to reduce both the operative risks and the ultimate complication by trying to completely eliminate the lesion. Even though these techniques are new and have not stood the test of time this paper would be incomplete if we did not at least mention them.

NEW PALLIATIVE TECHNIQUES

The problems and uncertainty of anastomoses in friable dissecting aortic tissue spurred research into techniques which were simpler and less haemorrhagic than the partial resection graft techniques. Dureau *et al.* (1978) from Lyon and Ablaza *et al.* (1978) in the United States simultaneously proposed the use of a prosthesis reinforced at both ends by a rigid ring in the form of an automobile wheel. Once the aneurysm is opened the graft is placed inside the aorta and the aortic tissue is drawn over the rims of the ring and tightened like a purse suture. We have no experience with this technique but the preliminary results are given in Dureau *et al.* (1978) and Ablaza *et al.* (1978).

Another palliative technique has been used by J. N. Fabiani of our service who solved the problem of acute ischaemia of the limbs in a patient with a type III dissection. He proposed to treat the ischaemia by axillo-femoral bypass which is an interesting solution in patients who cannot support a more radical intervention during the acute phase. In the same situation certain American surgeons have proposed the creation of re-entry openings in the iliac arteries (Wolfe and Moran, 1977).

RADICAL CURE OF AORTIC DISSECTIONS BY CIRCULATORY INVERSION AND PROGRESSIVE THROMBOSIS OF THE THORACIC AORTA

The previous cited techniques reduce the operatory mortality by reducing bleeding, but they are still palliative and do not affect the long-term mortality of 5–10% per year due to an evolution of the remaining aortic lesions. The technique which we propose herein is designed for radical cure, not by excision, but by exclusion of the diseased thoracic aorta and progressive thrombosis of the lesions. In addition, by avoiding sutures in friable aortic tissue, operative bleeding is considerably decreased. The technique is based on the following principles.

(1) The anastomoses are done in healthy tissue not in dissecting friable tissue and the aortic reconstruction is by bypass (Carpentier *et al.*, 1971).

(2) The placement of a permanent clamp on the aortic arch at a level dependent on the type of dissecting aneurysm produces a circulatory inversion in the dissected portion of the aorta.

(3) A progressive thrombosis of the thoracic aorta occurs beginning at the

clamp and progressing distally up to the aortic branches with high flow rates (main spinal and abdominal branches).

This technique was initially intended for dissections of the ascending aorta (types III C and III B) which had a high operative mortality rate due to retrograde dissection (Fig. 2, Table I). As opposed to De Bakey's technique this operation can be performed through a mid-line sternotomie and without extracorporeal circulation (Fig. 3). A bypass using a 25-mm Dacron graft is

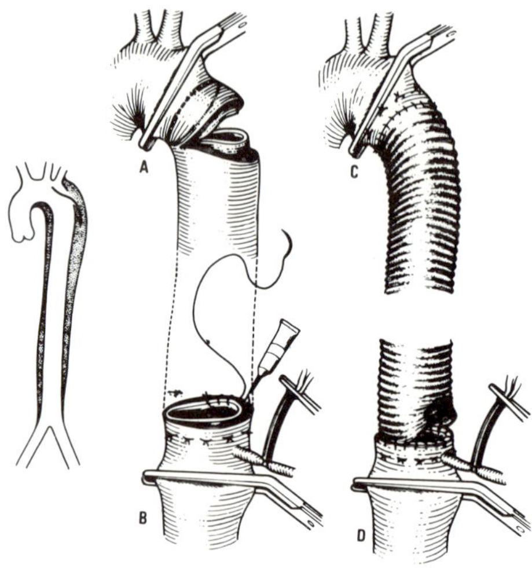

Fig. 2. Surgical treatment of type III C dissections. (A) Incision of the external cylinder showing the intimal tear. The dotted line shows the line of excision proximal to the intimal tear. (B) Aortic excision at T-9, gluing and suturing of the two cylinders. (C) Proximal anastomosis. (D) Distal anastomosis.

Table I. Hospital mortality.

	Surgical treatment			Medical treatment		
	Types I and II (%)	Type III (%)	Overall (%)	Types I and II (%)	Type III (%)	Overall (%)
De Bakey *et al.* (1965)			21[a]			
Austen (1970)	38	22				
Daily *et al.* (1970)	28	28		67	20	
Cooley (1970)			25			
Schumaker (1972)	17	22				
Dubost (1977)	30	56				
Girondin (1976)			72	100	60	81
Guilmet (1973)	28	25				

[a] Including chronic dissections.

performed between the ascending aorta which is clamped laterally and the abdominal aorta either sub-diaphragmatic or subrenal depending on the extent of the dissection. In the abdomen, the bypass passes in the posterior cavity of the omentum, then in the retroperiotoneal space. Once the bypass is completed, a permanent clamp is placed just distal to the subclavian artery, thus effectively reversing the circulation in the thoracic aorta. An arteriograph at three months shows a progressive exclusion of the dissected thoracic aorta by thrombosis. The progressive nature of the thrombosis allows for slow adjustment of the spinal circulation.

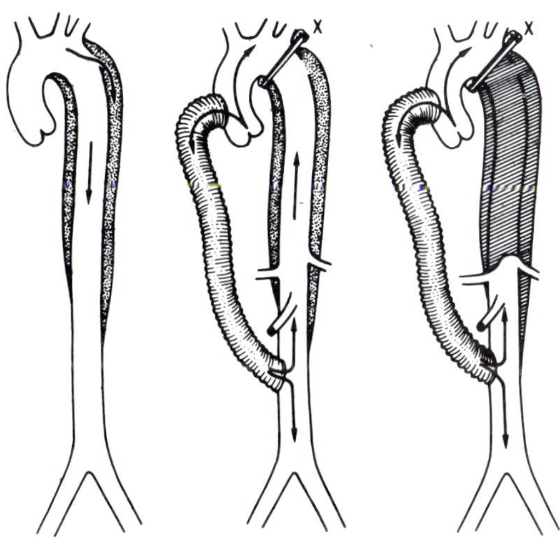

Fig. 3. Surgical treatment of type III C dissecting aneurysms by exclusion and thrombosis of the thoracic aorta. (Left) Lesions of the aorta. (Centre) Ascending aorta — abdominal aortic bypass with a permanent clamp (X) showing the inversion of the thoracic circulation. (Right) Progressive thrombosis of the dissecting thoracic aorta.

Afterwards, the same concept was applied to certain dissecting aneurysms involving the ascending aorta and the cervical arteries (Fig. 4). The approach is through a median sternotomie and laparotomie. A bypass is performed between the abdominal aorta (first step done without extracorporeal circulation) and the aortic orifice (second anastomose done under extracorporeal circulation and encircling the coronary ostia). The cervical great vessels are then re-implanted in the graft using a Dacron bifurcated graft (done without circulatory bypass). Here again, arteriography shows a progressive exclusion of the dissected aortic aneurysm.

RESULTS

Table I recapitulates the operative results found in the literature. Almost all the patients were treated by surgery using De Bakey's palliative technique

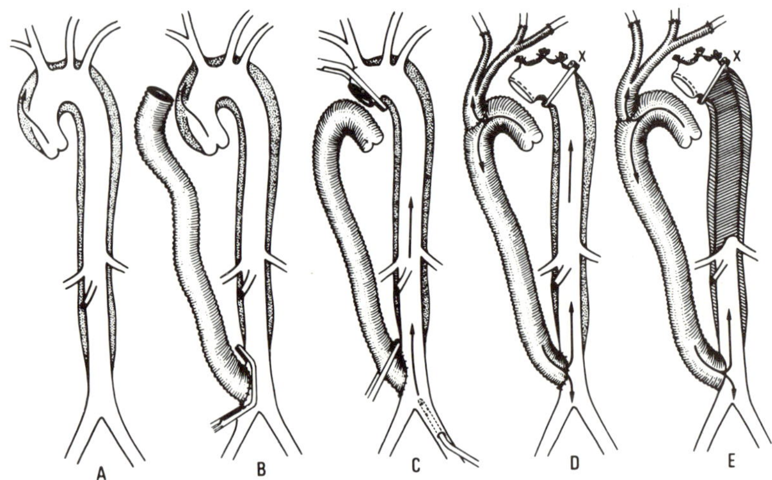

Fig. 4. Surgical treatment of type I A and I B dissecting aneurysms using progressive thrombo-exclusion of the dissected thoracic aorta. (A) Lesions. (B) Distal anastomosis with the abdominal aorta without extracorporeal circulation. (C) Proximal anastomosis to the aortic annulus at the level of the coronary ostia with extracorporeal circulation. (D) Without extracorporeal circulation, successive bypasses of the great cervical vessels followed by permanent aortic clamping (X). (E) Exclusion by progressive thrombosis of the thoracic aorta with spontaneous arrest at the level of high flow rate branches.

of partial resection and graft. Operative mortality has remained around 20–30%. It is surprising that type III dissections do not have a better operative prognosis especially since they are often operated on after the acute phase. The reason is that there is a high frequency of retrograde dissections starting at the aortic clamp or the proximal suture, or continuation of the dissection which interrupts the visceral circulation.

This surely justifies our exclusion thrombosis technique which anticipates and decreases the risks of rupture of the thoracic aorta, bleeding from suture points and retrograde dissections.

Few statistics have been established for long-term results, but it seems that the risks of complications after De Bakey's techniques is from 5% to 10% per year.

ACKNOWLEDGEMENT

This translation has been achieved by our excellent resident Michael Young.

REFERENCES

Ablaza, S. G., Gosh, S. C. and Grana, V. P. (1978). Use of a ringed intra luminal graft in the surgical treatment of dissecting aneurysms of the thoracic aorta. *Journal of Thoracic and Cardiovascular Surgery* **76**, 390.

Anagnostopoulos, E. E. (1975), "Acute Aortic Dissection". Baltimore University Park Press, Baltimore, Maryland.

Carpentier, A., Guilmet, D., Prigent, Cl., Gandjaack, I., Deloche, A., Lessana, A., Farge, Cl., Tricot, J., Morillo, F. and Dubost, Ch. (1971). Aneurysms of the aortic arch. *Thoraxchirurgie Vaskuläre Chirurgie* **19**, 5.

Daily, P. I., Trueblood, H. W., Stinson, E. B., Wuerflein, R. D. and Shumway, N. E. (1970). Management of acute aortic dissections. *Annals of Thoracic Surgery* **10**, 237.

De Bakey, M. E., Henly, W. S., Cooley, D. A., Morris, G. C., Crawford, E. S. and Beall, A. C. (1965). Surgical management of dissecting aneurysms of the aorta. *Journal of Thoracic and Cardiovascular Surgery* **49**, 130.

Dubost, Ch., Guilmet, D. and Soyer, R. (1971). "Les Anévrysmes de l'Aorte." Masson, Paris.

Dureau, G., Villard, J., George, M., Deliry, P., Froment, J. C. and Clermont, A. (1978). New surgical technique for the operative management of acute dissections of the ascending aorta. *Journal of Thoracic and Cardiovascular Surgery* **76**, 385.

Guilmet, D., Liebeaux, M., Dhainaut, J. F., Goudot, B., Francoual, M. and Bachet, J. (1977). Traitement chirurgical des dissections aigues de l'aorte ascendante. *Archives des Maladies du Coeur et des Vaisseaux* **70**, 639.

Wolfe, W. G, and Moran, J. F. (1977). The evolution of medical and surgical management of acute aortic dissection. *Circulation* **56**, 503.

TRAUMATIC RUPTURES OF THE AORTA: PATHOLOGY AND PATHOGENESIS

S. Sevitt

Birmingham, UK

Traumatic ruptures began to be separated from those due to underlying aortic disease only in the early part of this century. Only a few cases were reported in the British literature before the Second World War (Kemp, 1923; Shennan, 1929; Griffiths, 1931), and infrequent diagnosis is referred to by Strassman (1947) in his account of 72 cases and even by Marshall (1958) in his report on traumatic dissecting aneurysm. Most ruptures nowadays follow accidents on the road. However, tears have been found in air-crash victims (Haas, 1944; Teare, 1951), after falls from a height (Shennan, 1929; Fidler, 1949), in aircraft pilots falling to the ground (Wilson, 1946), following the free falling of lifts to the ground (Strassman, 1947; Parmley *et al.*, 1958), after direct blows on the chest not involving body deceleration (Kemp, 1923; Strassman, 1947; Parmley *et al.*, 1958), after a blow on the epigastrium (Forbes, 1944) and as a result of severe blast injury (Wilson and Tunbridge, 1943).

This account of a clinico-pathological analysis and of the underlying pathogenesis of the ruptures extends those previously reported (Sevitt 1977a, b). It deals with ruptures of the thoracic aorta, and examples are confined to those that occur after road traffic accidents. Occasional cases of traumatic rupture of the abdominal aorta have been referred to by Parmley *et al.* and others, but they are rare, and their origin is related to a displaced fracture or dislocation

Serono Symposium No. 44, "Peripheral Arterial Diseases: Medical and Surgical Problems", edited by S. Stipa and A. Cavallaro, 1982. Academic Press, London and New York.

of the dorso-lumbar spine similar to those that may occur in the distal half of the thoracic aorta.

PATHOLOGY

The ruptures are divided into three main groups according to the locations of the tears (Fig. 1).

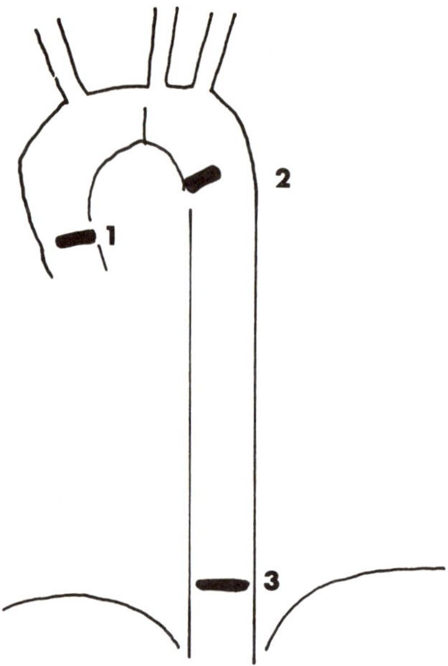

Fig. 1. Locations of major ruptures of the aorta found in road accident victims.

(1) Ruptures of the ascending aorta.
(2) Ruptures of the proximal descending aorta.
(3) Ruptures of the distal descending thoracic aorta.

Most cases have a single major rupture, but occasional examples of two large tears have been found such as those shown in Fig. 4 where the ascending aorta and the arch were separately torn.

RUPTURES OF THE ASCENDING AORTA

The ruptures are rarely visible externally but there is often some ecchymosis of the wall and sometimes some frank blood in the pericardial cavity.

When the aorta is opened from in front the ruptures present as transverse supravalvar tears of the intima and media situated 0.5–1.5 cm above the aortic cusps (Figs 2–4). This is also the main site of spontaneous aortic rupture. The

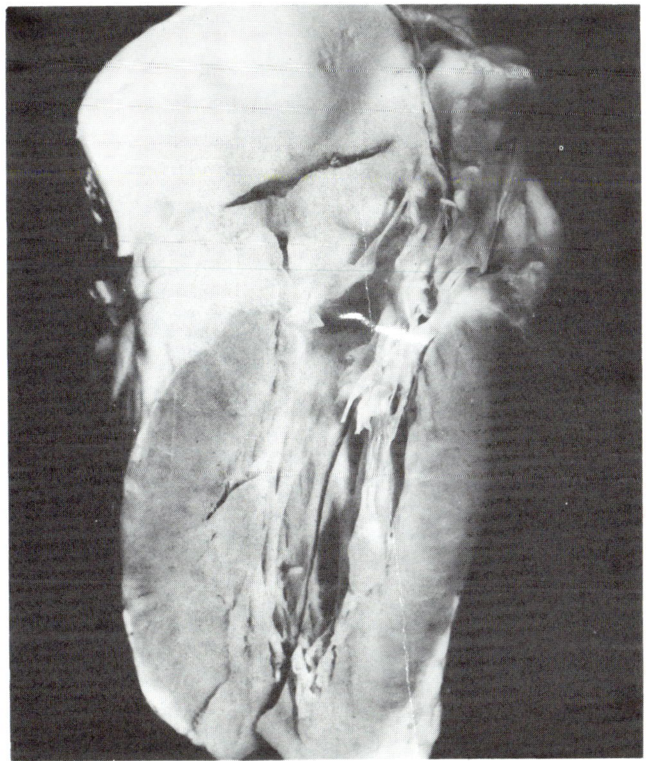

Fig. 2. Traumatic rupture of the ascending aorta. Note its posterior and supravalvar location.

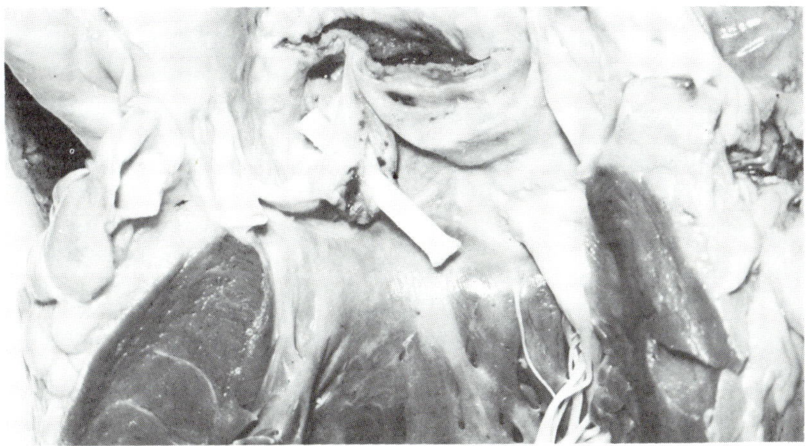

Fig. 3. Supravalvar rupture of the ascending aorta combined with rupture of a diseased valve cusp (Case 2).

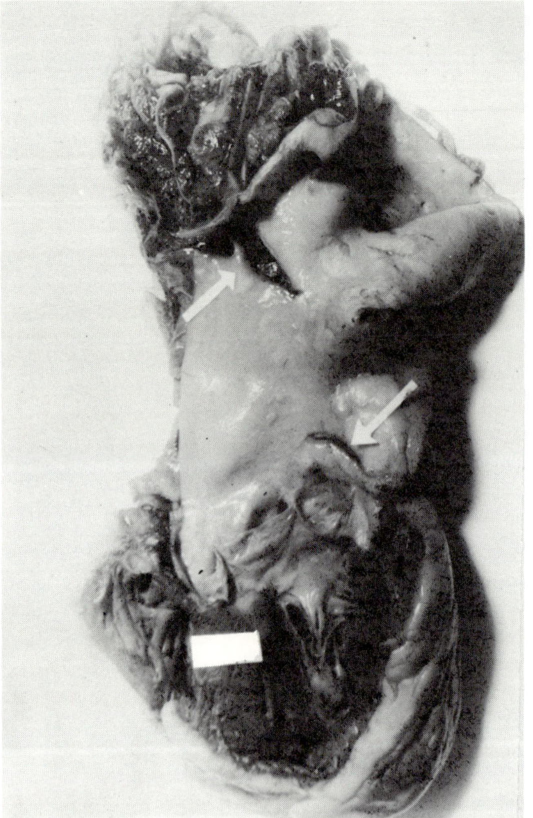

Fig. 4. Double aortic rupture, one in the ascending aorta and the other in the arch (arrows).

adventitia is not grossly torn though it is often infiltrated by haemorrhage. The ruptures measure 2.0 to 4 cm long and commonly involve between one-half and three-quarters of the aorta's circumference. Six of our seven cases were single ruptures — five on the posterior surface of the tube (Figs 2 and 3) and one anteriorly. Posterior location and incompleteness of rupture explain the absence of a haemopericardium in those without cardiac rupture. One of our cases had two ruptures (Fig. 4). Another had a rupture of a (thickened) aortic valve cusp (Fig. 3). Many had some degree of aortic atheroma reflecting their ages.

Most of the patients die rapidly after the accident, but this has as much or more to do with the severity and multiplicity of injuries, often including severe damage to the thorax. An example is cited below.

Case 1

A pedestrian suffered multiple bilateral fractures of the ribs, a fractured sternum, fracture dislocation of the upper thoracic spine with tearing of the spinal cord, fracture of the pubes and a small tear in the liver. The aorta showed a transverse supravalvar tear of three-quarters of its circumference. The right ventricle was also ruptured and a frank haemopericardium was present.

Some patients reach hospital alive only to die within the next few hours such as Case 2.

Case 2

A car driver succumbed 30 min after an injury caused by striking the steering wheel, with multiple fractures of the left ribs, laceration of the mesentery and 3.5 l of blood in the peritoneal cavity. The aortic rupture was located posteriorly. All three aortic cusps were thickened by chronic fibrous disease and the right coronary cusp had a short, recent, full-thickness rupture (Fig. 3). The aorta was severely atheromatous and the heart was enlarged from hypertension.

From experimental evidence (Moffatt *et al.*, 1966; Louhimo, 1967) ruptures of the ascending aorta from blows on the chest are likely to be caused by displacement of the heart downwards and into the left side of the thorax.

However, one of our subjects had no other evidence of thoracic (or abdominal) injury so a more indirect mechanism is also possible.

RUPTURES OF THE PROXIMAL DESCENDING AORTA

These are the majority of traumatic ruptures and include an important group which are or may be amenable to modern surgery. At necropsy most ruptures should be suspected on opening the chest because of extensive mediastinal ecchymosis or haemothorax, especially left-sided, or for both reasons. Then care needs to be taken to prevent further tears during removal of the thoracic contents *en bloc* by freeing the descending aorta posteriorly. The descending thoracic aorta is then opened longitudinally from behind.

The lesions are linear tears of the intima and media transverse to the long axis of the aorta and located 1–3 cm distal to the opening of the left subclavian artery. The adventitia is not grossly torn.

They can be divided into major and minor tears. Most attention is naturally paid to the major ones, but the minor ones are also of interest. They indicate the likely origin of the major ruptures and their essentially internal nature; but they also raise the question whether some of the major tears that terminate in massive haemorrhage, may arise as minor lesions and then extend under the influence of blood pressure, and also whether some may eventually and naturally heal.

Major Ruptures

Most are single linear ruptures located in the aortic isthmus and situated a little distal to the ostium of the left subclavian artery. All are transverse to the longitudinal axis of the aorta and most are gaping tears. Their lengths vary.

Some involve less than half the aortic circumference (Fig. 5), but more often up to three-quarters of the circumference is torn (Figs 6–8) and some ruptures are circumferential (Figs 9 and 10). Extension of initially partial to fully circumferential rupture seems possible.

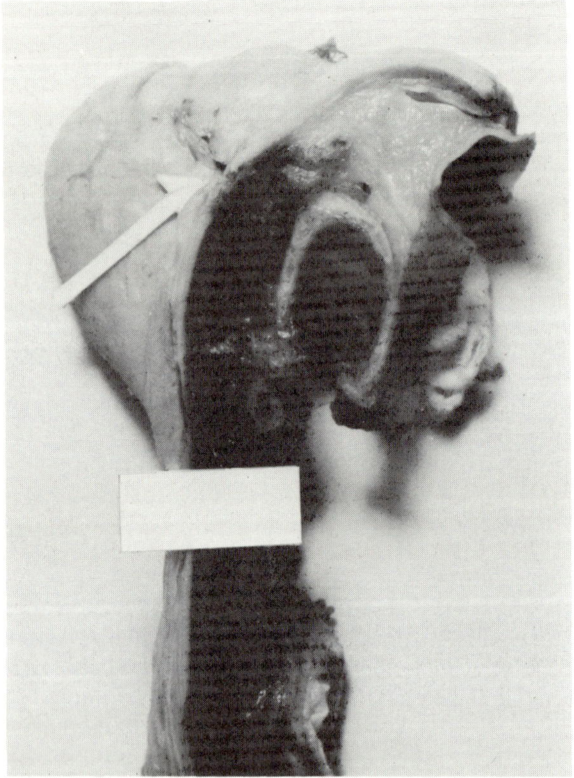

Fig. 5. Rupture of the anterior wall of the isthmus of the proximal descending aorta (arrow) with much periaortic haemorrhage tracking downwards. Rupture located above the opening of the first aortic intercostal artery.

Occasionally double tears are found, a feature observed in two of the 22 subjects with major ruptures in this region previously reported (Sevitt, 1977b). In one case the two large tears were located near one another (Fig. 11) and in the other case the ascending aorta was also ruptured (Fig. 4). A few also had minor subclinical tears.

Location of Rupture

The exact circumferential and longitudinal positions of the tears can help to determine their mechanism of origin. The circumferential positions of partial ruptures were assessed by reference to the openings of the right and left intercostal arteries which lie on the left posterior aspect of the aortic tube. The

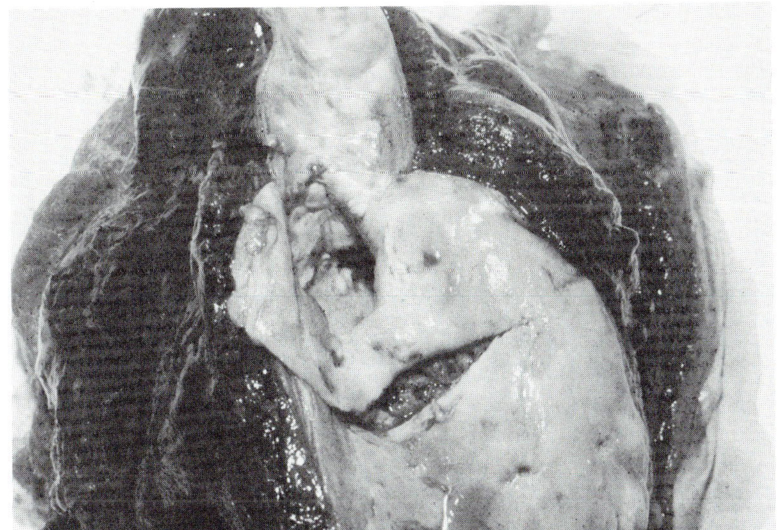

Fig. 6. Extensive rupture of the proximal descending aorta located 2 cm distal to the opening of the left subclavian artery and centred on the anterior wall. Aorta opened from behind.

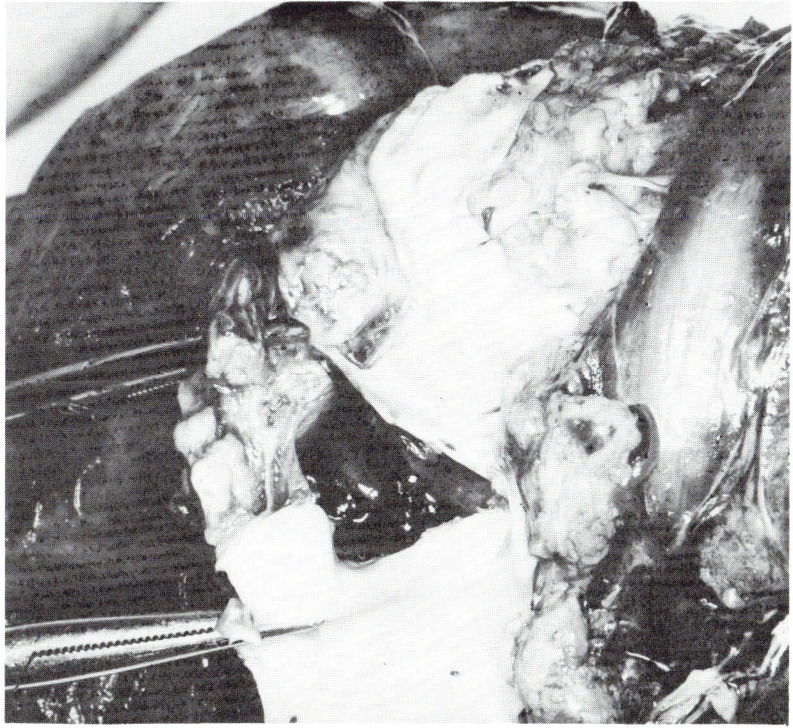

Fig. 7. False saccular aneurysm at the site of a traumatic rupture of the isthmus located between the levels of the first and second aortic intercostal arteries.

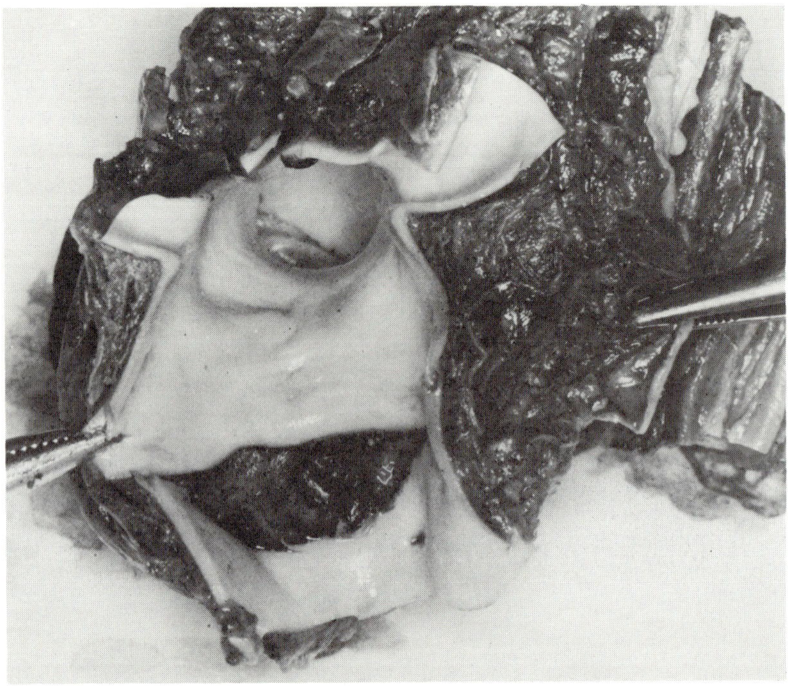

Fig. 8. Aortic rupture situated between the first and second aortic intercostal arteries with the formation of a local saccular aneurysm (Case 3).

majority were situated or centred anteriorly and a few anteriorly and somewhat to the right. These positions correspond to the inner or shorter curvature of the distal part of the arch, the part most liable to tear from overstretching.

It is also important to decide whether the ruptures lie proximal or distal to the ligamentum arteriosum (Botallo's ligament). This ligament binds part of the descending aorta to the left pulmonary artery and is closely related to the structures entering the root of the lung. The area of attachment is a fixed point acting like a hinge on which the aortic arch above and the distal aorta below it can move cranially or caudally depending on the forces applied.

The ligamentum arteriosum is situated to the level of the orifices of the first aortic intercostal arteries. In our series, most ruptures affecting the isthmus were above these orifices such as in Figs 5 and 9 for major tears and in Figs 12 and 13 for a minor one. However, in a few cases the rupture was at a level between the first and second aortic intercostal arteries (Figs 7 and 8) or just below the openings of the second aortic intercostal arteries, such as in Figs 10 and 14 for major and minor tears respectively. Thus, in our experience most ruptures were proximal to Botallo's ligament which suggests that the arch and proximal descending aorta had been overstretched in a cranial direction as indicated in Fig. 15. However a few were distal to this attachment and similar cases have been reported by Fidler (1949) and Voigt (1968). These point to a

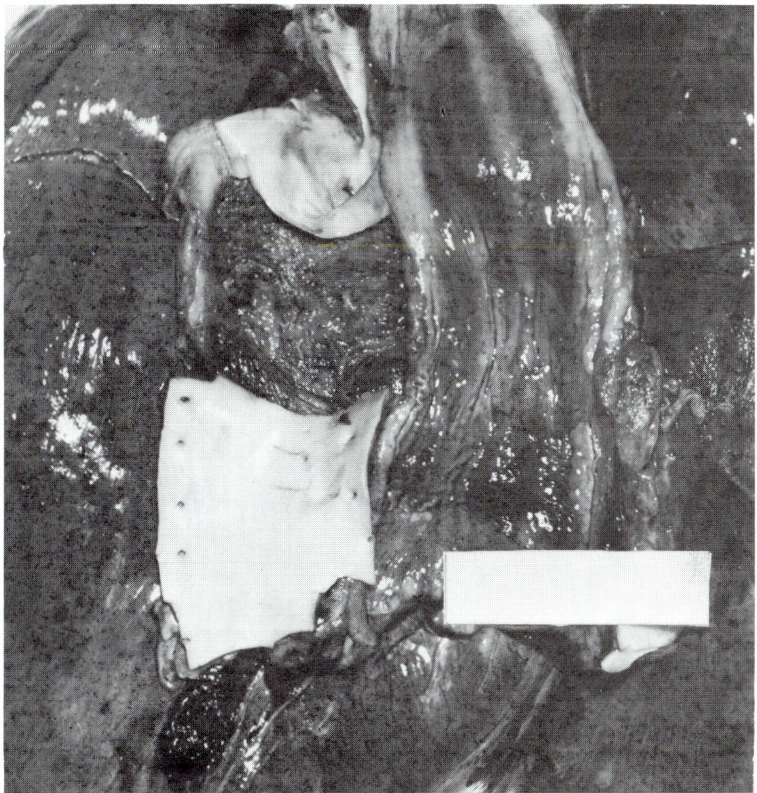

Fig. 9. Circumferential rupture above the level of the openings of the first aortic intercostal arteries. A fusiform false aneurysm had formed in the gap which was lined by adventitia and compressed blood clot (Case 4).

tearing tension directed caudally. Thus more than one mechanism is likely to cause similar tears. Presumably this is why the isthmus is the most frequent site of tearing.

Minor Ruptures

Several aortas with major ruptures also showed nearby minor non-haemorrhagic horizontal tears such as in Fig. 9. However in three cases the aortic tears were confined to minor splits, obviously subclinical. The smallest was only 5-mm long, non-haemorrhagic and located just beyond the arch (Fig. 12). Histologically the tear involved the intima and the inner third of the tunica media which were indented by pressure, so transforming the rupture into a micro-aneurysm (Fig. 13). Death was unrelated to the aortic lesion and occurred from cerebral injury 20 h after the accident. Another case showed three short subclinical tears in the classical site, and death occurred four days after a steering wheel injury from pulmonary thromboembolism.

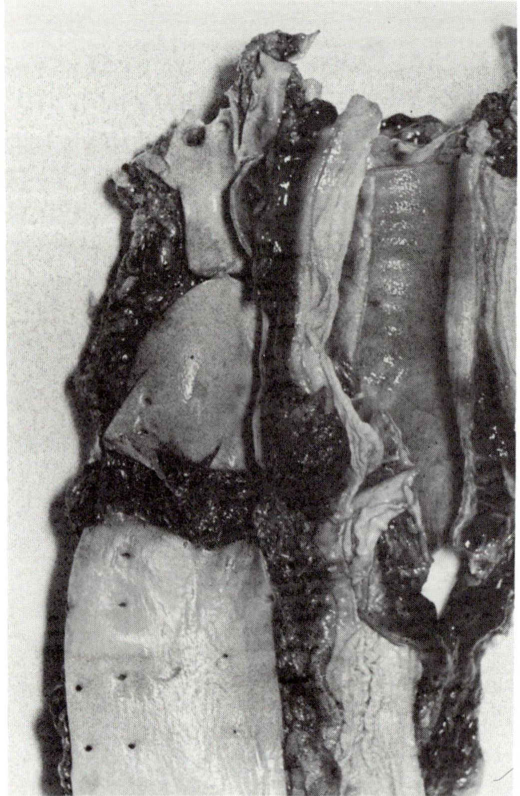

Fig. 10. Circumferential rupture located below the openings of the second aortic intercostal arteries.

Formation of False Aneurysms

Ten of our patients with *non-circumferential* tears had reached hospital alive, three surviving for between 5 and 16 h and four for between 1½ and 7 days after the accident. In six subjects, false saccular aneurysms lined by thrombus had formed at the rupture sites (Figs 7 and 8). Teflon grafting of the aorta was carried out in another subject but death occurred towards the end of surgery. Two of these patients died of causes seemingly unrelated to the rupture, such as Case 3.

Case 3

A 21-year-old motor cyclist admitted with fractures of both thighs and legs, was transfused urgently with blood. The left tibia was surgically plated and the right femur nailed. He failed to recover consciousness after anaesthesia and died in coma from classic fat embolism 3½ days after injury. A gaping aortic rupture with a false aneurysmal sac was found in the proximal descending

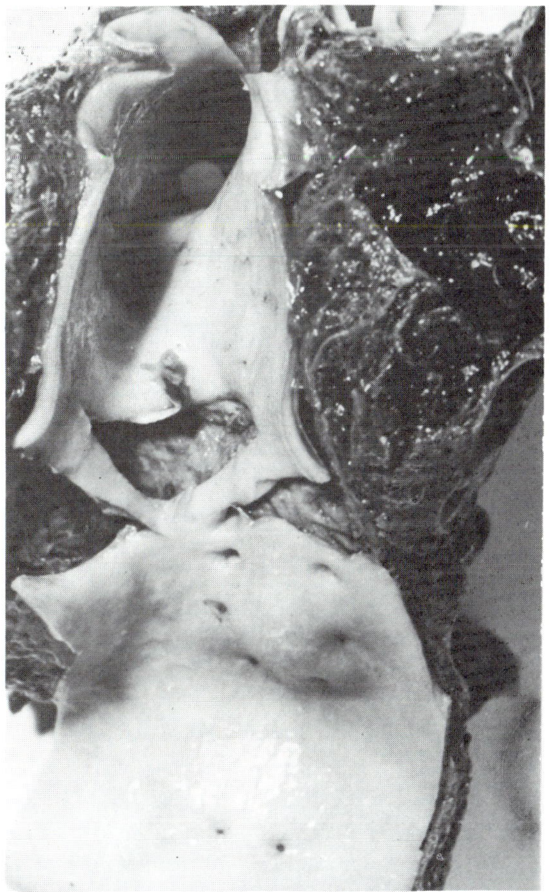

Fig. 11. Two major ruptures of the proximal descending aorta situated anteriorly and posteriorly. Aorta opened from in front in this case. Note gross mediastinal haemorrhage.

aorta (Fig. 8). Though haemorrhage had extended into the mediastinum and 0.5 l of blood was present in the left pleural cavity, his blood volume had been maintained by transfusion. The chest cage was intact.

Most subjects with *circumferential* tears die at the scene of the accident or soon after from massive haemorrhage but one patient survived for 11 days. The edges of the circumferential rupture had separated considerably (Fig. 9) but the adventitia was intact and a large fusiform false aneurysm had formed in the gap. Death occurred from massive haematemesis (Case 4).

Case 4

A 19-year-old motor cyclist collided with a lamp post and sustained a deep wound of the left thigh and groin, rupture of the femoral artery and fractures

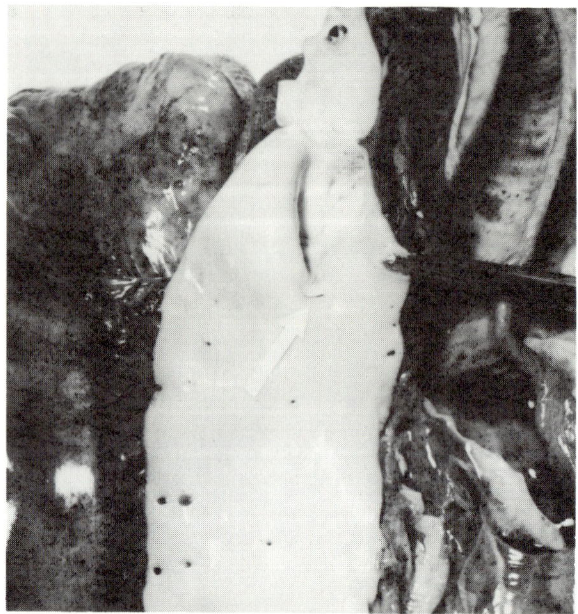

Fig. 12. Short minor rupture (arrow) in the anterior wall of the aortic isthmus above the level of the first aortic intercostal arteries.

of the left upper femur and pubic rami. The ruptured artery was grafted and a colostomy was performed on account of the groin wound. Radiologically the superior mediastinum became broadened for a time and he died from a massive haematemesis on the eleventh day. Necropsy revealed the circumferential false aneurysmal rupture. Extensive downward tracking of adventitial haemorrhage had occurred and had dissected into the wall of the oesophagus and stomach. There were also two minor tears. Haematemesis from traumatic rupture of the aorta must be exceptional.

Occasional cases persist for months or years after the accident without apparent effects or may present as chronic aneurysms without apparent cause. Cases of chronic aortic aneurysm dating back to an injury years previously have been reported (Keen, 1972). Probably the first necropsy description was by Vesalius (1557) of a man who had fallen from a tree two years previously. Probably the first clinical account was by Testa (1823), who described a pulsating thoracic aneurysm eroding a rib, which had followed a fall from a tree. Unsuspected and apparently stable chronic post-traumatic aneurysms have also been detected by routine radiography and successfully excised (Slaney *et al.*, 1966; Keen, 1972). Spontaneous healing of dissecting aneurysms has been described (Shennan, 1932; Sailer, 1942) and might also occur in those of traumatic origin.

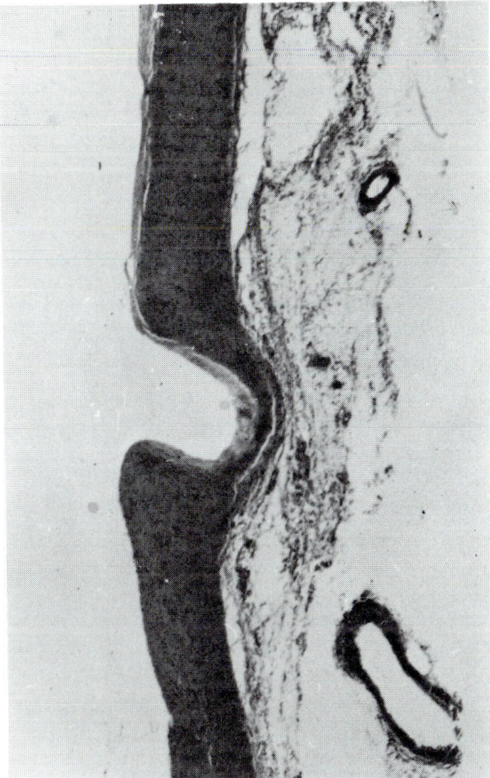

Fig. 13. Histology of the minor rupture shown in Fig. 12. The tear extends to the inner third of the tunica media and is indented by pressure into a micro-aneurysm.

RUPTURES OF THE DISTAL THORACIC AORTA

Anatomically these lesions are also transverse tears of the intima and media centred on the posterior wall of the aorta. They are related directly to dislocations or fracture dislocations of the dorsal spine. Unlike the ruptures in the other main sites, they seem confined to pedestrians hit by cars or motor cyclists involved in collisions. None of our six cases were found in occupants of motor vehicles. Multiple injuries were the rule and the aortic injuries were at least contributory to death in four subjects. The spinal injuries were of the hyperextension kind located between the levels of T5/6 and T12/L1. For example, one motor cyclist survived for 2 h after a head-on collision, and the aorta overlying the fracture dislocation at T10/11 showed a transverse tear 3 cm long on its posterior aspect with wide tracking of ecchymosis. In four subjects one or both pleural cavities contained 2 or 3 l of arterial blood. In one pedestrian, the rupture was minor and unrelated to death.

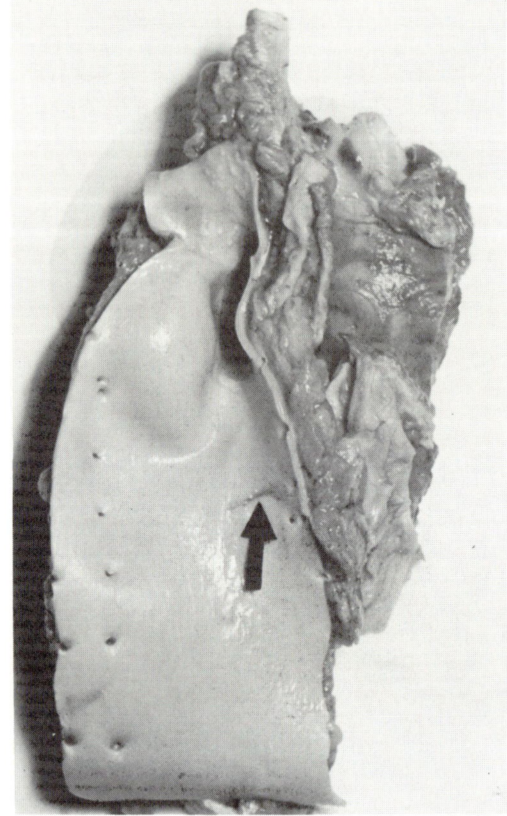

Fig. 14. Minor subclinical tear in the aortic isthmus located at a level between the openings of the second and third aortic intercostal arteries.

EPIDEMIOLOGICAL ASPECTS

In a study of 254 fatal road casualties occurring in the city of Birmingham (Sevitt, 1973), ruptures of the thoracic aorta were found more frequently among vehicle occupants than other road users. This was also the experience of Slätis (1962) and Lundevall (1964), though unlike the cases in Birmingham, they also reported cases among pedal cyclists. In Birmingham the incidence was 21% among 57 vehicle occupants (five out of 29 drivers and seven out of 28 passengers), 16% among 25 motorcyclists and 5.6% among 160 pedestrians killed. The overall frequency of ruptured aortas was 10% among the 254 road users but this was obviously influenced by the proportions of different road users. The difference between vehicle occupants and pedestrians was particularly evident in those who died within 1 h of injury: ruptured aortas were found in 39% of 31 vehicle occupants compared with 14% of 64 pedestrians who died by this time ($P < 0.001$). Rupture of the aorta, therefore, is

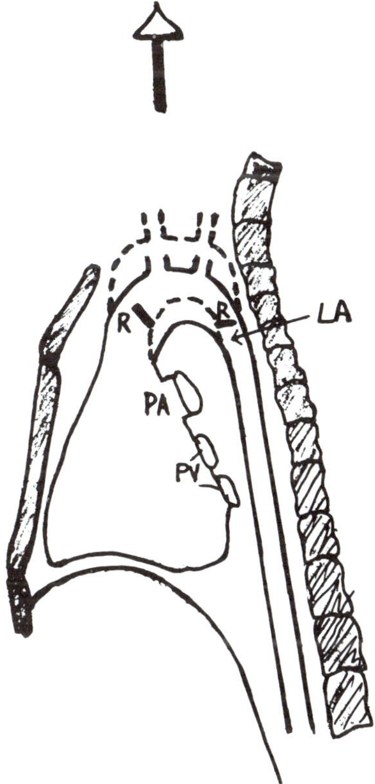

Fig. 15. Heart and aorta from the left with suggested mechanism of aortic rupture (R. R) from rapid deceleration of the body moving in a cranial direction (arrow). The superior aorta is tensed cranially (broken lines, see text). LA, ligamentum arteriosum; PA, pulmonary artery; PV, pulmonary veins.

one of the main causes of early death after accidents in drivers and passengers.

Analysis of the times of accidents showed a clear relationship between aortic rupture in vehicle occupants and accidents at night. Among 42 vehicle occupants (21 drivers, 21 passengers) who died after accidents between 6 p.m. and 6 a.m., 12 (29%) had aortic ruptures (seven were passengers and five were drivers). This compares with no aortic ruptures among 17 occupants (eight drivers) who died after accidents occurring from 6 a.m. to 6 p.m.

The same study revealed that consumption of alcohol by vehicle occupants was related to most aortic ruptures. Analysis of the blood alcohol levels found at post-mortem examination in fatally injured drivers and passengers was related to those with and without ruptures of the aorta. One out of 17 car occupants, dying without evidence of alcohol consumption had a ruptured aorta, whilst four out of seven of those with blood alcohol levels lower than 80 mg 100 ml^{-1} (the legal limit in Britain) and seven out of 18 of those with alcohol levels higher than this had traumatic ruptures of the aorta at necropsy. Alcohol consumption among many drivers probably leads to driving at excessive speed. The findings indicate that ruptured aortas in most vehicle occupants are a product of high-speed collisions at night in which alcohol drinking plays an important part.

PATHOGENESIS OF RUPTURE

Aortic ruptures have sites of predilection and explanations must take these into account. The vulnerability of special sites does not favour *direct* trauma to the aorta as a mechanism except for those in the distal half of the thoracic aorta. Moreover, the deep location of the proximal descending aorta would seem to protect it from rupture by anterior blows on the thorax. Furthermore, chest trauma is absent in some cases. Anatomical fixed points are relevant. Most ruptures affect the proximal descending aorta distal to the opening of the left subclavian artery. These tears are in the vicinity of the ligamentum arteriosum which fixes part of the aorta to the left pulmonary artery. Similarly, ruptures of the ascending aorta are located just above the semilunar valves, that is just distal to the ring-like attachment of the aorta to the heart.

Ruptures in the distal thoracic aorta or the abdominal aorta need not concern us further since they are directly related to a spinal dislocation directly behind them.

Ruptures primarily affect the intima and media. This means internal tearing. They are nearly all transverse, where points to longitundinal tension on the aortic tube. The aorta is a distensible stretchable tube and like a rubber tube when overstretched it has the potential of transverse tearing when sufficient longitudinal tension is applied. This is likely to be the final mode of rupture, possibly the common final pathway to tearing, whatever the precipitating means. This is also how many ruptures of other arteries, those referred to as "traction" injuries, occur. These are also transverse and internal, affecting the intima and media. The tunica adventitia often remains intact as in most aortic tears because the main strength of arteries resides in its strong collagenous nature.

Explanations of rupture must also take into account associated injuries to the victim or their absence, and the kinds of accidents with which they are associated. The accidents that cause most aortic ruptures fall into three main groups: those producing direct impact on the stationary chest, those producing rapid deceleration of the moving body without impact on the chest and those in which chest blows and deceleration are combined. The combination of blows on the chest and deceleration is the largest group and includes most subjects injured in traffic accidents.

Ruptures following jumping from a height, rapid fall of lifts to the ground or air crashes are often referred to as "deceleration" injuries. This may be so, but many of the victims have thoracic injury indicative of impact. On the other hand ruptures associated with impact on the chest while the body is stationary would seem to eliminate deceleration as a cause. This might not be so if the victim were thrown to the ground after the blow.

RUPTURES OF THE ASCENDING AND PROXIMAL DESCENDING AORTA

The main explanations of rupture put forward are as follows.

(1) Displacement of the heart downwards and to the left following impact on the sternum (ruptures ascending aorta).
(2) Upward displacement of the heart and mediastinum from a cranially directed impact on the lower chest (Voigt's "shovelling" mechanism) (ruptures proximal descending aorta).
(3) Acute deceleration of the moving body producing tension–stress on the wall of the aorta. The deceleration can be directed cranially or caudally or possibly horizontally (ruptures proximal descending aorta, and possibly ascending part).
(4) A combination of direct trauma to the thorax plus effects of deceleration, as in many drivers and front-seat passengers after frontal collisions of their vehicles (either rupture).
(5) An acute rise of intra-aortic pressure following a blow on the chest or deceleration (doubtful significance).

Blows on the Sternum and Displacement of the Heart

Ruptures have been found in stationary subjects struck violently on the chest by a heavy object as in the case reported by Kemp (1923) and some of those detailed by Strassman (1947). Deceleration cannot be invoked, unless the victims were thrown violently and received a second impact on the ground or elsewhere.

So far, ruptures of the isthmus have not been produced in experimental animals. On the other hand, blunt blows on the sternum without deceleration of the body can rupture the *ascending* aorta (Moffat *et al.*, 1966; Louhimo, 1967). Louhimo dropped heavy metal tubes from a height on to the sternum of young anaesthetized rabbits lying still on their backs. Midsternal blows regularly produced transverse supravalvular ruptures, and in a few animals also tears at the base of the innominate artery. Angiographic studies indicated that dislocation of the heart caudally and to the left played an important part in producing rupture. The frequency of rupture was not increased when horizontal deceleration of the body and blunt trauma to the thorax were combined, as occurrs during steering wheel impact.

Working with dogs sitting vertically and struck on the midsternum by a heavy steel impacter, Moffat *et al.* (1966) also produced transverse supravalvular tears. Like those produced by Louhimo (1967) and like ruptures in man, they were internal and posteriorly located in the aortic tube. In some animals the arch or the roots of its great vessels were torn. The animals were stationary when struck so body deceleration was absent. These workers also concluded that the heart was displaced downwards and into the left side of the chest by the impact, setting up tensile stresses in the aorta near to its origin which led to rupture.

A similar explanation is offered by Voigt and Wilfert (1969) for ruptures of the first part of the aorta in drivers following horizontally directed steering wheel impact on the chest, and heart and aorta displacement were demonstrated angiographically in compression tests on cadavers. However, drivers also suffer violent deceleration. Nevertheless this lesion was produced in a stationary cadaver subjected to a severe blow against the chest without deceleration (Coermann *et al.*, 1972).

It is reasonable to conclude that many ruptures of the ascending aorta associated with severe blows on the chest are produced by stretching tension following displacement of the heart downward and to the left. Should the aorta become transiently fixed by compression between the inwardly displacing sternum and the spine, the tension produced would be exaggerated. In short, the ascending aorta ruptures as the heart is pushed away from its aortic attachment.

However mechanisms not involving heart displacement must also be possible such as in the subject without evidence of injury to the chest or abdomen.

Voigt's "Shovelling" Mechanism

This phenomenon was described by Voigt as causing rupture of the proximal descending aorta in certain unrestrained front-seat occupants of cars involved in frontal collisions and struck heavily on the chest (Voigt, 1968; Voigt and Wilfert, 1969; Wilfert and Voigt, 1971). The impact however must be on the *lower* chest and directed in a *cranial* as well as a posterior direction. They are possible only in vehicles where the instrument panel is placed sufficiently high from the floor and there is a deep recess below it. With forward movement after a head-on collision, the knees of the front-seat occupant are able to pass below the instrument panel to strike the firewall. At the same time the pelvis moves forwards and downwards off the seat and the torso rotates backwards. The front of the body now faces upwards as well as forwards so that the blow against the steering wheel in the case of the driver, or against the instrument panel in the case of the passenger, comes to be directed cranially as well as backwards. The lower sternum is usually fractured and the lower ribs suffer bilateral anterolateral fractures. The sternal fracture buckles *outwards* as its lower fragment is displaced upwards and backwards. Cranial direction of impact is crucial because only then can the heart and mediastinum be displaced (shovelled) towards the head by the lower sternum. Cranial displacement puts a tensile stretch on the proximal descending aorta, which then ruptures near its fixed point to the ligamentum arteriosum.

The shovelling postulate was tested in cadavers by a pendulum struck in a cranioposterior direction against the lower chest wall. This produced ruptures at the classic site. Subsequent experiments on cadavers simulated drivers struck on the chest showed that the ruptures could be prevented (and other injuries reduced) by improving the design of the steering assembly and by lowering the instrument panel (Coermann *et al.*, 1972).

Role of the Body Deceleration

After sudden stopping of the body from rapid motion, internal organs and tissues continue moving for a fraction of a second and this can produce lesions. It is otherwise difficult to explain aortic ruptures in subjects with little or no evidence of injury to the chest (or abdomen) without involving indirect effects like those which can follow deceleration of the moving body. This is particularly relevant to ruptures of the proximal descending aorta but, as we have found, there are also occasional examples of rupture of the ascending aorta without evidence of injury to the thorax or abdomen (Case 3).

A postulated mechanism is illustrated in Fig. 15, viewing the aorta from the left (Sevitt, 1968). Deceleration in the cranial direction invokes sudden stretching tension of the superior aorta. Tears by this mechanism are most common just *proximal* to the attachment of the ligamentum arteriosum. Ruptures of the ascending aorta are less frequent, possibly because simultaneous movement of the heart in a cranial direction reduces the stress on the aortic ring. Simultaneous chest compression could enhance the danger of rupture by preventing heart displacement, thereby increasing tension on the superior aorta. Drivers and passengers become eligible when, after a head-on collision of their vehicle, they are thrown violently upwards as well as forwards, their heads striking the windscreen or its surround and evidence of this was found in a number of subjects in our series (Sevitt, 1977b). Pedestrians and motor cyclists become eligible when, after impact, they are thrown violently in a cranial direction. Body movement in drivers and passengers is suddenly decelerated by the impact on the head or chest or both within the vehicle, and in pedestrians and motor cyclists by hitting the ground or other hard objects. The arch of the aorta tends to displace towards the head, and the proximal aorta is placed under tension and may rupture (Fig. 15). Ruptures occur proximal to the attachment of the ligamentum arteriosum or, less likely, just distal to the heart. In our experience, the dominance of ruptures proximal to Botallo's ligament is consistent with the concept of cranially directed deceleration. This location does not favour horizontal deceleration as a mechanism. Furthermore, most ruptures are located on the anterior aspect of the proximal descending aorta and on the posterior aspect of the ascending aorta. These are continuations of the inner curvature of the arch, which is the shortest curvature, and, therefore, the most vulnerable to cranially directed stretching tension.

Deceleration from motion in a caudal direction would explain rupture of the proximal descending aorta found in cases of suicide and subjects jumping or falling from a height or in some persons thrown from a moving vehicle. This mechanism is also likely after a sudden fall of lifts to the ground and similar accidents. Fidler (1949) observed that the ruptures were situated a little distal to the aortic attachment of the ligamentum arteriosum. He concluded that they were caused by caudal movement of the abdominal and thoracic viscera after impact on the caudal end of the body, the force being transmitted to the aorta through arterial attachments. By this means the aorta is tensed caudally and is torn below Botallo's ligament and on its inner wall.

Some workers favour the notion of horizontal deceleration of the body after impact on the chest as the mechanism of rupture (Keen, 1972 and others) and envisaged forward displacement of the descending aorta below the ligamentum arteriosum as the underlying operative factor. However, intercostal bruising and tearing of intercostal arteries might then be expected but are not found at necropsy. Other workers envisage forward bending of the aortic arch as the mechanism after speed accidents with chest impact (Zehnder, 1956), and more complex mechanisms such as a torsion force tangential to the surface and a shearing force operative at the isthmus (Cammack *et al.*, 1959) or a combination of forces acting on fixed points including deceleration in a torsional plane on the aorta with a shearing force at the site of rupture (Murdock, 1957) have also been postulated.

CONCLUSIONS

The internal and transverse nature of all traumatic ruptures of the aorta indicates a stretching mechanism, and anatomical points of fixation largely determine location. The aortic attachment to the heart decides the supra-valvular site of rupture in the ascending aorta, and the attachment of the ligamentum arteriosum plays a vital part in locating ruptures in the proximal descending aorta, the isthmus.

Most ruptures are in the isthmus and they can be caused in several ways.

(1) By cranially directed deceleration after impact, producing transient stretching of the superior aorta.

(2) Through caudally directed deceleration after impact, as in those jumping from a height, producing caudal displacement of thoraco-abdominal viscera.

(3) By cranially directed displacement of the mediastinum following a cranially directed blow to the lower thorax (shovelling mechanism).

(4) Possibly by lateral displacement of the upper thorax after an appropriate blow.

(5) Possibly by horizontally directed deceleration.

More than one mechanism may be operative in individual cases, especially in victims of road accidents.

Most ruptures of the ascending aorta are caused by severe blows on the front of the chest whereby the heart is displaced downwards and to the left. Other mechanisms such as cranially directed deceleration must also operate, especially in subjects without chest injury.

Acute rises of aortic pressure induced by chest blows or deceleration are unlikely to be important for rupture but are still *sub judice*.

Ruptures of the distal descending aorta are associated with hyperextension injuries of the spine whereby the aorta is locally angulated forwards and tensed.

REFERENCES

Cammack, K., Rapport, R. L., Paul, J. and Baird, W. C. (1959). *Archives of Surgery (Chicago)* **79**, 244.
Coermann, R., Dotzauer, G., Lange, W. and Voigt, G. E. (1972). *Journal of Trauma* **12**, 715.

Fidler, K. (1949). *Canadian Medical Association Journal* **60**, 590.
Forbes, G. (1944). *British Medical Journal* **2**, 400.
Griffiths, S. J. M. (1931). *British Journal of Surgery* **18**, 664.
Haas, G. H. (1944). *Journal of Aviation and Medicine* **15**, 77.
Keen, G. (1972). *Annals of the Royal College of Surgeons of England* **51**, 137.
Kemp, P. R. (1923). *Lancet* **1**, 953.
Louhimo, I. (1967). *Acta Chirurgica Scandinavica* Suppl. 380.
Lundevall, J. (1964). *Acta Pathologica et Microbiologica Scandinavica* **62**, 34.
Marshall, T. K. (1958). *Journal of Clinical Pathology* **11**, 36.
Moffat, R. C., Roberts, V. L. and Berkas E. M. (1966). *Journal of Trauma* **6**, 666.
Murdock, C. E. (1957). *Archives of Surgery (Chicago)* **74**, 589.
Parmley, L. F., Mattingley, T. W., Manion, W. C. and Jahnke, E. J. (1958). *Circulation* **17**, 1086.
Sailer, S. (1942). *Archives of Pathology* **33**, 704.
Sevitt, S. (1968). *British Journal of Surgery* **55**, 481.
Sevitt, S. (1973). *Injury* **4**, 281.
Sevitt, S. (1977). *British Journal of Surgery* **64**, 166.
Sevitt, S. (1977). *Injury* **8**, 159.
Shennan, T. (1929). *Journal of Pathology and Bacteriology* **32**, 795.
Shennan, T. (1932). *Journal of Pathology and Bacteriology* **35**, 161.
Slaney, G., Ashton, F. and Abrams, L. D. (1966). *British Journal of Surgery* **53**, 361.
Slätis, P. (1962). *Acta Chirurgica Scandinavica* Suppl. 297.
Strassman, G. (1947). *American Heart Journal* **33**, 508.
Teare, D. (1951). *British Medical Journal* **2**, 707.
Testa, A. (1823). "Delle malattie del cuore, loro cagioni, specie, segni e cura" Patti Ed, Firenze.
Vesalius, A. Quoted by Sailer, S. (1942).
Voigt, G. E. (1968). *Hefte für Unfallheilkunde* **96**, 1.
Voigt, G. E. and Wilfert, K. (1969). "Mechanisms of injuries to unrestrained drivers in head-on collisions". *In* "Proceedings of the Thirteenth Stapp Car Crash Conference, New York." Society of Automotive Engineers, p. 295.
Wilfert, K. and Voigt, G. (1971). Mechanisms of injuries to unrestrained front seat passengers and their prevention by progressive instrument panel design". *In* "Proceedings of the Fifteenth Stapp Car Crash Conference, Coronada, California." Society of Automotive Engineers.
Wilson, J.V. (1946). "Pathology of traumatic injury", p. 111. Livingstone, Edinburgh.
Wilson, J. V. and Tunbridge, R. E. (1943). *Lancet* **1**, 257.
Zehnder, M. A. (1956). *Angiology* **7**, 252.

RUPTURED AORTA: CLINICAL EXPERIENCE

L. D. Abrams

Queen Elizabeth Hospital, Birmingham, UK

Aortic rupture is not as common in England as in the United States. My American colleagues say that this is because their cars are bigger and less controllable than those that we drive in Europe, where Italian influence has done so much to produce highly controllable cars.

Our series comprises 19 cases, 17 of which were operated on whilst in hospital for their initial injury and two presented some years later.

These two cases present the most important lessons to be learnt about the clinical features of aortic rupture. The first presented to me after routine chest X-ray had shown an aneurysm of the junction of the arch and descending aorta three years after a road traffic accident in which he had suffered a ruptured spleen and injury of the chest causing a large haemothorax. The spleen had been removed and his haemothorax drained. He had been very ill and the fact that he had a widened mediastinum on his original pictures had been overlooked. It was thought that fractured ribs were the source of intrapleural bleeding. At operation for his aneurysm it was apparent that he had suffered a partial rupture of the aorta. A short segment of aorta was resected and replaced with Dacron graft. The other patient was a pilot who during the last war was practising landing a light aircraft on a short runway fitted with arrester wires like an aircraft carrier. His plane was satisfactorily arrested and he came to a rather sudden stop and struck his face on the instrument panel. He suffered a slight nose bleed and went into the bar to have a drink to aid recovery. He did not seek medical attention. Seventeen years later he developed some slight discomfort in the chest and had his chest

Serono Symposium No. 44, "Peripheral Arterial Diseases: Medical and Surgical Problems", edited by S. Stipa and A. Cavallaro, 1982. Academic Press, London and New York.

X-rayed. This showed a large aneurysm in the classical situation so he was investigated by aortography on a Friday afternoon. His operation was scheduled for 9.00 a.m. on the following Tuesday morning but at 8.30 a.m. on that day his aneurysm ruptured. He was immediately transfused and taken to the operating theatre where it was found that his aneurysm arose from a complete transection of the aorta; the ends being separated by several centimetres in the aneurysmal sac. The aneurysm was resected and replaced. Although he had a satisfactory cardiovascular resuscitation his extreme hypotension had caused fatal cerebral injury.

These two cases present the essential lessons to be borne in mind if a diagnosis of aortic rupture is to be made. The first is that any patient who receives an injury either serious or trivial who has been stopped suddenly should have his chest X-rayed. That X-ray should be examined for evidence of widening of the superior mediastinum, especially on the left side. The sign most carefully looked for is that of pressure on the trachea causing a left-sided concavity. It is an exaggeration of the normal aortic arch impression. Unfortunately, this is not always present and I have had reported to me by a colleague a case of a man who had very slight mediastinal widening with a perfectly straight trachea who was thought not to have ruptured his aortic arch but in fact died a few days later from this condition.

Mediastinal widening can be caused by bleeding from other sources, such as fractures of the upper thoracic vertebrae, the back ends of the upper ribs and also by fracture of the sternum which may be extremely difficult to diagnose clinically.

The chest X-ray of a 69-year-old woman who was driving a car involved in a head-on collision wearing a safety belt, who was concussed and also suffered fractured clavicle ribs and lung contusion, showed widening of the mediastinum with a straight trachea. She had considerable breathing difficulties and although I thought she probably had not ruptured her aorta, I considered it essential that she should have an aortogram, which, fortunately, proved normal. She had slight tenderness over the upper part of the sternum but it was not until a week had elapsed that palpation of the sternum elicited slight crepitus, thus revealing her fracture and the cause of the mediastinal widening.

There are of course, clinical features directly attributable to the aortic lesions. The most notable of these is a "coarctation syndrome" in which the femoral pulses are weakened and the blood pressure in the arms raised. This occurred in two of the 17 cases in this series and it is important to remember that the lower half hypotension may cause interference with spinal cord function producing paresthesiae and weakness in the lower part of the body. Local haematoma may also interfere with the circulation in the left subclavian artery causing the pressure in the left arm to be significantly lower than that in the right.

The expanding haematoma may compress the oesophagus causing difficulty in swallowing, which in one of our cases was progressive. However, the great majority of our cases had no clinical findings directly attributable to the aortic rupture itself.

It is, therefore, of the utmost importance to remember that any patient who has been stopped suddenly may have suffered aortic rupture and that this should be suspected and sought after despite the severity of the patients' other injuries.

A young man who was riding a light motor bike came into collision with a car and suffered concussion, lacerations of his face, double fractures of both femorae, fractures of the tibia and fibular of one leg and fractures of the radius and ulnar of one arm. He was taken into hospital rather more than 50 miles from Birmingham where the surgical registrar did know that patients who stop suddenly should have their chests X-rayed. When he saw the X-ray with a wide mediastinum and concave tracheal shadow he arranged an aortogram and having seen the rupture, sent the patient to our care. He was, of course, appropriately transfused and arrived in good physical condition so his aortic rupture was sewn up and the succeeding 9 h was spent by one of our orthopaedic surgeons, carrying out internal fixation of his fractures. He was quite well at the end of his 11½-h anaesthetic but it was thought advisable to ventilate him overnight, so he was not extubated until the following morning after which he made an uninterrupted recovery.

His lesion was quite obvious on aortography and it should be noted that difficulty was experienced in passing the aortic catheter above the site of rupture although the tear was incomplete. Sometimes, the leak from the aorta is difficult to see despite excellent contrast in the aorta.

The operation itself is carried out through a long postero-lateral thoracotomy stripping the upper border of the fifth rib. My personal preference is to use a shunt from the heart to the lower half of the body, either through a cannula directed upwards in the left common femoral artery or placed pointing downwards in the lower part of the descending aorta. I think that it is important to pass the upper end of the shunt through the apex of the left ventricle into the ascending aorta. It is quite easy to feel the catheter in the ascending aorta and it does not interfere with the function of the aortic valve at all. It has the great advantage that perfusion of the lower half of the body continues throughout the cardiac cycle. A cannula placed in the left ventricular cavity only produces perfusion during systole and blood may even flow back from the lower half of the body into the ventricle during diastole which is, of course, by far the longest part of the cardiac cycle. I do not depend on a purse string in the apex of the left ventricle to hold the catheter in place but pass a narrow tape through the transverse sinus, bring it back down each side of the heart and tie it behind the collar on the cannula by the tip of the left ventricle. This holds the cannula in place securely without any risk of the purse strings tearing out. It is well known that success can be achieved in this operation without any bypass between the upper and lower halves of the body but it seems to me that this must increase the risk of spinal cord damage during the period of aortic cross clamping and in some patients this supply may be jeopardized before the operation begins.

Once the mediastinal pleura over the rupture is opened bleeding may start again so control of the aorta is essential. It is easiest to expose the descending aorta low in the chest first and then to start the incision in the mediastinal pleura as high as possible so that the left sub-clavician artery can be identified and followed down towards the aortic arch. The forefinger can then be run down the front of the subclavian artery and round behind the aortic arch, which is grasped between finger and thumb. The size of the haematoma in the mediastinum gives little indication of the extent of the rupture and when this is complete the aortic arch may be found to have retracted a considerable distance into the mediastinum. Bleeding from the lower end can be controlled by compressing the aorta against the spine. A majority of the cases in this series suffered incomplete rupture and the aorta was repaired by direct suture but in those cases in which the aorta was completely transected it was found so difficult to bring the ends close together that a 2-cm length of Dacron graft was used in order to make the operations simpler. It should be realized that the ends of the ruptured aorta are not absolutely clean cut by the injury and indeed the aorta may be split longitudinally as well as transversely.

Of the 17 cases operated on acutely, there have been three deaths. One of these was due to technical failure during the operation in that we never succeeded in gaining control of the aorta. There was practically no free blood in the pleural cavity and the haematoma was not very large but the ends of the aorta were 3 or 4 cm apart. The patient bled to death.

The second death was in a young man who also had a complete transection A graft was placed successfully in his aorta and he was little disturbed by the operation. Unfortunately, he had suffered severe deceleration injury of his lungs and in the course of 36 h both lungs became completely radio-opaque and he died within 48 h of injury because oxygenation was impossible.

The third death occurred some two weeks after the repair of an aortic rupture with a Dacron graft. This patient was known to have a widened mediastinum and also suffered from dysphagia. She was referred from another hospital ten days after her original injury and at operation it was found that the haematoma had caused considerable disruption of the wall of the oesophagus although it was thought that the mucosa was intact. However, this was probably not the case because she developed severe infection in the mediastinum and died from secondary haemorrhage due to infection of the aortic suture line.

Traumatic rupture of the aorta is a treacherous condition. If the patient survives the initial injury fatal bleeding may occur at any time afterwards. In a great majority of cases the diagnosis will not be obvious and must be carefully sought after.

Any patient who reports an injury of any sort and who has been stopped suddenly should have a chest X-ray which must be very carefully examined for signs of mediastinal widening. Whether there is no evidence at all of chest injury or in the presence of multiple injuries involving the chest and other parts of the body, if aortic rupture is suspected, aortography should be performed and the aorta repaired as soon as possible if the rupture is found. Our series shows that this can be undertaken with a very reasonable prospect of success.

RECONSTRUCTIVE SURGERY OF THE ARTERIES OF THE LOWER LIMBS BY MEANS OF THE BYPASS TECHNIQUE: PRESENT STATUS AND FUTURE DEVELOPMENTS

P. Fiorani, F. Speziale, M. Taurino, S. Bondanini and V. Faraglia

Cattedra di Chirurgia Vascolare dell'Università di Roma, Rome, Italy

The remarkable development of vascular surgery in the last 25 years was mainly due to the utilization of alloplastic prostheses, which significantly changed the prognosis of many arterial diseases, particularly those concerning the aorta and its branches, yielding increasingly favourable results. Clearly, the extensive use of vascular grafts has also resulted in some secondary complications, which, however, do not counterbalance the benefits arising from such a technique. Nevertheless, a careful prevention and a timely treatment is required.

Furthermore the operative mortality of aorto-iliac revascularization with the bypass technique has remarkably decreased in the last few years. Whilst in the early 1960s a mortality rate of 7.5% was apparent, now a 0.9% figure has been achieved, which corresponds with that indicated by the world-wide literature.

However, there still exist some problems in the implementation of revascularization interventions in the aorto-iliac-femoral area with synthetic prostheses, namely late complications such as the graft thrombosis, the prosthesis infection and the aortic anastomosis disease. As a matter of fact one of less unfrequent complications is the thrombosis, which seldom results in important problems, as it is possible to treat it with further applications.

The thrombosis is due, apart from technical imperfections, which on the

Serono Symposium No. 44, "Peripheral Arterial Diseases: Medical and Surgical Problems", edited by S. Stipa and A. Cavallaro, 1982. Academic Press, London and New York.

other hand are always possible, to the distal evolution of the atherosclerotic disease, with reduction of the "outflow", which in turn causes a slackening of blood flow in distal vessels and graft thrombosis.

Undoubtedly, the most dangerous complications are those caused by infections especially in the groin area, and by the aortic anasthomosis disease, which can either arise primitively or due to propagation of infection from other septic areas.

In our experience, an infective complications rate of 2.6% was observed, taking into account both the immediate and the late cases. This rate agrees with those recorded by foreign authors, who reported an infection rate ranging between 1% and 6% (Goldstone and Moore, 1974; Willwerth and Waldhausen, 1974; Lieckweg and Grenfield, 1977). However, these values may further decrease taking more adequate prophylaxis measures and a different approach to the problem.

Two different anathomo-clinical situations appear to be more frequently present during infections beyond those already well known. One of these is represented by a statistically significant increase of groin infections in patients who were submitted to early re-operations for several reasons.

In our experience (Pistolese *et al.*, 1981), based upon the observation of 400 consecutive revascularization of the aorto-iliac area, an infection rate of 8.6% was observed in reintervented patients, against the 1.2% figure appropriate to non-reintervented patients. The reintervention seems therefore to favour infections due to the increased possibility of cutaneous contamination, trauma of tissues and presence of haematoma (Jamieson *et al.*, 1975; Hammarsten and Holm, 1977). In practice, there are many cases when such an occurrence can be foreseen, especially when the "run-off" is not well settled, because in this case the operation may require several reinterventions to be successful.

Another well known situation is the high incidence of groin infection in patients submitted to aorto-femoral bypass graft in the presence of distal trophic lesions. In our experience, based upon 400 consecutive aorto-femoral revascularizations, five patients, over those 76 (6.5%) who had distal trophic lesions, developed infection; furthermore only four patients, over the remaining 324 (1.2%) developed infection.

The groin infection is a high local risk situation due to the possible diffusion of the infection along the graft and the consequent secondary affection of the aortic anasthomosis, which is well known to be the most dramatic situation that can be expected (Fiorani and Spagnoli, 1981). In situations with high local risk of infection, it has been an established practice for several years to perform an extra-anatomical bypass in provisional or permanent fashion.

This procedure has proven to be satisfactory not only because of the low mortality (about 1.6% in our experience) but also as far as patency is concerned (more of 55% being this figure recorded over 55 patients checked with an average follow-up period of 30 months, ranging from five months to nine years) (Pistolese *et al.*, 1981).

As far as the late aortic anastomosis disease without previous groin infection is concerned, in our experience a 0.6% figure was recorded over all possible aortic operations (emergency and elective abdominal aortic aneurysms, aorto-iliac revascularization, renal and visceral revascularization) and a 0.4% was recorded in aorto-femoral bypass (Fiorani *et al.*, 1980).

It is reasoned that in most circumstances an aortic false aneurysm, which eventually develops infection, may derive from a primitive aortic wall rupture with aneurismatic dilatation limited within the part of aorta close to the anastomosis, due to evolution of the atherosclerotic disease or following an exceedingly extended aortic TEA or dysplastic lesions (Fiorani *et al.*, 1980). Such a situation causes a dehiscence of the suture line, with consequent perianastomotic haematoma, which may develop as an infected false aneurysm, which in turn may generate complications such as rupture in the retroperitoneum or in the duodenum. Taking into account this possible evolution, this can clearly be avoided at the first operation by performing anastomosis on an atherosclerotic lesions indemn aorta section, possibly making an end-to-end anastomosis on indemn tissue.

However, a periodic and systematic check of the aorto-prosthetic area may be easily and reliably done by means of non-invasive measurements, such as echography and CAT. Whenever the presence of an aortic anastomosis disease may be suspected, the requirement for an angiography arises. Another method for improving the results of the bypass operations, is that of determining the anatomical situation of the femoral bifurcation, in order to eventually improve the "outflow" by means of an endarterectomy. A large consensus of opinions has not been reached on this subject as it is really artificious, beyond being difficult, to attribute to a single element the responsibility of an improved result without duly taking into account the presence of other factors in patients affected by occlusive arterial diseases of the lower limbs.

On this subject, 40 of 45 patients, reintervented because of a late graft thrombosis, were not submitted, at their first operation, to an endarterectomy of femoral bifurcation. It should be noted that in some cases the first operation had been performed by another surgical team (Pistolese *et al.*, 1981). These results should be interpreted taking into account the limitation of the originally available data; however, a recommendation for an extended use of the TEA procedure is evident.

Following the protracted experience of the bypass technique in the aorto-iliac area, the surgical indications for this operation have not been significantly modified, even though there has been a demand increase for the surgical treatment of second-stage arterial disease with respect to that relevant to the third and fourth stages. All this, despite the heavy mortality decrease, the prophylaxis of major complications and the improvement of the "run-off". This situation mainly derives from the fact that many factors which influence the late results are still not too clear. This suggests cautiousness when operating on young patients, who, on the other hand, need the help of a vascular surgeon more and more frequently.

In our experience, based upon the observation of 181 patients suffering from similar arterial lesions and risk factors, the patency rate of the bypass grafts, in a follow-up period ranging from six months to three years, shows a variation from the 62% of successful cases appropriate to patients younger than 40 years to the 76% appropriate to older people.

A method that has been used to try and explain this discrepancy is the observation of the anatomical lesions at the femoral bifurcation. According to our data, presently under processing, two are the main lesions which may be observed at the femoral bifurcation, for instance:

(1) The typical fibroatheromasic plaque, yellowish, rich of foam cells, with cholesterol inclusions. These cells following histoautoradiographic studies with ^{3}H-thymidine showed intense captation, which is an indication of evolutive lesions and represents a more recent lesion (Geer and Haust, 1974; Spagnoli *et al.*, 1980). This lesion can be observed in about 70% of young patients and only 55% of the older patients.

(2) The fibrotic lesion, whitish, which represents the more developed stage of stabilization of atherosclerotic lesions. This lesion is less frequent in young patients than in older patients.

When the revascularization is performed in a patient who has a fibrotic lesion at the femoral bifurcation, results are significantly better in young patients than in older ones, even though the number of observations made did not allow statistically meaningful values. As a matter of fact, in our series of 19 patients, under 40 years, checked over a follow-up period from six months to three years, in presence of whitish lesion, five successful cases were recorded over five interventions, whilst in presence of yellowish lesions, under the same conditions, there were three unsuccessful cases on a total of 14 operations.

The results obtained on 162 patients over 40 years suggest that, statistically significant data, in patients affected by yellowish lesions at the femoral bifurcation in whom a TEA has not been performed, the failure of the graft was observed in 30% of cases.

It is hoped that these data can be confirmed by further experience, with purpose of pre-operatively identifying the nature of the lesions, and of determining the indications, and possibly the techniques, which allow one to get a more effective result.

REFERENCES

Fiorani, P., Pistolese, G. R. *et al.* (1980a). L'addome acuto vascolare nel paziente con protesi aortica. Atti Società Italiana di Chirurgia, 82° Congresso, p. 573.

Fiorani, P., Pistolese, G. R., Faraglia, V. and Ventura, M. (1980b). Modern trends in surgical treatment of the aorto-iliac occlusive diseases in Italy. *Langenbecks Archiv für Chirurgie* **352**, 81.

Geer, J. C. and Haust, M. D. (1972). Smooth muscle cells in Atherosclerosis Monographs on Atherosclerosis. Karger, Basel.

Goldstone, J. and Moore, W. S. (1974). Infection in vascular prostheses. Clinical manifestations and surgical management. *American Journal of Surgery* **128**, 225.

Hammarsten, J. and Holm, J. (1977). Infections in vascular surgery. *Journal of Cardiovascular Surgery* **18**, 6.

Jamieson, G. G., De Weese, J. A. and Rob, C. G. (1975). Infected arterial grafts. *Annals of Surgery* **181**, 850.

Lieckweg, W. G. and Grenfield, L. J. (1977). Vascular prosthetic infections: collected experiences and results of treatment. *Surgery* **81**, 335.

Pistolese, G. R., Speziale, F., Taurino, M., Zaccaria, A. and Ventura, M. (1981). Considerazioni sulle indicazioni del by-pass axillo-femorale con particolare riferimento alle situazioni di alto rischio locale. *Archivo di Chirurgia Toracica e Cardiovascolare* **3**, 149.

Spagnoli, L., Faraglia, V., Villaschi, F., Taurino, M., Neri, L. and Fiorani, P. (1980). Autoradiographic studies on human occlusive arterial disease. XII World Congr. Angiology, Athens 7–12 Sept.

Willwerth, B. M. and Waldhausen, J. A. (1974). Infection of arterial prostheses. *Surgery Gynecology and Obstetrics* **139**, 446.

INTRA-OPERATIVE CHANGES IN VEINS USED FOR ARTERIAL REPLACEMENT WITH SPECIAL REFERENCE TO ENDOTHELIAL INJURIES AND THEIR REPAIR

R. Gottlob

Abteilung f. Experiment. Chirurgie, I. Chirurg. Univ. Klinik, Vienna, Austria

INTRODUCTION

After Kunlin did pioneering work on bypassing obstructed arteries by autogenous veins, this procedure became world-wide routine. Until now venous bypass procedures are regarded as the optimal way of replacing thrombosed arteries. Early patency rates are satisfactory, provided the inflow and outflow are sufficient and technical errors are avoided. Our investigations were stimulated by surgeons who claimed that they observed too many failures in extremities where the inflow or the outflow of the graft were sufficient. It was suggested that these failures might be due to endothelial changes in the grafts.

MATERIAL AND METHODS

For our experiments we used human saphenous veins, dissected in order to carry out a bypass procedure. In addition, we used saphenous veins of human cadavers and jugular veins of dogs.

Serono Symposium No. 44, "Peripheral Arterial Diseases: Medical and Surgical Problems", edited by S. Stipa and A. Cavallaro, 1982. Academic Press, London and New York.

Histological Procedures

The endothelial layer of the veins was examined in full thickness "*en face* preparations" after silver-staining and in "Haeutchen preparations".

For full thickness preparations the veins were carefully dissected and opened by thin scissors. Then the veins were pinned on cork plates, the intima layer facing the top. After rinsing with 5% glucose solution the veins were stained with 0.25% silver nitrate solution for 20 s. Then the veins were again rinsed, fixed in 5% formalin and dehydrated in increasing concentrations of ethanol. After clearing in wintergreenoil the veins were mounted between slide and coverglass and examined at 25–100 × magnification. This procedure permits the classification of the endothelial damage by an arbitrary scale from 0 to 8.

0: No damage (Fig. 1a). Only endothelial silver lines are seen, running predominantly in the axis of the vessel.

8: Complete desquamation of endothelia. Only silver lines pertaining to the media of the vessels are stained. They run predominately transversely to the axis of the vessel (Fig. 1b).

4: About 50% of the vessel is covered by endothelia while 50% is denuded (Fig. 1d).

1, 2, 3, 5, 6, 7 are intermediate classifications, 1 indicating minor changes, but not more than 12.5% of the observed area is damaged. 2 indicates that 12.5–25% of the surface is damaged — and so on.

Haeutchen preparations were obtained by soaking the dehydrated vessels as well as the slides — made of methylmethacrylate — in acetone. The vessels were then pressed with the endothelia against the slides in a vice. After drying the media and adventitia were pulled off so that merely an endothelial monolayer remained on the slide. This could be stained by hematoxilin and eosin so that the nuclei were displaced (Fig. 1c).

Dissection of the Veins

Conventional Dissection

In most instances vessels were dissected conventionally by skilled vascular surgeons who were asked to dissect the vessels as carefully as possible.

Endothelium-preserving Technique

Vessels were dissected by an endothelium-preserving technique by the author or by one of his co-workers so that any touching the vessels with forceps or with the hands of the surgeon or with swabs was avoided. These vessels were kept in place by holding sutures only and in case of bleeding the vessels were rinsed with saline containing small amounts of heparin and the fluid was sucked away at a place remote from the vessel. Similar manoeuvres were applied to stitching anastomoses. In all grafting procedures any retraction of the vein with conglutination of the lumina was strictly avoided by keeping the veins under tension by holding stitches which could then be used as the first stitches of the anastomoses.

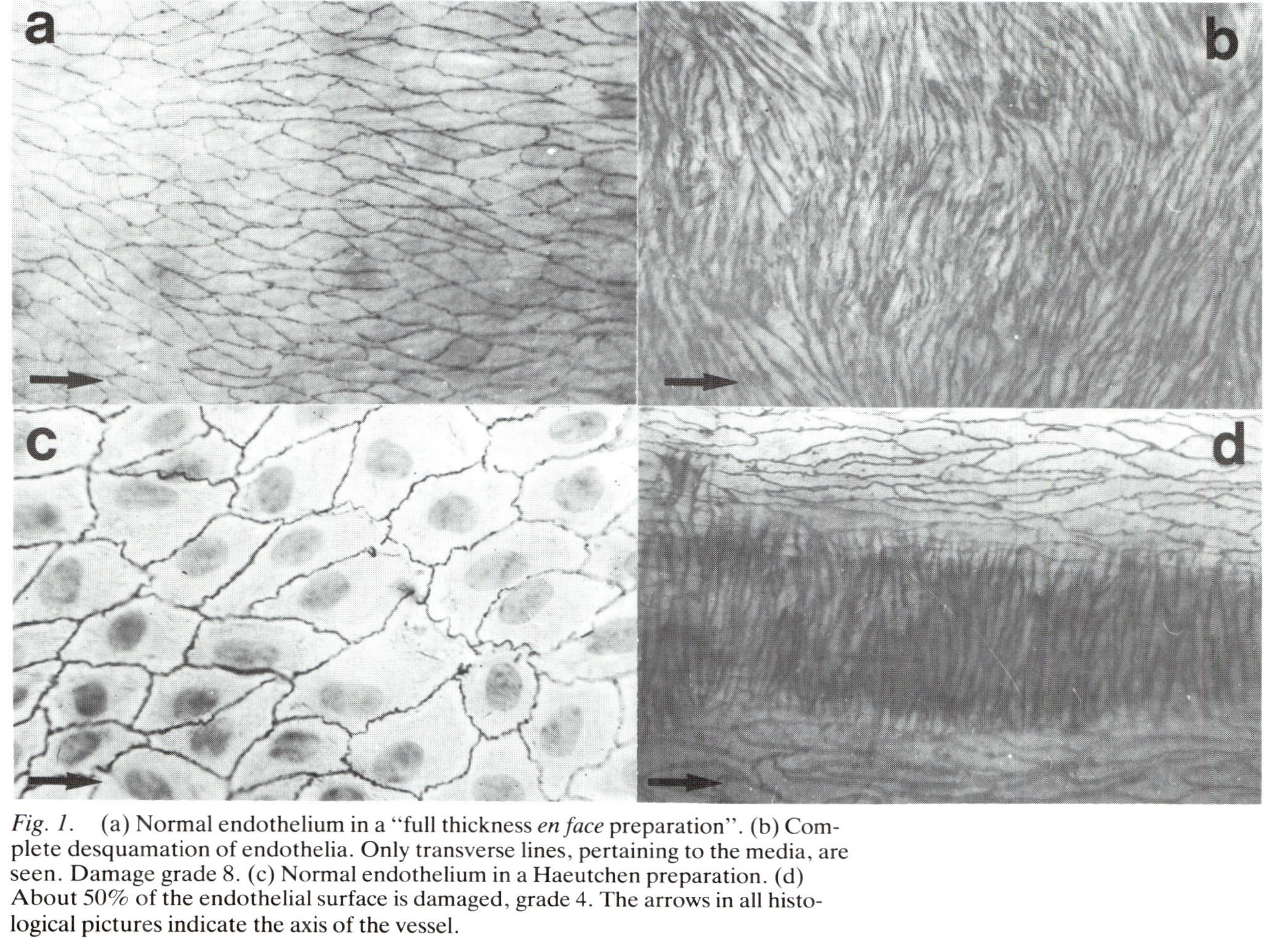

Fig. 1. (a) Normal endothelium in a "full thickness *en face* preparation". (b) Complete desquamation of endothelia. Only transverse lines, pertaining to the media, are seen. Damage grade 8. (c) Normal endothelium in a Haeutchen preparation. (d) About 50% of the endothelial surface is damaged, grade 4. The arrows in all histological pictures indicate the axis of the vessel.

RESULTS

Endothelial Changes Due to Dissection

Human veins, for use in grafting, were dissected, three by a conventional and three by an endothelium-preserving technique. Table I indicates the grade of damage. The figures indicate cross-sections examined. Severe damage was found in conventionally dissected veins, whereas in veins prepared by an endothelium-preserving technique much less damage was seen.

Table I. Human saphenous veins (grade of damage).

Conventional dissection	Endothelium preserving dissection
788888887	1120
67887	11035
215466	3000

Because only very little material was available from veins destined to serve as grafts in patients, in addition some veins of cadavers were dissected. The results are seen in Table II. One may note again the difference in the endothelial pattern and that we eventually learned to dissect cadaver veins without any damage (the last two veins).

Table II. Human cadaver veins (grade of damage)

Conventional dissection	Endothelium preserving dissection
77657	0200000
88878778	0000100
7766888887	22000
44632	11000
237	201000
6487	6432
86486	21220
644687	000000
67654	000000
66407	

Grafted Veins

In 11 dogs segments of the femoral veins, 4 cm in length, were grafted into the carotid arteries of the same animals. In one side a conventionally dissected vein was inserted whereas in the contralateral side a vein dissected by an endothelium-preserving method was grafted. After 1–20 days the animals were sacrificed and the veins were recovered and cut open after careful dissection. Table III represents the area, covered by an endothelium. One may note that in all instances after conventional dissection less endothelium was preserved than when an endothelium-preserving technique was applied. From the ninth day on, however, most parts of the intimal surface of both vessels were completely or subtotally covered by endothelia.

Table III. Arterialization of femoral veins of dogs by autografting (percentage intimal surface covered by endothelium).

Days after operation	Conventional dissection	"No touch—dissection"
1	30	75
2	*[a]	40
2	*[a]	90
3	25	50
4	80	70
6	30	100
8	5	80
9	90	90
12	100	100
14	70	90
20	100	100

[a] * indicates : obliterated.

There were distinct damages seen in vessels even after endothelium-preserving dissection. Our results were improved in a second series, devoted to a study of the rejection in homografts. No parietal thrombi were seen in the grafted veins in autologous control preparations between six and 70 days after the operation.

Anastomoses

When anastomoses were performed, using a careful but conventional technique, about 10 mm on both sides of the suture line were devoid of endothelia (Fig. 2b). When, however, an endothelium-preserving technique was applied the area devoid of endothelia could be reduced to about 1 mm or less (Fig. 2d).

Surgical Clamps

The question, to what extent endothelia are damaged by clamping the vessel, was examined together with Rauhs. We found that all types of metal clamps damage endothelia severely. Also clamps with small teeth cause considerable desquamation of endothelia, especially in areas between the teeth, where the vessel is exposed to frictional forces. Small areas, where the endothelial cells are merely compressed may show some endothelial covering immediately after clamping, however, the question whether these endothelia are viable remains open. Even microclips cause considerable endothelial

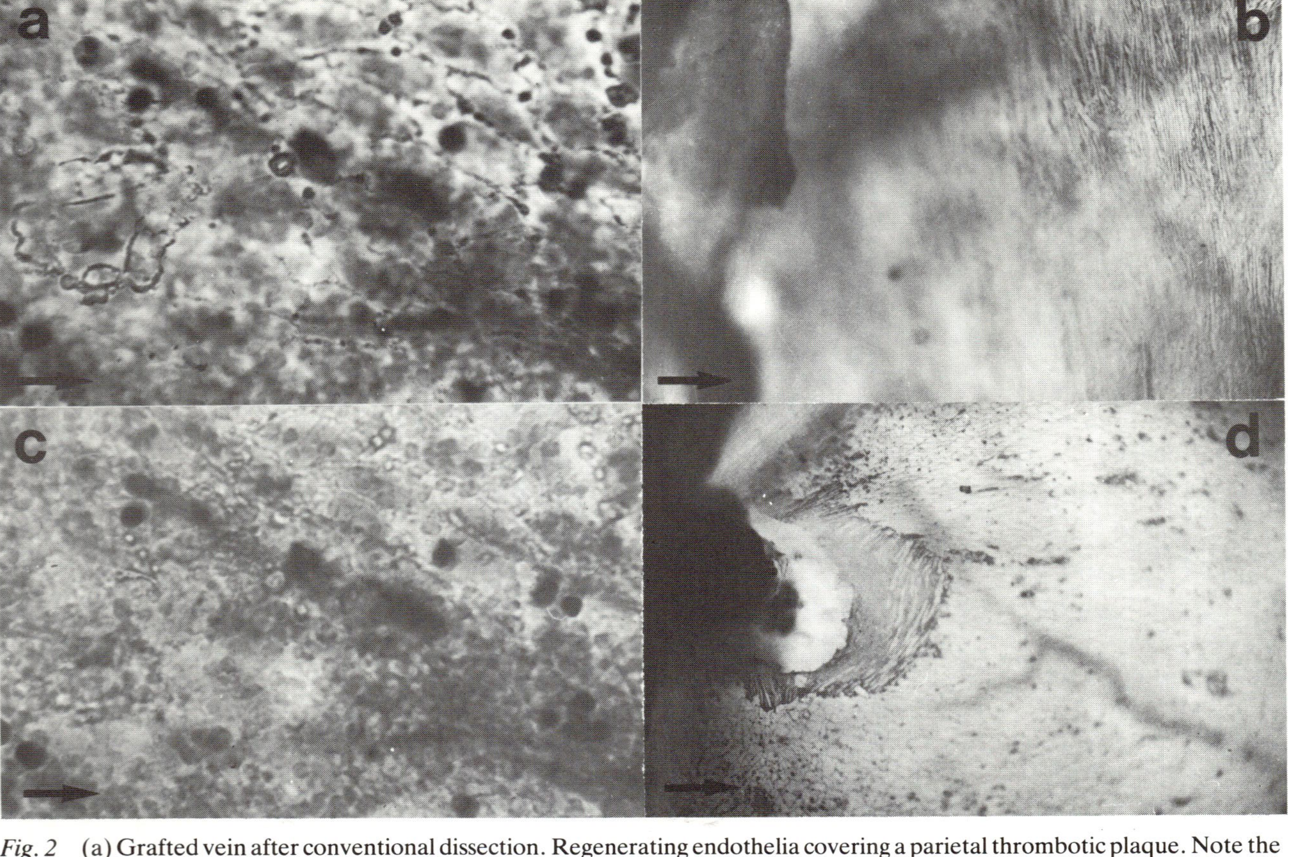

Fig. 2 (a) Grafted vein after conventional dissection. Regenerating endothelia covering a parietal thrombotic plaque. Note the delicate endothelial silver lines and the dissociation of the new endothelial cells. (b) An anastomosis sutured conventionally. No endothelial cells are found adjacent to the suture line (left). (c) The same field as seen in Fig. 3(a) but at a lower level. The parietal thrombus consisting of erythrocytes (ring structures), leucocytes and thrombocytes is seen. (d) Endothelium preserving technique. Endothelial cells are found close to the suture canal (left).

damage. The clamp with the least damage is the Hydragrip clamp of Fogarty, one of the branches of which is covered by a tube filled with fluid (Fig. 3a,b,c).

Because of these findings we abandoned the use of clamps, especially for the surgery of smaller vessels, whenever possible. Instead of clamping the vessels, the vessels were transfixed by sutures, leaving ample connective tissue or muscle between vessels and thread. For occlusion of the vessels the threads were pulled through a thin plastic tube and fixed under tension at the end of the tube by a small clamp.

Inflating the Vessels

When vessels were inflated by saline up to a pressure of 300 mgHg no endothelial changes were caused or mild changes only, consisting in a few linear tears in the intima (Fig. 3d).

Regeneration of Intra-operative Traumatic Lesions

Thrombotic Plaques

All areas deprived of their endothelia during operation are covered by parietal plaques consisting of thrombocytes, erythrocytes and a varying number of leucocytes. Two days after the operation one may notice that these plaques are being over grown by new endothelia arising from foci, where endothelia were preserved. These new endothelia are surrounded by silver lines more delicate than in normal vessels; they are spindle shaped or possess three or more processes. At the beginning these cells are dissociated. Eventually they form a continuous lining of endothelial cells, however, more permeable than normal endothelia, so that the underlying structures of the parietal thrombus are still discernable in the silver staining (Fig. 2a,c).

Regeneration Waves

When single endothelial cells or just small foci of endothelial cells are damaged, these cells become narrow and their cytoplasma is stained by silver nitrate, sparing the nuclei. In compensation the adjacent intact cells become broader so that narrow dark cells and broad unstained cells alternate. Occasionally some of the dark cells can be seen desquamating into the lumen of the vessel. Similar changes were seen when veins were compressed with clamps, the branches of which were covered by rubber tubings. We called this phenomenon "regeneration waves" (Gottlob *et al.*, 1976; Gottlob and Zinner, 1962) (Fig. 4a,b).

Multinucleated Endothelial Cells

At later periods some multinucleated endothelial cells are seen, but, only in such cases, where a conventional technique of dissection was applied. Multi-nucleated endothelial cells are seen frequently in man, especially in older individuals. In animals such multinucleated cells are rarely seen. We regard the formation of these multinucleated cells as a sign of regeneration in older individuals as well as after mild mechanical traumatization (Gottlob *et al.*, 1976; Gottlob and Zinner, 1962) (Fig. 5c).

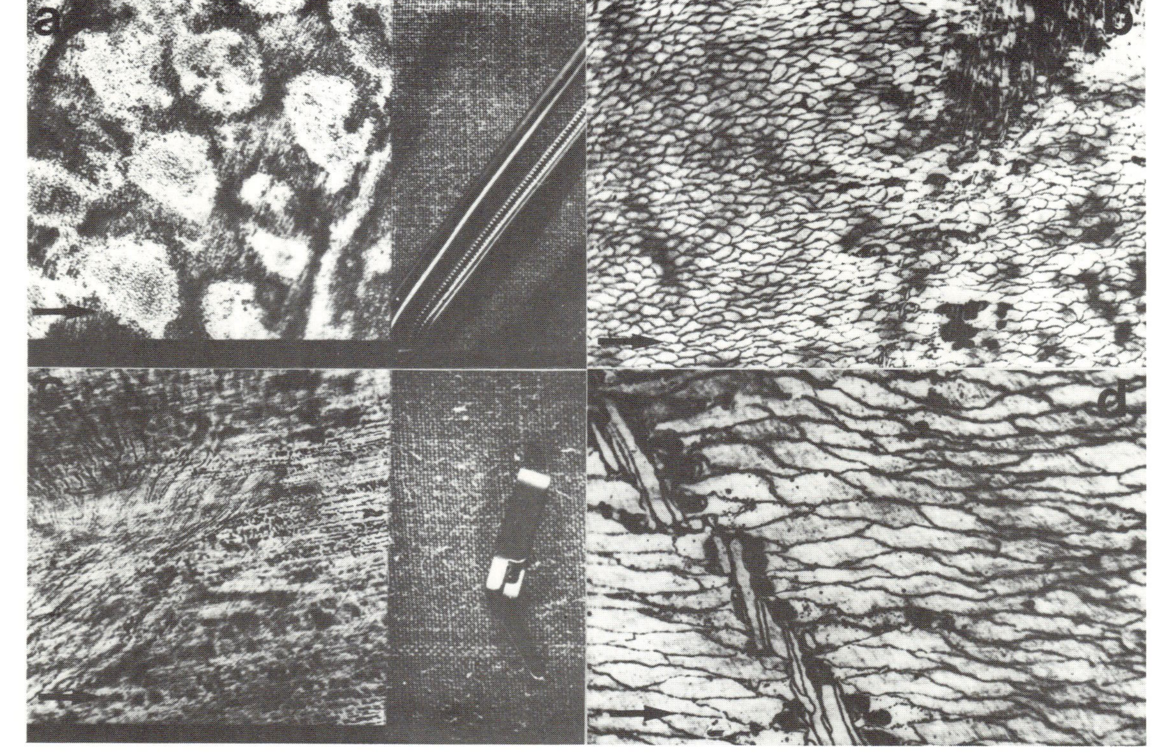

Fig. 3 (a) Damage caused by a conventional haemostatic vascular clamp with jaws covered by small teeth (right side of a). Note severe damage, especially between the areas compressed by the teeth where frictional forces were operative. (b) Moderate endothelial damage caused by Fogarty's Hydragrip clamp. (c) Distinct endothelial damage caused by the microclip (right side of c). (d) Moderate changes induced by inflating the vessel up to a pressure of 300 mgHg. Endothelial tears (left side of d) are seen but occasionally.

Vessels Dissected and Anastomosed by an Endothelium-preserving Technique

When an endothelium-preserving technique is applied the endothelia remain in place, parietal plaques, regeneration waves and multinucleated cells are seen rarely and if so, mostly close to the anastomotic region. Interestingly enough in our series the grafted veins retained the venous shape of the endothelia up to ten weeks (Gottlob *et al.*, 1976). Fonkalsrud *et al.* (1978) observed the preservation of the morphological characteristics of venous endothelium as long as five months after the operation. No permeability changes were seen in grafted veins when an endothelium preserving technique was applied (Fig. 5a).

Anastomoses

Parietal plaques consisting of erythrocytes, thrombocytes and leucocytes develop in the anastomotic area. This parietal thrombi can be detected arteriographically, especially when the anastomosis has been sutured conventionally. The thrombotic plaques were considerably reduced when an endothelium-preserving technique was applied for suturing the anastomoses.

Whereas the thrombotic plaques, found in the central areas of the graft, were as a rule overgrown by new endothelia after 7–12 days, the anastomotic areas remained devoid of endothelia for longer periods. In most instances the anastomotic region was covered by new endothelia 20 days after the operation, minor thrombotic plaques, however, were seen even on the 70th postoperative day.

Whereas the endothelia of the atraumatic grafted vessels are directed in the axis of the vessel, in most instances the endothelia, covering the anastomotic area, are situated in the transverse direction (Fig. 5b).

DISCUSSION

It was proven by our investigations that great portions of the endothelium are damaged when veins are dissected by conventional, though careful, methods. The endothelia can be preserved when the dissection is carried out "without touching" and these endothelia remain in place after insertion of the venous segments into an artery.

The endothelium-preserving dissection of a vein is painstaking and of longer duration than a conventional dissection. Another drawback is that in most instances long incisions are necessary for a dissection without touching. Many surgeons avoid long incisions by leaving in place skin-bridges in order to facilitate wound healing.

These drawbacks warrant a careful consideration whether this technique of endothelium-preserving dissection should be recommended for replacing peripheral arteries. The short-term patency of the graft depends not necessarily upon the intact endothelial lining, provided there exists an adequate inflow and outflow. In a series of investigations we could prove, however, that for replacement of veins the intact endothelial lining may be essential. In two series of experiments jugular veins of dogs and of rabbits were replaced by autogenous veins without creating arteriovenous fistulae and without post-

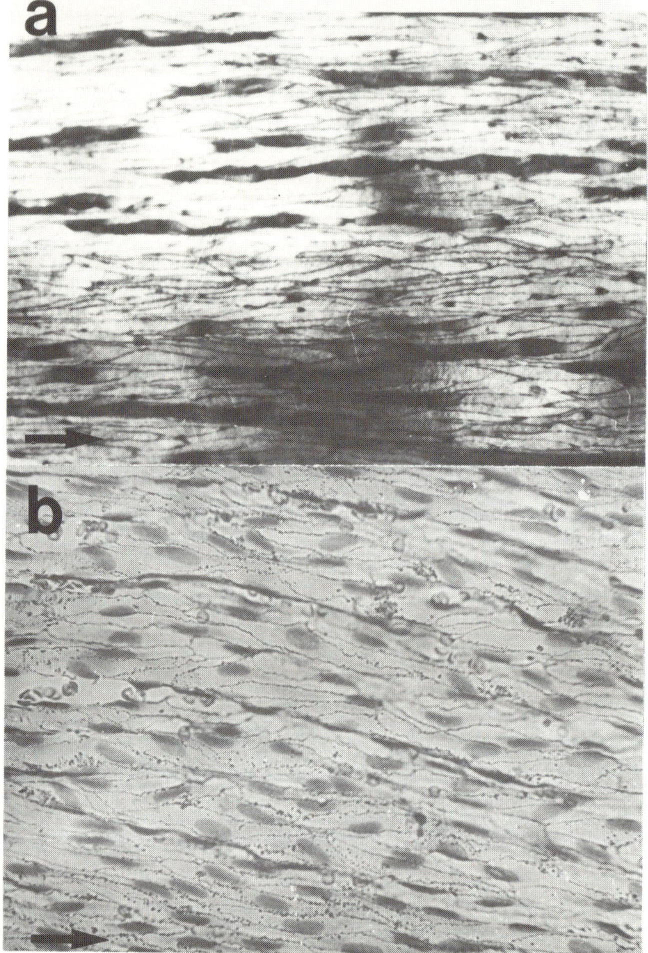

Fig. 4. (a and b). Regeneration waves: (a) in a full thickness preparation and (b) in a Haeutchen preparation 7 days after conventional dissection and grafting.

operative anticoagulant or antiaggregating treatment. May (1976) and Gottlob and May (1977) were able to improve the results of Palma operations when an endothelium-preserving technique was applied.

For arterial replacement we think that the endothelium-preserving technique should be used if there exists an impaired inflow or outflow or if very peripheral defects are to be bridged.

At the present time we cannot answer the question whether an endothelium-preserving technique might be advantageous even for routine bypass procedures, such as bridging defects in the region of the Hunter's channel or for aortocoronary bypass procedures. The short-term patency rate is quite satisfactory under these conditions. The long-term results, however, are not too favourable in some of the reports.

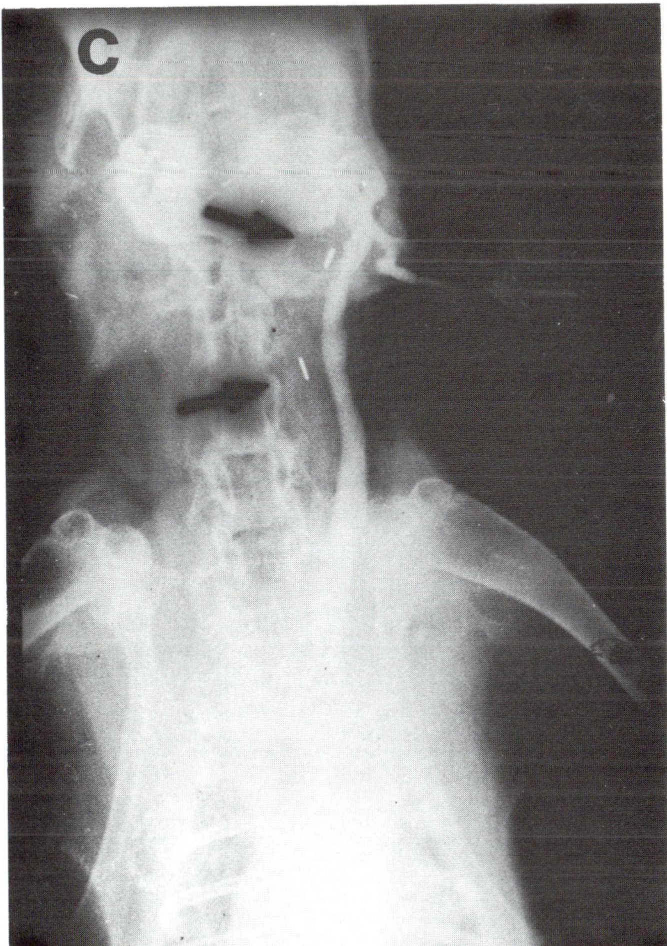

Fig. 4c. Veno-venous transplantation of a jugular vein of a rabbit. The arrows point to microclips indicating the level of the anastomoses.

There exist plenty of experimental evidence that atherosclerosis develops at sites of regenerated endothelial lesions. Björkerud and Bondjers (1971) concluded from their experiments that defective endothelia and increased permeability were one of the central atherogenetic factors. Bondjers and Björkerud (1973) found atherosclerotic lesions with defined morphological properties at sites of previous mechanical traumata in aortae of normolipidemic rabbits. Minick *et al.* (1980) maintain that there is clinicopathological and experimental evidence to indicate that arterial injury and the subsequent reactive changes may favour the accumulation of lipid at the site of injury and lead to atherosclerosis. Ross *et al.* (1974) described a platelet-dependent serum factor that stimulates proliferation of arterial smooth muscle cells *in vitro*. *In vivo* experiments of Fischer-Dzoga *et al.* (1974) as well

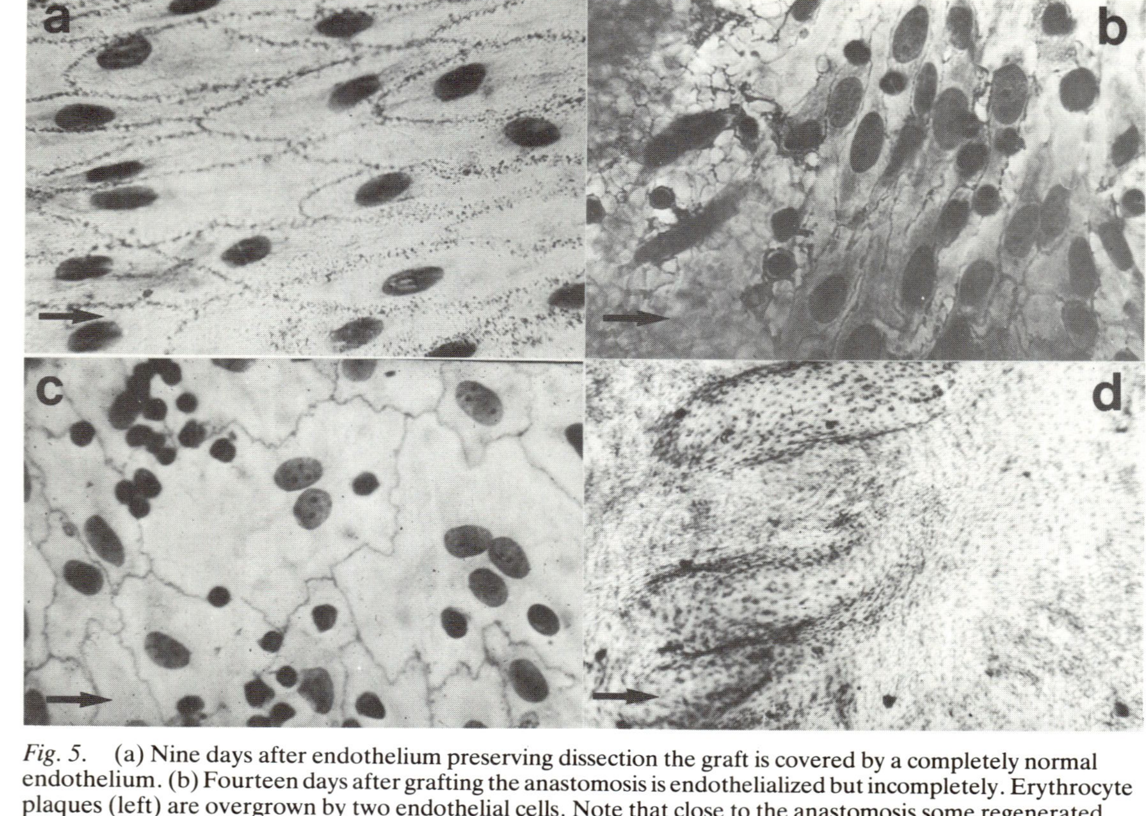

Fig. 5. (a) Nine days after endothelium preserving dissection the graft is covered by a completely normal endothelium. (b) Fourteen days after grafting the anastomosis is endothelialized but incompletely. Erythrocyte plaques (left) are overgrown by two endothelial cells. Note that close to the anastomosis some regenerated endothelia run transversely to the axis of the vessel. (c) After conventional dissection many multi-nucleated great endothelia are seen nine days after the operation. Note lymphocyte infiltration immediately underneath the endothelial layer. (d) Anastomosis, 27 days after grafting. Even the threads of the continuous suture are covered by new endothelia.

as of Friedman *et al.* (1977) support the hypothesis that the incorporation of thrombocytes at the site of previous defects stimulates subintimal smooth muscle cell proliferation.

Many authors describe arteriosclerotic or subintimal fibrotic lesions in veins, grafted into arteries (Barboriak *et al.*, 1974, 1978; Bondjers and Björkerud, 1973; Brody *et al.*, 1972; Ejrup *et al.*, 1961; Fuchs *et al.*, 1978; Gottlob *et al.*, 1975; Grondin *et al.*, 1979; Karayannacos *et al.*, 1978; McCann *et al.*, 1979, 1980; Szilagyi *et al.*, 1973; Wyatt and Gonzales, 1969). Our own experiments have proven that parietal thrombi containing a great amount of thrombocytes are incorporated into the vessel wall when endothelial lesions are repaired by overgrowth of parietal thrombi by new endothelia (Gottlob, 1977; Gottlob *et al.*, 1976). The observation that multinucleated endothelial cells are seen after repair of such lesions also indicates the possibility that these regenerated endothelia are less resistant to the development of sclerotic changes than the normal original endothelial lining.

Certainly it is not only the endothelial injury that might be responsible for the later subintimal proliferation and for the atherosclerotic changes. Ischaemia of the media may be an important factor as well (Fonkalsrud *et al.*, 1978; Fuchs *et al.*, 1978; Ramos *et al.*, 1976) and explain the diminution of smooth muscle fibres as observed by Szilagyi *et al.* (1973). In our experiments examining the full thickness preparations we obtained evidence that at least two days after the operation the vasa vasorum were again in connexion with the vascular system, they were dilated and filled with blood. A rapid establishment of the adventitional blood supply was observed by Wyatt and Taylor (1966). However, even a short duration of ischaemia might cause irreversible damage of the smooth muscles of the grafted veins.

Other factors involved in the degenerative changes of the grafted vein could be the arterial blood pressure in vessels not capable of tolerating continuous high pressures (Brody *et al.*, 1972; Fonkalsrud *et al.*, 1978; Karayannacos *et al.*, 1978; McCabe *et al.*, 1967). Also the accumulation of leucocytes in the wall of grafted vessels as observed by various authors (McCabe *et al.*, 1967; Stewart *et al.*, 1974) might contribute to degenerative changes in the graft. Endothelial desquamation due to surgical traumatization was observed also by Brody *et al.* (1972); Fonkalsrud *et al.* (1978); Reichle *et al.* (1973) and by Wyatt and Taylor (1966).

After our first recommendation a "no touch technique" for handling grafted veins was also advocated by various other authors (Fuchs *et al.*, 1978; Gundry *et al.*, 1980; Urschel *et al.*, 1972). Table IV displays our present

Table IV. Endothelium preserving technique for dissection of the grafts and for suturing anastomoses.

Value established	Procedure recommended	Value under discussion
For veno-venous transplants	For arterial replacement in cases with impaired inflow or outflow	For routine bypass grafts for prevention of late sclerotic changes

opinion about the indication for the use of an endothelium-preserving "no touch technique" in vascular surgery.

REFERENCES

Barboriak, J. J., Pintar, K. and Korus, M. E. (1974). Atherosclerosis in aortocoronary vein grafts. *Lancet* **2**, 621.

Barboriak, J. J., Pintar, K., Van Horn, D. L., Batayias, G. E. and Korus, M. E. (1978). Pathologic findings in the aortocoronary vein grafts. *Artherosclerosis* **29**, 69.

Björkerud, S. and Bondjers, G. (1971). Arterial repair and atherosclerosis after mechanical injury. *Atherosclerosis* **14**, 259.

Bondjers, G. and Björkerud, S. (1973). Cholesterol accumulation and content in regions with defined endothelial integrity in the normal rabbit aorta. *Atherosclerosis* **17**, 71.

Brody, W. R., Angell, W. W. and Kosek, J. C. (1972). Fate of venous coronary artery bypass in dogs. *American Journal of Pathology* **66**, 111.

Ejrup, B., Hiertonn, T. and Moberg, A. (1961). Atheromatous changes in autogenous vein grafts. *Acta Chirurgica Scandinavica* **121**, 211.

Fischer-Dzoga, K., Chen, R. and Wissler, R. W. (1974). Effects of serum lipoproteins on the morphology growth and metabolism of arterial smooth muscle cells. *Advances in Experimental Medicine and Biology* **43**, 299.

Fonkalsrud, W., Sanchez, M. and Zerubavel, R. (1978). Morphological evaluation of canine autogenous vein grafts in the arterial circulation. *Surgery* **84**, 253.

Friedman, R. J., Stemerman, M. B., Wenz, B., Moore, S., Gauldie, J., Gent, R., Trell, M. L. and Spaet, T. H. (1977). The effect of thrombocytopenia on experimental arteriosclerotic lesion formation in rabbits. *Journal of Clinical Investigation* **60**, 1191.

Fuchs, C. A., Mitchener, J. S. and Hagen, P. O. (1978). Postoperative changes in autologous vein grafts. *American Surgeon* **188**, 1.

Gottlob, R. (1977). The preservation of the venous endothelium by "dissection without touching" and by an atraumatic technique of vascular anastomosis. The importance for arterial and venous surgery. *Minerva Chirurgica* **32**, 693.

Gottlob, R. and May, R. (1977). Der Frühverschluß der Palma-Operation, Vorbeugung durch Anwendung einer endothelschonenden Operationstechnik. *Vasa* **6**, 263.

Gottlob, R. and Zinner, G. (1962). Ober die Regeneration geschädigter Endothelien nach hartem und weichem Trauma. *Virchows Archiv fur Pathologische Anatomie und Physiologie* **336**, 16.

Gottlob, R., Donas, P. and El Nashef, B. (1975). Untersuchungen am Endothel arterialisierter Venen I. Wirkungen einer atraumatischen Präparation. *Vasa* **4**, 243.

Gottlob, R., Donas, P., El Nashef, B. and Saghir, F. (1976a). Untersuchungen am Endothel arterialisierter Venen II. Morphologische Befunde bei autologen Venenimplantaten von Hunden. *Vasa* **5**, 111.

Gottlob, R., Donas, P. and El Nashef, B. (1976b). Untersuchungen am arterialisierten Venen III. Unterschiede zwischen autologen und homologen Transplantaten. *Vasa* **5**, 313.

Grondin, C. M., Campeau, L., Lespérance, J., Solyrnoss, B. C., Vouhé, P., Castonguay, Y. R., Meese, C. and Bourassa, M. G. (1979). Atherosclerotic changes in coronary vein grafts six years after operation. *Journal of Thoracic Cardiovascular Surgery* **77**, 24.

Gundry, S. R., Jones, M., Sshikara, T. and Ferraus, V. J. (1980). Optimal preservation techniques for human saphenous vein grafts. *Angiology* **21**, 729.

Karayannacos, P. E., Hosteller, J. R., Bond, M. G., Kakos, G. S., Williams, R. A., Kilman, J. W. and Vasco, J. S. (1978). Late failure in vein grafts. *Annals of Surgery* **187**, 183.

May, R. (1976). Surgical management of chronic venous occlusions of the extremities. *In* "XXV International European Congress, Society of Cardiovascular Surgery", p. 1. Belgrade.

McCabe, M., Cunningham, G. J., Wyatt, A. P., Rothnie, N. G. and Taylor, G. W. (1967). A histological and histochemical examination of autogenous vein grafts. *British Journal of Surgery* **54**, 147.

McCann, R. L., Hagen, P. O. and Fuchs, J. C. A. (1980). Aspirin and dipiryidamole decrease intimal hyperplasia in experimental vein grafts. *Annals of Surgery* **191**, 238.

McCann, R. L., Larson, R. M., Mitchener, J. S., Fuchs, J. C. and Hagen, P. O. (1979). Intimal thickening and hyperlipidemia in experimental primate vascular autografts. *Annals of Surgery* **189**, 62.

Minick, R. C., Falcone, D. J. and Hajjar, D. P. (1980). Endothelium in experimental atherosclerosis. *In* "Atherosclerosis" (A. M. Gotto, Jr., L. Smith and B. Allen, Eds), Vol. V. Springer, New York, Heidelberg, Berlin.

Ramos, J. R., Mansfield, P. B., Wechezak, A. and Sauvage, L. R. (1976). Histologic fate and endothelial changes of distended and non distended vein grafts. *Annals of Surgery* **183**, 205.

Reichle, F. A., Stewart, G. J. and Erra, J. (1973). A transmission and scanning electron microscopic study of luminal surfaces in dacron and autogenous vein bypass in man and dog. *Surgery* **74**, 945.

Ross, R., Glomset, J. A., Kariya, B. and Harker, L. A. (1974). A platelet-dependent serum factor that stimulates proliferation of arterial smooth muscle cells *in vitro*. *Proceedings of the National Academy of Sciences, United States of America* **71**, 1207.

Scott, H. W. Jr., Bolasny, B. L., Lanier, V. C., Younger, R. K. and Butts, W. (1970). Experimental atherosclerosis in autogenous venous grafts. *Archives of Surgery (Chicago)* **101**, 677.

Stewart, G. J., Titchie, W. G. M. and Lynch, P. R. (1974). Venous endothelial damage produced by massive sticking and emigration of leucocytes. *American Journal of Pathology* **74**, 507.

Szilagyi, D. E., Elliott, J. P., Hageman, J. H., Smith, R. F. and Dall'Olmo, C. A. (1973). Biologic fate of autogenous vein implants as arterial substitutes. *Annals of Surgery* **178**, 232.

Urschel, H. C., Razzuk, M. A., Wood, R. E. and Paulsen, D. L. (1972). Patency of autocoronary saphenous vein grafts. *Surgery* **72**, 1048.

Wyatt, A. P. and Gonzales, J. E. (1969). Atheromatous lesions in arterialized vein grafts. *British Journal of Surgery* **56**, 193.

Wyatt, A. P. and Taylor, G. W. (1966). Vein grafts: Changes in the endothelium of autogenous free vein grafts used as arterial replacements. *British Journal of Surgery* **53**, 943.

AUTOGENOUS VEIN FOR ARTERIAL BYPASS: ALTERNATIVES TO THE SAPHENOUS VEIN

D. R. Campbell and C. S. Hoar Jr.

Department of Vascular Surgery, New England Deaconess Hospital, Boston, Massachusetts, USA

It is now universally accepted that autogenous saphenous vein bypass grafting is the procedure of choice in suitable patients who present with disabling claudication, rest pain or gangrene. However, in as many as 25% of these patients, suitable autogenous saphenous vein is not available. Undoubtedly, as increasing numbers of patients undergo coronary artery bypass grafting, this will prove to be even more of a problem in the future. What to use when there is no suitable saphenous vein available remains a topic of heated debate among the experts, as this symposium will surely demonstrate, and a dilemma for the vascular surgeon practicing in the community.

With the advent of Dacron and Teflon grafts we started using them at the Deaconess Hospital whenever there was no adequate saphenous vein available. In 1973 we published our results comparing cloth grafts with saphenous vein grafting in diabetics (Fig. 1). I would comment that the Joslin Diabetic Clinic admits to the New England Deaconess Hospital in Boston, and so by far the greatest proportion of our patients are diabetics. The three-year cumulative patency for our cloth grafts was 59% versus 81% for the saphenous vein grafts. Initially, favorable reports in the literature also showed that the long-term failure rate was much higher than autogenous saphenous vein, particularly when the grafts were carried below the knee.

Serono Symposium No. 44, "Peripheral Arterial Diseases: Medical and Surgical Problems", edited by S. Stipa and A. Cavallaro, 1982. Academic Press, London and New York.

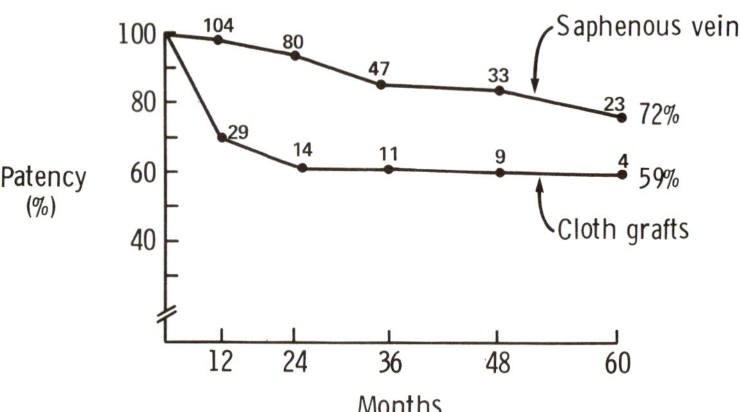

Fig. 1. Femoro-popliteal bypass grafts in diabetics (from Harman and Hoar, 1973).

Since then, two new graft materials have become available; namely, Polytetrafluoroethylene (PTFE) and glutaraldehyde tanned human umbilical cord vein (HUV). Early results with PTFE were so good that early workers even suggested that PTFE would prove to be better than autogenous saphenous vein. This has not been the case. Some of the better results have been obtained by Veith's group in New York. In 175 femoro-popliteal bypass grafts, there was a 62% cumulative patency at three years which was increased to 77% if one included those patients who occluded and were successfully re-operated on. Umbilical vein grafts also have their supporters. In a survey provided by Meadox Medicals, the cumulative patency of 519 femoral popliteal bypasses is 63.5% at 40 months. These operations were performed by Dardik and 16 other investigators from major university centers. These excellent results with PTFE and HUV, while inferior to autogenous vein, would suggest that either could be used when saphenous vein is unavailable. Not all investigators, however, have been so successful and many practicing surgeons have been unhappy with these new materials. In a recent report by Weisel and others from the University of Toronto the three-year patency of the 85 SV grafts was 75% compared with 34% for the 66 HUV grafts, and 33% for the 67 PTFE grafts. While it is always difficult to compare series because of unseen differences in patient selection, incidence of redo surgery etc. it does seem clear that the wide differences in results may reflect a need for extensive experience, which may limit these prostheses.

A number of animal studies have been published fairly recently which confirm the superiority of autogenous vein grafts, at least in dogs. Four-millimeter grafts were implanted in dogs for three to four months. Oblath *et al.* (1978) found the patency rate for HUV to be 53%, compared with 100% for autogenous vein. Hastings group found that 62.5% of the PTFE grafts remained patent. Feins *et al.* (1979) looked at HUV and found that a patency rate of 10% was significantly improved to 60% by treating the animals with Aspirin and dipyridamole. So, in animal studies at least, neither PTFE nor HUV matched up to autogenous vein.

In 1975 dissatisfaction with cloth grafts led us to start using alternative sources of autogenous vein, namely the arm veins, when there was no suitable saphenous vein available. The use of arm veins is not new, and there have been many anecdotal reports in the literature. In 1969 Kakkar looked at the physical characteristics of the cephalic vein in order to determine whether it would be a suitable conduit for bypass grafting. He dissected out the cephalic veins and the saphenous veins in 25 cadavers and looked at their length, diameter and ability to withstand pressure. The cephalic veins were of adequate length, had a greater diameter than the long saphenous vein when distended to 100 mgHg and they tolerated pressure well. None of the cephalic veins burst at a pressure of less than 430 mmHg, whereas the saphenous veins withstood pressures up to 600 mmHg. However, he noted that all the varicose saphenous veins burst at pressures of less than 100 mmHg. Interestingly, the cephalic vein had a greater diameter at the lower end than the long saphenous vein in all 25 cadavers studied. In 1970 Vellar and Doyle also looked at the length, diameter and pressure characteristics of arm veins and saphenous veins in ten cadavers. They noted that the average length of the cephalic vein was 50 cm and the basilic vein a little less. Both could withstand pressures greater than 300 mmHg without difficulty. The basilic vein, though adequate in all cases, was less distensible than the cephalic vein. These studies confirmed the suitability of arm veins as an alternative to saphenous vein.

In general, we have preferred not to use saphenous veins less than 4 mm in diameter, as these have been associated with increased graft failure. If the saphenous vein is deemed inadequate by reason of size or inadequate length, then we turn to the arm vein, preferring to leave the other leg intact, as it may be needed for a later procedure. In patients with previous saphenous vein ligation and stripping, or who have had the vein used in prior surgery, attention is immediately directed to the arm vein. In our first 18 cases eight patients had saphenous veins that were in part too small, so composite saphenous arm vein grafts were used. In four patients, the saphenous vein had been used for previous grafting; in three, the vein had been stripped and in one, the vein had multiple varicosities rendering part of the vein unsuitable.

When using arm veins we stress the importance of anticipating the need to use an arm vein. A history of previous surgery on the long saphenous vein is obviously important, though a previous history of an inadequate vein in the opposite leg is not necessarily indicative of an inadequate vein on the present side. If it is thought that an arm vein may be needed, the arms must be carefully examined to locate the best vein and that arm then spared of any further invasive testing, including venipuncture or intravenous placement. We have not used venography prior to surgery and do not consider it to be necessary.

At the operating table the arm is prepped in a similar fashion as the leg, and draped in a manner to allow free movement of the arm. Figure 2 demonstrates the anatomy of the superficial veins of the arm. The usual method of vein harvesting is to choose the largest most distal vein at the wrist and dissect proximally following the largest diameter vein. This usually results in the cephalic being taken, though occasionally the basilic is found to be more suitable. The arm veins are thinner walled than the saphenous vein, and one

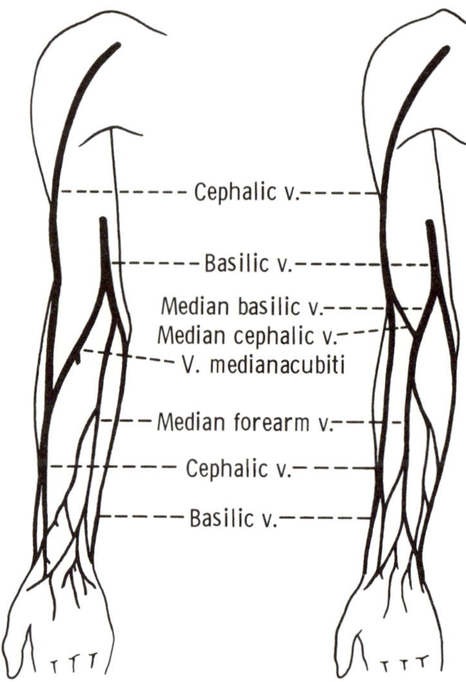

Fig. 2. The arm veins.

must be very meticulous and delicate in their dissection. For this reason, a continuous incision is made along the course of the vein, carefully isolating individual tributaries under direct vision. The individual branches are ligated with 4.0 silk. The ligatures should be placed 3–4 mm from the main vein to prevent constriction or dumb-belling of the main segment (Fig. 3). Larger tributaries are also suture ligated to prevent a blow out, which has occurred with ligation alone. Once the vein is harvested, it is reversed and gently distended with heparinized Ringer's solution to detect leaks, dumb-belling or stenotic segments. These stenotic segments have been found in a small number of cases, and presumably relate to previous trauma. They require excision and oblique end-to-end anastamosis. The vein is sewn in place with 6.0 monofilament suture using the standard technique. Again, it is stressed that meticulous handling of the arm vein is required, and for this reason, it is strongly recommended that magnifying glasses be used when constructing the anastomoses. Composite grafts with saphenous and arm veins are used in 40% of the patients, and when required, long oblique anastomoses are performed over a stent.

Kakkar (1969), Vellar and Doyle (1970) and Stipa (1972) all reported good results in a very small number of patients with a limited follow-up period. In 1976 Clayson and Dale reported on 11 patients in whom arm veins alone were used. Seven occluded within two years, though the authors point out that this was a particularly high-risk group, most of whom had had previous failures

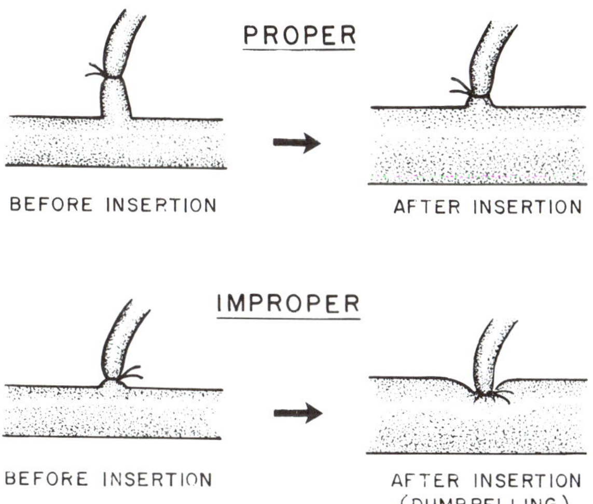

Fig. 3. Proper and improper placement of ligatures.

with autogenous saphenous vein, necessitating re-operation. We reported at the end of 1979 (Campbell *et al.*, 1979) 33 mostly diabetic patients who had under-gone femoro-popliteal or femoral–tibial bypass grafting, 20 of these having been followed for over a year (Table I). The one-year patency was 82%. Our series now totals 47 patients, and though our follow-up program is not completely up to date it is extremely encouraging. The more so when compared with our previously published results using autogenous saphenous vein and cloth grafts (Fig. 4). In a recent paper by Whittemore *et al.* (1981) from the Peter Brent Brigham in Boston on secondary femoro-popliteal reconstruction, the following results were obtained. Secondary reconstruction was performed using saphenous vein in 32 patients, arm vein in 16 patients, and a portion of the original vein graft in 18 patients. The differences in graft patency rates at five years among saphenous vein (37%), arm vein (34%) and original vein graft (36%) groups were not statistically

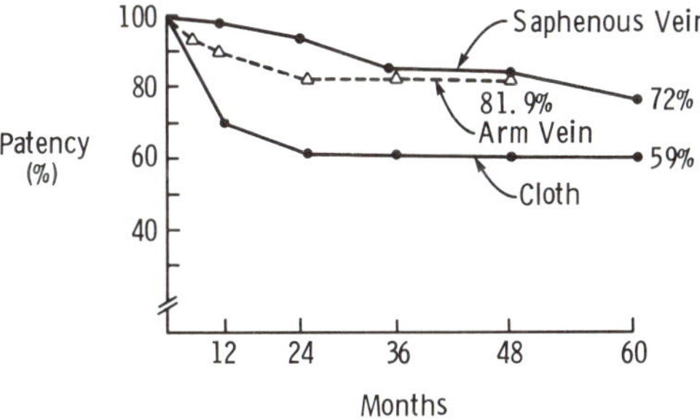

Fig. 4. Comparison of conduits for femoro-popliteal bypass grafts (from Campbell *et al.*, 1979).

significant. In contrast, all of 19 secondary procedures using prosthetic PTFE grafts had failed within three years.

As far as complications are concerned there are numerous reports of aneurysmal dilatation of cephalic veins used in coronary artery bypass grafting. This has not been noted when arm veins have been used in the femoro-popliteal position. In a series of 260 patients reports by Szilagyi in 1973, ten of 260 saphenous veins showed evidence of aneurysmal dilatation, so as more arm veins are used it is anticipated that some will undergo aneurysmal dilation. We found no problem with healing of the arm wound though one patient did develop a keloid.

Table I. Results of bypass grafts.

	Patient	Date of operation	Estimated length of arm vein	State of graft	Months of F/U
1	AM	12/75	30 cm C	Patent	41
2	DA	1/76	60 cm A	Patent	40
3	HM	1/76	30 cm C	Patent	40
4	IC	1/76	35 cm C	Patent	40
5	AP	1/76	40 cm C	Patent	39
6	MP	2/76	30 cm C	Patent	38
7	FG	3/76	40 cm A	Patent	38
8	LR	3/76	40 cm A	Failed	—
9	RK	4/76	30 cm C	Patent	37
10	JG	4/76	20 cm C	Patent	37
11	PG	4/76	30 cm C	Patent	36
12	AM	5/76	40 cm A	Patent	36
13	MD	5/76	35 cm C	Patent	34
14	DP	7/76	40 cm A	Patent	34
15	JS	8/76	20 cm C	Died	—
16	MR	8/76	60 cm A	Failed	—
17	MD	11/76	45 cm A	Failed	—
18	DP	3/77	45 cm A	Patent	26
19	VO	4/78	40 cm A	Patent	13
20	KS	4/78	18 cm C	Patent	13
21	LF	5/78	40 cm A	Patent	12
22	BF	5/78	16 cm C	Patent	12
23	VO	5/78	40 cm A	Patent	12
24	RS	6/78	30 cm A	Patent	11
25	WW	8/78	60 cm A	Died	—
26	AP	8/78	40 cm A	Patent	9
27	EV	9/78	30 cm C	Patent	8
28	ML	11/78	40 cm A	Patent	6
29	MV	12/78	40 cm A	Patent	5
30	MC	2/79	60 cm A	Patent	3
31	FB	3/79	40 cm A	Patent	2
32	EM	5/79	40 cm A	Patent	1
33	JG	5/79	40 cm A	Failed	—

A = arm vein alone; C = arm vein and saphenous vein composite graft.

With our good results reinforced by those from Brigham we now use arm veins whenever the saphenous vein is not available unless the length of time of the operation is a significant factor. I would stress again that careful handling of the vein and meticulous suture technique is essential if good results are to be obtained, and magnifying loops are very helpful. The chief disadvantage of using arm veins is the time it takes to harvest the vein, and this operation routinely takes us 4–5 h. However, with modern anesthesia this is not a problem. Therefore, we would recommend that any surgeon who is unhappy with the other alternatives to autogenous saphenous vein should try using arm veins. It may well be that in five years, we will have the perfect alternative to autogenous vein, but that point has not yet been reached.

REFERENCES

Campbell, D. R., Hoar, C. S. and Gibbons, G. W. (1979). The use of arm veins in femoral-popliteal bypass grafts. *Annals of Surgery* **190**, 740.

Clayson, K. R. and Dale, W. A. (1976) Arm veins for peripheral arterial reconstruction. *Archives of Surgery (Chicago)* **111**, 1276.

Feins, R. H., Roedersheimer, R. L., Green, R. M. *et al.* (1979). Platelet aggregation in human umbilical vein grafts and negatively charged bovine heterografts. *Surgery* **85**, 395.

Harmon, S. W. and Hoar, C. S. (1973). Cloth femoral popliteal bypass grafts in twenty-nine diabetic patients. *Archives of Surgery (Chicago)* **106**, 282.

Hastings, O. M., Krishna, M. J., Hobson, R. W. *et al.* (1978). A prospective randomized study of three expanded polytetrafluoroethylene (PTFE) grafts as small arterial substitutes. *Annals of Surgery* **188**, 743.

Kakkar, V. V. (1969). The cephalic vein as a peripheral vascular graft. *Surgery, Gynecology and Obstetrics* **128**, 551.

Meadox Medicals. "Dardik Biograft 36-Month Clinical Results". Vascular Rounds, Vol. I, April 1979.

Oblath, R. W., Buckely, R. O., Connelly, W. A. *et al.* (1978). Human umbilical veins and autogenous veins as canine arterial bypass grafts. *Annals of Surgery* **188**, 158.

Stipa, S. (1972). The cephalic and basilic veins in peripheral arterial reconstructive surgery. *Annals of Surgery* **175**, 581.

Szilagyi, D. E., Elliott, J. P., Hageman, J. H., Smith, R. F. and Dall'Olmo, C. A. (1973). Biologic fate of autogenous venous implants as arterial substitutes; clinical angiographic and histopathologic observations in femoro-popliteal operations for atherosclerosis. *Annals of Surgery* **178**, 232.

Vellar, I. D. and Doyle, J. C. (1970). The use of cephalic and basilic veins in peripheral vascular grafts. *Australian and New Zealand Journal of Surgery* **40**, 52.

Veith, F. J. and Gupta, S. K. (1981). Complications of expanded polytetrafluoroethylene grafts. *In* "Complications in vascular surgery". (Bernhard, V. M. and Towne, J. B., Eds), p. 585. Grune and Stratton, New York.

Weisel. R. D., Johnston, K. W., Baird, R. J. *et al.* (1981). Comparison of conduits for leg revascularization. *Surgery* **89**, 8.

Whittemore, A. D., Clowers, A. W., Couch, N. P. *et al.* (1981). Secondary femoro-popliteal reconstruction. *Annals of Surgery* **193**, 35.

FEMORO-POPLITEAL BYPASS GRAFTING WITH REVERSED AUTOLOGOUS SAPHENOUS VEIN: EXPERIENCE IN 98 CONSECUTIVE PATIENTS

S. Stipa, A. Cavallaro, V. Sciacca, M. Garofalo, A. Sterpetti and L. Di Marzo

IV Cattedra di Patologia Chirurgica dell'Università di Roma, Rome, Italy

MATERIAL AND METHODS

From November 1969 to December 1980, 104 femoro-popliteal bypass grafts were inserted into 98 patients (six of them being operated on bilaterally) utilizing autologous reversed saphenous vein.

During the same period, 39 additional femoro-popliteal bypasses were performed, using cephalic and/or basilic veins (seven), fresh homologous saphenous vein (two), expanded PTFE (20) and Dacron (10): they are not included in the present analysis.

The 98 patients were aged from 30 to 89 years (mean 63) and most of them (95) were male.

Only ten of them were free from significant associated disease, which were distributed as follows.

(A)	Heart	44 (44.8%)
	Diabetes	37 (37.7%)
	Hypertension	30 (30.6%)
	Kidney	26 (26.5%)
	Lung	19 (19.3%)
	CNS	10 (10.2%)
	Others[a]	33 (33.6%)

[a] Mostly duodenal ulcer 28/33 (84.8%).

Serono Symposium No. 44, "Peripheral Arterial Diseases: Medical and Surgical Problems", edited by S. Stipa and A. Cavallaro, 1982. Academic Press, London and New York.

(B)	No associated diseases	10 patients (10.2%)
	1 associated disease	28 patients (28.6%)
	2 associated diseases	28 patients (28.6%)
	3 associated diseases	22 patients (22.4%)
	More than 3 associated diseases	10 patients (10.2%)

Operative indication was claudication in 42 limbs (40.4%); the operation was performed for salvage in 62 limbs (59.6%).

Homolateral lumbar sympathectomy had been performed from one to 28 months in 18 limbs, with the following results.

Status quo	6 (33.5%)
Short-lasting improvement	5 (27.7%)
Worsening	7 (38.8%)

Procedures aiming at femoral inflow improvement had been performed in 13 limbs and the femoral-to-popliteal procedure was accomplished electively eight times (four in one stage with the proximal reconstruction and four at a distance of 15 days — 15 months from the former) and as an emergency procedure in five limbs.

Pre-operative study included routine angiographic examination under the form of aortography (either translumbar or by transfemoral catheterization) or femoral arteriography. Doppler ultrasonic evaluation was introduced into our clinical practice in late 1971 and has since become an essential step of pre-operative evaluation.

General anaesthesia was used in most cases; however in almost 30% of patients, local or preferably spinal anaesthesia was used.

The distal anastomosis was put always below the knee joint. The proximal anastomosis was taylored on the common femoral artery whenever possible; distribution of the bypass take-off sites was as follows.

Common femoral artery	85 (81.8%)
Deep femoral artery	10 (9.6%)
Endarterectomized proximal superficial femoral artery	7 (6.7%)
Dacron A–F prosthesis	2 (1.9%)

Veins with an inside diameter inferior to 4 mm were never used. The vein, once excised, was gently distended with heparinized normal saline.

Intra-operative angiography was seldom accomplished, mainly on account of technical problems, up to two years ago; then it became an almost routine procedure in leg arteries reconstructions especially with the purpose of studying the characteristics of the vascular bed distal to the site selected for establishing the end of the reconstruction (i.e. before the reconstruction itself was carried on); as a means of intra-operative control after the accomplishment of the bypass it is still scantly used; an evaluation of intra-operative Doppler flowmetry to detect eventual technical faults and to allow prognostic statements is actually being carried on.

Anticoagulation was used only during the operative procedure. Wide spectrum antibiotics were used in the post-operative course; a programme of pre- and intra-operative antibiotic prophylaxis, both general and topic, was given up after three years because the results were clearly not significant.

Follow-up studies were carried out by direct examination of the patient, relying on clinical and instrumental (mainly Doppler) data: control arteriography was performed very seldom and only when bypass failure was predictable on the basis of non-invasive examinations.

Results were analysed according to Cutler and Ederer (1958).

RESULTS

Immediate and Early Results

One patient died post-operatively (p.o.) from myocardial infarction; p.o. mortality was about 1%; 16 grafts failed within the first p.o. month.

Analysis of these failures gave the following results.

(1) One bypass, even if patent, did not succeed in relieving symptoms and BK amputation was unavoidable; the graft is still patent, after 84 months.

(2) In a quite similar case, the graft eventually thrombosed three months after amputation.

(3) One bypass carried on as an emergency procedure after failure of an aorto-femoral reconstruction, thrombosed after 24 h with resulting limb-threatening ischaemia; replacement by means of a Dacron graft with contralateral take-off was followed by long-term success.

(4) Infection played a significant role in three graft failures: two thromboses with subsequent AK amputation and one pseudo-aneurysm at the popliteal anastomosis which obliged us to extend the reconstruction down to anterior tibial artery, with long-term success.

(5) In the other ten limbs, graft failure was not reversible in spite of an aggressive trend to thrombectomy and rethrombectomy: AK amputation was unavoidable in three limbs operated on for salvage; return to pre-operative status was accepted in two limbs operated on for rest pain and in five limbs operated on for claudication.

Late Results

Fourteen patients died during the course of the follow-up period and 23 grafts failed. Survival according to clinical pre-operative status and diabetes is reported in Fig. 1.

Seven AK amputations were performed after graft failure. Amongst failing grafts are included two grafts patent but functionally useless: in one of them a BK amputation was performed. A new graft was attempted in three limbs:

(1) A femoro-popliteal bypass with fresh homologous vein (further occlusion after six months).

(2) Two femoro-tibial bypasses with one failure at one month and one extended patency.

Successful re-operations were also performed in one case of stenosis from

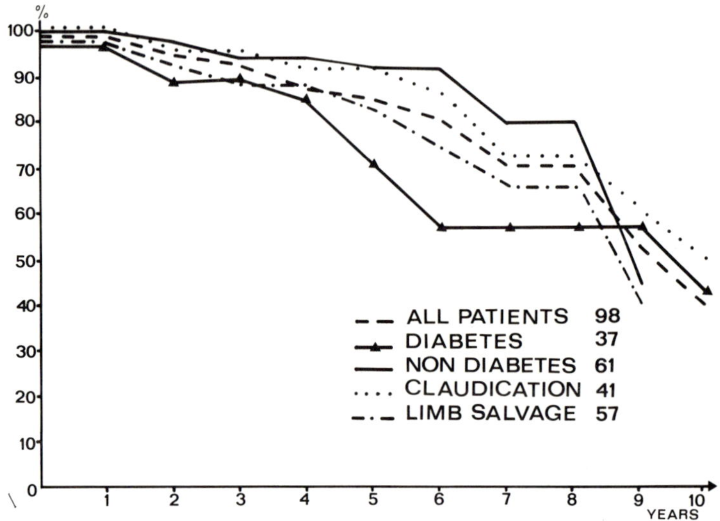

Fig. 1. Cumultative survival according to clinical status and presence/absence of diabetes.

subintimal fibrous hyperplasia and in one case of stenosis from calcified perigraft haematoma.

In Table I accumulative graft patency is reported.

The state at the end of the follow-up period is reported in Table II.

Claudication/Limb Salvage

In our experience (Table III) results in claudication patients were significantly better than in limb salvage ones ($P < 0.01$ from the third year of the follow-up period). Failure of grafts in claudicants brought to major amputation in two cases.

Diabetes/Non-diabetes

There was no difference in graft behaviour between these two groups (Fig. 2). Late mortality was higher amongst diabetics yet reaching statistical significance only at six, seven and eight years.

Outflow grading. It was possible in 82 limbs; outflow grading, on account of quality of radiograms, was roughly performed as:

I = three vessels patent
II = two vessels patent
III = one vessel patent or isolated popliteal artery

No significant difference was found in graft patency according to the division of patients into three groups (Fig. 3).

Table I. Accumulative patency of 104 femoro-popliteal vein grafts.

Interval	Grafts at risk	Failing grafts	Withdrawn from follow up		Interval failure rate (%)	Interval patency (%)	Accumulated patency (%)
			Death	End of follow up			
months							
0–1	104	16	1	0	15.4	84.6	84.6
1–6	87	9	0	4	10.5	89.5	75.7
6–12	74	1	0	1	1.3	98.7	74.7
12–24	72	4	3	4	5.8	94.2	70.3
24–36	61	7	1	11	12.7	87.3	61.3
36–48	42	1	1	2	2.5	97.5	59.7
48–60	38	0	1	9	0	100	59.7
60–72	28	1	2	3	3.9	96.1	57.3
72–84	22	0	3	6	0	100	57.3
84–96	13	0	0	2	0	100	57.3
96–108	11	0	2	4	0	100	57.3
108–120	5	0	1	2	0	100	57.3

Table II. State at the end of the followup (1–123 months; mean 46 months).

		Patent graft	No symptoms	Claudication	Ischaemia	AK amput.	BK amput.	Toe or TM amput.
Claudication	42	31 (74%)	30 (71%)	10 (24%)	–	2 (5%)	–	–
Limb salvage	61	33 (54%)	28 (47%)	5 (8%)	15 (24%)	10 (16%)	3 (5%)	6 (10%)

Table III. Accumulative patency according to clinical status and operative indication.

Interval	Grafts at risk	Failing grafts	Withdrawn from follow up		Interval failure rate (%)	Interval patency (%)	Accumulated patency (%)
			Death	End of follow up			
Months				Claudication			
0–1	42	7	0	0	16.6	83.4	83.4
1–6	35	2	0	1	5.8	94.2	78.5
6–12	32	0	0	0	0	100	78.5
12–24	32	0	1	2	0	100	78.5
24–36	29	2	0	3	7.2	92.8	72.8
36–48	24	0	1	1	0	100	72.8
48–60	22	0	0	5	0	100	72.8
60–72	17	0	1	2	0	100	72.8
72–84	14	0	2	4	0	100	72.8
84–96	8	0	0	1	0	100	72.8
96–108	7	0	1	1	0	100	72.8
108–120	5	0	1	2	0	100	72.8
				Limb salvage			
0–1	62	9	1	0	14.6	85.4	85.4
1–6	52	7	0	3	13.8	86.2	73.6
6–12	42	1	0	1	2.4	97.6	71.8
12–24	40	4	2	2	10.5	89.5	64.2
24–36	32	5	1	8	18.1	81.9	52.6
36–48	18	1	0	1	5.7	94.3	49.6
48–60	16	0	1	4	0	100	49.6
60–72	11	1	1	1	10	90	44.6
72–84	8	0	1	2	0	100	44.6
84–96	5	0	0	1	0	100	44.6
96–108	4	0	1	3	0	100	44.6
108–120	–	–	–	–	–	–	–

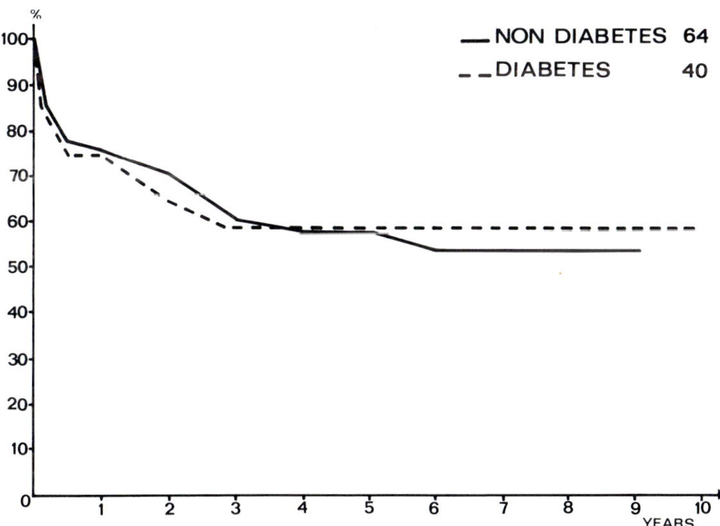

Fig. 2. Cumulative patency of femoro-popliteal vein grafts according to the presence/absence of diabetes.

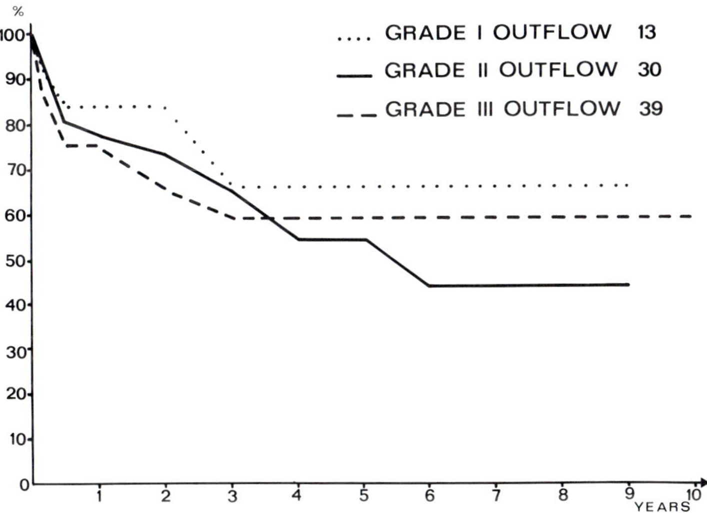

Fig. 3. Cumulative patency of femoro-popliteal vein grafts according to outflow grading.

Effect of age on graft patency. No difference was found between the patients above 63 years (43) and the younger ones (61) (Fig. 4).

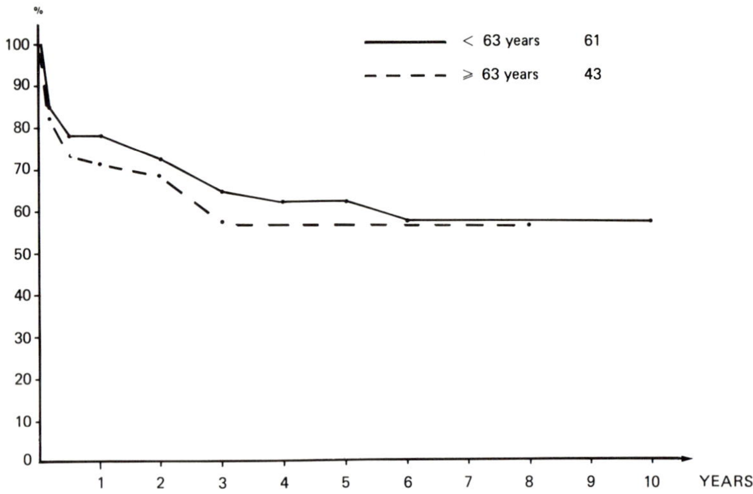

Fig. 4. Cumulative patency of femoro-popliteal vein grafts according to the age of the patients.

DISCUSSION

Early and Late Survival

Post-operative mortality, in our experience, compares favourably with that reported in other series; however, owing to the "bad quality" of these patients and the heavy incidence of associated diseases, we think it is only a matter of chance that our post-operative mortality was so low.

Late survival in peripheral vascular disease patients is much lower than in general population (Szilagyi *et al.*, 1979) especially when considering patients with ischaemic symptoms (King *et al.*, 1980): we could not do a comparison with the general behaviour of Italian population, owing to the wide range of age of our patients.

Early Patency

Early failure, in our series, exceeded 15%. This rather high percentage cannot be explained on the basis of patient selection, being similar in claudication and limb salvage patients as well as in diabetics and non-diabetics.

High incidence of early failure is also reported by Stephens and MacGowan, 1980 (14%); De Weese and Rob, 1977 (24%); Szilagyi *et al.*, 1979 (13%). In other series, early failure ranges from 2% (Sonnenfeldt and Cronestrand, 1980) to 6–8% (Darling and Linton, 1972; Kaminsky *et al.*, 1973; Cutler *et al.*, 1976).

Technical faults and wrong indication should account for the majority of early failures, in our as well as in others' experience (Ray *et al.*, 1970; Koontz and Stansel, 1972; Darling and Linton, 1972).

In particular, the need for amputation in spite of graft patency should mean that operative indication was not correct, being too extensive either the tissue loss at foot and/or leg level or the involvement of distal arterial bed (Szilagyi *et al.*, 1979).

Amongst the possibilities of technical faults, the use of small calibre veins has been probably overemphasized, being actually evident that the quality of the vein (LoGerfo *et al.*, 1977) and especially its wall thickness (Buxton *et al.*, 1980) bear a greater significance than the inside diameter.

In our experience, graft infection, as a cause of early failure, affected three limbs (2.8%): this high incidence—slightly superior to that reported by some other authors (Ray *et al.*, 1970; Myers *et al.*, 1978)—could not be correlated with the presence of open foot lesions.

Late Patency

Our results compare favourably with those reported by other centres: accumulated patency was 74.7% at one year, 61.3% at three years, 57.3% from the sixth year forward.

The five-year patency in a group of ten series reported from 1970 to 1980 by ten authors (Baddeley *et al.*, 1970; Fontaine *et al.*, 1970; Darling and Linton, 1972; Kaminsky *et al.*, 1973; De Weese and Rob, 1977; Harris and May, 1979; Mellière *et al.*, 1980; Perdue *et al.*, 1980; Sonnenfeldt and Cronestrand, 1980; Stephens and MacGowan, 1980) was 62.9%: the ten-year patency (Darling and Linton, 1972; De Weese and Rob, 1977; Szilagyi *et al.*, 1979; Stephens and MacGowan, 1980; Cranley and Hafner, 1981) ranges within 40% and 60%.

Graft patency is in general higher in claudication patients than in limb salvage ones (Darling and Linton, 1972; Kaminsky *et al.*, 1973; LoGerfo *et al.*, 1977; Naji *et al.*, 1978; Donaldson and Mannick, 1978; Codd *et al.*, 1979; Perdue *et al.*, 1980; Stephens and MacGowan, 1980); however, the difference reached rarely the statistical significance as it did in our experience.

Koontz and Stansel (1972) reported better results in ischaemia without trophic lesions than in claudication.

The quality of popliteal outflow did not appear to affect our results. The value of this parameter is debatable, being considered not relevant by some authors (Koontz and Stansel, 1972; Darling and Linton, 1972; Kaminsky *et al.*, 1973) and highly significant by others (Ray *et al.*, 1970; Buda *et al.*, 1976; De Weese and Rob, 1977).

Naji *et al.* (1978) find that outflow grading may affect results in limb salvage cases, not in claudication ones; this finding is not confirmed by Codd *et al.* (1979) who do not attribute any value to outflow grading in a series of limb salvage cases and by Cutler *et al.* (1976), who attribute an equally significant value in both groups of patients.

The latter authors report a beneficial influence of associated lumbar sympathectomy in case of impaired outflow and the same trend is followed by Stephens and MacGowan (1980).

The very good results obtained in case of isolated popliteal artery by Mannick *et al.* (1967) and by Saletta *et al.* (1980) appear to bring further into discussion the value of popliteal outflow grading which, in our opinion, should in any case rely not only on pre-operative angiography but be confirmed by intra-operative angiography, owing to the frequent incompleteness of the former as for the details of distal arterial tree branches.

When outflow grading is optimally performed, correlation between outflow quality and graft patency is reported to reach the significance of linearity (Nicholas and Latshaw, 1979).

Diabetes does not affect the results of femoro-popliteal grafting as for patency, even if there is general agreement on a higher incidence of complications and a reduced long-term survival in diabetics.

CONCLUSIVE REMARKS

During the last decade indications to femoro-popliteal grafting were clearly restricted in favour of the increasing practice of femoro-tibial grafting and of the procedures aiming to enhance blood flow through the profunda femoris artery: however, femoro-popliteal bypass remains a widely diffused reconstructive procedure.

In claudication cases, surgical indication should be quite restrictive, limited only to patients complaining of really disabling symptoms.

Even if the results of femoro-popliteal grafting in claudicants are very satisfactory, the persisting incidence of major amputations as a consequence of graft failure should be kept in mind.

Naji *et al.* (1978a) report an incidence of three major amputations within five years in a group of 100 claudicants submitted to femoro-popliteal grafting; Stephens and MacGowan (1980) report no amputation in claudication cases. These data should compare favourably against the incidence of 0.5% amputation per year in non-operated claudicants included in the Framingham study (Peabody *et al.*, 1974).

We believe that a careful surveillance should anticipate timely the passage from simple claudication to disabling claudication or rest pain; in any case, claudication patients should be operated on *only* if the best chances are assured: good general conditions, experienced surgeon, optimal vein, good popliteal artery.

The results obtained in limb salvage cases fully justify the indications to surgery, mainly when they are evaluated in terms of extended limb salvage and not only of extended graft patency (Baddeley *et al.*, 1970: LoGerfo *et al.*, 1977; Codd *et al.*, 1979; Perdue *et al.*, 1980).

Graft failure or unsuccessful surgical exploration could jeopardize the possibility of a BK amputation, as reported by Stoney (1978) and by Kazmers *et al.* (1980): however, we do not agree with these authors on the opportunity of resorting directly to BK amputation in order to save knee joint; we believe that every effort should be made to save and restore the function of the entire limb, also in sight of the frequently bilateral involvement of limb circulation.

REFERENCES

Baddeley, R. M., Ashton, F., Slaney, G. and Barnes, A. D. (1970). Late results of autogenous vein bypass grafts in femoropopliteal arterial occlusion. *British Medical Journal* **1**, 653.

Buda, J. A., Weber, O. J., McAllister, F. F. and Vorhees, A. B. Jr. (1976). Factors influencing patency of femoropopliteal artery bypass grafts. *American Journal of Surgery* **132**, 8.

Buxton, B., Lambert, R. P. and Pitt, T. T. E. (1980). The significance of vein wall thickness and diameter in relation to the patency of femoropopliteal saphenous vein bypass grafts. *Surgery*, **87**, 425.

Codd, J. E., Barner, H. B., Kaminsky, D. L., Ramey, A. E., Garvin, P. J., Kaiser, G. C. and Willman, V. L. (1979). Extremity salvage by revascularization. *Vascular Surgery* **13**, 95.

Cranley, J. J. and Hafner, C. D. (1981). Newer prosthetic material compared with autogenous saphenous vein for occlusive arterial disease of the lower extremity. *Surgery* **89**, 2.

Cutler, B. S., Thompson, J. E., Kleinsasser, L. R. J. and Hempel, G. K. (1976). Autologous saphenous vein femoropopliteal bypass: analysis of 298 cases. *Surgery* **79**, 325.

Cutler, S. J. and Ederer, F. (1958). Maximum utilization of the life table method in analyzing survival. *Journal of Chronic Diseases* **8**, 699.

Darling, R. C. and Linton, R. R. (1972). Durability of femoropopliteal reconstructions. Endarterectomy versus vein bypass grafts. *American Journal of Surgery* **123**, 472.

De Weese, J. A. and Rob, C. G. (1977). Autogenous venous grafts ten years later. *Surgery* **82**, 775.

Donaldson, M. G. and Mannick, J. A. (1980). Femoropopliteal bypass grafting for intermittent claudication. Is pessimism warranted? *Archives of Surgery (Chicago)* **115**, 724.

Fontaine, R., Fontaine, J. L., Lampert, M. and Grosse, A. (1970). Personal experience with reconstructive arterial surgery in femoro-popliteal obstructions. *Journal of Cardiovascular Surgery* **11**, Suppl. 3, 89.

Harris, J. and May, J. (1979). A comparison between saphenous vein and dacron velour grafts for femoropopliteal bypass. *Australian and New Zealand Journal of Surgery* **49**, 211.

Kaminsky, D. L., Barner, H. B., Dorighi, J. A., Kaiser, G. C. and Willman, V. L. (1973). Femoropopliteal bypass with reversed autogenous vein. *Annals of Surgery* **177**, 232.

Kazmers, M., Satiani, B. and Evans, W. E. (1980). Amputation level following unsuccessful distal limb salvage operations. *Surgery* **87**, 683.

King, R. B., Myers, K. A., Scott, D. F., Devine, T. J., Johnson, N. and Morris, P. J. (1980). Femoropopliteal vein grafts for intermittent claudication. *British Journal of Surgery* **67**, 489.

Koontz, T. J. and Stansel, H. C. Jr. (1972). Factors influencing patency of the autogenous vein-femoropopliteal bypass graft: an analysis of 74 cases. *Surgery* **71**, 753.

LoGerfo, F. W., Corson, J. D. and Mannick, J. A. (1977). Improved results with femoropopliteal vein grafts for limb salvage. *Archives of Surgery (Chicago)* **112**, 567.

Mannick, J. A., Jackson, B. T., Coffman, J. D. and Hume, D. M. (1967). Success of bypass vein grafts in patients with isolated popliteal artery segments. *Surgery* **61**, 17.

Mellière, D., Bertin, J., Olivier, J. J., Lasry, G., Danis, R. K., Gilliet, G. and Vasile, N. (1980). Les pontages veineux inversés de l'axe fémoro-poplité. *Nouvelle Presse Medicale* **9**, 681.

Myers, K. A., King, R. B., Scott, D. F., Johnson, N. and Morris, P. J. (1978). Surgical treatment of the severely ischaemic leg: II — salvage rates. *British Journal of Surgery* **65**, 779.

Naji, A., Barker, C. F., Berkowitz, H. D., Chu, J. and Roberts, B. (1978). Femoro-popliteal vein grafts for claudication: analysis of 100 consecutive cases. *Annals of Surgery* **188**, 79.

Naji, A., Chu, J., McCombs, P. R., Barker, C. F., Berkowitz, H. D. and Roberts, B. (1978). Results of 100 consecutive femoropopliteal vein grafts for limb salvage. *Annals of Surgery* **188**, 162.

Nicholas, G. G. and Latshaw, R. F. (1979). Femoropopliteal bypass grafting: predictive value of preoperative angiography. *American Journal of Surgery* **138**, 672.

Peabody, C. N., Kannel, W. B. and McNamara, P. M. (1974). Intermittent claudication: surgical significance. *Archives of Surgery (Chicago)* **109**, 693.

Perdue, G. D., Smith, R. B. III, Veazey, C. R. and Ansley, J. D. (1980). Revascularization for severe limb ischaemia. *Archives of Surgery (Chicago)* **115**, 168.

Ray, F. S., Lape, C. P., Lutes, C. A. and Dillihunt, R. C. (1970). Femoropopliteal saphenous vein bypass grafts. Analysis of 150 cases. *American Journal of Surgery* **119**, 385.

Saletta, C., Hopkins, W., Littooy, F. N. and Baker, W. H. (1980). Femoral-isolated popliteal bypass: selected use in severe limb ischemia. *American Surgeon* **46**, 436.

Sonnenfeldt, T. and Cronestrand, R. (1980). Factors determining outcome of reversed saphenous vein femoropopliteal bypass grafts. *British Journal of Surgery* **67**, 642.

Stephens, R. B. and MacGowan, W. A. L. (1980). Review of 210 autogenous vein by-pass operations. *Journal of Cardiovascular Surgery* **21**, 143.

Stoney, R. J. (1978). Ultimate salvage for the patient with limb-threatening ischemia. Realistic goals and surgical considerations. *American Journal of Surgery* **136**, 228.

Szilagyi, D. E., Hageman, J. H., Smith, R. F., Elliott, J. P., Brown, F. and Dietz, P. (1979). Autogenous vein grafting in femoro-popliteal atherosclerosis: The limits of its effectiveness. *Surgery* **86**, 836.

FEMORO-TIBIAL BYPASS GRAFTING WITH REVERSED AUTOLOGOUS SAPHENOUS VEIN: EXPERIENCE IN 61 CONSECUTIVE PATIENTS

S. Stipa, A. Cavallaro, A. Alessandrini, M. Garofalo, A. Sterpetti and A. Mingoli

IV Cattedra di Patologia Chirurgica dell'Università di Roma, Rome, Italy

MATERIAL AND METHODS

From November 1969 to February 1981, 61 patients (61 limbs) were submitted to femoro-tibial reconstruction by means of reversed autologous saphenous vein: the number of bypasses totalled 75, being ten patients operated on two times and two patients operated on three times.

During the same period, 51 additional tibial reconstructions with the bypass technique were performed on 38 patients, in which graft material other than autologous saphena was used (cephalic and/or basilic vein 3; Dacron + autologous vein 2; expanded Polytetrafluoroethylene 46): these are not included in the present report.

At the time of operation (or first operation) age ranged from 28 to 87 years (mean 59); most patients (54 = 88.5%) were male.

Incidence of significant associated diseases was relevant.

Diabetes	24 (39.3%)
Heart	23 (37.7%)
Lung	12 (19.6%)
Kidney	9 (14.7%)
CNS	6 (9.8%)

Serono Symposium No. 44, "Peripheral Arterial Diseases: Medical and Surgical Problems", edited by S. Stipa and A. Cavallaro, 1982. Academic Press, London and New York.

Only 17 patients (27.8%) were free from associated diseases, being:

19 (31.3%) affected by one associated disease
20 (32.7%) affected by two associated diseases
5 (8.2%) affected by three associated diseases

Eight patients had been submitted, at other institutions, to homolateral lumbar sympathectomy, from one to 12 months, with the following results:

Status quo	5
Worsening	1
Short-lasting improvement	2

In two patients, a contralateral lumbar sympathectomy had been performed with long-term improvement.

Reconstructive surgery aiming to improve inflow to deep femoral artery, was performed in eight limbs: six times aorto-femoral grafting, performed 1–12 months before, did not succeed in relieving ischaemic symptoms, in spite of good anatomical results; in two limbs, iliaco-femoral TEA was performed in one stage with femoro-tibial grafting.

In three patients, failure or complications of a saphenous vein femoro-popliteal bypass graft, performed by us respectively 1.6 and 30 months before, prompted us to reoperate, changing into a femoro-tibial bypass.

In five cases, the technique of jump-bypass was used.

(1) Two times electively and in one stage, the tibial branch taking-off from a femoro-popliteal bypass.

(2) Three times in two stages (emergency 2, election 1), the distal branch arising from a femoro-tibial bypass.

Operative indication, in 61 limbs was:

Disabling claudication	5 (8.2%)
Rest pain	20 (32.8%)
Gangrene	36 (59.0%)

Pre-operative evaluation included angiography under the form of aortography (either by the translumbar route or according to Seldinger's technique) or of femoral arteriography and, from the end of 1971, CW Doppler ultrasound.

In five patients, the diagnosis of rickettsial arteritis was suspected on account of positivity of serological tests (Rickettsia Burnettii 3, RQ18 2) according to Babudieri and Zardi (1952); in one case the circulatory impairment derived from iatrogenic trauma; in all other cases typical atherosclerotic lesions were evident.

The operation was performed under general (58 times), local (six times) or spinal (11 times) anaesthesia.

The site for distal anastomosis was selected on the basis of pre-operative angiography and Doppler findings as well as of direct examination of the artery and intra-operative distal arteriography.

Distribution of distal anastomosis in 75 procedures was:

Tibio-peroneal trunk	4 (5.3%)
Peroneal artery	6 (7.9%)
Post-tibial artery (upper third)	3 (3.9%)
Post-tibial artery (middle third)	6 (7.9%)
Post-tibial artery (lower third)	27 (36.3%)
Medial plantar artery	2 (2.6%)
Anterior tibial artery (popliteal space)	10 (13.0%)
Anterior tibial artery (anterior tibial compartment)	16 (21.8%)
Pedal artery	1 (1.3%)

Approach to tibial vessels was accomplished by the medial route for popliteal trifurcation, posterior tibial and peroneal arteries; through the anterolateral aspect of the leg for anterior tibial artery.

The proximal anastomosis was put on common femoral artery whenever possible; the bypass take-off sites are distributed as follows:

Common femoral artery	57 (76.2%)
Deep femoral artery	7 (9.3%)
Endarterectomized superficial femoral artery	2 (2.6%)
Limb of Dacron A–F graft	1 (1.3%)
Popliteal artery	3 (4.0%)
Femoro-popliteal bypass	2 (2.6%)
Femoro-tibial bypass	3 (4.0%)

In most cases, the internal saphena, excised from the malleolar level to its termination, was long enough to bridge the distance between proximal and distal anastomoses; in eight cases it was necessary to compound the graft from two or more pieces of vein, from both legs. The vein, once excised, was gently distended with heparinized normal saline; veins with diameter inferior to 4 mm were discarded.

The proximal anastomosis was taylored with a running 5-0 suture; the distal one with running 6-0 suture; many times, however, a series of interrupted stitches was used to optimally mould the distal corner of the lower anastomosis.

The bypass route was in general anatomic in reconstructions ending on tibioperoneal trunk, posterior tibial and peroneal arteries; mainly subcutaneous in those ending on the anterior tibial artery beyond the interosseous membrane.

Anticoagulation was used only during the operative procedure.

Intra-operative angiography was used sometimes to control the state of the bypass, more often to choose the best site for implantation of the bypass termination.

The follow up was performed by direct examination of the patients, both clinical and instrumental (CW Doppler); control arteriography was performed in few cases and usually when misfunction of the graft was evident.

Analysis of results was made following Cutler and Ederer (1958).

RESULTS

Early Results

Post-operative mortality was 4.9%: three patients.

Two patients died from heart failure after thrombosis of a second graft; one died from diabetic coma with second graft patent.

Early failure affected 20 grafts in nine limbs of surviving patients and three grafts in three limbs of patients subsequently died after a second graft attempt.

Of the nine limbs unsuccessfully submitted to surgery, seven were amputated at AK level (in two of them a transmetatarsal amputation had been attempted when the graft was still patent).

Early failure was evident, in most cases, 24–36 h after the operation, only in five limbs there was a satisfactory function of the bypass for one to two weeks: in two of these, infection with skin disruption leading to uncovered graft at anastomotic sites, was the evident cause of failure.

Late Results

Seven patients died during the course of the follow up and six grafts failed: no graft failure was observed from the 36th month forward.

Late graft failure was attributable two times to iatrogenic trauma.

(1) One false aneurysm with ensuing thrombosis followed a control angiography erroneously performed by Seldinger's technique on the limb bearing the bypass.

(2) A subcutaneous bypass, misdiagnosed as "pulsating varix" was submitted to sclerotherapy.

In one case thrombosis followed a sustained hypotension and in another one an exaggerated and prolonged knee flexion (long trip by car). Three of these patients were submitted to AK amputation, after an unsuccessful attempt of re-operation.

In two other patients, with positive serology for rickettsiae, late bypass closure did not affect the positive result of the reconstructive procedure, coinciding with spontaneous recanalization of popliteal artery in the former and development of an effective collateral flow through the superior genicular artery in the latter.

In Tables I and II the cumulative patency and the status at the end of the follow up are reported.

The percentage of limb salvage was slightly superior to that of limb with patent graft and obviously superior to that of graft patency (Figs 1 and 2).

Toe or transmetatarsal amputation was performed on 19 limbs with patent graft; eventual graft failure in five limbs led to major amputation in two cases of early failure and in one out of three cases of late failure.

No difference was observed as for graft patency between diabetic and non diabetic patients (Fig. 3); late survival was significantly reduced in diabetics (Fig. 4).

Table I. Accumulative patency of 75 femoro-tibial vein grafts (61 patients, 75 grafts)[a]

Interval	Grafts at risk	Failing grafts	Withdrawn from follow up: Death	Withdrawn from follow up: End of follow up	Interval failure rate (%)	Interval patency (%)	Accumulated patency (%)
months							
0–1	75	23	3	0	31.2	68.8	68.8
1–6	49	1	1	6	2.2	97.8	67.3
6–12	41	3	1	2	7.6	92.4	62.2
12–24	35	0	0	0	0	100	62.2
24–36	35	2	0	4	6.1	93.9	58.4
36–48	29	0	1	5	0	100	58.4
48–60	23	0	1	4	0	100	58.4
60–72	18	0	1	7	0	100	58.4
72–84	10	0	1	4	0	100	58.4
84–96	5	0	1	0	0	100	58.4
96–108	4	0	0	0	0	100	58.4
108–120	4	0	0	0	0	100	58.4

[a] Ten patients operated on twice, two patients operated on three times.

Table II. State at the end of the follow-up (1–128 months, mean 48 months).

Patients	58	
Limbs	58	
Patent graft		43 (74.1%)
Saved limb		48 (82.7%)
No symptoms		22/48 (45.8%)
Claudication		24/48 (50.0%)
Rest pain		2/48 (4.2%)

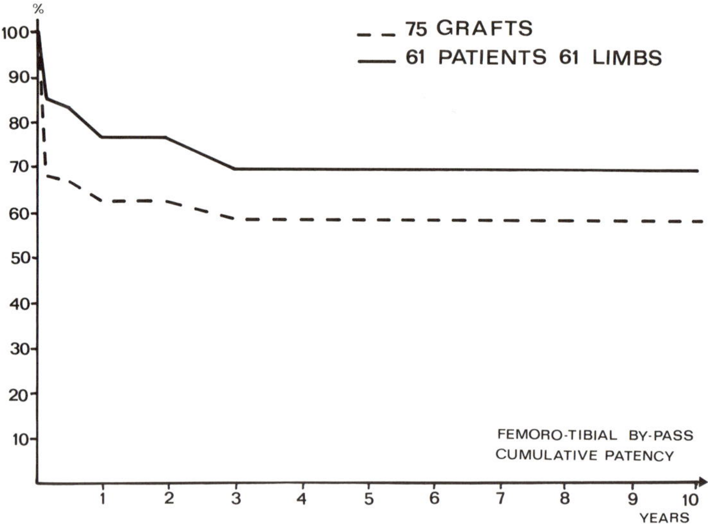

Fig. 1. Cumulative patency of 75 femoro-tibial vein grafts performed on 61 limbs.

No difference was found in graft patency according to the site of distal anastomosis and, in particular, bypasses ending on peroneal artery behaved quite similarly as those ending on posterior or anterior tibial arteries; the more or less proximal position of lower anastomosis did not affect the results. Our first tibial reconstruction, patent from 128 months, was a femoro-peroneal bypass. Both grafts on medial plantar artery failed; the graft on pedal artery is patent from more than 30 months. Of the five bypass constructed by the jump technique:

(1) One performed electively, in one stage (femoro-popliteal + posterior tibial) is patent from six years.

(2) The second one similarly performed, failed almost immediately.

(3) In the three cases of tibial + jump tibial bypass performed in two stages, there were one early failure, one failure after three months, one extended patency.

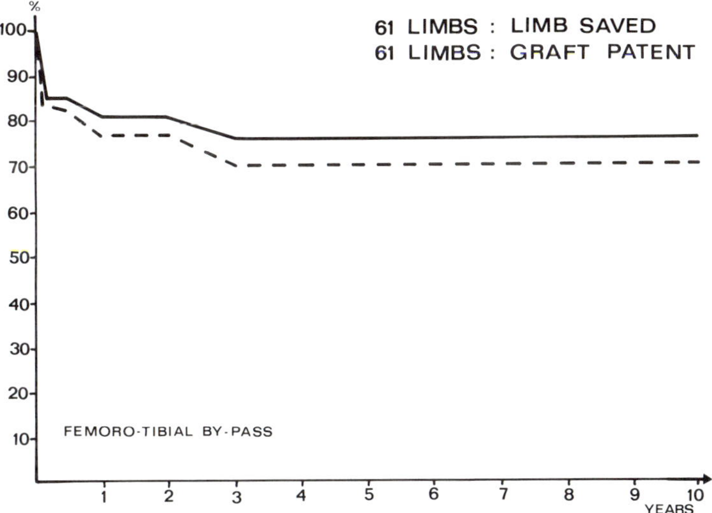

Fig. 2. Cumulative behaviour of the 61 limbs operated on, as for definite salvage and graft patency (dotted line).

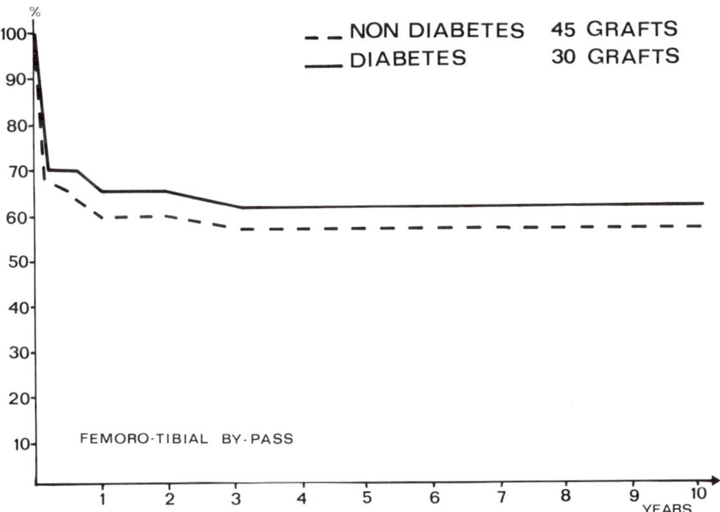

Fig. 3. Cumulative graft patency according to the presence/absence of diabetes.

COMMENT

Our results can be compared favourably with those reported by other authors (Imparato *et al.*, 1973; Szilagyi *et al.*, 1979); Reichle *et al.* (1979) report a five-year patency of about 47%.

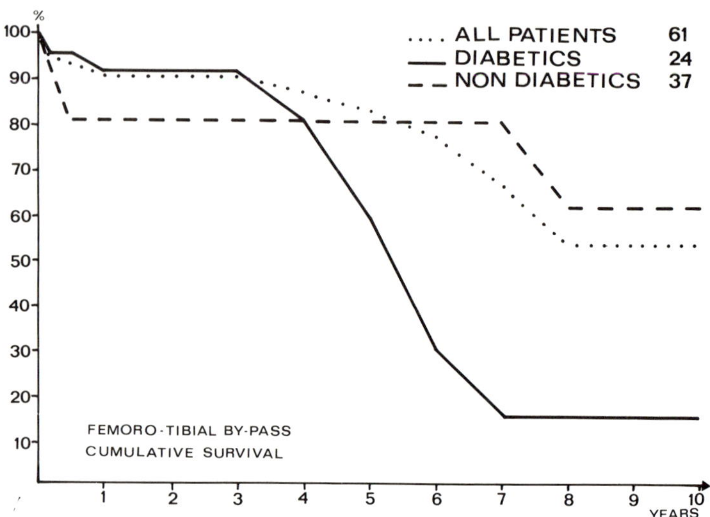

Fig. 4. Cumulative survival of the entire patient population and according to the presence/absence of diabetes.

Worth of mention, late patency, in ours as well as in others' experience, is rather constant after an impressively high incidence of failures within the first year.

Technical faults and wrong indication should account for the majority of early failures: in our experience, the latter should bear a greater importance, being our philosophy to "try" the bypass, when the only alternative is a major amputation, even in very prohibitive local conditions, and the constant failure of our early re-grafting procedures should indicate as not correct our attitude: however, the extended success scantly achieved in "desperate" cases should act in favour of our trend, yet tedious and anti-economic.

The lack of difference in results according to the artery used for distal anastomosis is also reported by other authors (Jausseran *et al.*, 1977); the role of peroneal artery remains however controversial: Szilagyi *et al.* (1979) and Dardik *et al.* (1979) report a lower patency, both early and late, with femoro-peroneal bypass; contrarily, very good results are reported by Graham and Hanel (1981) and the fundamental role of peroneal artery, when both tibial arteries are occluded, is stressed by Hirai *et al.* (1980); in the experience of Reichle *et al.* (1980) results of peroneal reconstructions are slightly inferior to those of the tibial ones only within the first two years: thence forward the behaviour of both types of bypasses is quite similar.

Prescinding from eventual technical difficulties, the patency of a tibial graft is probably a matter of outflow quality and not of site and calibre of artery, as tested also by the good results achievable through bypasses ending on pedal artery (Van Gestel *et al.*, 1977; Heimann and Schanzer. 1979) and through complex (sequential bypass, jump-bypass) or multiple revascularization procedure (Flinn *et al.*, 1980; Jarrett *et al.*, 1980; Ip *et al.*, 1980).

Diabetes does not appear to influence significantly the behaviour of tibial grafting procedures, in ours as well as in others' experience (Ferguson *et al.*, 1978; Reichle *et al.*, 1980).

In conclusion, when facing major amputation, femoro-tibial grafting appears a quite acceptable procedure, in spite of the high percentage of early failures, mainly if one considers that extended limb salvage rates are in general superior to patency rates (Tingaud *et al.*, 1978).

REFERENCES

Babudieri, B. and Zardi, O. (1952). Ricerche diagnostiche sulla febbre Q. *Giornale di Malattie Infettive e Parassitarie* **4**, 190.

Cutler, S. J. and Ederer. F. (1958). Maximum utilization of the life table method in analyzing survival. *Journal of Chronic Diseases* **8**, 699.

Dardik, H., Ibrahim, I. M. and Dardik, I. I. (1979). The role of the peroneal artery for limb salvage. *Annals of Surgery* **189**, 189.

Ferguson, I. A., Rosengarten, D.S., Stuchbery, F. E. and Barnett, A. J. (1978). Arterial reconstruction extending below the popliteal bifurcation. *British Journal of Surgery* **65**, 410.

Flinn, W. R., Flanigan, D. P., Verta, M. J. Jr., Bergan, J. J. and Yao, J. S. T. Jr. (1980). Sequential femoral-tibial by-pass for severe limb ischemia. *Surgery* **88**, 358.

Graham, J. W. and Hanel, K. C. (1981). Vein grafts to the peroneal artery. *Surgery* **89**, 264.

Heimann, T. and Schanzer, H. (1979). Popliteal-to-dorsalis pedis by-pass for limb salvage: a case report. *Vascular Surgery* **13**, 125.

Hirai, M., Ohta, T. and Shionoya, S. (1980). The role of the peroneal artery in arterial occlusive disease of the leg. *Vascular Surgery* **14**, 78.

Imparato, A. M., Kim, G. E., Madayas, M. and Haveson, S. (1973). Angiographic criteria for successful tibial arterial reconstructions. *Surgery* **74**, 830.

Ip, M. W., Le Veen, H. H. and Piccone, V. A. (1980). Limb salvage by inverted "Y" grafts to below knee arteries. *Journal of Cardiovascular Surgery* **21**, 329.

Jarrett, F., Berkoff, H. A. and Crummy, A. B. (1980). Segmental femoro-tibial by-pass: clinical results. *Canadian Journal of Surgery* **23**, 78.

Jausseran, J. M., Reggi, M., Dubouloz, M. and Courbier, R. (1977). Les pontages fémoro-jambiers. Appréciation des résultats à distance. *Angeiologie* **29**, 135.

Reichle, F. A., Martinson, H. W. and Rankin, K. P. (1980). Infrapopliteal arterial reconstruction in the severely ischemic lower extremity. A comparison of long-term results of peroneal and tibial by-passes. *Annals of Surgery* **191**, 59.

Reichle, F. A., Rankin, K. P., Tyson, R. R., Finestone, A. J. and Shuman, C. R. (1979). Long-term results of 474 arterial reconstructions for severely ischemic limbs: A fourteen year follow-up. *Surgery* **85**, 93.

Reichle, F. A., Rankin, K. P., Tyson, R. R., Finestone, A. J. and Shuman, C. R. (1979). Long-term results of femoroinfrapopliteal by-pass in diabetic patients with severe ischemia of the lower extremity. *American Journal of Surgery* **137**, 653.

Szilagyi, D. E., Hageman, J. H., Smith R. F., Elliott, J. P., Brown, F. and Dietz, P. (1979). Autogenous vein grafting in femoro-popliteal atherosclerosis: the limits of its effectiveness. *Surgery* **86**, 836.

Tingaud, R., Quancard, X., Masson, B., Mamere, L., Dumas, P. J., Desplantez, J. and Serise, J. M. (1978). Les pontages jambiers. Bilan de 67 observations. *Chirurgie* **104**, 162.

Van Gestel, R., Casaer, Y. and De Canniere, P. (1977). La greffe veineuse sur les artères du pied. *Angeiologie* **29**, 219.

A FIVE-YEAR CONSECUTIVE STUDY OF THE SAPHENOUS VEIN USED FOR ARTERIAL BYPASS *IN SITU*

A. M. Karmody, D. M. Shah and R. P. Leather

Department of Surgery, Albany Medical College, Albany, New York, USA

INTRODUCTION

The idea of using the saphenous vein *in situ* as an infrainguinal arterial bypass was first suggested by Rob 20 years ago (May *et al.*, 1965) and the first series of these procedures was reported by Hall in 1962. Although conceptually very attractive, this procedure has however been used only sparingly throughout the world. In the North American literature its results have both been praised (Connolly and Stemmer, 1970) and villified (Barner *et al.*, 1969). Hall (1978) and Gruss *et al.* (1980) working in Europe have continued to report good results with this technique. Because of these favorable experiences, the authors have been encouraged to undertake a prospective attempt at the application of the saphenous vein arterial bypass *in situ*. In contrast to valve fracture as suggested by May *et al.* (1965) and valve excisions by Hall (1962), the authors have used the method of valve incision which was developed and previously described by Leather *et al.* (1979). This report will present the results of a five-year consecutive experience of saphenous vein arterial bypass *in situ*.

CLINICAL MATERIALS AND METHODS

Of 344 consecutive attempts to use the saphenous vein *in situ* for arterial

Serono Symposium No. 44, "Peripheral Arterial Diseases: Medical and Surgical Problems", edited by S. Stipa and A. Cavallaro, 1982. Academic Press, London and New York.

bypass, it was possible to complete 323 bypasses of which 308 were carried out for limb threatening ischemia. Only these patients will be further considered in this paper. Of the patients in this limb salvage category, 120 were women (37%), 132 were insulin-dependent diabetics (41%) and over 80% were in the seventh and eighth decades of life. The site of the distal anastomoses are shown in Fig. 1. Of the 173 bypasses to the popliteal artery, 17 terminated in isolated segments of this artery. One-hundred-and-thirty-five reconstructions were carried out below the level of the popliteal artery to single tibial arteries or the tibio-peroneal trunk. In eight of these procedures the recipient tibial artery showed no direct angiographic communication with the plantar arterial arch of the foot. Proximal anastomoses were constructed at the level of the common femoral artery in 294 of the 308 bypasses and in 127 of the 135 infrapopliteal bypasses. Approximately 26% of the veins used in the entire series and 40% of the veins used in the infrapopliteal bypasses were 3.5 mm or less at their distal ends.

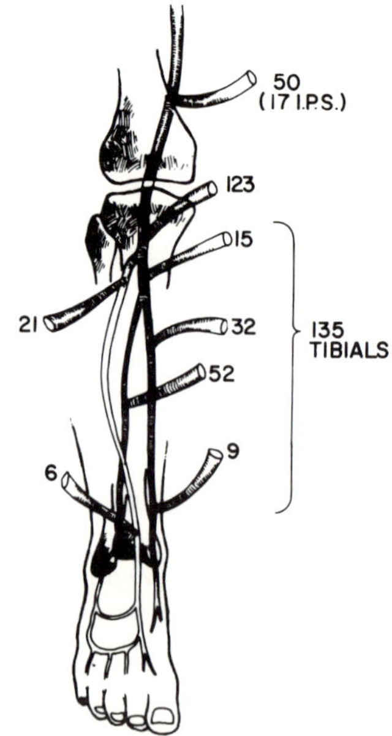

Fig. 1. Sites of distal insertion of bypasses. One-hundred-and-seventy-three were inserted into the popliteal artery of which 17 were isolated popliteal segments. A majority of the tibial bypasses can be seen to be inserted into the peroneal artery.

TECHNIQUE

Although the essential elements of the techniques used are the same as that previously reported, certain modifications have been introduced which further simplify the procedure of valve incision. Micro-scissors of varying lengths have been designed for this purpose and are introduced through the proximal end of the saphenous vein after its detachment from the common femoral vein or through a side branch 2 cm or more proximal to the site of the valve (Fig. 2) (Leather *et al.*, 1981). The authors have also successfully used a

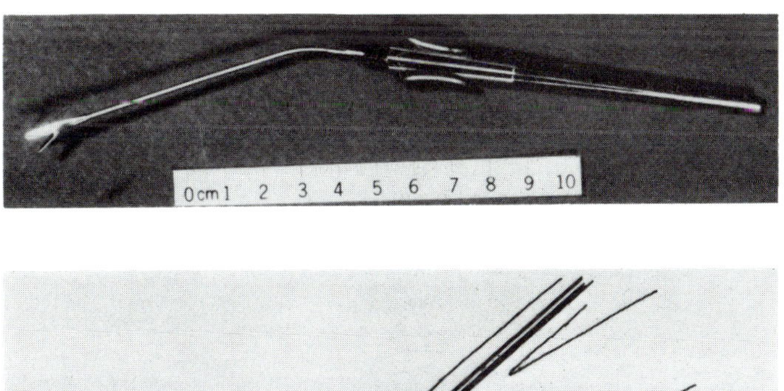

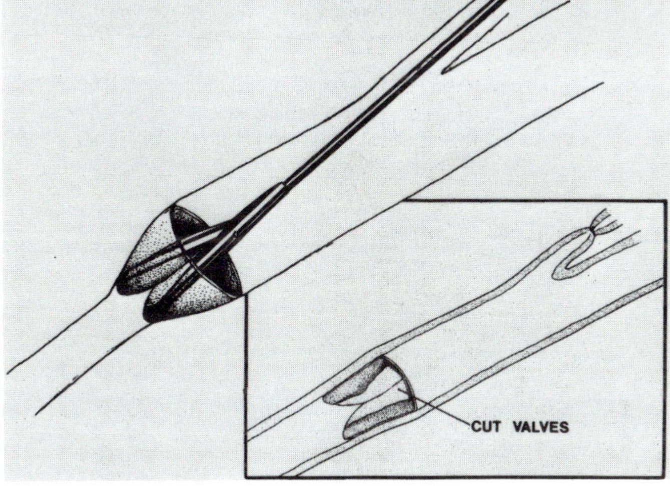

Fig. 2. Original design of micro-scissor made for insertion through a 1-mm side branch proximal to the valve closed by fluid or arterial pressure. The scissor engages the valve and cuts across the fibrous cusps rendering incompetence.

modified long-shafted scissor (25 cm) for valve incision through the open proximal end of the vein to the mid-thigh level (Fig. 3) (Shah and Buchbinder, 1981). In addition, a valvulotome has been specifically designed for achieving valve incision via retrograde passage either through the distal end of the vein or through a suitably placed side branch distal to the valve site (Fig. 4). During both proximal and distal anastomoses the mobilized free segments of saphenous veins were cooled with a cold heparanized Dextran 70 solution to minimize any potential endothelial ischemia and pathological platelet deposition (Leather *et al.*, 1981).

In making the distal arterial exposure, it has been found useful to place the skin incision posterior to the vein which thus remains attached to the upper (tibial) skin flap (Fig. 5). This fixes its position relative to the artery and aids in the achievement of optimal spatial relationships. When the vein has been left

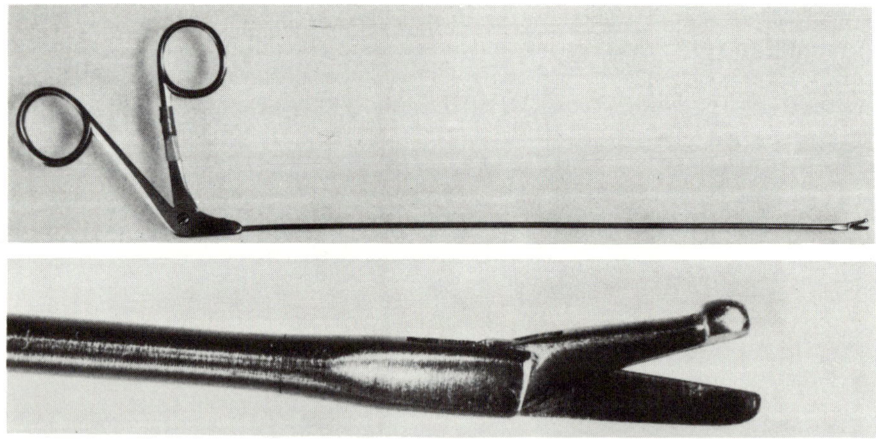

Fig. 3. Later design of the scissor that consists of a long 2-mm shaft, 23 cm in length. Note the blunted edges of the tips to prevent endothelial damage during passage and engagement of the cusps. This scissor is inserted through the open end of a detached saphenous vein and is used for valve incision down to the mid-thigh level.

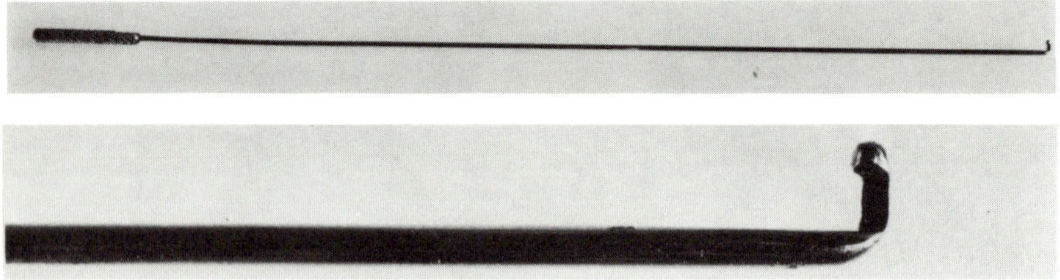

Fig. 4. (a). Valvultome shown in full with inset of the rounded ball end with cutting blade between the shaft and tip.

attached to the posterior tissue flap, this has sometimes resulted in distortions in length and rotation during its anastomosis to the distal artery. After the three or four proximal valves have been incised, usually to the mid-thigh level, the proximal end of the saphenous vein is anastomosed to the femoral artery. Thereafter, arterial pressure is used to dilate the vein and to determine the site of the next distal valve. In lean patients, this is readily identifiable by digital determination of cessation of the subcutaneous venous pulse at the site of a competent valve. This valve site is then exposed through a suitably placed skin incision so that the orientation of the valvotomy scissors or valvulotome within the vein can be clearly seen. We strongly recommend that all manipulations for defunctioning of valves be carried out under direct vision because the most common areas of endothelial damage are caused during this step (Fig. 6). In patients with thick subcutaneous tissue, in whom it may not be possible to feel pulsation in the vein, the valve sites can be determined either by continuous incision along the course of the vein or by passage of a 3 French

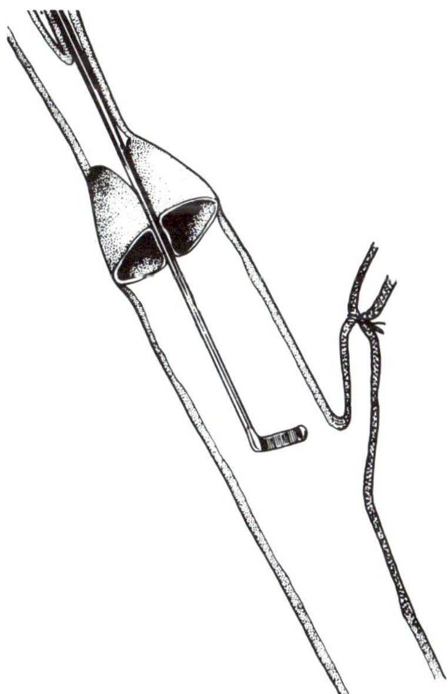

Fig. 4. (b) This instrument is passed through a side branch distally or through a distal open end of the vein. It is self-centering on the cusp and when the sharp edge engages the cusp incises it cleanly.

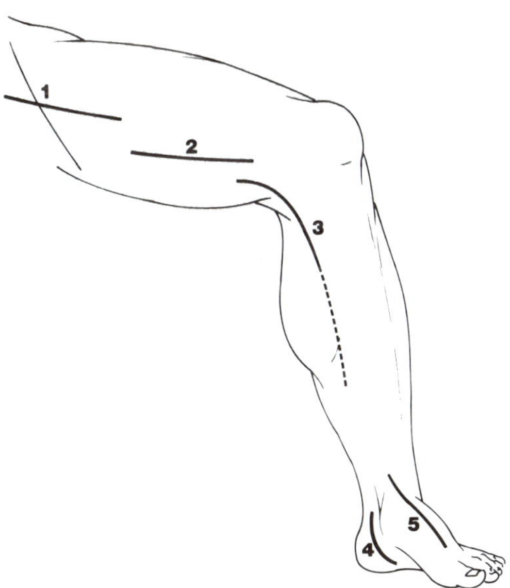

Fig. 5. Incisions used for exposure of the veins and arteries. The dotted line on the calf shows extension of this incision for exposure of the posterior tibial and the peroneal arteries.

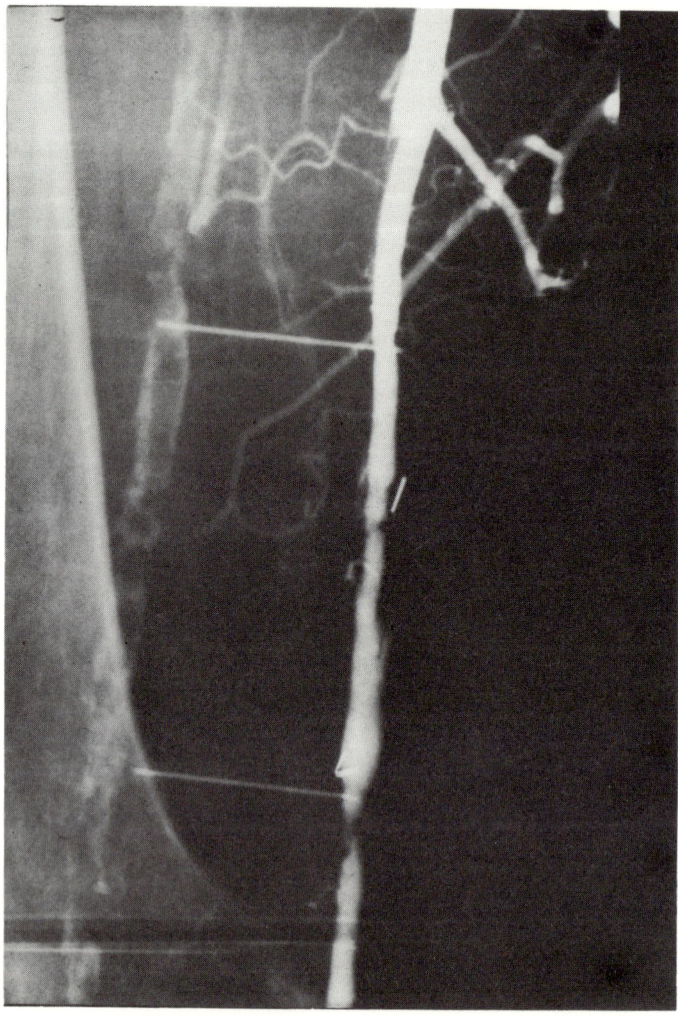

Fig. 6. The vein is left attached to the upper skin flap below the knee because this aids in spacial orientation and prevents twisting. If necessary, a continuous incision over the vein can be made provided undo dissection of the wall is not carried out. Platelet deposition if there is endothelial damage. These injured venous segments need to be widely opened, the platelet removed and a vein patch carried out.

balloon catheter from the proximal open end of the vein or convenient side branch until it impacts on the next competent valve which has been brought into the closed position by arterial pressure or fluid pulsation. The length of the catheter is used to determine the site of a valve and the vein is visualized at this point. This procedure of valve incision is continued until pulsatile flow is achieved through the open distal end of the vein. The tourniquet method of doing the distal anastomosis as described by Bernhard *et al.* (1980) has been extensively used and found to be very efficient. In all other respects the operation has remained the same as conventionally practiced and previously described.

It is now customary for us to use a 3-mm micro Doppler probe (Bach-Simpson) applied intra-operatively directly to the vein and arteries in order to determine the quality of flow to identify hemodynamically significant fistulas. When one of these is present, there may be diminished pulsations in the free segment of vein and the flow signal is characteristically of a soft and low pitch as opposed to a continuous high pitch proximal to or at the site of the fistula. Although the flow probe has been helpful in locating arteriovenous fistulas, the routine use of operative angiography when the anastomoses have been completed is still considered to be essential for the identification and interruption of all functioning arteriovenous fistulas and determination of distal anastomotic problems (Fig. 7).

RESULTS

In the post-operative period all patients have been examined at specific intervals by the authors and only two have been lost to follow up. These post-operative examinations consist of Doppler ultrasound examination along the course of the bypass and pulse volume recordings at rest and following exercise on the treadmill. Pulsations in the bypass were readily determined with certainty by digital examination over the posterio-medial aspect of the knee joint because of the subcutaneous position of the vein in this area. This obviates any confusion concerning palpation of submuscular graft pulses and doubt about the source of flow signals heard in this area with an ultrasound stethoscope.

In 344 consecutive attempts to apply this method, the procedure has had to be abandoned in 21 cases, 16 because of an inadequate vein and five for technical reasons. This has provided a vein utilization rate of 93.9%. This high rate of utilization has been possible because this procedure *in situ* has allowed the use of veins as small as 2 mm in distal diameter. Approximately 40% of the infrapopliteal bypasses were performed with veins of 3.5 mm or less in diameter. Life-table analysis of 308 procedures performed for limb salvage is graphically displayed in Fig. 8, and compared with the results reported by Naji *et al.* (1975). The specific group of 135 bypasses to arteries below the level of the popliteal artery has also been examined by life-table analysis. This is shown in graphic form in Fig. 9, together with the life-table analysis of the cases reported by Reichle and Tyson (1975). There were seven deaths within the peri-operative period (2.3%). A total of ten major amputations were necessary in the 308 limbs at risk. Nine were below the knee and one was above the knee. The cumulative limb salvage at 48 months by life-table analysis is 89.8%. There were ten residual arteriovenous fistulas that required surgical interruption ten days to three months later. These procedures consisted of interrupting the fistulous branch under local anesthesia as an out-patient. Five isolated stenotic lesions were detected on follow-up

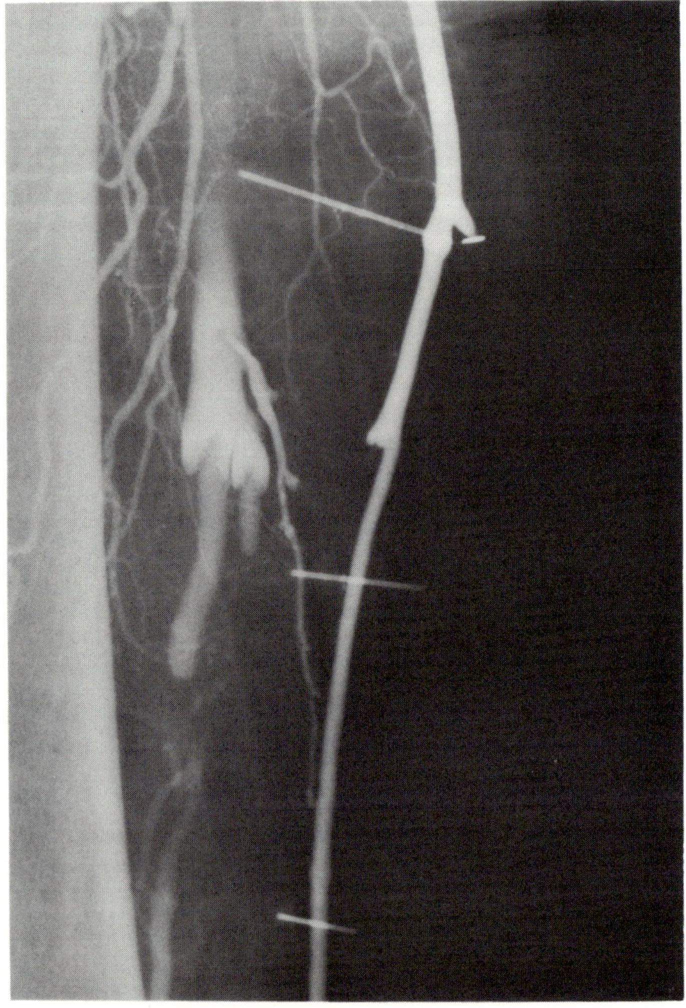

Fig. 7. Small but significant arteriovenous fistula as shown on operative angiogram. The needles mark the position of the fistula that is significant because it communicates directly with the femoral vein and will be a source of increase in the femoral venous pressure.

examination. They were manifested by qualitative changes in pulse wave contour on PVR examination and the development of a pressure gradient within the bypass. All were found to be present at valve sites at which subendothelial hyperplasia had occurred. These lesions were successfully corrected by vein patch angioplasty.

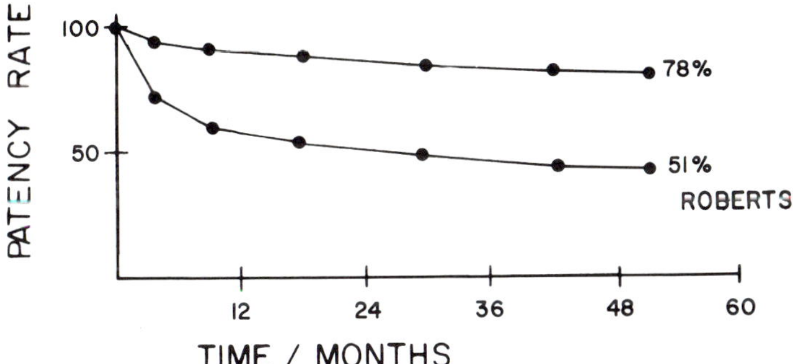

Fig. 8. Life-table analysis of all limb salvage cases. The five-year cumulative patency is 78% versus 51% from the series by Roberts (Naji *et al.*, 1975). This is typical of most reversed vein bypass series.

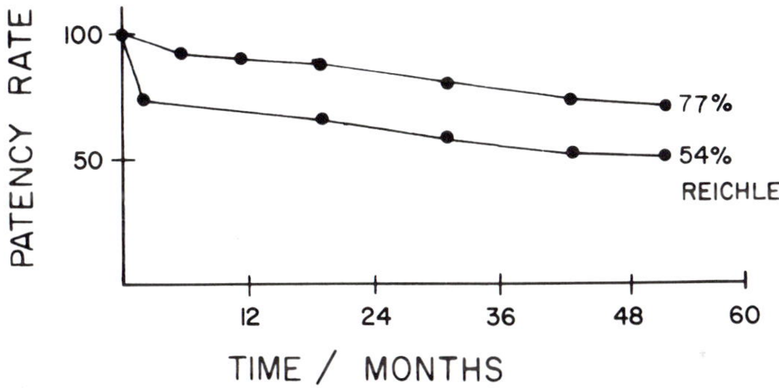

Fig. 9. Separate analysis of 135 infrapopliteal bypasses. These are compared with Reichle's figures (Reichle and Tyson, 1975) which are the best for these operations. Note in both Figs 8 and 9 the sharp fall-off within the first 12 months and then the parallel grafts thereafter.

DISCUSSION

The two problems which are specific to this procedure as opposed to that of harvested reversed vein bypass are those of the presence of venous branches as potential arteriovenous fistulas and the venous valvular obstructions. Most of the side branches of the vein are identified during the visualization of each valve site and mobilization of the proximal and distal ends (Samuels *et al.*, 1968). Operative angiography and the use of micro-probe has helped to identify the rest intra-operatively. On average, only two to three fistulous venous branches will require interruption in continuity after the arterial anastomoses have been performed and in no instance has an arteriovenous fistula jeopardized the patency of the bypass distally.

However, it is clear from our experience to date that the most important feature of this procedure is the efficient and atraumatic defunctioning of venous valves. To achieve this, we wish to stress again that it is imperative that the valve site be visualized in all instances so that it can be incised under direct vision. This can be done most efficiently if the leaflets are brought into the closed position by arterial pressure or proximal fluid pulsations. The cutting instrument should engage the valve leaflets accurately along the free edge of the cusp and 90° to its plane of closure. As previously described by Samuels, this plane is almost always parallel to the skin (Samuels *et al.*, 1968).

These requirements impose certain design features on any instrumentation that has or is being developed for these purposes. The shape of all cutting edges should be so designed that only the valve is exposed to the sharp edge, i.e. there should be no risk of damage to the vein wall from the cutting edge of the instrument. All parts of the instruments that are likely to impinge on the vein wall should be rounded or gently curved and blunt. Two types of "valve incisions" scissors have been designed with blades that meets these requirements. With respect to the modified micro-scissors, the size of the blades and the stem on which they are carried have been made as small as possible so that they can be introduced through a 1- to 2-mm side branch. To accommodate the wide variation in proximal vein diameters and the corresponding valve dimensions, two pairs of scissors have usually been used to reach valves in the mid-thigh region from the open end of the detached saphenous vein. The blades of this instrument are ball-tipped to achieve their bluntness. A valvulotome has also been designed with these features so that its tip is a round ball and the edge between the shaft and this ball has been carefully sharpened under a microscope. It is self-centering on the valve cusp and direct inspection of these valves have shown cleanly divided cusps.

From the above description of principles of instrument design for efficient valve defunctioning without traumatizing the venous endothelium, it is clear that our philosophy has been averse to the use of instruments which pass or are pulled along the vein wall thus tearing the valve down this passage. This is particularly true of instruments which fit snugly against the vein wall itself. These include all the instruments that are passed from the distal end of the vein and are then withdrawn from the proximal vein in a distal direction. Such instruments that cause valve fracture have been designed by Skagseth and Hall (1973) and used by himself and by Gruss *et al.* (1980) and that designed and used by J. Cartier (personal communication) of Montreal on which work has never yet been published to our knowledge. One of the difficulties of these particular instruments has also been that the size of the vein at the distal end is limited to 3.5–4 mm since the present instruments are not made any smaller than these sizes. Since a very high percentage of the veins used by us for single tibial bypass are below this and since stretching of small veins by dilating instruments are inimical to their integrity, we have not made prolonged attempts to use these devices. Samuels *et al.* (1968) have also designed an instrument along the lines similar to the ones mentioned above. We have tried to use this instrument by courtesy of the designer and also a Hall valve-stripper which has been made to our modifications with cutting edges. However, we have become concerned about their performance and propensity for endothelial damage. In addition, the poor results reported by Barner *et al.* (1969) concerned a technique of prograde valve fracture and all of these intruments in fact achieve valvular dysfunction by means of forceful fracture. Valve incision as described above has, therefore, remained our standard technique for these procedures and appears to comfortably satisfy these technical requirements.

Even casual inspection of the life-table plots show that after six months, the attrition rates in both the *in situ* and reversed saphenous vein bypass are similar if not identical. This is in agreement with well-documented work that a stable endothelial surface is slowly achieved in reversed veins only after an interval of several weeks (Szilagyi *et al.*, 1973). The difference in patency between these two methods of use of the saphenous vein is clearly determined by their performance within the first six months and appear to be related to the maintenance of a normal endothelium in the arterialized vein *in situ*. This is reflected in an almost total lack of thrombogenicity even when the flow rates that can be obtained in these conduits are very low. This is exemplified by the long-term patency of procedures *in situ* in which very limited outflow tracts are used. In collaboration with B. Y. Lee, in such patients we have measured resting flow rates in tibial bypasses as low as 23 ml min^{-1}. This finding should not be surprising because medieval surgical writings have recorded that a completely stagnant intravenous column of blood will remain fluid for many weeks if the endothelial surface has not been disturbed (living test tube). In this respect, Sauvage has also shown in his studies on external velour Dacron grafts that with the formation of a stable endothelial surface, the "thrombogenicity index" of these artificial grafts will rise dramatically from 30 s at the time of implantation to 2 h when the tissue lining of the graft is fully established (Sauvage *et al.*, 1974). Hence, the importance of an intact endothelial lining for arterial conduits cannot be overestimated. This lack of thrombogenicity of the bypass *in situ* is further shown by our experiences with two patients, one of whom had occlusion of the outflow tract for three days and the other for ten days. In both of these patients the conduit *in situ* continued to pulsate and the blood within them remained fluid thus allowing their use as inflow sources for more distal arterial reconstructions. Angiograms of these two patients also showed that an unexpected bonus of a small degree of outflow was provided by the intact vasa vasorum of the vein wall.

These conclusions based on clinical observations are strengthened by our canine experimental data, which show that at one-, four-, eight-, sixteen- and 24-week intervals scanning electron micrographs of the endothelial surface of arterialized bypass *in situ* has showed consistently normal appearances (Fig. 10) while the endothelial surface of a cooled reversed vein (Abbot *et al.*, 1974) is edematous, considerably denuded of endothelium and scarred by fibroblastic ingrowth (Fig. 11). Those experiments show that within the first few weeks of arterialization the endothelium is preserved in the bypass *in situ*, whereas that of the reversed vein is seriously compromised (Buchbinder *et al.*, 1981). In general, at least 16 weeks were required before a stable endothelium surface was achieved in the excised reversed vein in this experimental model.

Although the procedure of saphenous arterial bypass *in situ* by the method of valve incision requires greater technical skills and experience, the continued demonstration of superior patency and greater vein utilization rates

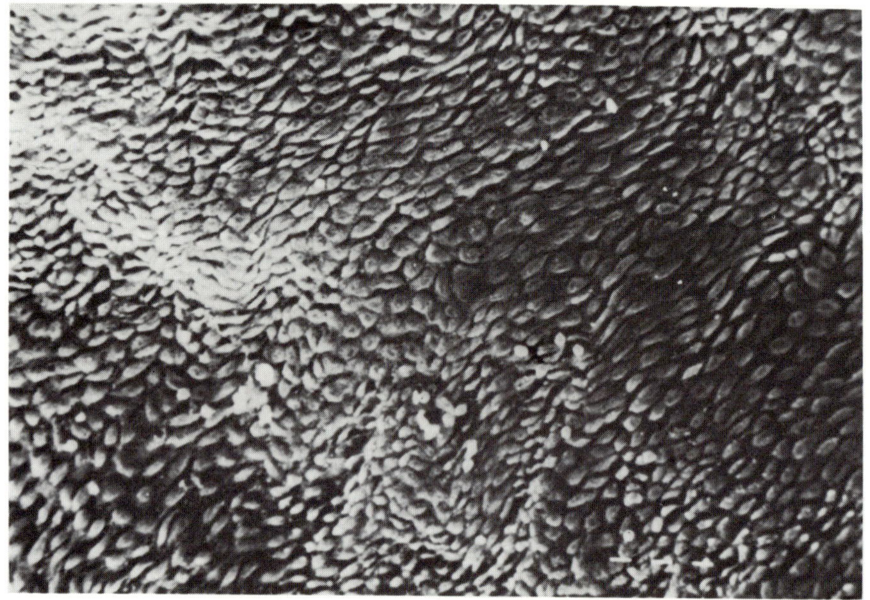

Fig. 10. Smooth normal endothelial surface of vein *in situ* at three- and six-month intervals. There is no sign of endothelial deterioration and the wall is not exposed.

when compared with reversed vein justifies continued application and further development of this method of arterial reconstruction.

REFERENCES

Abbott, W., Wieland, S. and Austen, W. G. (1974). Structural changes during preparaton of autogenous venous grafts. *Surgery* **76**, 1031.

Barner, H. B., Judd, D. R., Kaiser, G. C. *et al*. (1969). Late failure of arterialized "In-Situ" saphenous vein. *Archives of Surgery (Chicago)* **99**, 781.

Bernhard, V. M., Boren, C. H. and Towne, J. B. (1980). Pneumatic tourniquet as a substitute for vascular clamps in distal bypass surgery. *Surgery* **87**, 709.

Buchbinder, D., Singh, J. K., Karmody, A. M., Leather, R. P. and Shah, D. M. (1981). Comparison of patency rate and structural changes of *in situ* and reversed vein arterial bypass. *Journal of Surgical Research* **30**, 213.

Connolly, J. E. and Stemmer, G. A. (1970). The non-reversed saphenous vein bypass for femoral-popliteal occlusive disease. *Surgery* **68**, 602.

Gruss, J. D., Karadedos, C., Bartels, D. and Tsafandakis, E. (1980). Experience with the in-situ saphenous vein graft for femoropopliteal bypass. *In* "Arterial Reconstruction of the Lower Limb, Proceedings of an International Symposium". Leuven, Belgium, 7th June 1980. Medical Education Services, Oxford.

Hall, K. V. (1962). The great saphenous vein used "In-Situ" as an arterial shunt after extirpation of the vein valves. *Surgery* **51**, 492.

Hall, K. V. (1978). The saphenous vein used "In-Situ" as an arterial bypass. *American Journal of Surgery* **136**, 123.

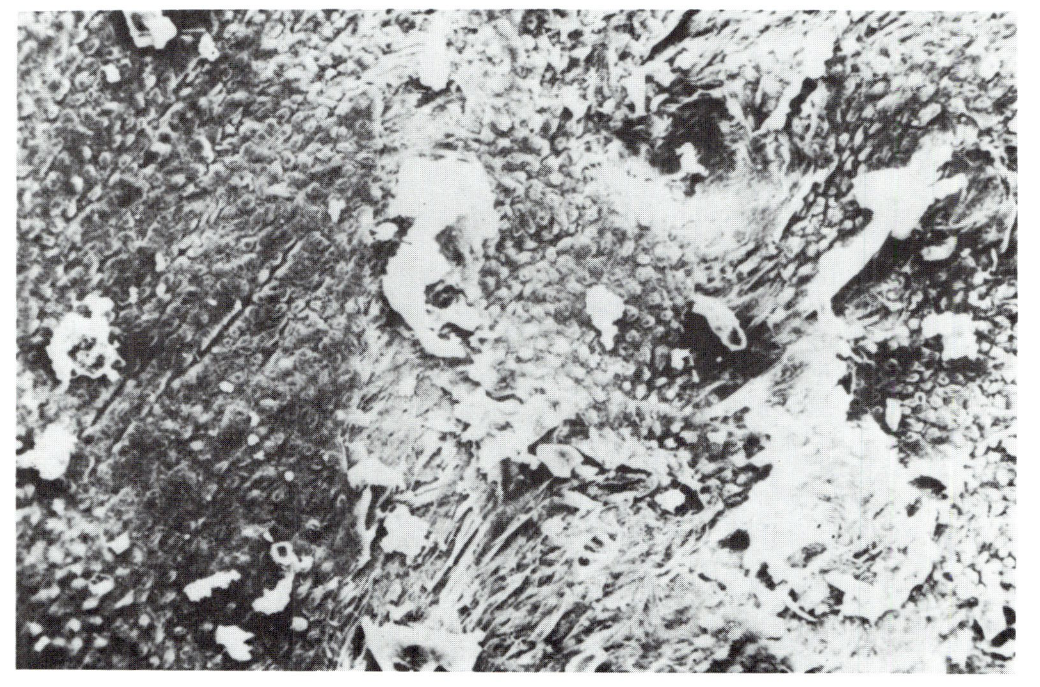

Fig. 11. Contrast to Fig. 10 at three months. The areas of denudation of endothelium are still present, there is much swelling and the wall is exposed thus rendering the vein very thrombogenic.

Leather, R. P.., Powers, S. R. and Karmody, A. M. (1979). A reappraisal of the "In-Situ" saphenous vein arterial bypass: its use in limb salvage. *Surgery* **86**, 453.
Leather, R. P., Shah, D. M., Buchbinder, D., Annest, S. J. and Karmody, A. M. (1981). Further experience with the saphenous vein used *in situ* for arterial bypass. *American Journal of Surgery* **142**, 506.
May, A. G., DeWeese, J. A. and Rob, C. G. (1965). Arterialized "In-Situ" saphenous vein. *Archives of Surgery (Chicago)* **91**, 743.
Naji, A., Chu, J., Roberts, B. *et al.* (1975). Results of 100 consecutive femoropopliteal vein grafts for limb salvage. *Annals of Surgery* **191**, 162.
Reichle, F. A. and Tyson, R. R. (1975). Comparison of long term results of femoropopliteal or femorotibial bypasses for revascularization of severely ischemic lower extremities. *Annals of Surgery* **182**, 449.
Samuels, P. G., Plested, W. G., Cincotti, J. J. *et al.* (1968). "In-Situ" saphenous vein arterial bypass. *American Surgeon* **34**, 122.
Sauvage, L. R., Berger, K. E., Wood, S. J., Yates, S. G. II, Smith, J. C. and Mansfield, P. B. (1974). Interspecies healing of porous arterial prostheses observations 1960–74. *Archives of Surgery (Chicago)* **109**, 698.
Shah, D. M. and Buchbinder, D. (1981). Modified technique to produce valvular incompetence in the "In-Situ" saphenous vein arterial bypass. *Archives of Surgery (Chicago)* **116**, 356.
Skagseth, E. and Hall, K. V. (1973). In-Situ vein bypass. *Scandinavian Journal of Thoracic Cardiovascular Surgery* **7**, 53.
Szilagyi, D. E., Elliott, J. P., Hageman, J. H. *et al.* (1973). Biologic fate of a autogenous vein implants as arterial substitutes. *Annals of Surgery* **178**, 232.

THE NATURAL HISTORY OF FEMORO-POPLITEAL AUTOGENOUS VEIN GRAFTS

D. E. Szilagyi

Department of Surgery, Henry Ford Hospital, Detroit, Michigan, USA

Far from being an inert pipeline, the human artery is a very highly complicated physiologic machine. Each histologic component of the wall — the endothelium, the elastic laminae, the smooth muscle, the vasa vasorum and the ground substance — has its specific and important function. To satisfy these diverse and complex physiologic demands, the ideal "arterial substitute" would obviously have to be another artery of the same donor derivation. But the supply of such grafts is extremely limited and the technique of their procurement complex. In fact, because of its narrow scope, the clinical experience with the use of autogenous arterial grafts is almost negligibly small. If one must take out of consideration autogenous arteries, on grounds of general biologic consideration the most satisfactory compromise for the replacement of an artery would be an autogenous vein. Its superficial location, its physiologic expandability and its physical qualities render it eminently suitable for this purpose.

In this presentation I will attempt to describe briefly the qualities of the greater saphenous vein that make it a satisfactory arterial substitute, the changes it undergoes after implantation, the results achieved with its use and some practical details the observance of which may enhance its usefulness. The background of these remarks is largely my personal experience.

The histologic structure of the greater saphenous vein is characterized by an abundance of smooth muscle elements and the presence of adequate amounts of collagenous and elastic elements. This structure, which assures a tensile

Serono Symposium No. 44, "Peripheral Arterial Diseases: Medical and Surgical Problems", edited by S. Stipa and A. Cavallaro, 1982. Academic Press, London and New York.

strength equal or superior to that of an artery of comparable size, has been one of the revolutionary changes in human anatomy. With upright posture the hydrostatic pressure in a lower extremity vein approaches 100 mmHg, and during acts of physiological effort this value may be considerably higher. In its superficial position, the wall of the greater saphenous vein must contain this pressure without assistance from surrounding tissue elements such as the cushioning effect of musculature. It should be noted that even though the greater saphenous vein, and to a lesser degree the deep veins of the lower extremity, show excellent structural characteristics at birth, it takes a decade or more of upright posture before the vein reaches its full development. Young children's saphenous veins lack this quality and are not suitable for transplantation under arterial hemodynamic conditions.

In 1973–1974 we investigated the post-implantation behaviour of autogenous vein grafts after femoro-popliteal reconstructive arterial surgery by serial angiograms in 260 cases and by histologic study in 31 recovered specimens. The cases had been followed both angiographically and clinically. A scrutiny of the post-operative angiograms in the 260 cases disclosed six types of morphologic abnormality of clinical significance, which can be described briefly as follows (Table I). Intimal thickening consisted of progressive concentric narrowing of the lumen of the graft. In most cases these lesions seemed to originate in the fibroblastic organization of layers of sequential mural thrombi, but at times they represent the angiographic manifestation of subendothelial fibroblastic hyperplasia.

(1) *Atheromatous intimal and mural changes* closely imitated the roentgen appearances of atherosclerotic lesions as seen in the arterial system.
(2) *Fibrosis of venous valves* was seen as a narrow segment of stenosis.
(3) *Traumatic fibrosis* appeared to result from instrumental damage and led to a narrowing a few millimeters in length. Suture stenosis usually appeared as a ring-like stricture.
(4) *Aneurysmal dilatation* was probably a manifestation of advanced atherosclerosis but it may also have resulted from other causes.

The interpretation of the morphologic changes seen in roentgenograms was based on their correlation with findings obtained from the gross and microscopic examination of anatomic specimens. Thirty-one such specimens were recovered (Table II). Nearly one-third of all the recovered grafts showed atherosclerotic changes and these changes appeared to occur more frequently the longer the implant had been in place.

The gross appearance of a well-incorporated vein graft on inspection after recovery four years after implantation shows no visible flaw. On gross examination this vein may be mistaken for a freshly removed surgical specimen. In the microscopic section thick intima was noted made up of mature connective tissue and covered with a smooth endothelium-like layer. The media was thin and the smooth muscle cells markedly diminished. The lack of any cellular infiltrate indicating adverse immune reaction was striking. This was a persistent finding even in those grafts that had undergone atherosclerotic alterations or showed the other changes described earlier.

Because of limitation of space, only the two most important types of

Table I. Autogenous (saphenous) vein implants: roentgenologic structural changes in 220 femoro-popliteal and 40 femoro-infrapopliteal grafts.

Type of lesion	Total number	Mean time of onset (months)	Percentage showing progress	Outcome							
				Observed				Re-operated			
				Open		Closed		Open		Closed	
				No.	%	No.	%	No.	%	No.	%
Intimal thickening	21	16.2	66.6	15	75.0	5	25.0	1	All	–	–
Artherosclerosis	20	45.2	95.0	12	92.3	1	7.7	7	All	–	–
Fibrotic valve	15	14.0	73.3	4	36.4	7	63.6	4	All	–	–
Fibrotic stenosis	11	19.1	90.0	1	11.1	8	88.9	2	All	–	–
Suture stenosis	8	9.0	75.0	3	37.5	5	62.5	0	–	–	–
Aneurysmal dilatation	10	28.0	50.0	9	90.0	1	10.0	0	–	–	–
Total	85	23.9	65 (76.5)	44	(62.0)	27	(38.0)	100.0		–	–

Table II. Autogenous (saphenous) vein implants: incidence of structural change in 31 histologic specimens.

Length of implantation (months)	Atherosclerosis	Fibrotic valve	Fibrotic stenosis	Intimal thickening	Multiple	Normal
12	–	1	2	3	–	1
13–24	1	3	1	2	–	–
25–36	–	1	1	–	–	2
37–48	1	–	–	–	–	–
49–60	2	1	–	–	–	1
61–96	4	–	1	–	–	–
97–146	2	–	–	1	–	–
Total	10	6	5	6	–	4

morphological alterations will be described in detail: atherosclerosis and intimal thickening.

Intimal thickening appears as a somewhat wavy concentric narrowing of almost the entire length of the vein. This diffuse stenosis may be caused by two pathological processes, both leading to thickening of the intima and narrowing of the lumen.

One of the causes of the intimal thickening is the deposition of sequential layers of thrombi. The cause of this lamination of mural clots is undoubtedly a decreased velocity of flow. This is an early phase of the process that eventually will lead to loss of patency in most of the grafts with poor outflow tracts. In the second variant of intimal thickening the principal change is the marked increase in the smooth muscle and connective tissue elements of the sub-endothelial layer. This phenomenon may well be a response of the venous intima to the altered intra-luminal hemodynamic conditions, and is frequently seen in venous bypasses in the coronary position.

The first irregularities of the luminal contour may appear as early as three months post-operatively. The changes are slowly progressive but eventually threaten the function of the graft.

Angiographically the alterations closely resemble atherosclerosis in arteries. On gross inspection ulcerative and stenotic plaques of the intima are present, and in microscopic section typical atheromata are seen. In angiograms the crude incidence of these post-implantation changes is rather high. However, many of these defects were minor. Many were man-made and preventable, and others were sharply localized and operable. Only two lesions appear to be unavoidable and appear refractory to surgical correction: atherosclerosis and intimal thickening (forming altogether 16.7% of the total). The relevant data regarding the natural history of the anatomic changes are summarized in Table I. The most important findings relate to the progression and ultimate fate of these lesions. One can see that all the lesions were progressive but to varying degrees. As regards the ultimate result, if no prior attempt was made to correct the defects, very few lesions maintained patency for long. On the other hand, all the lesions that were deemed remediable and were repaired yielded excellent results.

The ultimate test of the functional value of an arterial substitute is, of course, the rate of cumulative patency maintained over a period of observation exceeding at least two but preferably five years.

In a recent study we surveyed 531 patients with 597 operations utilizing autogenous vein grafts for femoro-popliteal atherosclerosis between January 1963 and December 1977. Both the early and late patency rates were ascertained by angiographic studies. The follow-up period extended from 30 days to 15 years, 23% of the patients having been followed for more than five years. The purpose of the study was to test the effectiveness of femoro-femoral, femoro-popliteal and femoro-infrapopliteal autogenous vein grafting in terms of the effects of a variety of factors on early and late patency rates. The factors scrutinized were as follows: degrees of severity of occlusive disease, the anatomical location of the surgical procedure, the presence of diabetes and the quality of the vein graft. Among the more important findings were the following.

The immediate post-operative results showed patency rates that varied from 85.7% for femoro-femoral to 70.4% for distal femoro-infrapopliteal operations. A comparison of the clinical state of the patient with patency rates in the immediate post-operative period bore out the close correlation between patency and clinical status.

The overall trend of late patency rates, that is the trend of patency rates in all classes of cases, showed the greatest decrease in patency during the first year after operation, when it dropped by nearly 20%. Thereafter, the attrition was very gradual and quite stable, varying between 2% and 4% annually.

When the late cumulative patency rates between femoro-femoral reconstruction (that is, with the distal anastomosis above the knee) and femoro-popliteal (that is, with the distal anastomosis below the knee) showed relatively slight differences, with some advantage to the less extensive operation, the difference between the comparative patency rates of femoro-popliteal and femoro-infrapopliteal operations was statistically significant and varied from 13% to 20% in favor of the less complex procedure. The comparative patency rates in distal infrapopliteal operations were much less satisfactory with a mean duration of patency of 15.5 months.

A most significant finding was that in the evaluation of the effects of the physical qualities of the vein graft, the implants classified as "excellent" or "good" showed distinctly superior late cumulative patency rates. The five-year patency rate with good or excellent grafts was 58.4% and that with fair or poor vein grafts was 26.9%; the respective ten-year patency rates were 47.1% and 18.6%.

In summary, therefore, these observations confirm the status of the greater saphenous vein as an excellent arterial substitute in anatomical locations for which its dimensions are appropriate. It has shown complete immunological compatibility, flawless histologic acceptance and the maintenance of adequate tensile strength. As a bypass, both in the femoro-popliteal and in an infrapopliteal anatomical regions, it has made possible the achievement of patency rates in terms of five to ten years far superior to those obtained by any other reconstructive technique or with the use of any other arterial substitute. The greater saphenous vein as an arterial graft is subject to certain types of structural degeneration due both to extrinsic and intrinsic causes. The most important changes due to intrinsic causes are atherosclerosis and intimal thickening.

Although by angiographic examination one-third of the implants show some structural change, about two-thirds of these lesions are of minor character. It seems well proven, however, that all these changes are progressive and whenever possible they should be corrected as soon as detected. One-fourth of these changes can be prevented by careful surgical technique and about one-fourth, once noted, can be corrected by relatively simple surgical means. These aspects of the post-implantation history of the greater saphenous vein grafts emphasizes the importance of a very careful post-operative follow-up period.

It is reasonable to assume that with improved techniques of harvesting and temporary storing the saphenous vein grafts the incidence of some of the post-implantation changes may be reduced.

SAPHENOUS VEIN ALLOGRAFTS

G. M. Williams, A. Ter Haar, J. V. Sitzman and J. J. Ricotta

Division of Transplantation and Vascular Surgery Service,
The Johns Hopkins University School of Medicine,
Baltimore, Maryland, USA

INTRODUCTION

One of the remarkable features of clinical renal transplantation is the high rate of patency of renal artery and vein and the absolute lack of aneurysmal dilatation. Renal artery problems have been reported to occur in 1–10% of transplant recipients and are produced by three principal factors: (1) fibrotic constriction 1–2 cm beyond the anastomosis; (2) kinking and twisting of the vascular segments and (3) anastomotic narrowing. Thrombosis of the renal artery or vein unaccompanied by rejection of the kidney itself is invariably the result of technical failure. Considering the results with just these vessels, they are equivalent or even superior to the long-term results achieved with autologous saphenous vein grafts, even when these grafts are placed into the high-flow renal system.

These observations led us to studies we have reported in 1975 (Williams *et al.*). Exploiting the fact that the endothelium from females contains sex chromatin bodies readily determined in Hautchen preparations, we found that in the rat, dog and man arterial homografts lost their native endothelium and new endothelial cells appeared which were of recipient type. Further, the fibrous reaction occurring around the adventitia of the vessel was very intense and explained why aneurysm dilatation failed to occur. On the basis of these experiments we reasoned that if rejection could be modified to result in the

Serono Symposium No. 44, "Peripheral Arterial Diseases: Medical and Surgical Problems", edited by S. Stipa and A. Cavallaro, 1982. Academic Press, London and New York.

slow loss of donor endothelium and its repopulation by the host, long-lasting vascular patency could be achieved. This simple hypothesis has been tested in experimental animals and in man, and three principal problems remain, which will be discussed.

THROMBOSIS IN UNMODIFIED HOSTS

It is now well established that vascular tissues are antigenic and that rejection is inevitable in mismatched donor–recipient pairs. While in certain high-flow positions viable vascular homografts have remained patent for long periods of time, the histopathological changes are similar in all species and the results uniformly poor when these grafts are subjected to low-flow situations. In our own experience and that of others, carotid artery homografts have only a 33% rate of patency at six months. In man, the extensive experience of Ochsner and colleagues (Ochsner *et al.*, 1971) have demonstrated the fact that thrombosis is the rule with virtually all grafts becoming occluded by 1½ years.

Two avenues of research have been pursued in an attempt to improve patency rates: antirejection therapy and anticoagulation. Small doses of Imuran (1 mg kg^{-1}) improved carotid homograft patency to 89% at six months. Histological examination of the grafts at this time point showed that the majority of the endothelial surface was repopulated by cells from the recipient, despite the immunosuppressive therapy. These findings clearly demonstrated the promise that mild immunosuppression might "take the edge" off the rejection process, allowing for orderly repopulation.

Additional studies have been carried out with antiplatelet agents. Because of the prohibited expense of long-term studies, we have chosen the femoral vein location for our model of vascular allograft acceptance or rejection. In the dog, we have never had a femoral vein allograft placed in the venous system remain patent for more than three weeks (Ricotta *et al.*, 1979). However, the combination of Aspirin and Dipyridamole regularly resulted in four-week graft patency. Only one of seven grafts was occluded at six weeks and one graft was patent at ten months. These results permit an optimistic view that combined immunosuppressive and antiplatelet therapy will result in an orderly process of endothelial rejection and repopulation.

THE CHRONICITY OF THE HEALING PROCESS

Studies in the rat, dog and man have demonstrated that inflammatory changes associated with fibrin platelet clot persist for long periods of time in vascular allografts. Healing is still not complete in the aortic location in the rat after six months. Likewise, the dog carotid was not healed completely after four months. In human transplant recipients, absent endothelium and foci of inflammatory cells and clot are present in the renal artery and its branches for as long as 1½ years after transplantation. In the rat we found that treatment with immunosuppressive agents improved patency but retarded the repopulation process. Thus, we have been forced to conclude that therapy designed to modify the rejection process and prevent clotting must be continued for protracted periods of time.

In order to confront this problem, therapy must be benign and basically free of its own complications. Treatment of recipients with small doses of azathioprine (1 mg kg^{-1} day^{-1}). Dipyridamole and Aspirin fulfil this criteria.

AVAILABILITY

The lack of immediate availability of saphenous vein allografts is the greatest practical problem to greater application in our opinion. The patient with intermittent claudication is not really a candidate for reconstruction by means of venous allografts. Rather, it is the patient with gangrene or severe intractable rest pain that requires a bypass to a small distal tibial vessel and needs the normal endothelium to maintain patency. It is chiefly for this reason that our clinical experience has been limited to three cases. All were treated with Imuran 50 mg day^{-1}, aspirin 600 mg day^{-1} and dipyridamole 200 mg day^{-1}.

In all three cases bypasses to the lower one-third of the leg were carried out using normal freshly harvested saphenous vein allografts. Early patency was achieved in all cases and symptoms were relieved in all cases. Healing of gangrenous digits was achieved with minor amputations in two of the three patients. One graft clotted at eight months, a second remained patent until the death of the patient at two years after grafting. The third was ligated because of anastomotic rupture related to sepsis at the distal anterior tibial anastomosis. This case will be summarized briefly, because it dramatizes the problem of ready availability.

The patient was a 71-year-old physician who presented in desperation because of intractable right foot rest pain. He had had an aortofemoral endarterectomy ten years previously, which had remained patent. Left and right saphenous vein grafts were carried out eight and seven years ago, each being placed to the distal popliteal artery. About 1½ years prior to admission, the patient became symptomatic in the right leg and, despite worsening of symptoms, refused amputation. Arteriography demonstrated patency of a small anterior tibial artery, which continued down to the level of the ankle but could not be followed further. He was placed on a waiting list for an ABO compatible graft.

Our search for a cadaver saphenous vein was intensive and extensive and lasted 4½ weeks before consent was obtained. During that period of time, consent was obtained to remove kidneys from one cadaver donor, but the family declined removal of the saphenous vein. The patient or a member of his family called us daily. When a graft was obtained and transplanted, the early results were salutary. The patient was at home when serious drainage was noted to appear at the suture line in the lower third of the leg. *Pseudomonas* was cultured and, despite antibiotic therapy, anastomotic rupture occurred at ten weeks. This was repaired by placing a 4-inch segment of remaining autologous saphenous vein, the placement of catheters in the wound, irrigation with antibiotic solutions and systemic antibiotics.

Nevertheless, rupture occurred again and an above-knee amputation was performed. The vein graft had necrotic endothelium with some thrombus formation at the sites of valves.

CRYOPRESERVATION

Because it was intolerable for patients, family and physician to wait for the acquisition of fresh saphenous vein, recent attempts have been devoted toward a more practical system. Several investigators have achieved good patency rates with frozen and stored vein grafts in experimental animals (Calhoun *et al.*,1977; Weber *et al.*, 1975; Malone *et al.*, 1980) and Ochsner has noted better results with frozen grafts than with fresh grafts in man. In current studies, the jugular vein was excised, placed into tissue culture media containing 10% Dimethylsulphoxide (DMSO) and allowed to equilibrate at room temperature for 1 h. Thereafter, the vein was rapidly frozen in liquid nitrogen and stored at −70° for periods of at least one week. Thawing was achieved by simple equilibration at room temperature. These techniques were selected because of their simplicity and ready availability.

These grafts placed into the venous system consistently demonstrated higher patency rates equal to femoral vein grafts. Extended patency was achieved using Dipyridamole and Aspirin alone.

CONCLUSION

(1) The viable venous homograft is fraught with the problem of rejection but the rejection process may be harnessed under the right circumstances as an aid to prevent aneurysm formation.

(2) An enlightened public will provide the only solution to the short supply of these veins for use.

(3) Cryopreservation by freezing in DMSO is promising as it may allow for the banking of veins and their prompt distribution.

REFERENCES

Calhoun, A. D., Baur, G. M., Porter, J. M. *et al.* (1977). Fresh and cryopreserved venous allografts in genetically characterized dogs. *Journal of Surgical Research* **22**, 687.

Malone, J. M., Moore, W.S., Kischer, C. W. *et al.* (1980). Venous cryopreservation: endothelial fibrinolytic activity and histology. *Jounal of Surgical Research* **29**, 209.

Ochsner, J. L., DeCamp, P. T. and Leonard, G. L. (1971). Experience with fresh venous allografts as arterial substitute. *Annals of Surgery* **173**, 933.

Ricotta, J., Schaff, H. and Gadacz, T. (1979). Effect of aspirin and dipyridamole on the patency of allograft veins. *Journal of Surgical Research* **26**, 262.

Weber, T., Dent, T. *et al.* (1975). Viable vein graft preservation. *Journal of Surgical Research* **18**, 247.

Williams, G. M., Ter Haar, A., Krajewski, C., Parks, L. and Roth, J. (1975). Rejection and repair of endothelium in major vessel transplants. *Surgery* **78**, 694.

FABRICATION AND TESTING OF VASCULAR PROSTHESES

R. W. Snyder

Bard Implant Division, Billerica, Massachusetts, USA

INTRODUCTION

Since 1952 when Voorhees *et al.* reported the use of Vinyon-N* cloth for the repair of arterial defects, a number of materials have been investigated for arterial prostheses. Both polymers and metals have been considered. Early work centered on the use of the textile structure as a suitable replacement.

Two polymer yarns emerged from this early period as the materials of choice. Polytetrafluoroethylene (PTFE) in the form of Teflon and Polyethylene Terephthalate (PET) in the form of Dacron. Currently, PET in a textile structure has become the material of choice. This choice of material is based upon over 25 years of successful use.

STRUCTURE

Dacron textile prostheses are currently available in a number of different structures. These structures have different applications in regard to the handling and host acceptance. Figure 1 shows the luminal surface of a woven structure. Note that the yarns run continuously in the longitudinal and circumferential direction. The longitudinal yarns are known as the ends or the warp. The circumferential yarns are termed picks or the weft.

*Vinyon-N, Teflon and Dacron are trademarks of E.I. DuPont de Nemours.

Serono Symposium No. 44, "Peripheral Arterial Diseases: Medical and Surgical Problems", edited by S. Stipa and A. Cavallaro, 1982. Academic Press, London and New York.

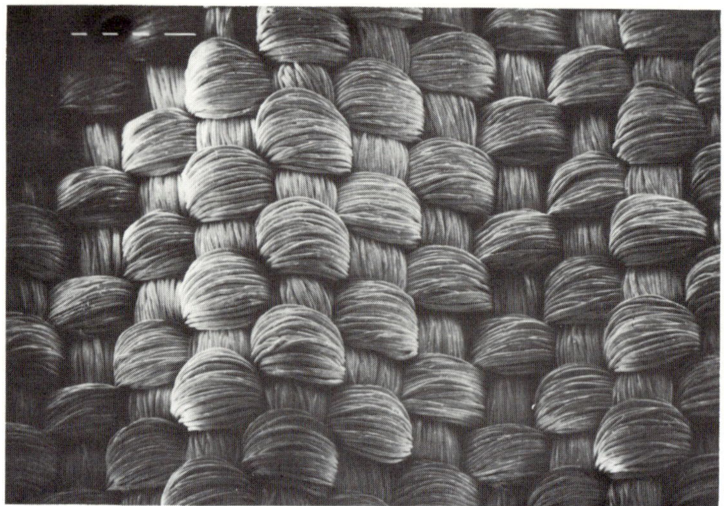

Fig. 1. Inner surface of USCI surgical products 12 mm DeBakey woven Dacron vascular prosthesis (×20) (implant lot No. 742130, sterile lot No. 10L04081; USCI and DeBakey are trademarks of C. R. Bard, Inc.).

Arterial prostheses are also available in various knit structures. One such structure is the weft knit structure. Knits can also be fabricated in a warp construction. The luminal surface of a Sauvage BIONIT prosthesis is shown in Fig. 2. Note that, although the yarns bend and twist in both directions, they are predominantly in the longitudinal or warp direction. Warp knit products are in general more complex than weft knit structures. Figure 3 shows the adventitial surface of the same structure.

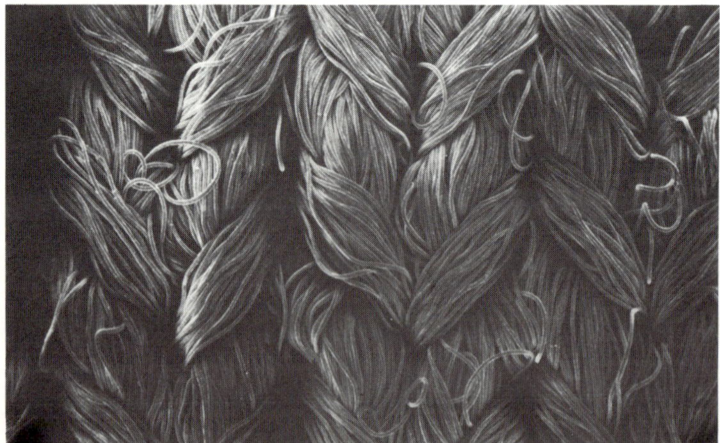

Fig. 2. Inner surface of USCI surgical products 12 mm Sauvage Bionit (warp) knit Dacron vascular prosthesis (×20) (implant lot No. 749511, sterile lot No. 10I04061; Sauvage is a trademark of C. R. Bard, Inc.).

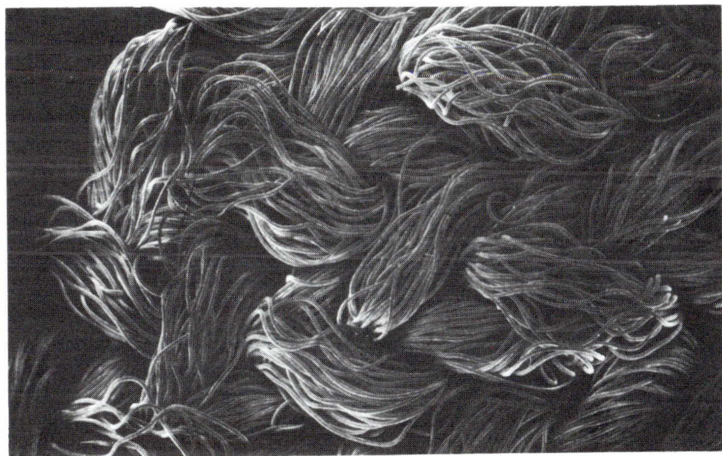

Fig. 3. Outer surface of USCI surgical products 12 mm Sauvage Bionit (warp) knit Dacron vascular prosthesis (×20) (implant lot No. 749511, sterile lot No. 10I04061; Sauvage is a trademark of C. R. Bard, Inc.).

CHARACTERISTICS

In the design of the vascular prosthesis, the bioengineer must keep in mind three things: surgeon acceptance, host acceptance and product longevity. These criteria manifest themselves in three basic parameters: prosthesis handling, prosthesis material and porosity and prosthesis strength. As shown in Fig. 4 these three parameters are somewhat dependent functions of each other. For, the two basic types of textile prostheses, woven and knit, the structure affects each of these parameters somewhat differently.

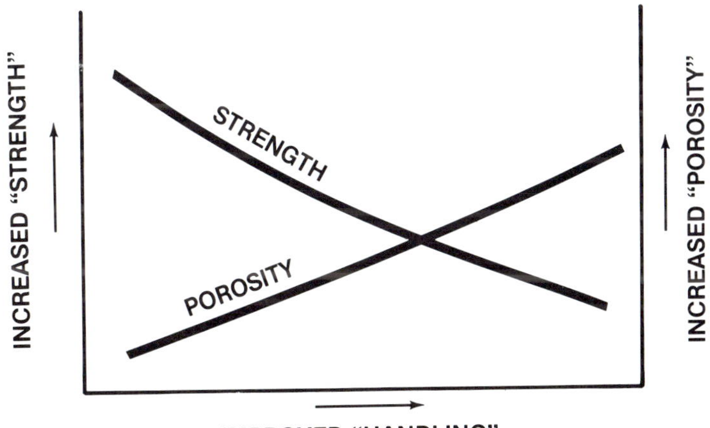

Fig. 4. Parameteric relationship between strength, porosity and handling in non-biological vascular prostheses.

Shown in Fig. 5 is a woven structure in both a stretched and unstretched configuration. In terms of prosthesis strength, if the direction of the blood flow is from left to right, the stresses due to pressure would be supported by the vertical yarns. Longitudinal tensile strength will be a function of the strength of the yarns running from left to right. Unless one set or the other of the yarns are packed very close together, inducing sharp bends in the other set of yarns, this structure will be extremely strong.

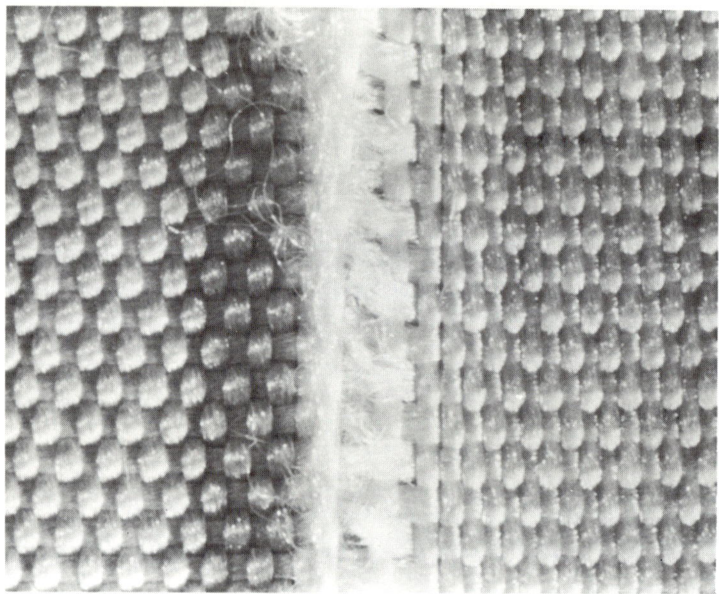

Fig. 5. Woven structure unloaded (left) and loaded (right).

Most of the forces will translate into tensile stress in the direction of the yarn. In fact, the bursting strength of a woven prosthesis with a moderate packing factor is nearly related to the strength of the yarn.

However, in terms of handling, if one were to bend or fold this product to conform with the artery, it is necessary to bend the individual yarns making the product feel stiff. Suturing can also be difficult because, if the yarns are close together, a needle will likely hit one of the strands of yarn and resist puncture. Also, if the stitches are taken too close to the end of the fabric, the transverse yarns may pull out causing fraying. However, in this configuration, it is possible to put the yarns very close together and achieve a low porosity.

On the other hand, in this typical weft knit structure shown in Fig. 6, the load must be transferred from loop to loop. No yarn goes across the fabric in a straight line. Furthermore, the load causes the filaments to bend increasing the stresses in the individual yarns. In such a structure, it is typical for the bursting pressure to translate into approximately 60–70% of the yarn tensile strength. In this type of structure, it is difficult to get the yarns as close together as in the woven structure due to the fact that a needle is used to form

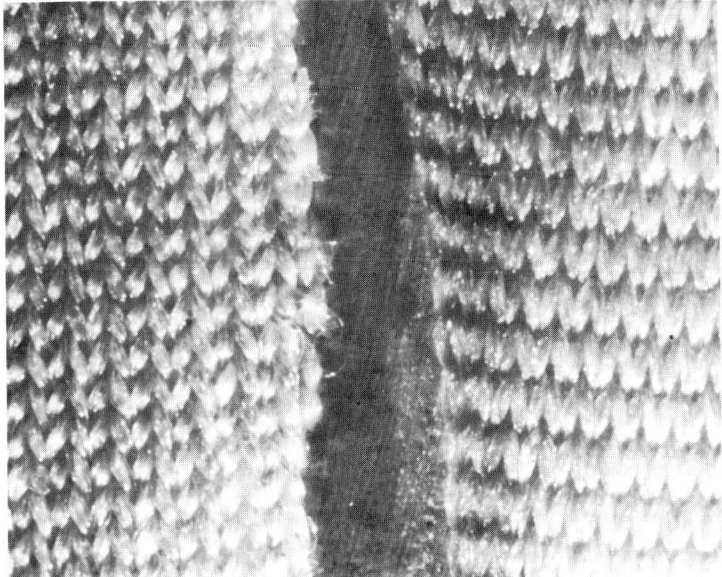

Fig. 6. Weft knit structure unloaded (left) and loaded in tension (right).

each stitch which provides a lower limit to the size of the stitch and due to the sharp bends in the yarns. This further decreases the tensile strength by decreasing the number of yarns per centimeter available to support the load. This also results in a higher porosity prosthesis. This higher porosity, however, improves suturability.

Finally, if one bends a knit fabric, the yarns pivot on each other rather than bending. This yields a softer feeling material which conforms more easily to the natural artery. Thus, improved handling has been achieved at the expense of higher porosity and lower strength. However, this is not necessarily a bad trade-off for many applications.

It should be noted that, with warp knitting, a wide variety of patterns are possible. The comments made previously concerning the weft knit prosthesis hold also for this structure; although, it is much more difficult to relate bursting pressure to yarn strength. Also, because of the higher number of yarns in a given stitch, the porosity tends to be somewhat lower. Finally, in such a structure one must be careful to provide more than one yarn to transfer the load between rows of stitches. This type of structure yields a slightly stiffer prosthesis with an increase in strength over the weft knit structure; however, these values do not approach that which is possible in a woven prosthesis. Other types of warp knit structures may not enjoy any advantage over a weft knit structure, as the type of warp knit pattern and the yarn also affect these parameters.

Handling in a vascular prosthesis is really made up of a number of considerations. The ease with which the prosthesis can be cut and made to conform to an artery can be an important part of handling. Needle puncture force and suture drag, as well as suture tear-out force also impact upon the handling characteristics of a prosthesis. Finally, one must consider the preparation required prior to implantation. The product should not require any preparatory steps to render it nontoxic. Pre-clotting, which is an integral part of the preparation of the prosthesis, must be as consistent as possible within patient variation.

The optimum porosity of a textile vascular prosthesis (measured as defined in Fig. 7) depends upon its applications, material and structure. In thoracic surgery or with patients for which it is necessary to minimize blood loss, a low porosity vascular prosthesis is recommended. However, many of these low porosity vascular prostheses do not demonstrate the type of long-term tissue encapsulation that is necessary for high patency rates in the more demanding smaller diameter prosthesis applications. Wesolowski (1962) demonstrated that the porosity of a vascular prosthesis was related to a calcification index representing tissue necrosis and thus to the long-term survival of the neo-intima. Thus, he proposed his Gossamer concept.

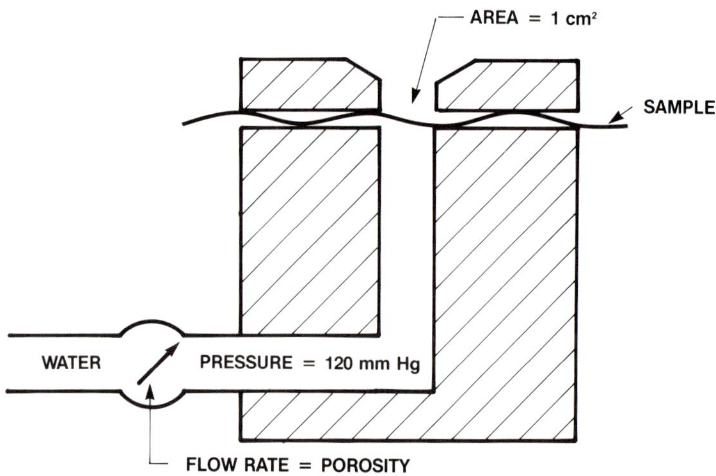

Fig. 7. Method for measuring porosity in a textile vascular prosthesis (Wesolowski, 1962).

It has been demonstrated, however, by several investigators including Sauvage *et al.* (1971) that the velour prostheses with their lower porosity yield the same healing characteristics as the higher porosity knit products. In addition, the presence of velour increases the pre-clotting efficiency beyond that achieved by simply decreasing the porosity. It is thought that the improvement in healing characteristics may be partially due to the fact that the velour component stabilizes the structure and protects the ingrowing tissue; thus preventing the tufts rhexis described by Wesolowski (1962).

In considering the longevity of a vascular prosthesis, several failure modes must be studied. The stability of the structure, i.e. its resistance to dilatation and the long-term breaking strength of the material itself must both be considered. It is as important to prevent long-term dilatation as it is to prevent rupture of the fabric.

Three separate phenomena lead to the dilatation of a textile vascular prosthesis. First, as the crimps are removed either by stretching or pressurization, the prosthesis diameter increases. Second, if the basic polymer is loaded beyond its elastic limit, the material will stretch and the prosthesis will dilate as well as increase in length due to the longitudinal forces. Finally, a knit textile structure, particularly one with a high porosity, can be rearranged. That part of the yarn which runs in the longitudinal direction can slip causing that part of the stitch in the circumferential direction to lengthen (Fig. 6). The result is a graft which increases in diameter but shortens in length. Many of the dilatations reported in high porosity simple knit prostheses were in this type.

Data published by Edwards *et al.* (1978) and by Guidoin *et al.* (1980) demonstrate that Dacron vascular prostheses lose less than 25% of their initial strength shortly after implantation. However, beyond this period, the strength stabilizes. Data from Edwards *et al.* (1978) is shown in Fig. 8. Grafts that have been implanted up to 18 years still retain adequate strength. Recent data is described by Snyder *et al.* (1981) for three years of canine implant.

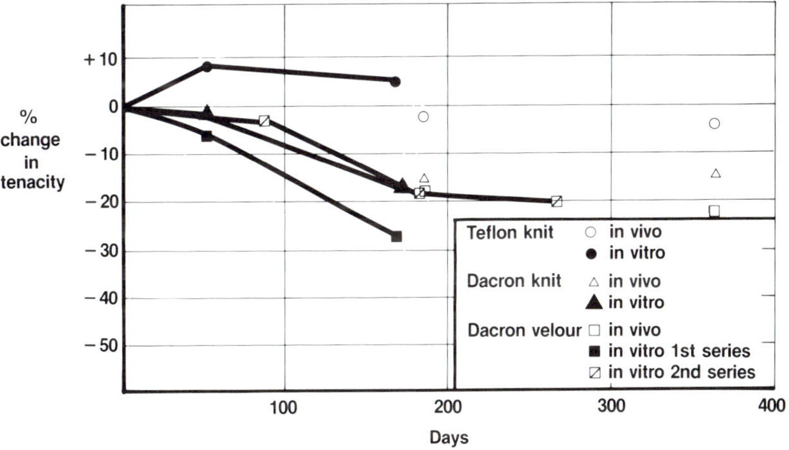

Fig. 8. Percentage change in tenacity for Teflon and Dacron knit prostheses versus time on life tester or as canine implants (Edwards *et al.*, 1978).

As recently discussed by Berger and Sauvage (1981), Dacron vascular prostheses do fail. As noted in a recent Utah Biomedical Test Laboratory study for the FDA (Mortensen, 1981) this is uncommon. As noted by Berger and Sauvage (1981) and Botzko *et al.* (1981), although Dacron has exhibited the necessary longevity for a vascular prosthesis, it can be a fragile material. Dacron vascular prostheses can be damaged by clamping, needle punctures, autoclaving etc. As manufacturers improve their techniques and increase the longevity of these products, surgeons must also be aware of proper handling techniques.

TESTING

In order to maintain the design parameters chosen by the bioengineer, a number of tests on each batch of vascular prostheses is necessary. Positive identification and testing of all materials, not just the Dacron material used in a prosthesis, must be carried out. Traceability must be maintained from the lot of material used to fabricate the prosthesis through to the final step in processing the prosthesis. Dimensions of the finished prosthesis such as the inflated diameter and the usable length need to be measured for each batch of products.

In addition, since the structure of the prosthesis is as important as its material, water porosity tests, shown schematically in Fig. 7 or some equivalent test, must be made on each batch of prostheses. In order to ascertain that the process has not harmed the prosthesis; in addition to the records kept on each process parameter, strength testing of each batch of prostheses must be performed.

CONCLUSION

The bioengineer must optimize handling characteristics, material, porosity and strength. This can be done by careful selection of the proper textile structure. The optimum structure depends upon the application for the vascular prosthesis. The surgeon must handle the prosthesis carefully, optimize the anastomoses and prosthesis location, carefully pre-clot the prosthesis and minimize the effects of thrombogenicity by monitoring run-off and blood chemistry intra- and post-operatively. Finally, the patient also contributes both involuntarily through progression of disease and other conditions such as overall health and diabetes and voluntarily through changes in living habits.

REFERENCES

Berger, K. and Sauvage, L. R. (1981). Late fiber deterioration in Dacron arterial grafts. *Annals of Surgery* **193**, 477.

Botzko, K. M., Clark, C., Turnquist, C. and Snyder, R. (1981). The effects of trauma on Dacron vascular prostheses. "Seventh Annual Meeting of the Society for Biomaterials". May 1981.

Edwards, W. S., Snyder, R. W., Botzko, K. and Larkin, J. (1978). Comparison of durability of tensile strength of Teflon and Dacron grafts. *In* "Graft Materials in Vascular Surgery" (H. Dardik, Ed.), p. 169. Yearbook Publishers, Chicago, Illinois.

Guidoin, R., Gosselin, C., Roy, J., Gagnon, D., Marois, M., Noel, H. P., Roy, P., Martin, L., Awad, J., Bourassa, S. and Rouleau, C. (1980). Structural and mechanical properties of Dacron prostheses as arterial substitutes. *In* "Mechanical Properties of Biomaterials" (G. W. Hastings and D. F. Williams, Eds), p. 547. Wiley, New York.

Mortensen, J. D. (1981). "Final Report Vascular Replacements; A Study of Safety and Performance". UBTL Division, TR 5-533-011 February 1981.

Sauvage, L. R., Berger, K., Wood, S. J., Nakagawa, Y. and Mansfield, P. B. (1971). An external velour surface for porous arterial prostheses. *Surgery* **70**, 940.
Snyder, R. W., Edwards, W. S., Botzko, K. M. and Larkin, J. (1981). Dacron and Teflon prostheses: a three year implant study. "Seventh Annual Meeting of the Society for Biomaterials". May 1981.
Voorhees, A. B., Jaratski, A. and Blakemore, A. H. (1952). The use of tubes constructed from Vinyon-N cloth in bridging arterial defects. *Annals of Surgery* **135**, 332.
Wesolowski, S. A. (1962). "Evaluation of Tissue and Prosthetic Vascular Grafts". Thomas, Springfield, Illinois.

EXTERNAL VELOUR WEFT-KNITTED COMPOSITE FIBRIN/DACRON PROSTHESES (NONSUPPORTED AND SUPPORTED) FOR FEMORO-POPLITEAL BYPASS

L. R. Sauvage

Cardiovascular Reconstruction Division,
Bob Hope International Heart Research Institute,
the Providence Medical Center, and the Department of Surgery,
University of Washington School of Medicine, Seattle, Washington, USA

In my practice of clinical vascular surgery, which dates back to 1960, I have come to the following conclusions regarding the use of Dacron prostheses for femoro-popliteal bypass.

(1) No prosthesis is as acceptable as a segment of autogenous saphenous vein which is of uniform 5- to 6-mm diameter, of good quality and which has been carefully harvested to preserve its endothelial flow surface.

(2) The porous Dacron prosthesis should be regarded as a framework over which fibrin is deposited prior to implantation by a process best described as "autofibrinization" (rather than "pre-clotting"). This forms a composite fibrin/Dacron prosthesis which then possesses the surface characteristics of an acceptable autogenous substance and the strength of a strong, relatively inert, synthetic fiber framework.

(3) This composite fibrin/Dacron graft is highly thrombogenic because the formation of fibrin is dependent upon the action of thrombin. An inevitable side-effect of this action is the elaboration of two powerful platelet activators, thromboxane A_2 and ADP. Thrombin is the potent enzymatic end-point of both the intrinsic and extrinsic coagulation systems, and

Serono Symposium No. 44, "Peripheral Arterial Diseases: Medical and Surgical Problems", edited by S. Stipa and A. Cavallaro, 1982. Academic Press, London and New York.

catalyses the conversion of fibrinogen to fibrin. In addition, thrombin activates platelets to release thromboxane A_2, which converts within minutes to thromboxane B_2, a less active but more stable compound which is still capable of attracting and activating platelets. The entrapment of red blood cells in the fibrin mesh and the trauma of the autofibrinizing process lead to red cell injury and release of ADP, also a potent platelet activator.

For the composite fibrin/Dacron graft to be useful as a conduit for bypass of small peripheral arteries, these powerful prothrombotic agents must be removed from its flow surface. Our objective is to reduce the thrombogenicity of the flow surface to that of pure cross-linked fibrin, uncontaminated by either thrombin or other platelet activators.

(4) Inactivation of thrombin on the flow surface of the composite fibrin/Dacron prosthesis is accomplished in the fourth (and final) step of our autofibrinizing process by the union of heparin-activated antithrombin III with thrombin.

(5) The methodology to remove the other powerful platelet activators (thromboxane A_2, B_2 and ADP) from the flow surface has not been worked out, and needs much study. Currently, we are evaluating the efficacy of washing the autofibrinized graft with Ringer's lactate until its colour has changed from red to white. Preliminary research suggests that this simple method has merit as a means to remove these activators.

(6) A composite fibrin/Dacron conduit that crosses the knee joint is vulnerable to both kinking and compression when the joint is flexed.

(7) A crimped flow surface causes unacceptable turbulence in small-caliber prostheses, increasing the likelihood of thrombotic occlusion of the graft. In contrast, a noncrimped flow surface is free of bloodstream turbulence, but is more prone to kinking and compression with flexion of the knee joint.

(8) The noncrimped Dacron fiber framework can be rendered resistant to kinking and compression by heat-fusing a coil of polypropylene to its outer wall. This support coil reinforces the graft wall, yet allows it to curve easily and assume an "S" shape in response to flexion of the knee.

(9) However, adding such an external support coil introduces a new set of special problems for the femoro-popliteal graft during flexion of the knee. These problems are more severe for the below-knee than for the above-knee graft. Contrary to nonsupported composite fibrin/Dacron grafts, which tend to kink when the knee is flexed, supported grafts do not. The supported graft and popliteal artery must adapt to the shortened distance of the flexed position by altering the straight-line position they assume when the knee is extended. The forces engendered by the flexed position compel the supported graft to assume an S-shaped configuration and simultaneously act to cause the infra-anastomotic popliteal artery to do the same if it has the freedom to move. But if the artery does not possess adequate freedom, the forces of the flexed position will cause the infra-anastomotic popliteal artery to kink and obstruct flow.

(10) The addition of an external velour component to the weft-knitted Dacron prosthesis facilitates pre-implant autofibrinization and subsequent graft healing.

(11) Composite externally supported (EXS) fibrin/Dacron prostheses can be used with a high degree of success for above-knee femoro-popliteal bypass, and with a lower (but still good) degree of success in the below-knee position if the graft, lower anastomosis and distal popliteal artery are capable of adjusting their positions without kinking when the knee is flexed.

With these points as background, I shall now review the experiences I have had with composite fibrin/external velour weft-knitted Dacron prostheses for femoro-popliteal bypass since I first used this design in 1970. My experience until 1978 involved only unsupported Dacron prostheses; 114 of these were placed to, but not beyond, the knee joint. Since 1978, 46 polypropylene-supported (EXS) prostheses have been placed, 30 above and 16 below the knee joint.

DESCRIPTION OF PROSTHESES

An external velour weft-knitted Dacron design has been employed throughout the 11-year period of this study, crimped and unsupported in the 1970 to 1978 period and noncrimped, supported (termed EXS) in the 1978 to 1981 period. Surface and cross-sectional views of these prostheses are shown in Figs 1 and 2. As mentioned previously, the EXS prosthesis was developed to overcome the main problems associated with the use of crimped Dacron grafts beyond the knee joint: (1) increased thrombogenicity caused by a washboard flow surface and (2) tendency of the flexed knee to both kink and compress an unsupported prosthesis.

In overcoming these limitations, our first step (in conjunction with USCI of Billerica, Massachusetts, United States) was to eliminate the crimp, and our second was to render the prosthesis resistant to both kinking and compression by heat-fusing a coil of polypropylene to its outer velour surface. The outgrowth of this effort has been the development of a family of "site-specific" externally supported Dacron prostheses known as "EXS" for use in axillo-femoral, femoro-popliteal and femoro-tibial locations (Fig. 3).

The EXS femoro-popliteal external velour weft-knitted Dacron prosthesis is an integral tube that is fabricated differentially to have three distinct sections, a lower section 10 cm long which is noncrimped and nonsupported, a mid-section of length 30 cm or 45 cm which is noncrimped and supported, and an upper section 20 cm long which is crimped but not supported. The noncrimped nonsupported lower portion of the prosthesis is designed to facilitate ease of suturing to the popliteal artery. The anastomosis should be begun about 3 mm distal to the junction with the supported body of the prosthesis. Hence, only a short segment of the proximal part of the nonsupported lower section of the prosthesis is actually retained. The main part of the prosthesis is the noncrimped supported middle section, which provides a smooth flow surface to the blood and a wall that is kink- and compression-resistant to its environment. The crimped nonsupported upper end of the prosthesis enables easy adjustment in the length of the prosthesis, retaining only a segment adequate to join to the femoral artery without undue tension. The EXS

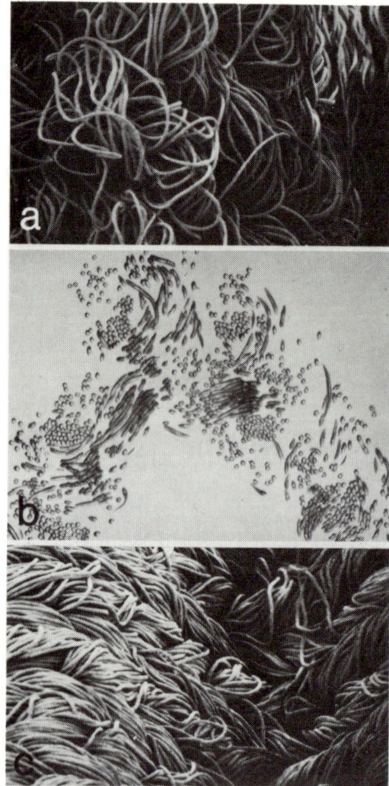

Fig. 1. External (SEM × 36), cross-sectional (SEM × 35) and internal (SEM × 32) views of the USCI Sauvage filamentous velour prosthesis used clinically during the decade of the 1970s. Note filamentousness of external surface and comparative smoothness of inner flow surface. Outer filaments serve as a trellis for cellular attachment and ingrowth, whereas the inner surface is comparatively smooth but sufficiently textured to allow fibrin to securely attach to it.

femoro-popliteal prosthesis is made in two lengths, one 60 cm in overall length with a 30-cm supported body for use as an above-knee bypass and one 75 cm in overall length with a 45-cm supported body for use as a below-knee bypass. Both of these lengths are provided in 5 mm and 6 mm sizes.

FORMATION OF COMPOSITE FIBRIN/DACRON PROSTHESIS BY PRE-IMPLANT AUTOFIBRINIZATION OF DACRON FIBER FRAMEWORK RECEIVED FROM MANUFACTURER

Precise pre-implant autofibrinization of knitted Dacron prostheses is important to both their short- and long-term success. The basic four-step method we have described previously (Yates *et al.*, 1978) for use with non-

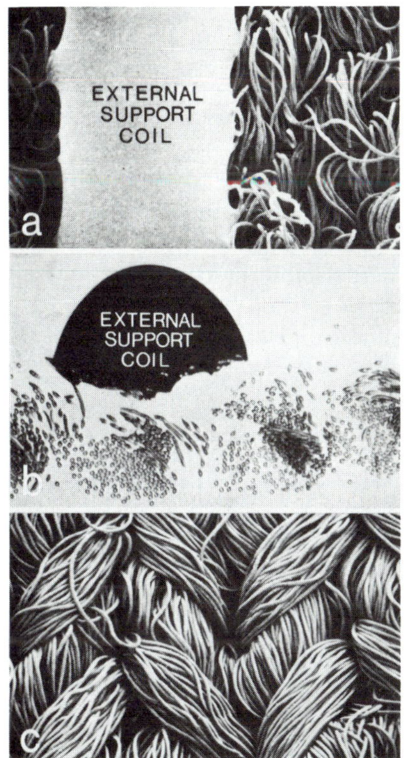

Fig. 2. (a) External (SEM × 32), (b) cross-sectional (LM × 35) and (c) internal (SEM × 36) views of the USCI Sauvage EXS Dacron graft. The filamentous nature of the outer wall and the attachment of the support coil to the velour surface is shown in (a) and (b). The comparatively smooth inner wall is shown in (c).

supported grafts is also used for autofibrinizing the EXS prosthesis, with the modification shown in Fig. 4. A balloon-tipped catheter is used to remove blood from the lumen of the EXS prosthesis after each step. An assistant is required to perform this maneuver quickly and properly. It is necessary to work rapidly after introducing nonheparinized blood in steps two and three; otherwise, cross-luminal fibrin strands will tend to form. To be certain that the graft will be impervious, I often add another exposure to nonheparinized blood — a "3_b" step, so to speak.

The fourth and final step of our protocol employs heparin-activated anti-thrombin III to inactivate thrombin. To leave the graft saturated with this potent thrombogenic enzyme implies either a lack of concern for, or understanding of, thrombogenicity. Upon completion of our four-step method for autofibrinization, the flow surface of the composite fibrin/Dacron prosthesis should be impervious, smooth and depleted of thrombin. As indicated in my introductory conclusion (numbers three, four and five), there is much more to

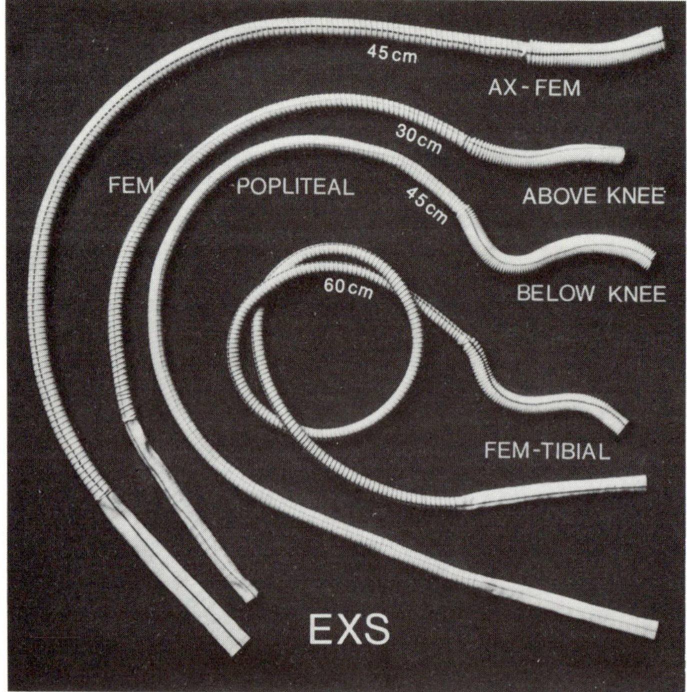

Fig. 3. Family of USCI Sauvage EXS prostheses. Note "site-specific" configurations, with lengths of supported segments varying according to need of implant site. The numbers refer to the length of the supported section of the prosthesis.

achieving a hypothrombogenic flow surface than inactivating thrombin, albeit both a very powerful procoagulant and a potent platelet activator. We have only recently begun to address ourselves to a study of means for removing thromboxane A_2, B_2 and ADP from the flow surface of the composite fibrin/Dacron graft prior to implantation. This is an exciting area for investigation, and I am optimistic that much will be learned which will prove of positive value in reducing the thrombogenicity of the flow surface to that of pure cross-linked fibrin uncontaminated by residual prothrombotic enzymes or activators.

It is worthy of emphasis that the composite fibrin/Dacron prosthesis must be blood-tight at the completion of the autofibrinizing process. If it is not, the process must be repeated, using topical thrombin to initiate fibrin formation and insure that the wall is impervious.

The autofibrinized fibrin/Dacron graft should be regarded as a protein autograft which derives the necessary strength for dimensional stability from the Dacron framework buried within its substance. Although it may sound a bit extreme, I feel that if the surgeon is unable to spend the few minutes required to properly construct the fibrin component of the EXS composite fibrin/Dacron prosthesis, *he should not use this prosthesis*. The time spent in

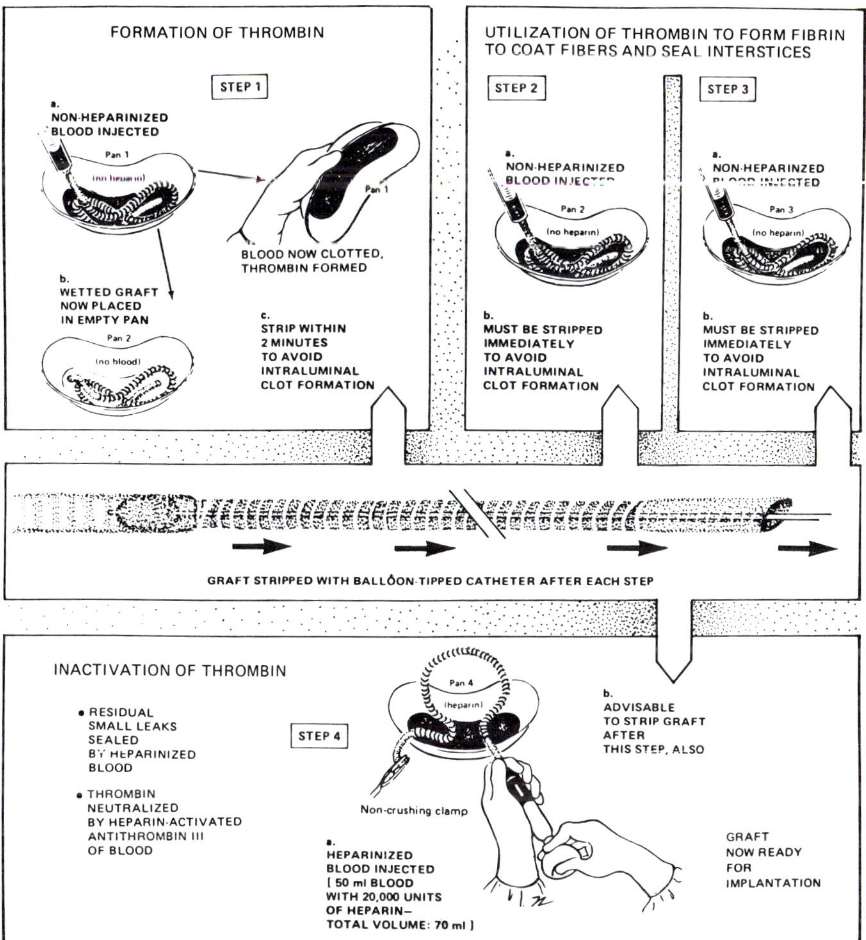

Fig. 4. Four-step method for autofibrinization of EXS prostheses. The prosthesis as received from the manufacturer is but a skeleton upon which the surgeon, through the autofibrinization process, constructs an autogenous protein conduit that derives the necessary strength for dimensional stability from the Dacron framework buried within its substance. At the completion of the fourth step, the flow surface is rendered impervious, smooth and hypothrombogenic.

properly fibrinizing the EXS prosthesis will likely be rewarded by increased patency rates, both short- and long-term. There must be no compromise in striving to produce the finest possible fibrin flow surface before implantation. To do less than this will limit the success of the EXS composite fibrin/Dacron prosthesis for femoro-popliteal bypass. We can gain inspiration for our efforts to make the finest prosthesis possible by recalling that fibrin is one of nature's chief means for covering a denuded vascular surface as a prelude to healing.

PROPER POSITIONING OF THE PROSTHESIS

The nonsupported composite fibrin/Dacron graft we used in 1970–1978 for above-knee femoro-popliteal bypass was routed subcutaneously through the lower thigh and there turned to join the above-knee popliteal artery. This technique at least partially compensates for upward movement of the above-knee portion of the popliteal artery during knee joint flexion to help prevent kinking of the graft, as shown in Fig. 5. The lower part of the graft, when positioned in this manner, will tend to move like a pendulum, swinging up with flexion and down with extension of the knee.

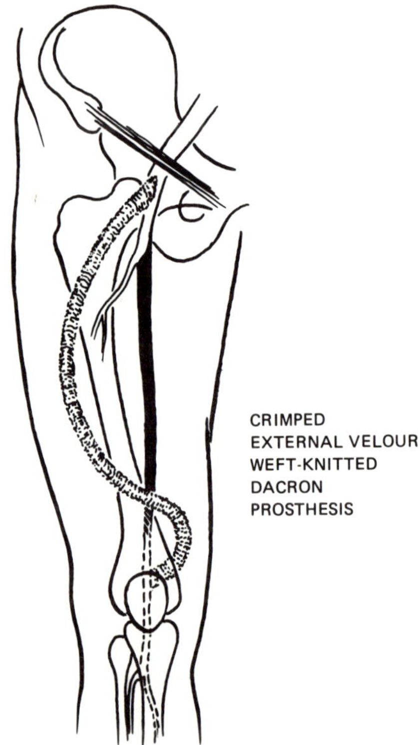

Fig. 5. Position of above-knee crimped nonsupported Dacron grafts implanted in the 1970 to 1978 period. This position in part compensates for the upward movement of the above-knee popliteal artery in response to flexion of the knee.

On the contrary, the EXS composite fibrin/Dacron graft should not be run superficially when used for femoro-popliteal bypass, even in the above-knee position. This prosthesis is designed to be run deep, parallel to the artery, in the manner shown in Fig. 6. This prevents angulation of the nonsupported distal end against the supported body of the graft during joint flexion.

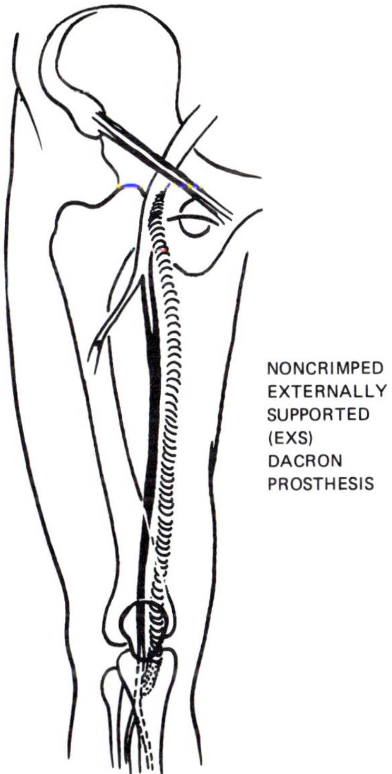

Fig. 6. Position of below-knee supported (EXS) femoro-popliteal prosthesis employed in the 1978 to 1981 period. The EXS graft is both kink- and compression-resistant. This graft should be run deep, parallel to the artery. If it is run in the manner shown in Fig. 5, there is danger of angulation at the junction of the supported body with the short nonsupported segment used for the distal anastomosis.

SYSTEMIC HEPARINIZATION DURING GRAFT IMPLANTATION

We have used systemic heparin intra-operatively for all patients receiving composite fibrin/Dacron femoro-popliteal bypass grafts, aiming to prevent distal bed thrombosis and to prevent blood in the field from clotting and contaminating the graft with thrombin. We use 200 units of heparin per kilogram of body weight during graft implantation to elevate the activated clotting time (ACT) to more than 400 s.

Additionally, our experimental work has shown that delaying heparin neutralization for 15–20 min following clamp release increases the patency rate of porous Dacron fabric grafts in the canine carotid artery (Yates *et al.*, 1978). The initial high flow of heparinized blood across the fibrin flow surface washes prothrombotic enzymes and activators away, and likely deposits a layer of albumin on the surface to further passivate it.

Over the years, we have become more sophisticated in the use of protamine sulfate, and now monitor the ACT closely during heparin reversal by protamine, aiming to keep it just above the pre-operative levels. We seldom give more than 0.5 mg of protamine for each 100 units of heparin administered. It is probable that excessive doses of protamine create a hypercoagulable state by neutralizing both endogenous and exogenous heparin. Hence, we have no quarrel with those who use smaller amounts of heparin systematically and do not use protamine at all, allowing the heparin to dissipate naturally.

OTHER ASPECTS PERTINENT TO SUCCESSFUL IMPLANTATION OF THE COMPOSITE EXS FIBRIN/DACRON FEMORO-POPLITEAL GRAFT

Selecting Prosthesis of Proper Length and Diameter

Femoro-popliteal EXS prostheses are constructed in 5-mm and 6-mm diameters and in supported lengths of 30 cm and 45 cm. The length and caliber of graft used depend upon the size of the popliteal artery and the distance to be spanned by the graft.

Proper length of the graft is determined in relation to the distance to be spanned. The crimped upper end of the prosthesis is 20 cm long and the noncrimped nonsupported lower end is 10 cm long. The length of the supported section must not be longer than the distance to be transversed. Instead, it should be from 2 cm to 3 cm shorter but it can be as much as 20 cm shorter. I recommend that the lower end of the supported section should be positioned within 3 mm of the heel stitch of the lower anastomosis. Selection of the proper length of graft assures that its upper end will be at least 2–3 cm away from the site of anastomosis to the common femoral artery. This length of crimped, nonsupported upper section serves to prevent angulation of its junction with the supported body of the graft when the hip is flexed.

For an above-knee femoro-popliteal bypass, the 30-cm length of supported central section is adequate to span any distance between 32 cm and 50 cm (including the 30-cm supported section, plus 20 cm of the crimped nonsupported upper end). For a below-knee femoro-popliteal bypass, the 45-cm supported section is adequate to span any distance between 47 cm and 65 cm. For a short-legged patient, the 30-cm support section prosthesis may be adequate for a below-knee femoro-popliteal bypass.

Perform the Lower Anastomosis First to Position the Supported Body in the Most Advantageous Location

The composite EXS fibrin/Dacron femoro-popliteal prosthesis is properly positioned when the lower support coil of the body is within 3 mm of the heel stitch of the distal anastomosis. Only by performing the distal anastomosis first can one with certainty place the lower support coil in this precise location. The noncrimped supported section, with its ability to resist kinking and compression, is used to best advantage when placed in this position.

The properly implanted EXS femoro-popliteal graft consists of (a) a short length of the noncrimped nonsupported lower section anastomosed to the popliteal artery; (b) the full length of the supported central section, extending distally to within 3 mm of the heel stitch of the popliteal anastomosis and (c) a length of the crimped nonsupported proximal section that varies according to the distance of the supported body from the site of anastomosis to the femoral artery.

Proper Length of Distal Anastomosis

After three years of experience with the EXS prosthesis, I am convinced that it is best to make the distal anastomosis approximately three times as long as the diameter of the prosthesis (but not longer). For example, if a 6-mm EXS graft is being used, the incision in the popliteal artery should be about 18 mm long. If the anastomosis to the popliteal artery below the knee is more than three times the diameter of the graft, a problem may arise during flexion of the knee (Fig. 7). The portion of artery included in the anastomosis tends to shorten during knee flexion, but the fabric component of the fibrin/Dacron prosthesis can only buckle, predisposing to occlusive thrombosis.

In the past, I made the distal anastomosis four times as long as the diameter of the graft, but now believe this to be too long. My current technique is as follows: I first incise the artery, making the incision three times the diameter of the graft. Then I cut the distal portion of the graft as shown in Fig. 8. From a point 3 mm distal to the lower support ring, I make a concave cut into the graft, aiming to reach a 40% depth at a distance equal to the diameter of the prosthesis. This cut is then continued distally at this 40% depth for a considerably longer distance than needed, and there the graft is transected.

The distal anastomosis is then performed with interrupted stitches, placing the first stitch at the apex of the heel of the anastomosis. The interrupted stitches are then brought out on each side of the anastomosis in an alternating manner. At a point one graft diameter from the end of the arteriotomy, the graft is cut in convex manner to form a rounded end that nicely fits the remaining open space of the arteriotomy. The anastomosis is then completed in a precise manner with interrupted stitches to avoid any constriction of the lumen.

Mandatory Changes that must Occur with Flexion of the Knee in the Straight-line Orientation of Both the Below-knee EXS Femoro-popliteal Graft and the Popliteal Artery below the Anastomosis

When the knee is flexed the tibia rotates posteriorly and superiorly on the femoral condyles, shortening the vertical distance from groin to popliteal artery (Fig. 9). Both the graft and popliteal artery must accommodate to this shortening. Accommodation of the EXS graft could at least in theory occur in three ways: (1) by contraction of the graft (not possible), (2) by kinking (neither possible nor desirable) or (3) by assuming an S-shaped position (both feasible and desirable with the EXS graft, as shown in Fig. 10).

The shortening forces of flexion also bear on the infra-anastomotic popliteal artery. Seldom does the aged artery have the elasticity to accommodate

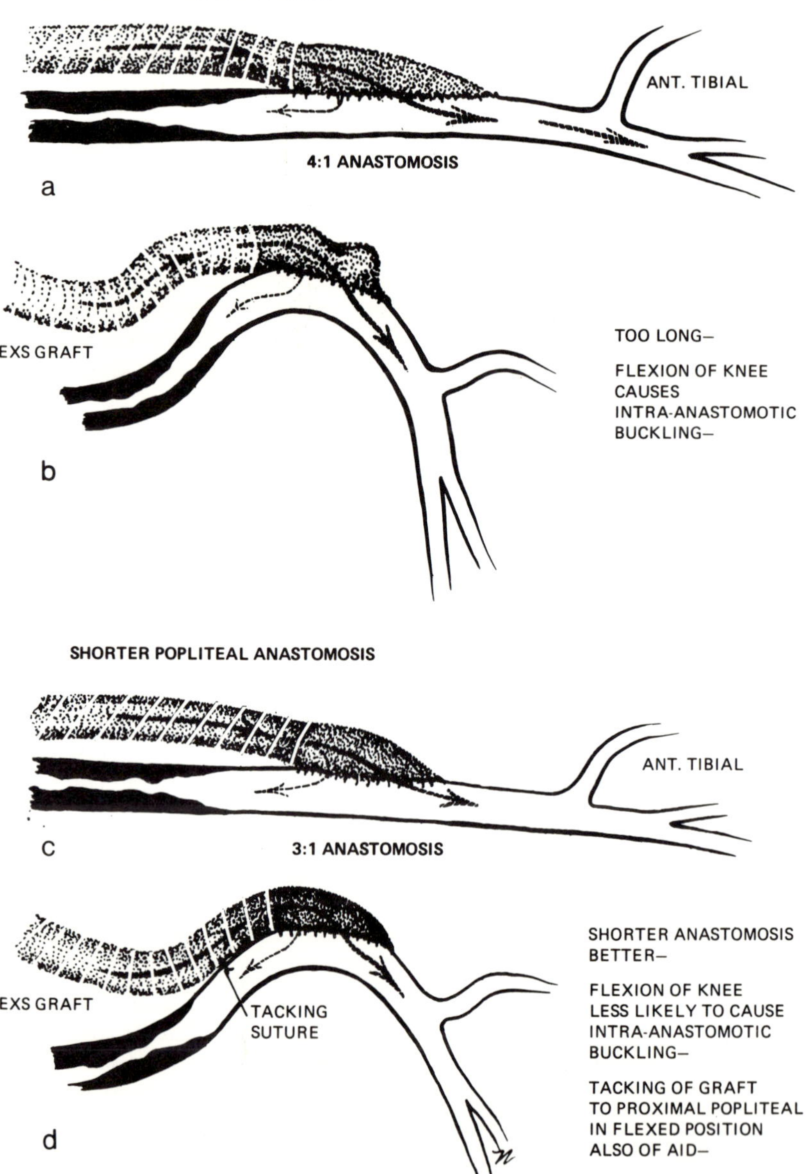

Fig. 7. Optimal length for EXS popliteal anastomosis. Length of anastomosis four times diameter of graft (a) is too long, as fabric tends to buckle during flexion of knee (b). Length of anastomosis three times diameter of graft (c) is less likely to buckle during flexion of knee (d). Tacking of proximal support ring to adventitia of artery with knee flexed is of further aid in preventing distortion of anastomosis with flexion of knee.

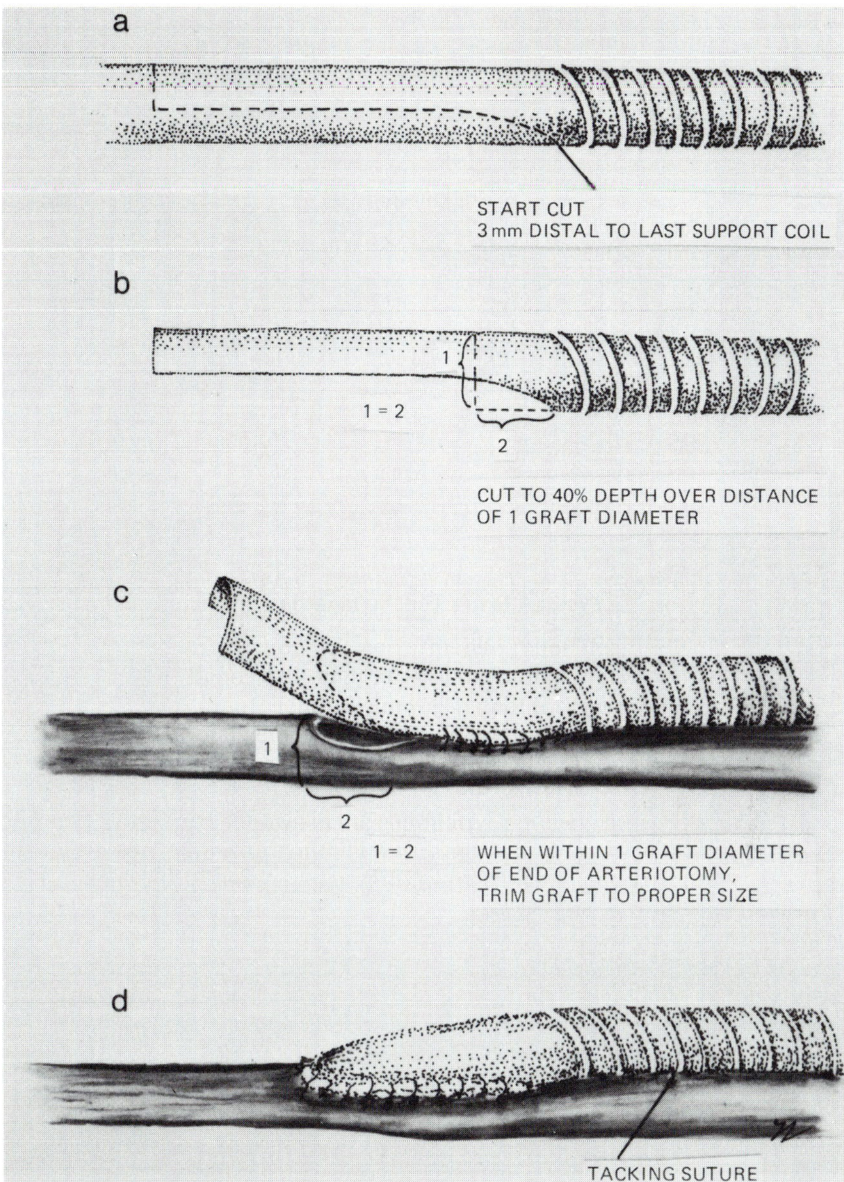

Fig. 8. Simplified method for cutting graft for distal anastomosis. The graft is cut in concave fashion with curved scissors to a depth of 40% over a distance equal to the diameter of the graft. This cut is then continued with straight scissors at the 40% depth for a distance well in excess of the proposed length of the anastomosis. Suturing is begun at the heel and continued toward the toe of the anastomosis. When the suturing has progressed to within one diameter of the end of the arteriotomy, the graft is trimmed with the curved scissors in convex fashion to round the end off to proper length.

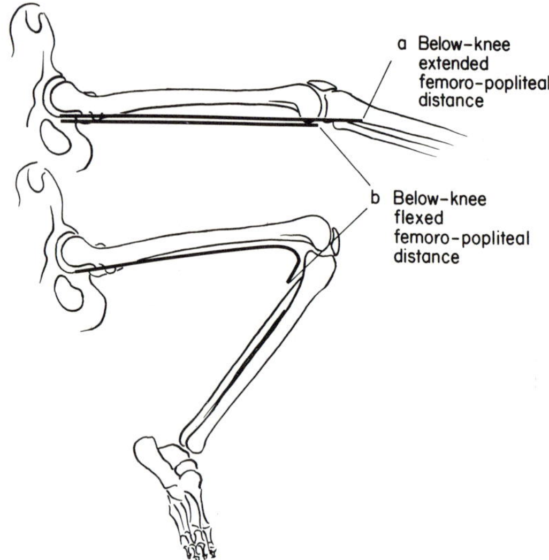

Fig. 9. The considerable magnitude of shortening of the vertical distance between the site of attachment of the graft to the common femoral artery above and to the popliteal artery below with flexion of the knee. This illustration was drawn from a human skeleton and measurements taken. These measurements revealed the "graft" length in the extended knee position to be 45 cm and in the flexed position to be 40 cm. This approximate 10% shortening must be accommodated by both the graft and the infra-anastomotic popliteal artery which independently may either assume the desirable S-shaped position or the undesirable kinked position.

this change by actual shortening through elastic recoil. Instead, it too must either assume a mini-S-shaped position or kink. The artery will assume the desirable S configuration if it has the freedom to move (Fig. 10). If it does not, it will be forced into a kinked position (Fig.11) likely to obstruct flow. By severely flexing the knee at surgery, one can determine whether the artery can assume a nonobstructed mini-S-shaped position and, if it cannot, which structures must be divided to give it this freedom. I now divide the soleal tendon and/or any other nonvital structure or bands or small veins that restrict motion of the artery beyond the anastomosis with flexion of the knee.

CLINICAL RESULTS

Above-knee Femoro-popliteal Bypass

Our results with 114 crimped nonsupported (Fig. 12) and 30 noncrimped supported (Fig. 13) composite fibrin/Dacron prostheses are shown. The comparative performance of the EXS prosthesis at three years (Fig. 14) is superior (86% patency versus 64% in this series), but definitive assessment of

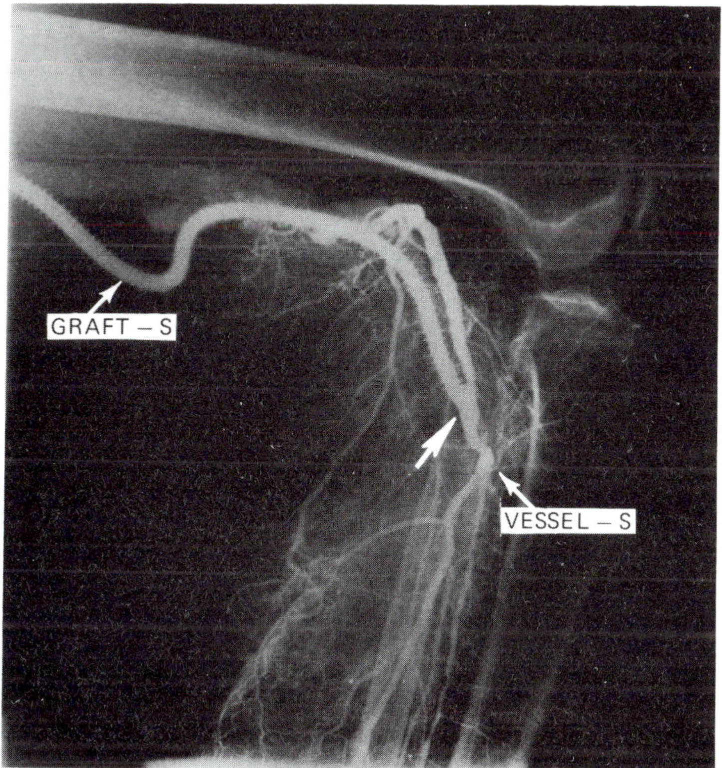

Fig. 10. Arteriogram showing below-knee EXS femoro-popliteal graft in flexed position. Note the large S position assumed by the EXS graft and the small S position assumed by the infra-anastomotic popliteal artery to accommodate to the 10% shortened length of the flexed position.

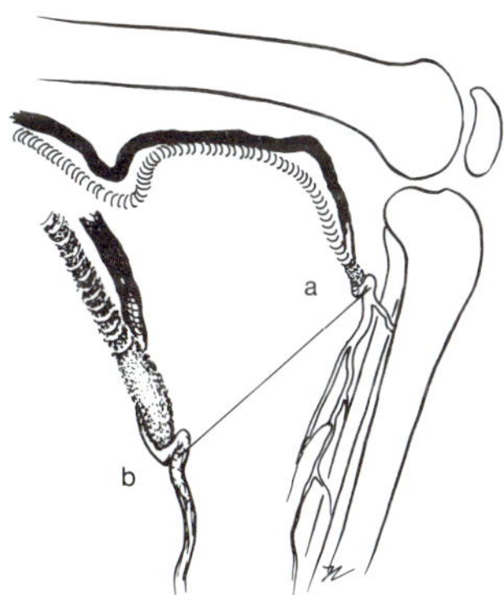

Fig. 11. Kinking of the infra-anastomotic popliteal artery with flexion of the knee when the artery has insufficient freedom to move. The closer the anastomosis is to the soleal tendon, the greater is this tendency. Division of the soleal tendon is of value to give mobility to the distal popliteal artery.

Patients	Grafts	Closures	Open	Mean Implant	Patency
92	114	44		24 mo.	61%
			70	55 mo.	

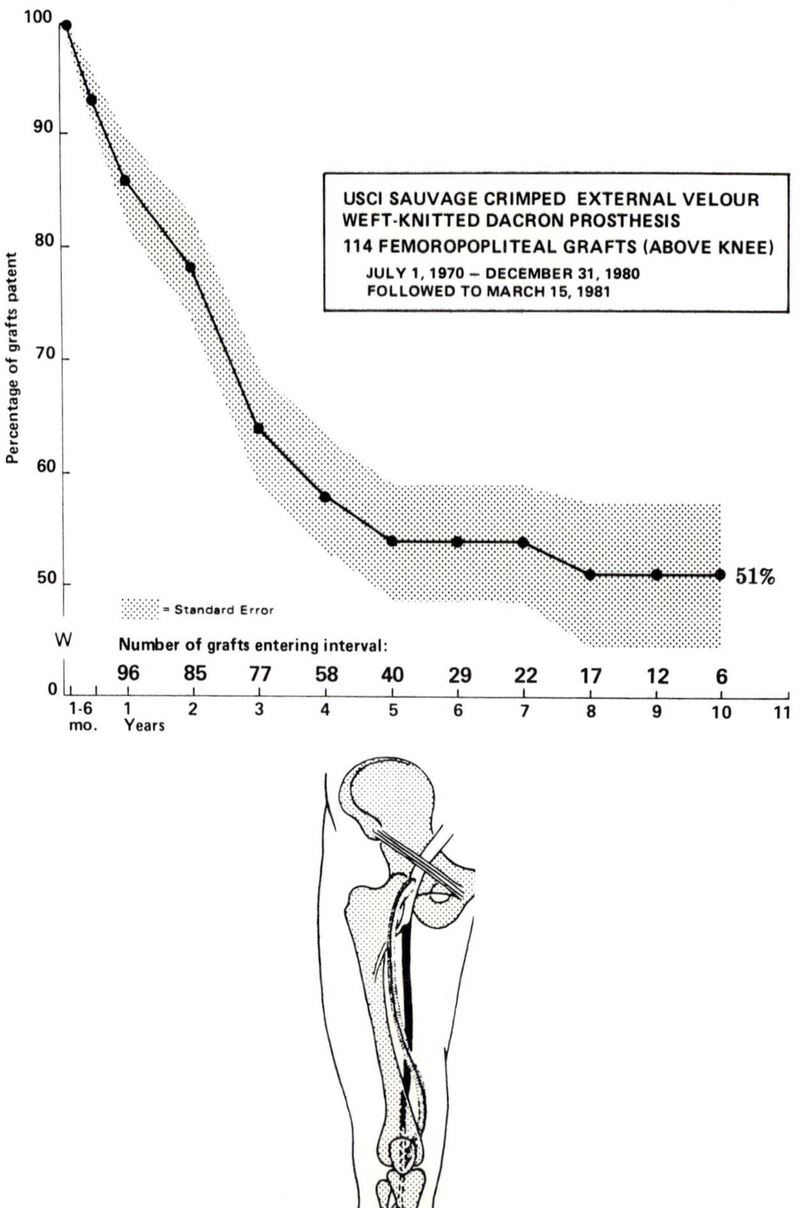

Fig. 12. Life-table results for 114 USCI Sauvage external velour weft-knitted Dacron above-knee femoro-popliteal grafts implanted during the 1970 to 1980 period with a follow-up period to 15 March 1981. The progressive fall-off in the early years contrasts with the relative stability of the grafts surviving the fifth year.

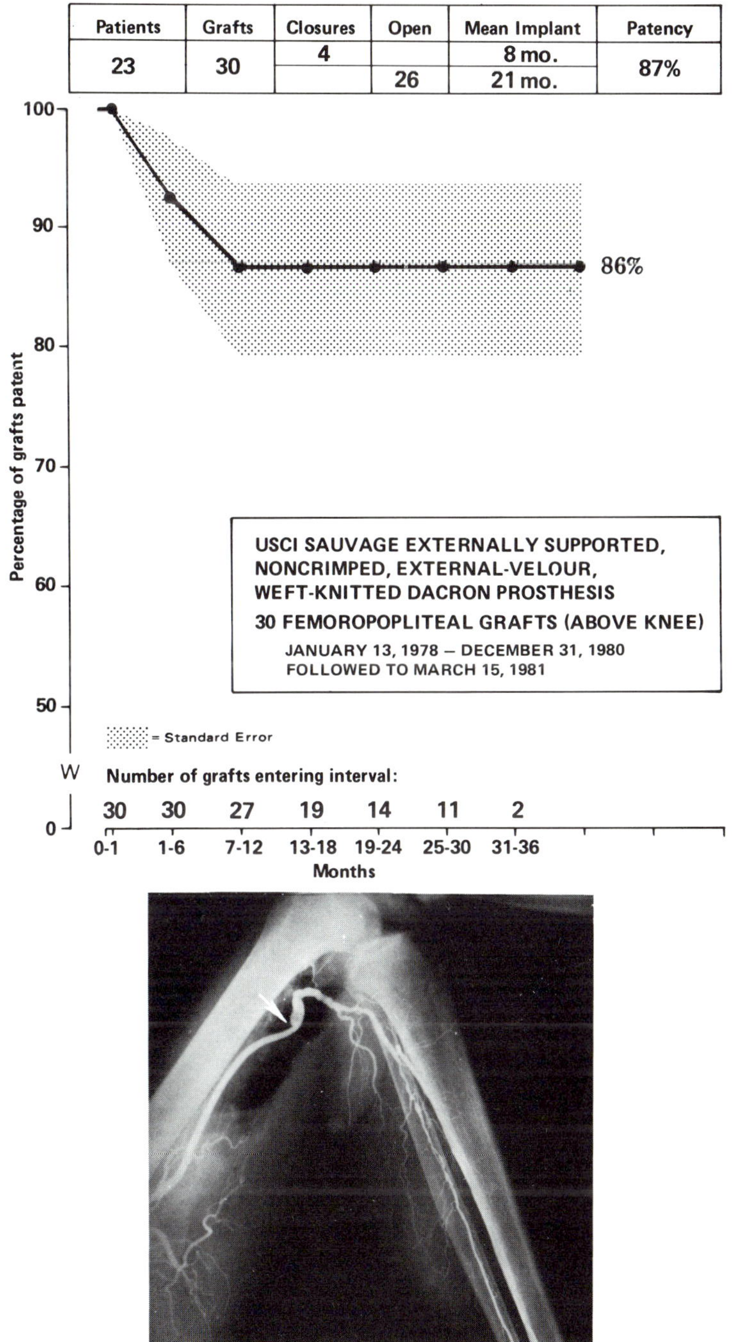

Patients	Grafts	Closures	Open	Mean Implant	Patency
23	30	4		8 mo.	87%
			26	21 mo.	

Fig. 13. Life-table results for 30 USCI Sauvage EXS above-knee femoro-popliteal grafts implanted during the 1978 to 1980 period with a follow-up period to 15 March 1981. Note that after a modest early fall-off, the patency of these grafts has been maintained at 86% out of 36 months.

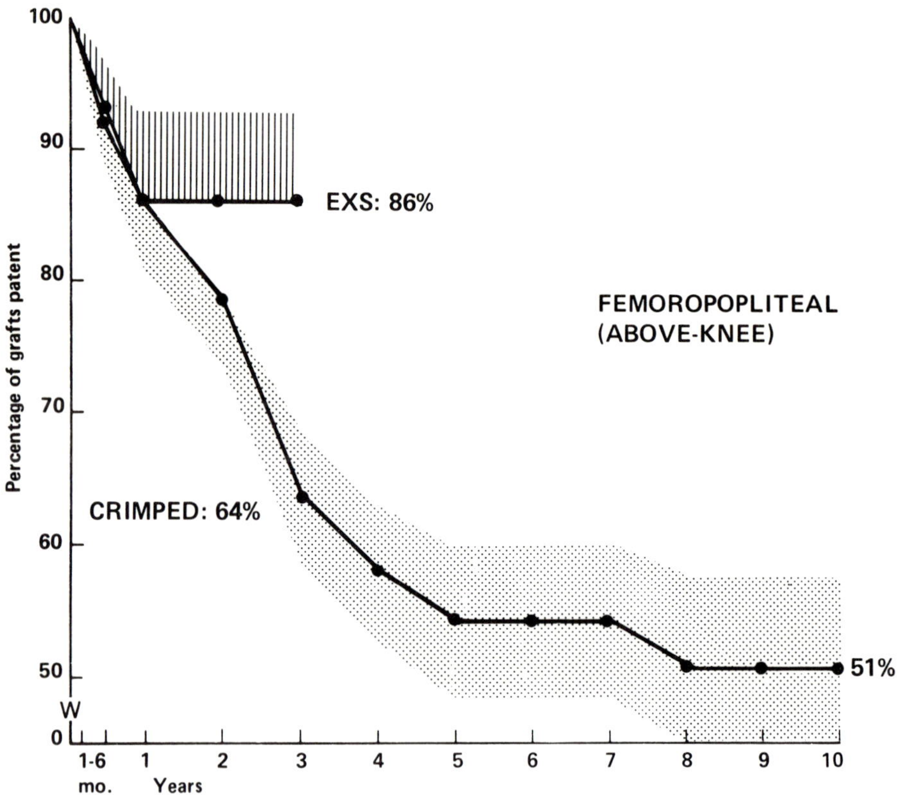

Fig. 14. Superimposition of life-table results of crimped nonsupported and EXS grafts implanted as above-knee femoro-popliteal grafts. There is improvement in the patency results with the EXS prosthesis at three years (86% patency versus 64%).

this graft must await the passage of more time. At this moment, the comparison clearly favours the EXS graft.

Below-knee Femoro-popliteal Bypass

Since we have not used the crimped nonsupported prosthesis for below-knee femoro-popliteal bypass, our results are limited to EXS prosthesis implantations. These are few in number (16) and have been followed for a relatively short time (mean implant of 18 months) with a life-table patency at three years of 62% (Fig. 15). I believe it reasonable to anticipate improvement of patency as we apply to subsequent cases what we have learned in this early experience, especially as regards assuring that the popliteal artery below the anastomosis has adequate freedom to assume a mini-S-shaped configuration with flexion of the knee.

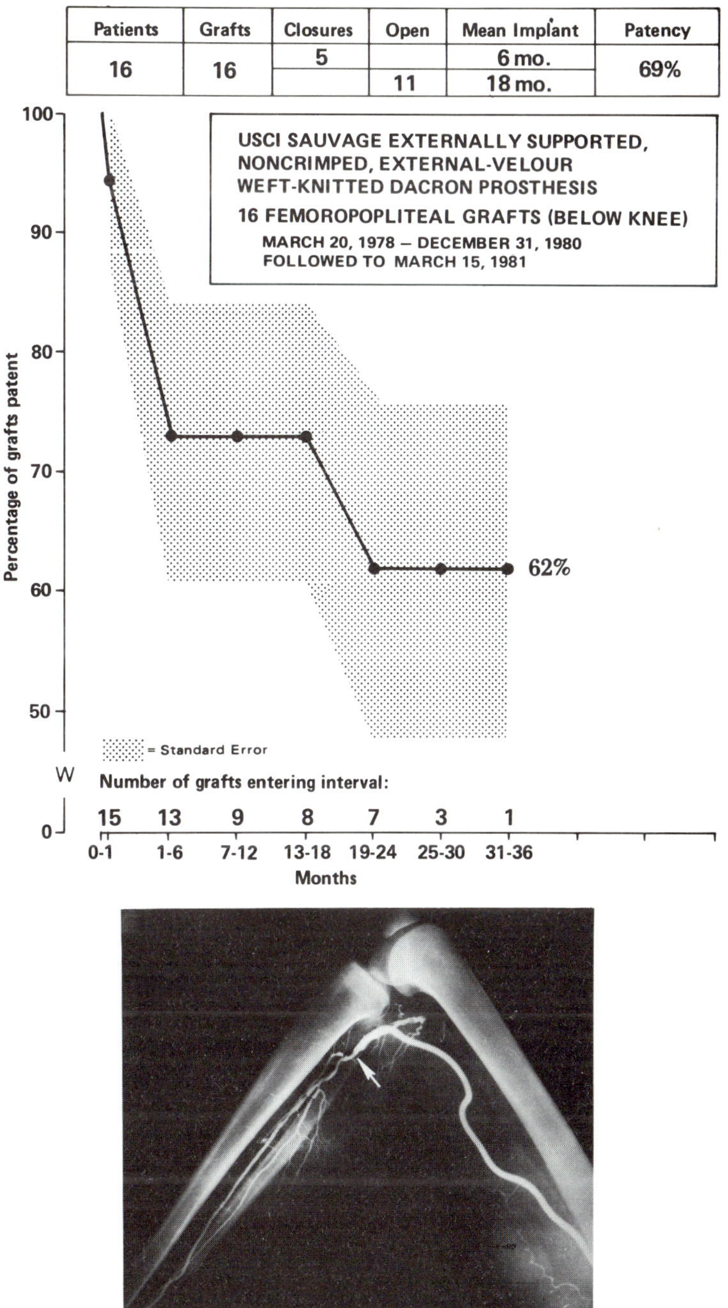

Fig. 15. Life-table results for 16 USCI Sauvage EXS below-knee femoro-popliteal prostheses implanted in the 1978 to 1980 period, with a follow-up period to 15 March 1981. There has been a learning curve in the use of the EXS prosthesis below the knee (Figs 7–11). More cases followed for longer periods are required to gain an accurate estimate of the long-term performance of EXS prostheses used for below-knee femoro-popliteal bypass.

DISCUSSION

The relatively good long-term (11-year) success rate of 51% for above-knee crimped external velour weft-knitted composite fibrin/Dacron prostheses is noteworthy. These results are a challenge to other types of grafts that have been added more recently to the surgical armamentarium for use in femoro-popliteal bypass.

Our results suggest that the noncrimped EXS prosthesis is superior to its predecessor, the crimped nonsupported prosthesis for above-knee femoro-popliteal bypass (three-year life-table patency of 86% versus 64%). Our below-knee EXS result of a 62% life-table patency at three years is encouraging but not a reason for complacency.

While our experimental results show the composite fibrin/Dacron EXS prosthesis to outperform Gore-Tex and the umbilical vein Biograft (Kenney *et al.*, 1980; Sauvage *et al.*, 1979), proper assessment of the comparative clinical value of EXS prostheses for below-knee femoro-popliteal bypass must await more EXS cases followed for longer periods.

I believe that post-operative platelet suppression programs should be used for most patients who have received composite EXS fibrin/Dacron femoro-popliteal bypass grafts. A first recommendation is that patients should be vigorously encouraged to stop smoking as part of their pre-operative instruction. Chances of having the patient stop smoking following surgery are significantly increased if due attention has been given to this important subject pre-operatively. There are many papers documenting the adverse effects of smoking on the long-term patency of prosthetic grafts, even including those of large caliber (Auerback *et al.*, 1965; Ahmedd *et al.*, 1976). It is probable that smoking causes sufficient vasoconstriction to produce a stop–start flow pattern in small arteries. V. V. Kakkar (personal communication) has shown a measurable increase in beta thromboglobulin levels in individuals smoking a single cigarette, indicating activation of platelets with a subsequent "release response".

The flow rates in femoro-popliteal bypass grafts may be below the thrombotic threshold velocity (TTV) of the fibrin flow surface of the composite fibrin/Dacron EXS prosthesis. This velocity is defined as that at which thrombus formation begins. This concept is illustrated in Fig. 16.

If the ability of the platelets to be activated by the flow surface is decreased, the TTV has in effect been lowered, i.e. the surface can be exposed to lower flows without activating either Factor XII (intrinsic system) or platelets. Hence, it seems reasonable that a platelet suppression program should add to the long-term patency of synthetic below-knee femoro-popliteal bypass grafts in most patients. Though without adequate data, we believe in general that if the flow velocity through a composite EXS fibrin/Dacron graft is less than 8 ml cm^{-2} graft cross-sectional area per second, thrombotic occlusion is likely after a period of several months unless the patient is protected by an effective platelet suppression program. For a 5-mm EXS femoro-popliteal prosthesis, this means a minimal flow of about 100 ml min^{-1}, and for a 6-mm prosthesis of about 144 ml min^{-1}.

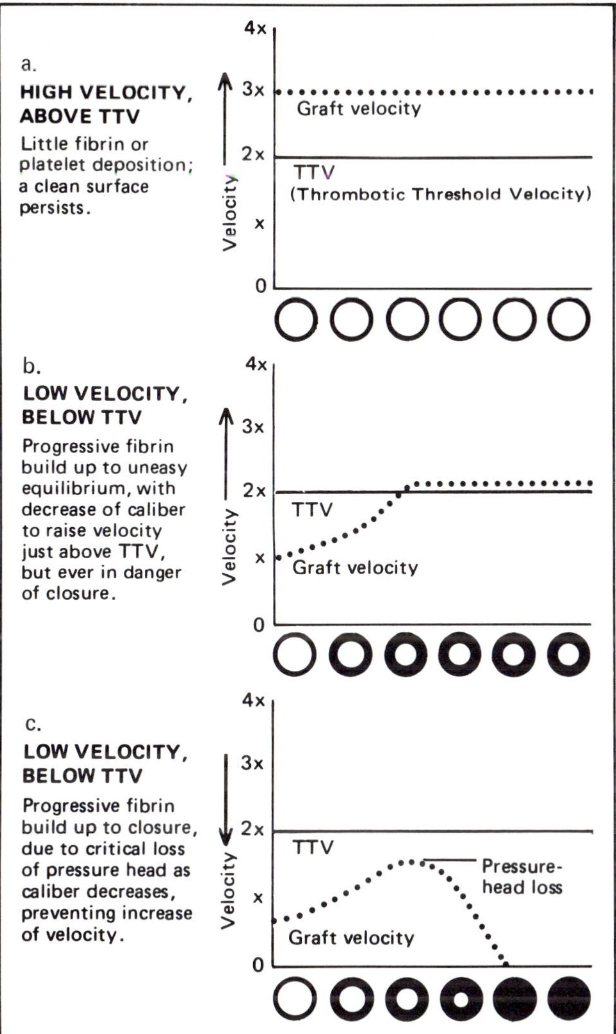

Fig. 16. Flow-surface thrombus deposition in relation to velocity of blood flow. Our concept is that for every surface, there is a velocity above which thrombus deposition cannot occur, and below which it must occur. The velocity at which thrombus formation just begins is termed the thrombotic threshold velocity, or TTV. (a) If the initial flow velocity is above the TTV, no significant flow-surface deposition occurs. (b) If the initial flow velocity is below the TTV, fibrin deposition must occur. This deposition continues until the decrease of caliber of the flow channel raises the flow velocity to just above the TTV, thereby halting further fibrin deposition. (c) If the initial flow rate is so low that the build up of fibrin and/or platelets on the flow surface is unable to raise the velocity to above the thrombotic threshold due to pressure head loss within the graft, deposition continues relentlessly to total occlusion.

If flow rates of this magnitude are not achievable, a long-term platelet suppression program is advised. Under these circumstances, we routinely give 100 ml of Dextran 40 before clamp release and continue this agent at 20 ml h^{-1} for 72 h. Our current post-operative regimen includes 50 mg vitamin B_6 daily, 400 IU of vitamin E daily (Cox *et al.*, 1980) and one pediatric aspirin (75 mg) morning and evening for a total dosage of 2.5 mg kg^{-1} day^{-1} (McCollum *et al.*, 1980). The total cost of these medications is about 10 cents per day. Doses of aspirin above 5 mg kg^{-1} day^{-1} have been shown to inhibit prostacyclin formation by platelets, whereas smaller doses (2.5–3 mg kg^{-1} day^{-1}) do not block prostacyclin formation but are sufficient to block thromboxane A_2 formation (Masotti *et al.*, 1979).

In the past, we have also used 100 mg of Persantine daily, but now believe this to be unnecessary, since pyridoxal-5′-phosphate, a metabolite of vitamin B_6, appears to perform a similar antiplatelet function (Ahmedd *et al.*, 1976).

SUMMARY

Our experience with crimped external velour weft-knitted composite fibrin/Dacron grafts for above-knee femoro-popliteal bypass shows a life-table patency of 51% at 11 years. Our mid-term life-table results at three years for noncrimped EXS external velour weft-knitted composite fibrin/Dacron grafts above the knee are superior to those of the crimped nonsupported grafts (86% patency, compared with 64%). I recognize that many factors other than the intrinsic attributes of the prostheses may have influenced these results. Our three-year below-knee femoro-popliteal life-table patency of 62% for the EXS is less desirable. This lower patency may in part reflect a learning curve in our proper use of this prosthesis for below-knee femoro-popliteal bypass, as discussed in the text. Although showing considerable promise in this location, longer follow-up periods of more cases will be required before a definitive evaluation of the value of the composite EXS fibrin/Dacron graft for below-knee femoro-popliteal bypass can be made in relation to that of other currently available prostheses.

REFERENCES

Ahmedd, S. S., Moschos, C. B., Lyons, M. M., Oldewurtel, H. A., Coumbis, R. J., Regan, T. J. and Jenkins, B. (1976). Cardiovascular effects of long-term cigarette smoking and nicotine administration. *American Journal of Cardiology* **37**, 33.

Auerback, O., Hammond, E. C. and Garfinkel, L. (1965). Smoking in relation to atherosclerosis of the coronary arteries. *New England Journal of Medicine* **273**, 775.

Cox, A. C., Rao, G. H. R., Gerrard, J. M. and White, J. G. (1980). The influence of vitamin E quinone on platelet structure, function, and biochemistry. *Blood* **55**, 907.

Kenney, D. A., Berger, K., Walker, M. W., Robel, S. B., Boguslavsky, L., Ray, L. I., Lischko, M. M. and Sauvage, L. R. (1980). Experimental comparison of the thrombogenicity of fibrin and PTFE flow surface. *Annals of Surgery* **191**, 355.

McCollum, C. N., Crow, M. J., Rajah, S. M. and Kester, R. C. (1980). Anti-thrombotic therapy for vascular prostheses: an experimental model testing platelet inhibitory drugs. *Surgery* **87**, 668.

Masotti, G., Poggesi, L., Galanti, G., Abbate, R. and Neri Serneri, G. G. (1979). Differential inhibition of prostacyclin production and platelet aggregation by aspirin. *Lancet* **2**, 1213.

Sauvage, L. R., Walker, M. W., Berger, K., Robel, S. B., Lischko, M. M., Yates, S. G. and Logan, G. A. (1979). Current arterial prostheses. Experimental evaluation of implantation in the carotid and circumflex coronary arteries in the dog. *Archives of Surgery (Chicago)* **114**, 687.

Yates, S. G., Barros, D'sa, A. A. B., Berger, K., Fernandez, L. G., Wood, S. J., Rittenhouse, E. A., Davis, C. C., Mansfield, P. B. and Sauvage, L. R. (1978). The preclotting of porous arterial prostheses. *Annals of Surgery* **188**, 611.

UMBILICAL VEIN GRAFTS: TECHNIQUES AND RESULTS FOR LOWER EXTREMITY REVASCULARIZATION

H. Dardik

Vascular Surgical Service, Englewood Hospital, Englewood, New Jersey, USA

Reliable and readily available alternatives to the autologous saphenous vein for lower extremity revascularization continue to be a major goal for vascular surgeons. Since 1974 umbilical cord vessels have been employed clinically as vascular conduits (Dardik *et al.*, 1976). Prior attempts using these structures without aldehyde tanning resulted in predictable failure (Nabseth *et al.*, 1960; Yong and Eiseman, 1962; Dardik and Dardik, 1975). Current processing involves acquisition of cords from obstetric delivery suites and then processing with glutaraldehyde in a complex series of steps. Previous work from our laboratory demonstrated the absolute necessity for tanning and the superiority of glutaraldehyde over dialdehyde starch (Dardik and Dardik, 1975; Dardik *et al.*, 1976). The grafts are covered with a polyester Dacron mesh and stored in alcohol*. Extensive investigations employing biochemical, physical and electrical parameters have demonstrated these grafts to be biocompatible and thromboresistant.

TECHNIQUE

Gentle handling of the graft is critical. Clamping or rough manual handling

---

*Biograft,™ Meadox Medicals, Inc., Oakland, New Jersey.

Serono Symposium No. 44, "Peripheral Arterial Diseases: Medical and Surgical Problems", edited by S. Stipa and A. Cavallaro, 1982. Academic Press, London and New York.

will result in intimal fracture and dissection. This is particularly liable to occur if excessive traction is employed with Silastic vessel loops or if standard vascular clamps are applied tightly. Intra-luminal balloon tamponade may be the safest method to achieve vascular control. Thickness and thinness of the wall has no relevance to the effectiveness of the material. It may introduce differences in the ease with which the graft can be sutured but, in fact, makes very little difference. Thick grafts become thinner with arterial pressure once the proximal anastomosis is completed. External tissue shreds may occasionally be seen. They can either be simply snipped off or ignored. One should not pull on these tissue fragments. Prior to implantation the graft must be irrigated thoroughly to wash out alcohol and aldehyde residues. Hufnagel (1978) has described the use of an undiluted heparin rinse after irrigation and prior to implantation that may, by surface bonding, result in increased thromboresistance at the flow surface. Cranley and Hafner (1980) prefer low molecular weight dextran. We employ the former technique but await further data regarding the need and efficacy of these additional pre-implant maneuvers.

Systemic heparinization is employed using 1.25 mg kg^{-1} and is monitored intra-operatively by the activated clotting time test (Mabry *et al.*, 1979). We usually do the proximal anastomosis first, but the distal anastomosis can be performed initially if the surgeon prefers. It is essential that the tunnelling of the graft be performed through a metallic or plastic tunneller. Damage to the graft can occur if it is simply pulled through the tissue tunnel, due to friction between the outer Dacron mesh and the tissues. An alternative technique is to coat the graft just prior to placement in the tunnel with a sterile water soluble lubricant. For the distal anastomosis, interrupted suture technique with fine monofilament suture material is employed at the ends of the arteriotomy. A continuous technique is employed along the lateral margins. We endeavour to make this anastomosis approximately 22–25 mm long which has been shown by intra-operative arteriography, to give a smoother and better taper. The interrupted suture method may also preserve the compliance of the graft at the anastomosis. Intra-operative arteriography is routine to identify any technical fault and to demonstrate the run-off, including the pedal arch (Dardik *et al.*, 1978).

The medial approach was employed to gain access to the popliteal and posterior tibial arteries at all levels. The anterior tibial artery is dissected from the intermuscular cleft of the anterior compartment by a long anterolateral incision. Fasciotomy is always performed. A laterally based incision with partial fibulectomy is preferred to the medial approach for exposure of the peroneal artery throughout its entire course. Close attention to a number of technical details is essential in order to secure success. These include meticulous handling of all tissues and particularly the arteries. If calcification exists, fracturing of these vessels must be avoided.

Post-operative graft thrombosis presents the surgeon with several options. Firstly, he may do a thrombectomy or he may simply ignore the graft thrombosis and permit the situation to continue and observe the clinical course of the patient. Finally, the surgeon may replace the original graft with a new one altogether and in this situation the original graft may or may not be removed.

The decision as to which alternative to select depends in turn on a number of factors. These include the time of thrombosis with regard to when it occurs since the graft was implanted, the mechanism for thrombosis and finally the extent. Early thromboses, defined by those that occur in the immediate or early post-operative period are usually due to one of two factors: (1) technical mishap, (2) extremely poor run-off. In the latter instance, intra-operative arteriography is helpful to define this problem and the decision could be made to either ignore the thrombosis and accept the situation as a failure or to consider the possibility of performing an adjunctive arterio-venous fistula (Ibrahim *et al.*, 1980). Technical mishaps which might not have been appreciated or recognized on the intra-operative arteriogram might be recognized at re-exploration of the graft. These can be corrected depending on the exact mechanism such as removal of plaque distal to the distal anastomosis and peforming vein patch angioplasty, correction of an unrecognized inflow problem by endarterectomy or proximal bypass or other such techniques. Our management in such circumstances consists of re-exploration of the graft distally and securing control of the graft and the distal vessel. After heparinizing the patient an arteriotomy is established along the longitudinal axis of the graft overlying the site of the distal anastomosis. If necessary the opening in the graft is extended across the distal anastomosis at the apex and then distally into the artery itself. Since we ordinarily perform an interrupted suture technique at this level, an unraveled suture line is never a problem. Any firm thrombosis is usually located at this point and can be removed manually. Distal exploration with a balloon catheter is performed and the distal circulation further assessed. At this point the status of the proximal portion of the graft must also be appreciated. Generally there is no pulse and if none can be restored by simple and gentle manual massage from above, a balloon catheter is introduced from below with great care being taken not to overly inflate the balloon. More often however, we open up the upper wound and manually compress the thrombus downward so that the patients own blood pressure will extrude the clot. We will then pass the balloon catheter from below upward making certain that all thrombus is removed and then proceed with closure of the distal arteriotomy. However, since catheter balloons can be easily compressed by firm thrombus, we do not hesitate securing control of the upper portion of the graft, doing a small arteriotomy at this point and then proceed with manual extraction of thrombus or irrigation of the entire graft with heparinized solution prior to balloon catheter extraction of any residual thrombus. Once these techniques have been completed the upper arteriotomy can be closed primarily as well as the lower one. If the distal arteriotomy extends across the artery, we will apply a saphenous or umbilical vein patch to prevent stricture. Late graft closures usually present a slightly different problem in that the dissection of the graft may be quite difficult particularly at anastomotic areas. In several instances we have explored the graft remote from the anastomosis and performed very simple balloon catheter extractions. This, of course, is fraught with risk and should be limited only to patients who might otherwise not be candidates for extensive reconstructions. In those patients in whom the dissection can be performed in the anastomotic region, maneuvers similar to those described for early thrombosis are performed. Many grafts can thereby be salvaged even where the graft has been closed for periods exceeding four weeks. In those cases where the dissection of the graft is virtually impossible or if there is concern with regard to the status of the graft, either because of changes following implantation or because of damage following maneuvers to extract thrombus, we have not hesitated to simply implant a new graft placed at either a similar level or at a more proximal level for the proximal anastomosis and distal to the previously performed distal anastomosis. We usually remove whatever segments of graft are readily seen in the operative field.

The most important feature for Biograft thrombectomy is extreme gentleness when manipulating the graft. When using a balloon catheter overinflation must be avoided. On many occasions it may be preferable, prior to ballon catheter extraction of thrombus, to try to extrude the graft by gentle external massage or by direct irrigation of the graft after performing proximal and distal arteriotomies. Openings in the graft may be made vertically at the proximal and distal anastomotic areas. In the body of the graft a transverse opening is preferable in order to avoid stricture. At the distal anastomosis, if the arteriotomy is carried across the anastomosis into the artery, a vein patch should be applied. If there is concern with the structural integrity of the graft or difficulty with the dissection, one should not hesitate placing a new graft. Finally, it is our routine to perform an intra-operative arteriogram at the time of original surgery. This cannot be overly emphasized. The information obtained will be useful in the event of subsequent thrombosis and is essential to guide the surgeon in making appropriate decisions regarding thrombectomy.

INDICATIONS

The indications employed for selecting cases for bypass in this series were based on the following: (1) limb salvage manifest by a pre-gangrenous state and/or progressive lesions of the foot or leg that would otherwise lead to imminent limb amputation, (2) rest pain and/or nonhealing lesions but the limb is not imminently at risk, (3) disabling claudication and (4) prophylactic for asymptomatic popliteal aneurysms. Our experience with the glutaraldehyde-stabilized human umbilical cord vein graft now consists of 552 implantations in the lower extremity performed over the five-year period, 1975 to 1980. There were 286 popliteal, 169 tibial and 97 peroneal reconstructions. Two hundred and thirty-three of the popliteal reconstructions were infrageniculate. Patients who had peroneal reconstructions were predominantly older and there was a high incidence of diabetes mellitus in this group (72%). Many patients had already undergone vascular reconstructions. Approximately one-half of the group having tibial and peroneal reconstructions had undergone some form of prior bypass that had failed and then required an extended or complex procedure in order to save the limb. The most common previous procedure was femoro-popliteal bypass with autologous saphenous vein.

A variety of biophysical and chemical tests have been employed in studying explant materials. The testing program included internal reflection spectroscopy (IRS), critical surface tension (CST), morphological evaluation by light and electron microscopy and various mechanical and biochemical parameters. In addition, structural analysis of function grafts *in vivo* was obtained by serial post-operative arteriograms.

CLINICAL RESULTS

Operative mortality rates for popliteal, tibial and peroneal reconstructions were 3.5, 3.0 and 4.1% respectively. The cumulative graft patency rates for each of the three types of reconstruction are shown in Figs 1 and 2. There is no statistical validity for the final two-year figures since the numbers of cases are small. Figure 3 summarizes the cumulative patency rates for popliteal reconstructions according to location of the distal anastomosis (above or below the knee), the presence or absence of diabetes mellitus and the influence of the run-off. As might be predicted, the presence of diabetes mellitus, poor run-off and reconstructions extending distally initially lead to worse results than if these factors are not present. However, these differences appear to diminish with time.

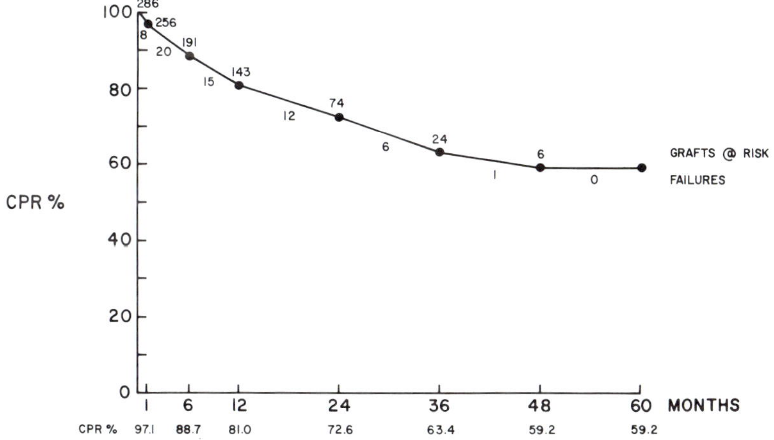

Fig. 1. Cumulative patency rates for all femoral popliteal reconstructions. Figures above curve represent numbers of patients entering that particular time interval. Figures below curve are number of patients with failed grafts in a particular time interval. CPR, cumulative patency rate.

Factors that were related to most failures included the quality of the artery into which the distal anastomosis was performed as well as the run-off beyond this vessel. Calcification was associated with a higher incidence of ultimate graft closure. The absence of a pedal arch was associated with early graft closure in almost all instances. Early failures were usually due to inappropriate case selection with the factors previously identified being present. Late failures were usually due to progressive disease, particularly in the distal

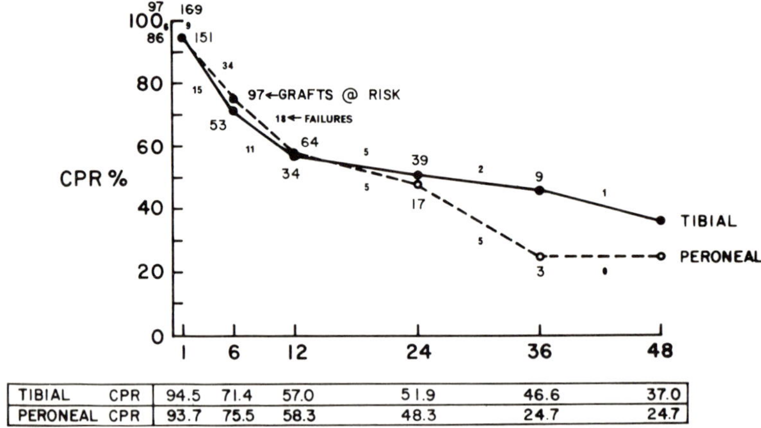

TIBIAL CPR	94.5	71.4	57.0	51.9	46.6	37.0
PERONEAL CPR	93.7	75.5	58.3	48.3	24.7	24.7

Fig. 2. Cumulative patency rates for tibial and peroneal reconstructions.

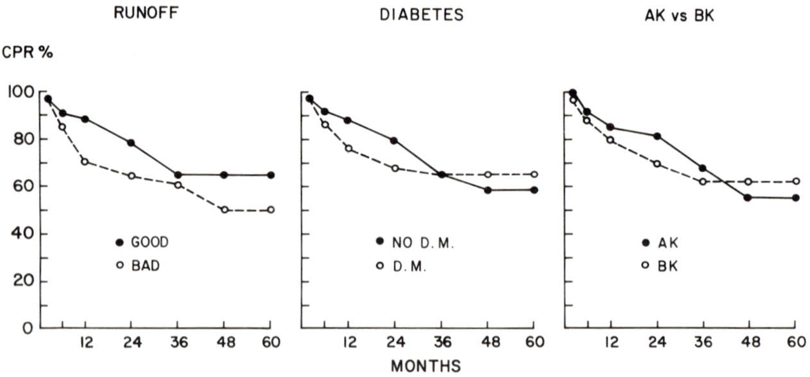

Fig. 3. Cumulative patency rates for femoral popliteal reconstructions according to site of distal anastomosis, presence or absence of diabetes and state of run-off circulation.

circulation. In some patients an accelerated progression of the atherosclerotic process was also observed in the inflow circulation. The actual number and percentages of thrombectomies performed for each of the reconstruction groups is depicted in Fig. 4. Successful thrombectomies were obtained in less than 10% of the popliteal and peroneal reconstructions and 14% of the tibials. Many of the failed thrombectomies would today not have even been attempted. Fourteen infections (2.5%) occurred in this series of which 11 (2.0%) failed. Ten required removal and one thrombosed *in situ*. There were no instances of biodegradation either by aneurysm formation or by myointimal proliferation. Only one graft showed segmental ectasia at 20 months. Three false aneurysms occurred early in the series and were probably due to faulty technique. Cumulative limb salvage is depicted in Fig. 5. These

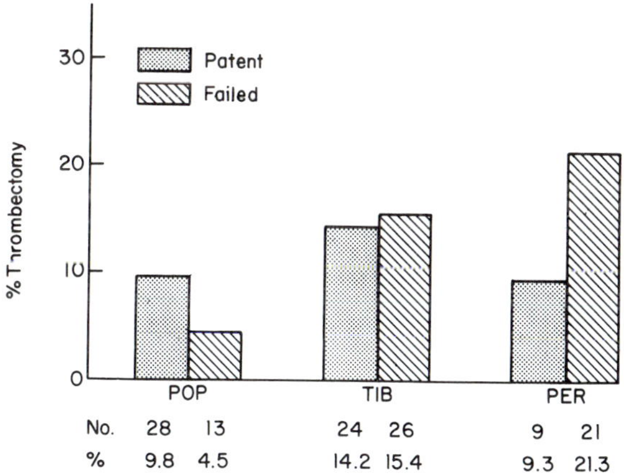

Fig. 4. Number and percentage of thrombectomies required for each of the reconstruction groups. Most of the thrombectomies performed that ultimately failed would today not even be attempted based on the results of either pre-operative or intra-operative arteriography.

results confirm the effectiveness even of peroneal reconstruction in securing limb salvage despite later closure of the graft. The actual number and type of amputations performed is shown in the histogram portion of Fig. 5.

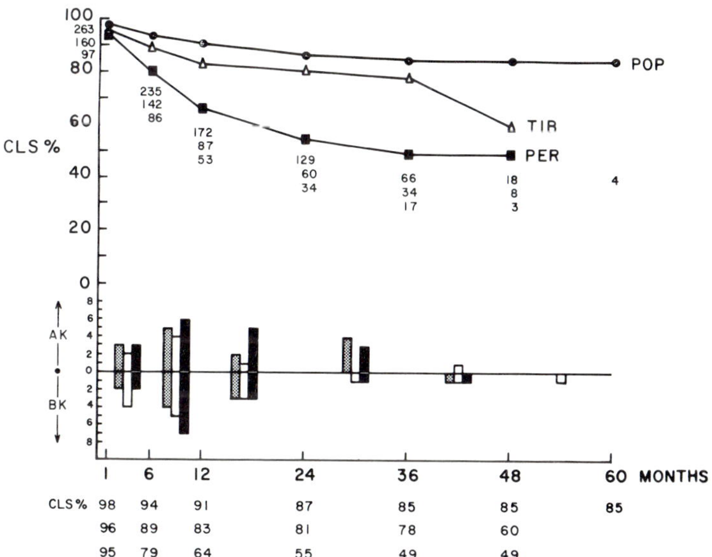

Fig. 5. Cumulative limb salvage rates following popliteal, tibial and peroneal reconstruction. The actual numbers of amputations are indicated in each time interval in the histogram portion of this figure. Amputations above or below the knee are indicated relative to the horizontal axis.

DISCUSSION

The results of the cumulative patency rates obtained in reconstructions of the popliteal, tibial or peroneal arteries were similar to those obtained by ourselves and others using autologous saphenous veins in comparable cases (Dardik *et al.*, 1979, 1980; DeWeese and Rob, 1977; Cutler *et al.*, 1976; LoGerfo *et al.*, 1977; Naji *et al.*, 1978; Szilagyi *et al.*, 1979). Analysis of the failures in this series indicates that the majority were due to faulty case selection. Using today's criteria, most of these patients would not now be considered suitable for operation, for example, those with absence of the pedal arch and extensive calcification of the run-off vessels. Preliminary investigation employing adjunctive arteriovenous fistulas for remote tibial and peroneal bypasses under circumstances of actual or predictable failure have been encouraging (Ibrahim *et al.*, 1980). Most graft failures are due to progression of the disease, usually in the distal circulation, but sometimes in the proximal inflow circulation as documented by serial arteriography.

This graft requires expert surgical technique and a short period of thorough irrigation to eliminate aldehyde and alcohol residues. The early and long-term experience has been sufficiently gratifying to warrant its continued use for reconstructions involving the popliteal, tibial and peroneal segments. In addition, the post-operative morphologic data reported here further confirm the biodurability of these grafts. Evidence of biodegradation has been exceedingly minimal, without any significant incidence of aneurysmal degeneration, calcification or intimal hyperplasia. Lipid deposition has been noted by light and electron microscopy as well as by infrared spectrographic analysis. This observation may, however, be more related to the type of lipid metabolism indigenous to the particular patient rather than to the graft itself. High lipid levels at an early post-operative stage were manifest in patients with evidence of progressive atherosclerotic involvement in other systems. Many of these patients died early of myocardial infarction or strokes. Late and minimal lipid deposition occurred in patients with relatively stable systemic atherosclerosis. These patients showed no progression. An interesting phenomenon associated with glutaraldehyde was the marked increased resistance of these graft materials to infection. The exceedingly low rate of infection is a manifestation of this resistance. Additionally, graft dissolution and hemorrhage did not occur in the presence of graft infection.

From its inception and even to the present day, the umbilical cord vein project has been surrounded by skepticism and at times incredulity. Review of our results, however, suggests that in fact the glutaraldehyde stabilized umbilical vein prosthesis can serve as an attractive alternative to the saphenous vein. Although this study is primarily concerned with a particular graft material, it is evident that the success to failure ratio is complex. Experience, judgement and meticulous technique are prerequisites to durable graft patency. No graft material can make up for lack of these principles nor should the surgeon blame his failures on the particular material employed. The use of glutaraldehyde-stabilized umbilical vein simply makes these operations easier by providing a reliable material that is nonantigenic, mechanically equivalent to normal vascular structures and biocompatible as determined by physical and chemical modalities.

REFERENCES

Cranley, J. J. and Hafner, C. D. (1980). Current status of the umbilical vein graft. Complications in Vascular Surgery. (V. Bernhard, Ed.), p. 597. Grune & Stratton, New York.

Cutler, B. S., Thompson, J. F., Kleinsasser, L. J. *et al.* (1976). Autologous saphenous vein femoropopliteal bypass: analysis of 298 cases. *Surgery* **79**, 325.

Dardik, H. and Dardik, I. (1976). Successful arterial substitution with modified human umbilical vein. *Annals of Surgery* **183**, 252.

Dardik, I. and Dardik H. (1975). The fate of human umbilical cord vessels used as interposition arterial grafts in the baboon. *Surgery, Gynecology and Obstetrics* **140**, 567.

Dardik, H., Ibrahim, I. M., Baier, R., Sprayregen, S., Levy, M. and Dardik, I. (1976a). Human umbilical cord: a new source for vascular prosthesis. *JAMA* **236**, 2859.

Dardik, H., Ibrahim, I. M. and Dardik, I. (1979). The role of the peroneal artery for limb salvage. *Annals of Surgery* **189**, 189.

Dardik, H., Ibrahim, I. M., Jarrah, M., Sussman, B. and Dardik, I. (1980). Three-year experience with glutaraldehyde stabilized umbilical vein for limb salvage. *British Journal of Surgery* **67**, 229.

Dardik, H., Ibrahim, I. M., Koslow, A. and Dardik, I. (1978). Evaluation of intra-operative arteriography as a routine for vascular reconstructions. *Surgery, Gynecology and Obstetrics* **147**, 853.

Dardik, H., Ibrahim, I. M., Sprayregen, S. and Dardik, I. (1976b). Clinical experience with modified human umbilical cord vein for arterial bypass. *Surgery* **79**, 618.

DeWeese, J. A. and Rob, C. G. (1977). Autogenous venous grafts ten years later. *Surgery* **82**, 775.

Hufnagel, C. A. (1978). Heparin-bonded surfaces in prostheses and biografts. *In* "Graft Materials in Vascular Surgery" (H. Dardik, Ed.), p. 191. Yearbook Publishers, Chicago, Illinois.

Ibrahim, I. M., Sussman, B., Dardik, I., Kahn, M., Israel, M., Kenny, M. and Dardik, H. (1980). Adjunctive arteriovenous fistula with tibial and peroneal reconstruction for limb salvage. *American Journal of Surgery* **140**, 246.

LoGerfo, F. W., Corson, J. D. and Mannick, J. A. (1977). Improved results with femoropopliteal vein grafts for limb salvage. *Archives of Surgery (Chicago)* **112**, 567.

Mabry, C. D., Thompson, B. W. and Read, R. C. (1979). Activated clotting time (ACT) monitoring of intraopeative heparinization in peripheral vascular surgery. *American Journal of Surgery* **138**, 894.

Nabseth, D. C., Wilson, J. T., Tan, B., McDonough, E. F., Weiner, J. and Child, C. G. (1960). Fetal arterial heterografts. *Archives of Surgery (Chicago)* **81**, 929.

Naji, A., Jennifer, C., McCombs, P. R. *et al.* (1978). Results of 100 consecutive femoropopliteal vein grafts for limb salvage. *Annals of Surgery* **188**, 162.

Szilagyi, D. E., Hageman, J. H., Smith, R. F., Elliott, J. P., Brown, F. and Dietz, P. (1979). Autogenous vein grafting in femoropopliteal atherosclerosis: the limits of its effectiveness. *Surgery* **86**, 836.

Yong, N. K. and Eiseman, B. (1962). The experimental use of heterologous umbilical vein grafts as aortic substitutes. *Singapore Medical Journal* **3**, 53.

STRUCTURAL CHARACTERISTICS, FABRICATION, HISTOLOGIC RESPONSE AND ADVANTAGES OF EXPANDED REINFORCED PFTE VASCULAR GRAFTS (ERPTFEVG)

B. Boyce and J. A. Cannon

Research and Development Section, Medical Products Division
W. L. Gore & Associates, Inc., Flagstaff, Arizona, USA

INTRODUCTION

The expanded reinforced polytetrafluoroethylene prosthetic vascular graft (ERPTFEVG) is the result of a process invented by Robert W. Gore in 1969. The possibilities of the material in vascular applications were recognized by W. L. Gore, and a tube produced from expanded PTFE was first tried experimentally and clinically by Ben Eiseman, Professor of Surgery, University of Colorado Medical School (Soyer *et al.*, 1972). The Gore-Tex* vascular graft has since been used extensively, especially for arterial bypass procedures in the lower extremities.

STRUCTURAL CHARACTERISTICS AND FABRICATION

Polytetrafluoroethylene is a synthetic polymer consisting of replicated molecules formed by the bonding of two carbon atoms with four fluorine atoms in a linear chain-like configuration, and is characterized by a strongly

*Gore-Tex is a registered trademark of W. L. Gore & Associates, Inc.

Serono Symposium No. 44, "Peripheral Arterial Diseases: Medical and Surgical Problems", edited by S. Stipa and A. Cavallaro, 1982. Academic Press, London and New York.

negative surface charge and an extreme degree of chemical inertness, once synthesized (Fig. 1). The expansion process allows a solid wall tube (essentially full density) of chemically pure PTFE to be expanded in the longitudinal direction, so that the PTFE material is dispersed into a node and fibril configuration. There is a resulting void space in the node–fibril structure, which comprises approximately 85% of the tube wall by volume (Fig. 2b).

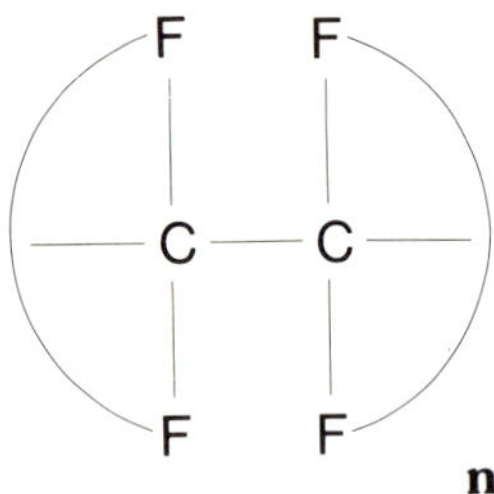

Fig. 1. Chemical structure of PTFE. The basic unit of this polymer is two carbon and four fluorine atoms with $n = 1$ million or more.

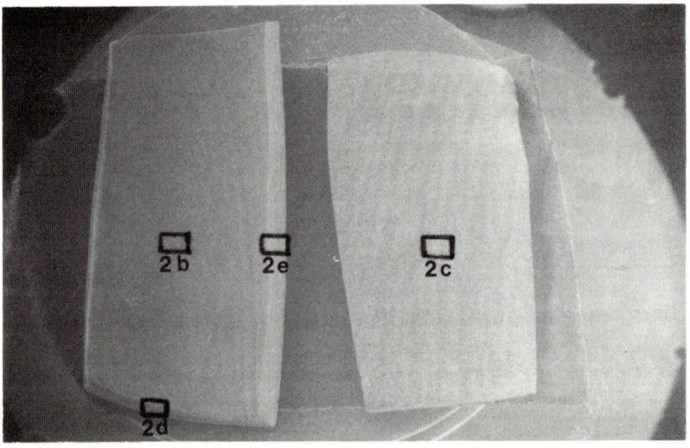

Fig. 2a. Orientation photographs (× 6.4) with squares indicating sites on luminal surface, wall, longitudinal section and transverse section, presented at higher magnification (× 832) in (b–e).

The commercial product is manufactured so that the fibril length roughly averages 30 μm. The wall structure produced, because of the hydrophobic nature of PTFE and the relative size of the internodal spaces, will allow the passage of gas through the wall but not aqueous fluids, at pressures under 150 mmHg.

It was discovered early that, whereas the longitudinal tensile strength of expanded PTFE is many times stronger than any physiologic vascular requirement, the circumferential or hoop strength is not. This deficit was corrected by the addition of an expanded PTFE film with the fibrils oriented at right

Fig. 3. A five-day Gore-Tex vascular graft human implant, with protein, fibrin and scattered cell nuclei in the graft wall, and blood elements on the luminal surface (right). (H & E, × 250.)

Fig. 4. A convenient method of cutting beveled ends of a Gore-Tex vascular graft using a hemostat and a #11 blade scalpel.

Fig. 5a. An empty, unpressurized Gore-Tex vascular graft curved around a US dime (approximately 18 mm diameter). Note kinking.

Fig. 5b. A pressurized Gore-Tex vascular graft curved around a dime. Note smooth contour. The graft is pressurized to 2 psi or 100 mmHg.

Fig. 6. A post-operative arteriogram of a Gore-Tex femoro-popliteal below-knee graft, showing the leg flexed at the knee approximately 110°. Note absence of kinking.

Fig. 7. The external appearance of a standard 20 mm × 10 mm internal diameter bifurcated Gore-Tex vascular graft.

Fig. 8. A typical segment removed from a Gore-Tex vascular graft canine implant, to be submitted for longitudinal sectioning or SEM scan.

Fig. 9. Histological appearance of a one-year Gore-Tex vascular graft femoro-popliteal implant. Examples at × 250 of stains used for the histologic examination of retrieved Gore-Tex vascular grafts. Figure 9a shows a hematoxylin and eosin stain used to delineate cell nuclei. Blue-stained cell nuclei can be seen on the outer tissue layer and in the graft wall. Figure 9b shows a trichrome stain used to identify collagen and fibrous tissue, which stain blue-green. Figure 9c shows a fibrin stain used to identify fibrin and protein on a graft flow surface. Figure 9d is an overview of the one-year human implant. Flow surface is on the right (× 100).

Fig. 10. Examples of 2½ (Figure 10a), 3½ (Figure 10b), and 4½ (Figure 10c) year Gore-Tex vascular graft femoro-popliteal human implants, show various degrees of tissue incorporation into the graft wall. All show a stable flow lining (trichrome, × 100).

Fig. 11. A two-month canine implant to demonstrate the tissue response to crimped, knitted Dacron. Note the thick fibrous flow surface to the right, and the thick fibrous capsule on the outer surface. Tissue has penetrated between, but not into, the fiber bundles (trichrome, × 100).

Fig. 12. Example of flow linings on Gore-Tex vascular grafts, as viewed with the scanning electron microscope. Figure 12a depicts the appearance of the surface of a short-term clinical graft inserted as an A-V fistula for dialysis access. Fibrin, platelets and other blood elements are noted (× 5000). Figure 12b—Blood elements on the luminal surface of a short-term canine implant (× 2500). Figure 12c—Confluent endothelial-like cells on the luminal surface of a long-term canine implant Gore-Tex vascular graft. Such healing has not been observed in the human (× 1250).

Fig. 13. A well-healed dialysis access puncture site from a functioning human Gore-Tex A-V fistula (trichrome, × 100).

Fig. 14. A section of an infected Gore-Tex vascular graft implanted in the human as an A-V fistula. Such infections are generally localized to the area of needle puncture. (Brown-Brenn bacterial stain, × 2500.)

Fig. 15. A thin section through a false aneurysm above the site of multiple dialysis needle punctures in a Gore-Tex vascular graft A-V fistula. Note fragmented graft wall, lower left and upper right. Fibrin has accumulated within the pseudoaneurysm capsule (trichrome, × 25).

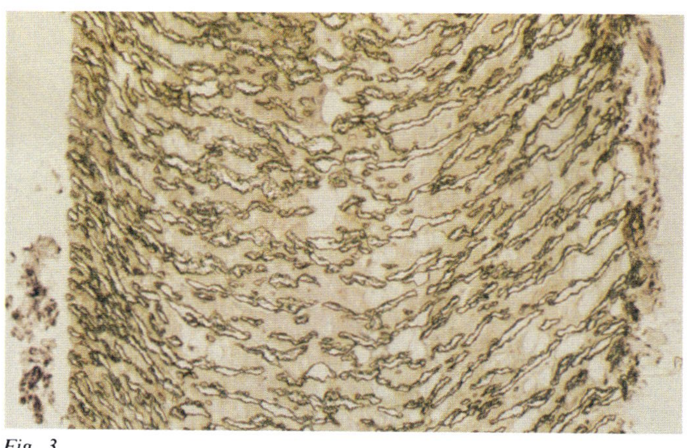

Fig. 3

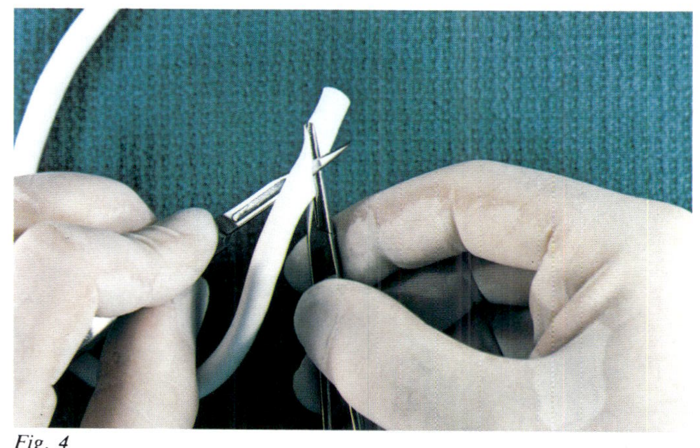

Fig. 4

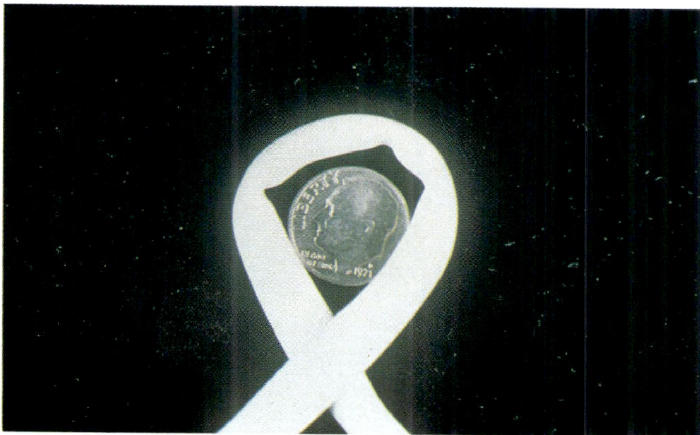

Fig. 5a

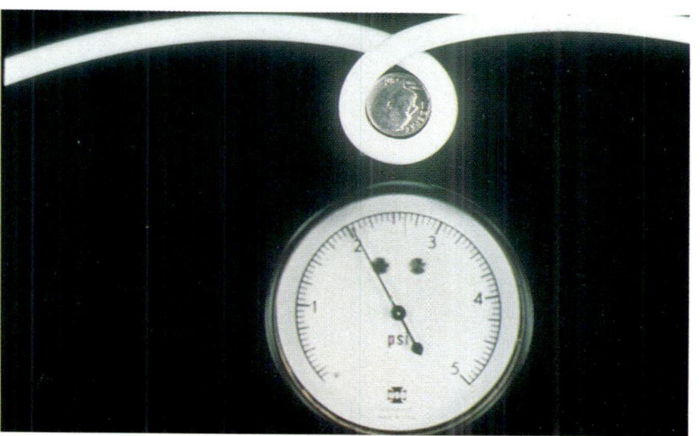

Fig. 5b

Fig. 6

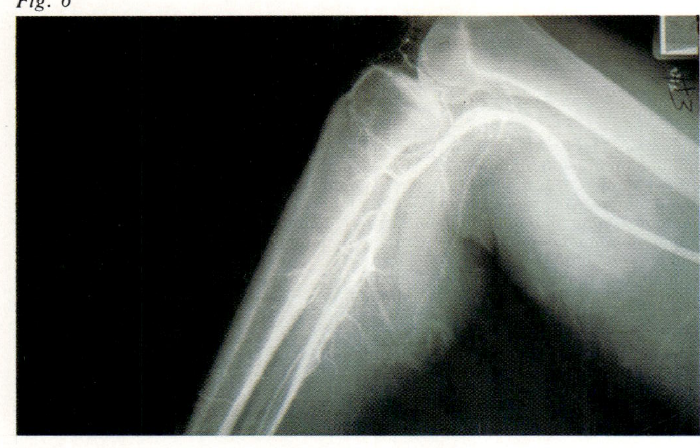

Fig. 7

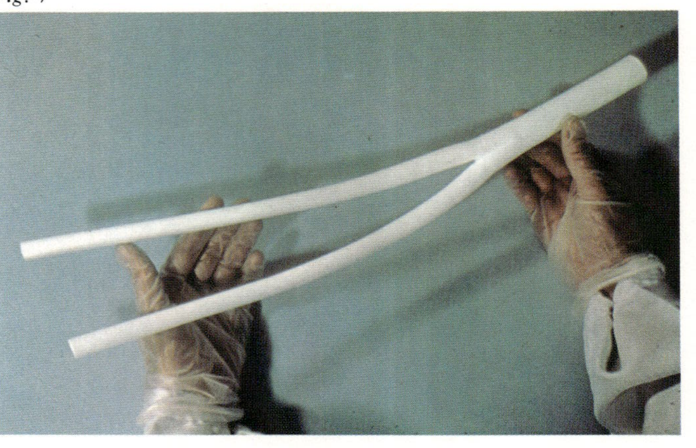

Fig. 8

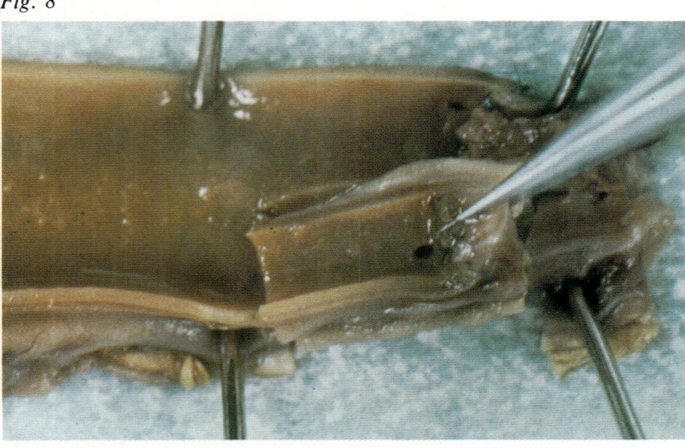

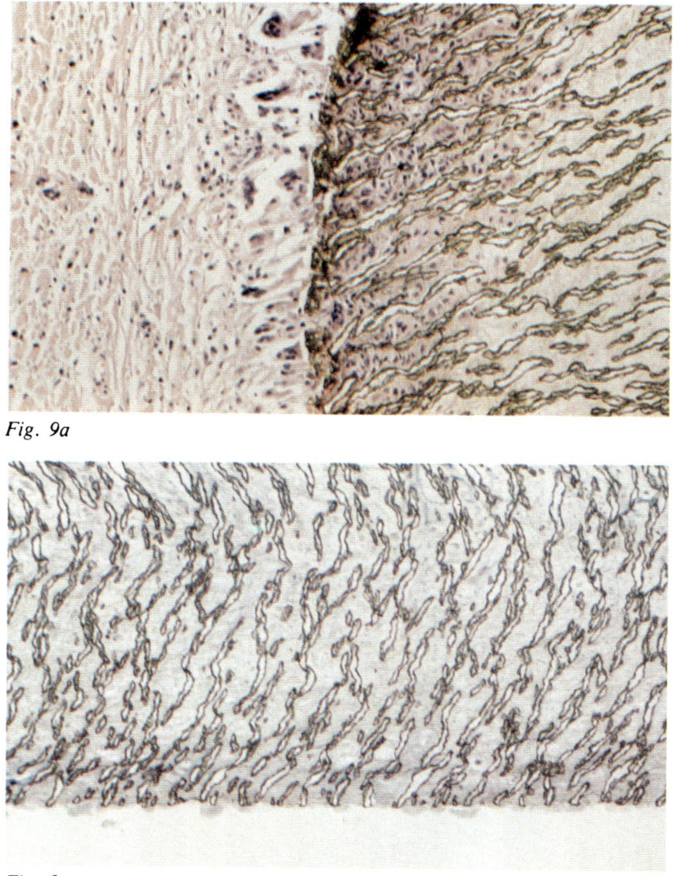

Fig. 9a

Fig. 9c

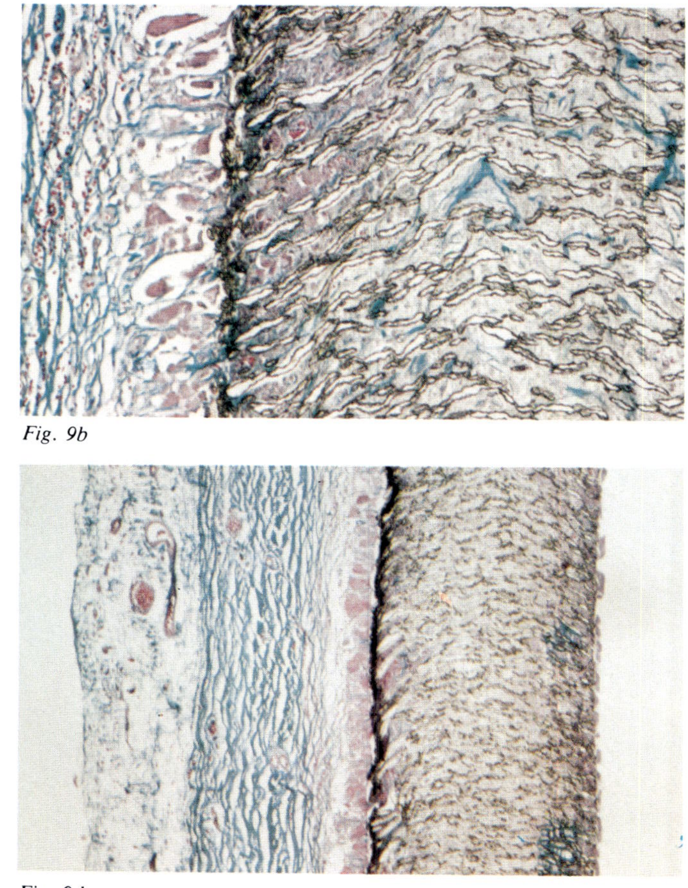

Fig. 9b

Fig. 9d

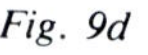

Fig. 10a

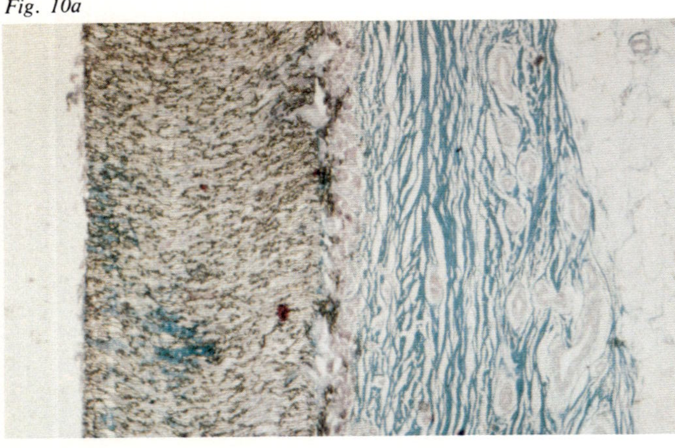

Fig. 10b
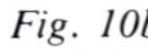

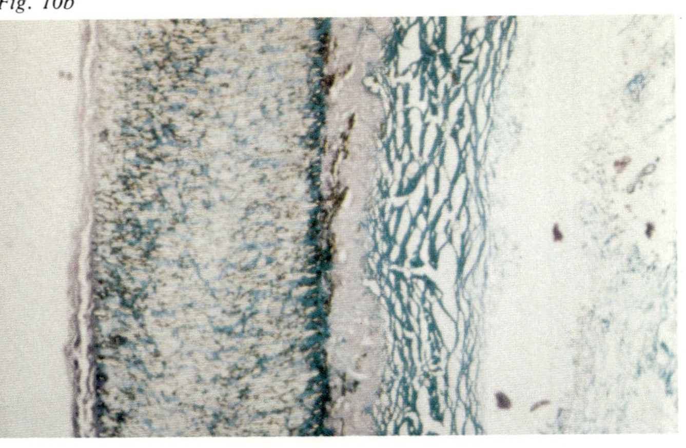

Fig. 10c

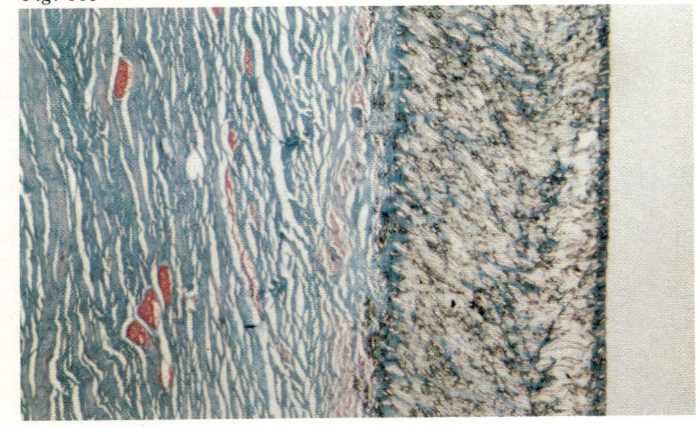

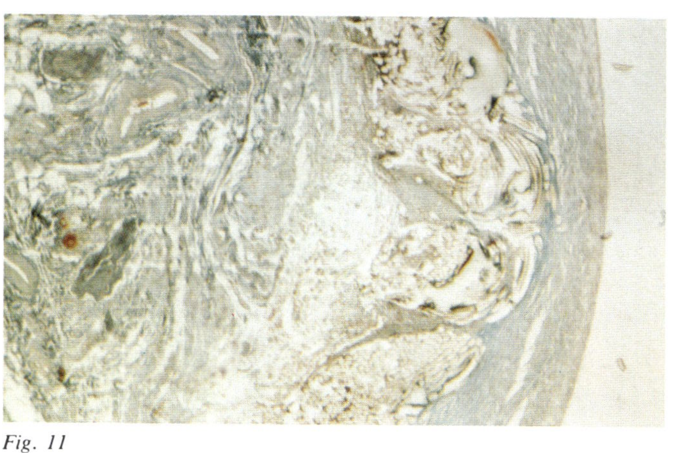

Fig. 11

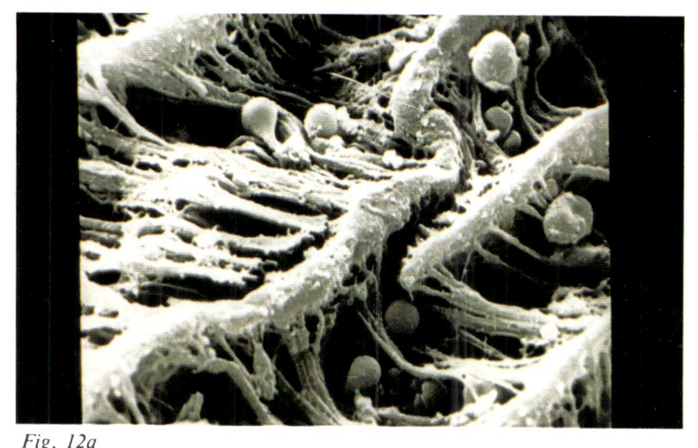

Fig. 12a

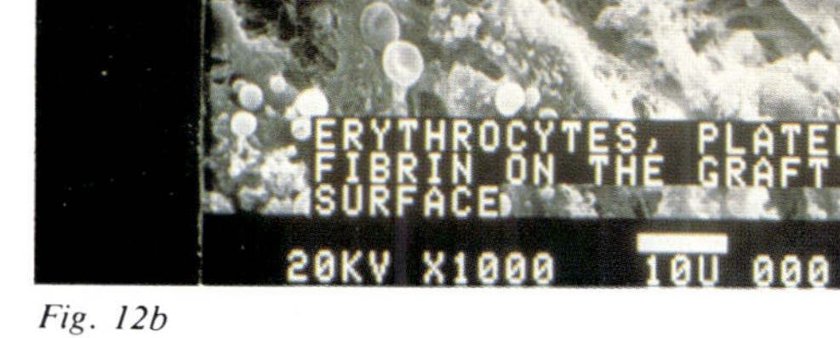

Fig. 12b

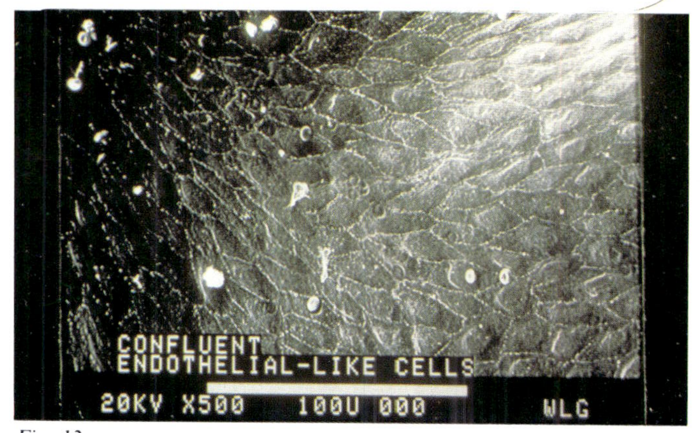

Fig. 12c

Fig. 13

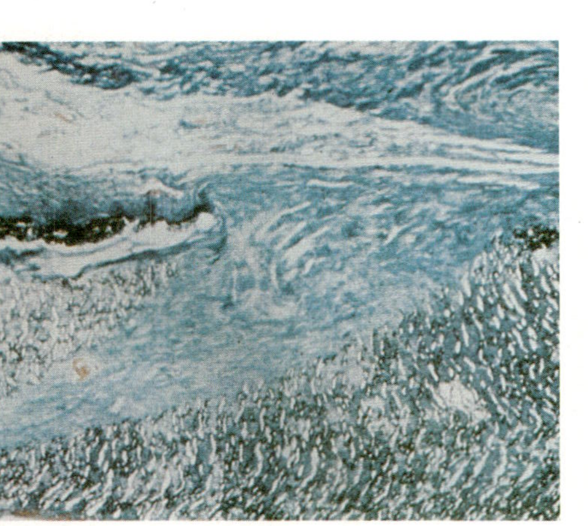

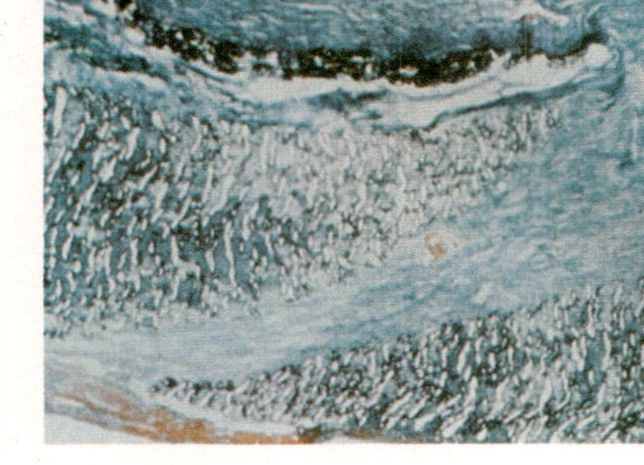

Fig. 14

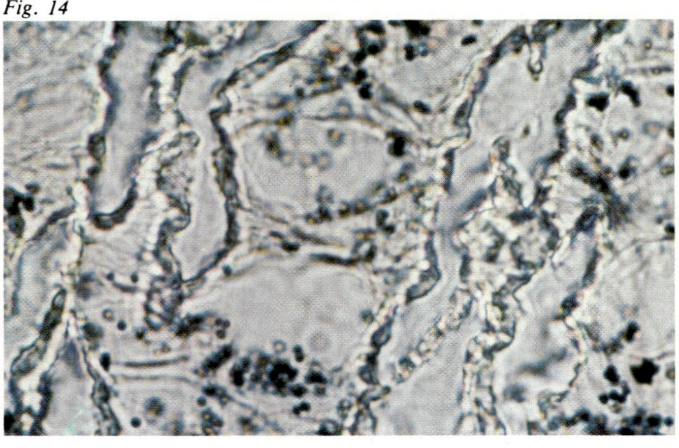

Fig. 15

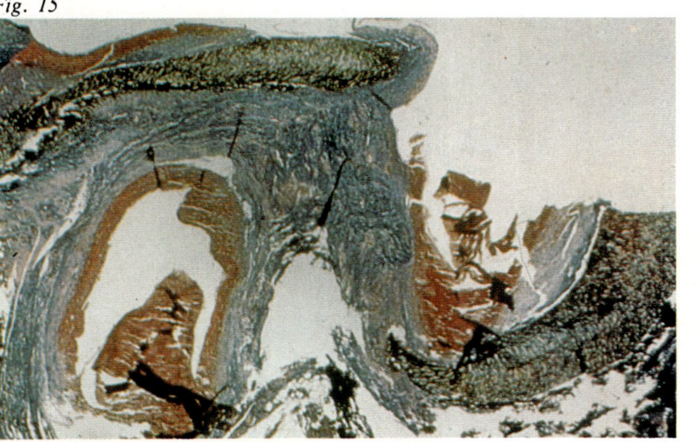

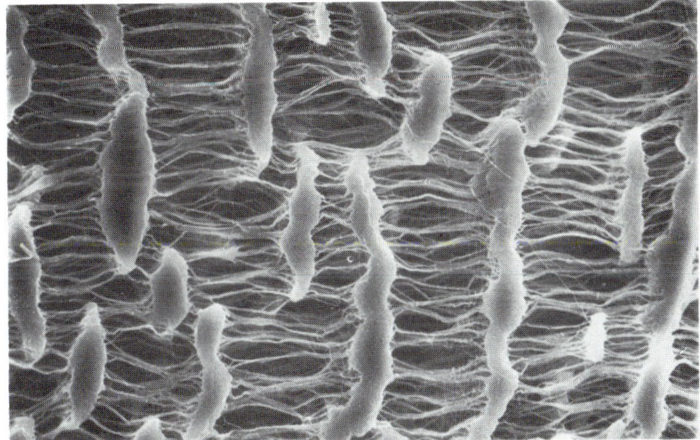

Fig. 2b. Standard Gore-Tex vascular graft luminal surface. Note node–fibril structure (× 832).

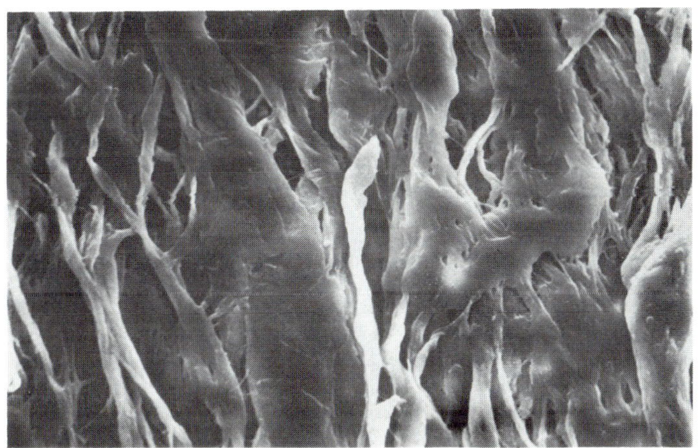

Fig. 2c. Standard Gore-Tex vascular graft outer surface (× 832). The node–fibril structure of the reinforcing film is always oriented at right angles to the node-fibril orientation of the base tube.

angles to the fibrils within the wall of the base tube. The resulting tubular structure remains chemically pure expanded PTFE but will withstand burst pressures of 70 psi or approximately 3600 mmHg (Fig. 2a–c).

The ERPTFEVG is thus a synthetic vascular conduit which upon implantation creates no inflammatory or allergenic response and becomes incorporated on its external surface by surrounding body tissue. The graft luminal surface presents a negative charge and is relatively nonthrombogenic, and although promptly coated with an extremely thin layer of protein, no thrombus is propagated as long as a minimum flow rate is maintained. After

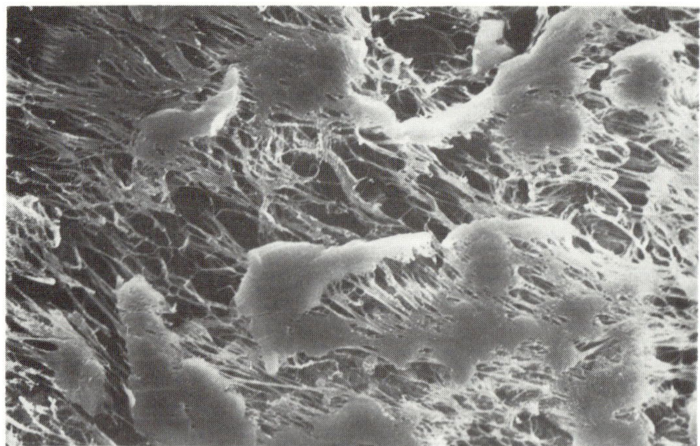

Fig. 2d. Transverse wall section standard Gore-Tex vascular graft (× 832). Transversely, the nodes appear flat and somewhat plate-like.

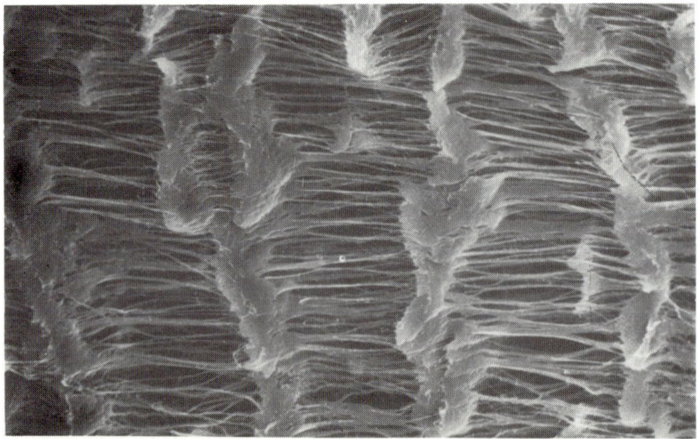

Fig. 2e. Longitudinal wall section standard Gore-Tex vascular graft (× 832). Longitudinally, the nodes appear thin and oblong.

two to four days of implantation, the wetting agents in the body tissue and serum cause the graft wall to become hydrophilic. The result is penetration of the wall with serum proteins and a sparse infiltration of erythrocytes, neutrophilic leukocytes and, ultimately, fibroblasts (Fig. 3).

The addition of the reinforcing film has totally prevented the formation of intrinsic aneurysms and has significantly increased suture retention. Although the film is bonded firmly enough to the base tube so that no separation is encountered after implantation, it has been found that the film can be disrupted from the wall if the graft is cut with other than a very sharp instrument. If scissors are used for cutting the graft, the blade should be freshly sharpened and the pivot screw firmly tightened. If a scalpel blade is used it should be fresh, and cutting should be accomplished with the graft on a firm flat base. A convenient way of cutting the graft is to apply a straight or curved hemostat adjacent to the length desired, making the cut flush with the jaws of the hemostat (Fig. 4).

When the ERPTFEVG is handled in the unpressurized condition, it shows a tendency to kink easily when bent. However, when pressurized to physiologic levels, it becomes highly flexible and a 6-mm internal diameter graft can easily be formed into a 360° curve around a circle as small as 1.5 cm in diameter (Fig. 5a,b). Thus, the graft is suitable for cross-joint or below-knee applications, and there is no evidence that patency duration is affected *per se* by joint flexion (Fig. 6).

The expanded reinforced PTFE graft material is available in a convenient selection of diameters, lengths, and configurations. It is supplied in internal diameters from 3 mm to 24 mm, in lengths up to 100 cm, in tapers and in a bifurcated configuration (Fig. 7).

HISTOLOGIC RESPONSE

The most common current application of the Gore-Tex vascular graft is for femoro-popliteal bypass. In order to interpret the histological slides, it is important to understand the manner in which the material is prepared for light and scanning electron microscopy analyses. The gross specimens, preferably fixed in glutaraldehyde, are photographed and described. Two side-by-side representative longitudinal sections are removed from selected areas for respective microscopy (Fig. 8). The histologic response to femoro-popliteal implants at 1, 2½, 3½ and 4½ years is depicted in Figs 9 and 10.

Longitudinal sections, approximately 5–7 μm thick are stained with three different stains depicted in Fig. 9(a–c). A graft implanted in the femoro-popliteal position for one year is used to illustrate the histological stains. The H & E stain (Fig. 9a) illustrates adherent fibrous tissue on the outer surface (indicated by the reinforcement) with blue-stained cell nuclei present in the graft wall. The Trichrome stain (Fig. 9b) illustrates limited collagen infiltration into the graft wall. The Fibrin stain (Fig. 9c) shows a thin stable fibrin–protein flow lining. Fig 9(d) shows an overview of a one-year femoro-popliteal implant. In contrast, the 2½-year femoro-popliteal implant (Fig. 10a) shows a deeper penetration of collagen into the graft wall. A 3½-year femoro-popliteal implant (Fig. 10b) illustrates even greater collagen penetration. At 4½ years (Fig. 10c) this femoro-popliteal implant shows a consistent fairly dense collagenous matrix throughout the graft interstices. Note that a stable thin flow lining is present on all implants and that erythrocytes and proteinaceous material are present in differing degrees in all implants.

By contrast, a crimped Dacron prosthesis also viewed in longitudinal section (Fig. 11) shows a more extensive connective tissue response on the outer surface, in the graft wall and on the luminal surface. Note, however, that the wall structure, comprised of Dacron yarn, shows no evidence whatsoever of collagen penetration into the yarn interstices. These spaces do contain protein and are large enough to admit bacteria but not leukocytes.

Scanning electron microscopy (SEM) is utilized to study blood components and cellular growth onto the luminal surface of implanted vascular grafts. Figure 12(a–c respectively) illustrates a thin fibrin flow lining, erythrocytes and platelets and endothelial cells on the graft luminal surface. The endothelial cells shown are present on the luminal surface of a Gore-Tex vascular graft implanted in a canine.

It is to be noted that endothelial coverage of a clinically implanted Gore-Tex vascular graft has not been observed to progress further than approximately 2 cm from either anastomosis. To our knowledge, this behaviour is true of all clinically implanted synthetic or biosynthetic grafts.

The second most common use of the Gore-Tex vascular graft is for A-V fistula construction for vascular access. The histologic response is essentially the same. The needle puncture sites are routinely healed with connective tissue within a short period of time (Fig. 13). The tissue progresses from the outer surface to the luminal surface with little penetration into the surrounding wall, and with variable spread around the entry site on the luminal surface. Complications can occur if rigid asepsis is not followed during dialysis (Fig. 14), or if the graft is repeatedly punctured in a localized area. When such trauma occurs, localized hemorrhage resulting in the formation of a pseudoaneurysm capsule may necessitate graft revision or removal (Fig. 15).

ADVANTAGES OF THE EXPANDED REINFORCED PTFE VASCULAR GRAFT

Polytetrafluoroethylene is the most chemically inert of any synthetic material currently or historically utilized for vascular grafting. In contrast, Nylon, by hygroscopic action, loses much of its tensile strength in one or two years. Dacron is more resistant to this action, beginning to lose its tensile strength in eight to ten years. Polytetrafluoroethylene appears to be totally resistant to any form of chemical denaturization and is completely stable at temperatures of 250° or lower. The material is degraded by high-energy radiation and therefore cannot be sterilized by this method (Imperial Chemical Industries Limited, 1978).

The material has a thoroughly documented history of biocompatibility, carries a highly electronegative surface charge and is nonthrombogenic. The Gore-Tex vascular graft does not require pre-clotting. The material cuts well, providing sharp instruments and proper cutting techniques are utilized, as described previously. The graft material is highly flexible and accepts sutures with ease. At physiologic pressures and temperatures, the graft becomes a highly flexible conduit. Thus, the graft can be passed across joints with little tendency to kink, even in areas of acute flexion, i.e. knee joints. With the knee acutely flexed, there is no evidence of decreased ankle to brachial pressure ratios in the flexed compared with the unflexed position (Burnham *et al.*, 1980). The smooth outer surface of the graft allows easy passage through tissue tunnels.

As a blood conduit, the ERPTFEVG is yielding the best patency duration rates in the relatively small diameters and long lengths in which it is commonly used (i.e. internal diameter 6 mm, length 60 cm) of any synthetic or biosynthetic graft available. In these smaller diameters the Gore-Tex vascular graft is second only to autologous saphenous vein in overall performance.

In the event that thrombosis is encountered with a Gore-Tex vascular graft, the graft is more easily thrombectomized than any other graft including autologous saphenous vein, and a gratifying ensuing success rate can be accomplished.

Patency duration rates are graphically illustrated in Figs 16 and 17 and now are extending throughout four years. The figures show comparative results for lower extremity bypasses for claudication and for limb salvage. The cumulative first-time thrombosis rate of the ERPTFEVG in the arteriovenous fistula position is presented in Fig. 18.

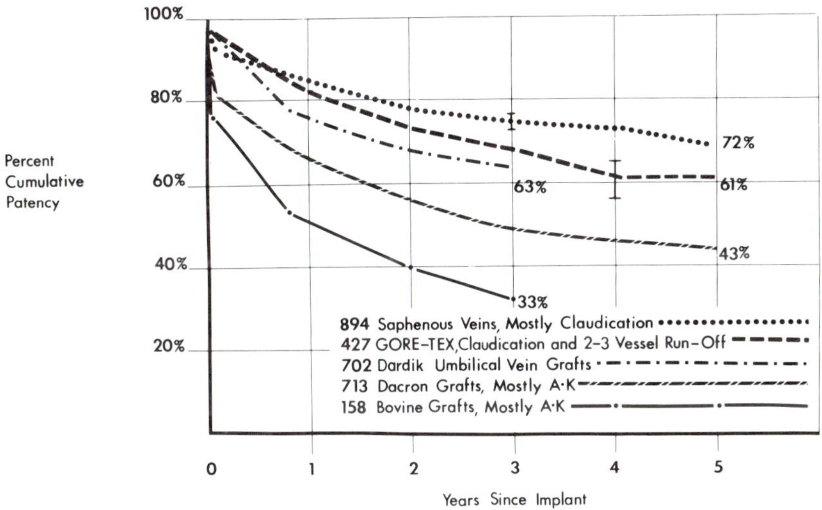

Fig. 16. Life-table patencies: femoro-popliteal bypass, comparing saphenous vein, Gore-Tex, umbilical vein, Dacron and bovine hetero graft for claudication, 2–3 vessel run-off. Note that the curves for Dacron grafts and bovine grafts represent grafts in the femoro-popliteal above-knee position. The curves for Dardik umbilical vein grafts cannot be designated for certain as referring to patients suffering from claudication only, since the designations are not described in the available published data.

SUMMARY AND CONCLUSIONS

The chemical and physical characteristics of the ERPTFEVG are presented. The biocompatibility of this synthetic graft is emphasized. The histologic response to the graft after various periods of implantation is described and depicted. Patency duration life-table curves are graphically illustrated.

In conclusion, the ERPTFEVG is the graft material of choice second only to available adequate saphenous vein for arterial reconstruction procedures,

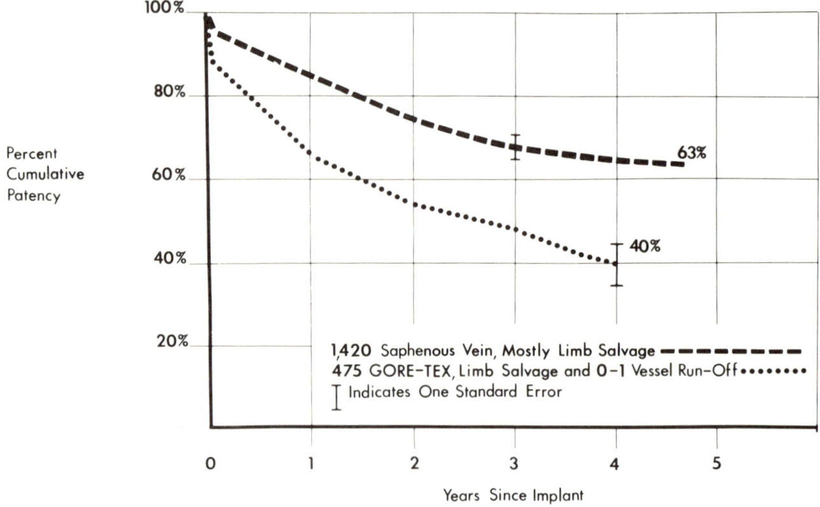

Fig. 17. Life-table patency curves comparing saphenous vein with Gore-Tex vascular grafts in the femoro-popliteal position for limb salvage.

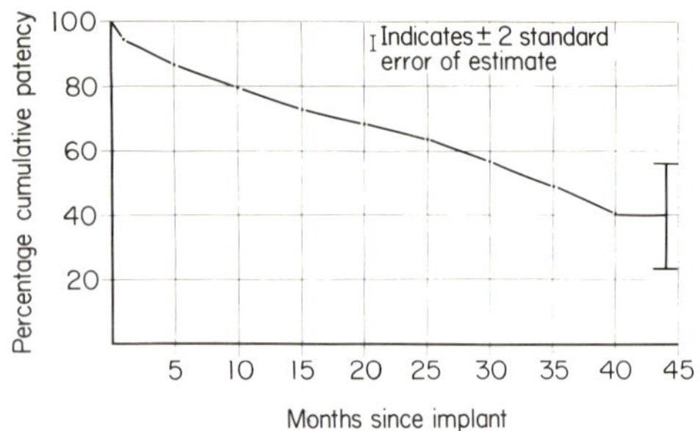

Fig. 18. Life-table curve for Gore-Tex vascular grafts (mostly 6 mm internal diameter) implanted as A-V fistulae for hemodialysis vascular access. (Number at risk: worldwide — 4685. Approximately 900 surgeons.)

especially in the femoro-popliteal and vascular access A-V fistula positions. Histologic examination of retrieved clinically implanted grafts illustrates clearly that the graft material is biocompatible and becomes incorporated by the surrounding tissue. Patent grafts develop a stable flow lining even throughout 4½ years of implantation, the maximum thus far observed histologically.

REFERENCES

Burnham, J., Flannigan, D., Goodreau, J., Yao, J. and Bergan, J. (1980). Ankle pressure changes in distal bypass grafts during knee flexion. *Surgery* **87**, 652.

Imperial Chemical Industries Limited, Plastic Division (1978). "Physical properties of Unfilled and Filled Polytetrafluoroethylene". Technical Service Note, F12/13. Hertfordshire, 1978.

Soyer, T., Lempinen, M., Norton, L. and Eiseman, B. (1972). A new venous prosthesis. *Surgery* **72**, 864.

EXPERIENCE WITH THE PTFE* GRAFT IN FEMORO-POPLITEAL BYPASS SURGERY AND VASCULAR ACCESS FOR HEMODIALYSIS

M. Haimov and J. H. Jacobson II

Department of Surgery, Division of Vascular Surgery, Mount Sinai School of Medicine, New York, New York, USA

The PTFE graft became available to our group in July 1975. Experience with 226 grafts placed in the femoro-popliteal position and 218 grafts used for the construction of vascular access for hemodialysis will form the basis of this report.

METHOD

Two-hundred-and-twenty-six grafts were implanted in 190 patients in the femoro-popliteal position. The average age of these patients was 68 years; 114 patients were males (60%) and 76 were females (40%); 78 patients were hypertensive (41%) and 76 patients were diabetics (40%). Indications for surgery were severe disabling claudication in 99 patients (52%), and rest pain or gangrene in 91 patients (48%). In 26% of the patients, the surgery was secondary, i.e. a previous femoro-popliteal bypass had failed. The distal run-off was classified as good if one or more distal vessels were patent in continuity with the popliteal segment and for distance extending to the ankle

*PTFE is expanded polytetrafluoroethylene.

Serono Symposium No. 44, "Peripheral Arterial Diseases: Medical and Surgical Problems", edited by S. Stipa and A. Cavallaro, 1982. Academic Press, London and New York.

level. It was considered poor if a blind popliteal segment was present or the tibial vessels were patent only for the proximal one-third of the leg.

In accordance with the classification, 133 limbs (59%) had poor run-off, and 93 limbs (41%) had good run-off. All operations were done under general inhalation anesthesia. In 79 bypasses, the distal anastomosis was done to the popliteal artery above the knee and in 147 bypasses it was placed in the popliteal artery below the knee joint.

Two-hundred-and-eighteen grafts were used as a vascular substitute in the construction of vascular access in patients with end-stage renal disease on hemodialysis. The indication for the use of the prosthesis in these patients was the unavailability of suitable arteries or veins for the construction of a standard arteriovenous fistula.

RESULTS

The patency of the grafts was determined by examination of distal pulses, segmental pressure measurements, direct percutaneous evaluation of graft flow using a Doppler flow meter and angiographically when indicated. Cumulative percentage patency was calculated by the life-table method. The graft was considered closed if a second operation was required to re-establish patency. Results with femoro-popliteal graft procedures are summarized in Table I. The cumultative patency rate was 89% at three months; 76% at 12 months; 68% at 24 months; 55% at 36 months and 52% at 48 and 60 months. There was no significant difference in the patency rates of grafts placed below and above the knee. Poor run-off or secondary surgery was associated with significantly higher rates of failures during the first 12 months, 59% and 45% respectively ($P < 0.001$). Twenty-five grafts required thrombectomy with or without revision to re-establish patency. Results with these grafts are summarized in Table II. Twelve-months patency rate for these grafts was 67% and 24-month patency rate was 51%.

Table I. PTFE femoro-popliteal bypasses — patency.

Interval (months)	Total grafts at risk	# Open	# Closed	Interval patency (%)	Cumulative patency (%)
3	226	202	20	89	89
6	202	190	12	94	83
12	172	158	14	92	76
18	121	117	4	96	73
24	77	72	5	93	68
30	58	54	4	93	63
36	35	31	4	88	55
48	23	22	1	95	52
60	12	12	0	100	52

Table II. PTFE femoro-popliteal grafts — patency following thrombectomy.

Interval (months)	Total grafts at risk	# Open	# Closed	Interval patency (%)	Cumulative patency (%)
3	25	20	5	80	80
6	20	19	1	95	76
12	19	17	2	89	67
18	16	15	1	93	63
24	11	9	2	82	51
30	5	5	0	100	51
36	5	4	0	80	41
48	1	1	0	100	41

COMPLICATIONS OF FEMORO-POPLITEAL GRAFTS

Eleven patients died during the first three months following surgery (5.7%). All deaths were cardiac in patients with severe generalized arteriosclerotic disease, with the exception of one. This last patient died from bleeding following removal of an infected prosthesis. Eight patients developed false aneurysms, five of these associated with graft infection. The aneurysms were repaired in five patients and the five infected grafts were removed. In two additional patients who developed graft infection which was localized, healing was achieved with antibiotic treatment without graft removal. There were 18 above or below knee amputations all associated with graft failures, both early and late. Five patients developed serous collections around the graft which required repeated aspiration. None of these grafts became infected or was lost because of this complication. No true aneurysms developed in the PTFE grafts used in the femoro-popliteal position, although 50 of these grafts were of the nonreinforced type.

PTFE GRAFTS FOR VASCULAR ACCESS

Two-hundred-and-twenty-six grafts were placed in the arm or forearm as arteriovenous communication to serve as vascular access for hemodialysis. Results with this type of application of the graft are summarized in Table III. The cumulative patency rates for these grafts were 97% at three months; 86% at 12 months; 78% at 24 months; and 75% at 36 months. The causes of failure in these grafts were in order of frequency: graft thrombosis, secondary graft infection during the course of hemodialysis treatment, aneurysm formation and primary graft infection.

DISCUSSION

Our experience with the PTFE graft, as well as data reported by others, warrant cautious optimism (Haimov *et al.*, 1979; Veith *et al.*, 1978a). The

Table III. PTFE grafts for vascular access.

Interval (months)	Total patients at risk	# Open	# Closed	Interval patency (%)	Cumulative patency (%)
0–3	218	211	7	97	97
3–6	211	209	2	99	96
6–9	189	181	8	95	51
9–12	171	162	9	94	86
12–18	142	136	6	95	82
18–24	108	103	5	95	78
24–30	89	86	3	96	75
30–36	63	63	0	100	75
36–48	33	30	3	90	68

experience is currently passing the five-year mark and it seems to indicate the prosthesis is comparable to the autogenous saphenous vein although one still has to wait for the judgment of time with larger number of patients.

The graft has been applied successfully to clinical situations where no other well-tested better alternatives are currently available (Veith *et al.*, 1978b). It certainly appears to be superior to the marginal or poor quality saphenous vein, although in cases where a good autogenous vein is available in a patient with reasonable life expectancy, the last should be the prosthesis of choice.

Technically the graft possesses some, although not all, of the characteristics of the ideal prosthesis, i.e. easy availability, good tissue incorporation, low tendency to thrombosis and bleeding and low tendency to infection. Except for the occasional serous collections, there are no graft specific complications. Aneurysmal dilatations which have occurred with the nonreinforced graft have not been reported with the reinforced one. One advantage of this graft over the autogenous saphenous vein is the ease of thrombectomy. The experience mentioned in this report is encouraging, since satisfactory long time patency rates seem to be achievable after thrombectomy and graft revision (Veith *et al.*, 1980).

From the technical point of view, the graft can be used employing standard surgical techniques. Since it has no elasticity, the length needed should be carefully ascertained to avoid redundancy and kinking or undue tension on the suture line. There is a tendency for bleeding from the needle puncture holes which can be minimized by using fine suture material.

Results with the use of the graft for vascular access are better in our hands than those with the autogenous saphenous vein or the modified bovine heterograft. Based on this experience, we feel that our earlier conclusions are correct and that continued cautious applications of this new vascular prosthesis is justified.

REFERENCES

Haimov, M., Giron, F. and Jacobson, J. H. (1979). The expanded Polytetrafluoroethylene graft. Three years' experience with 362 grafts. *Archives of Surgery (Chicago)* **114**, 673.

Veith, F. J., Moss, C. M., Fell. S. C. *et al*. (1978a). Comparison of expanded Polytetrafluoroethylene and autologous saphenous vein grafts in high risk arterial reconstruction for limb salvage. *Surgery, Gynecology and Obstetrics*, **147**, 749.

Veith, F. J., Moss, C. M., Daly, V. *et al*. (1978b). New approaches to limb salvage by extended extra-anatomic bypasses and prosthetic reconstructions to foot arteries. *Surgery* **84**, 764.

Veith, F. J., Gupta, S. and Daly, V. (1980). Management of early and late thrombosis of PTFE femoro-popliteal bypass grafts. Favorable prognosis with appropriate reoperations. *Surgery* **87**, 581.

EARLY COMPLICATIONS OF AUTOGENOUS SAPHENOUS VEIN BYPASS

H. M. Becker and V. Sciacca

Surgical University Hospital, München, Munich, West Germany

Early complication in using autogenous venous bypass is first of all post-operative haemorrhage, infection and early thrombotic occlusion (Stipa *et al.*, 1972, 1977) (Tables I and II). Most of these complications are of iatrogenic

Table I. Early complications: autogenous saphenous bypass.

Femoro-popliteal saph. bypass	*n*	Complication rate (%)
Post-operative haemorrhage	5	0.6
Infection	17	2.1
Occlusion (within 30 days post-operation)	104	13.0
Total: 802 operations	126	15.7

Table II. Early complications: autogenous saphenous bypass.

Femoro-popliteal bypass	*n*	Early thrombotic occlusion
Stage II: claudication	97	5 (5.2%)
Stage III: rest pain	310	41 (13.2%)
Stage IV: acral necrosis or ulcers	395	58 (14.7%)
Total	802	104 (13.0%)

Serono Symposium No. 44, "Peripheral Arterial Diseases: Medical and Surgical Problems", edited by S. Stipa and A. Cavallaro, 1982. Academic Press, London and New York.

origin either by wrong indication or faults in surgical technique, rather than by inadequate post-operative care (Brener *et al.*, 1975; Charlesworth *et al.*, 1975; Cooley and Wukasch, 1979; Craver *et al.*, 1973; Flinn *et al.*, 1980; Gordon *et al.*, 1975a, b; Gundry *et al.*, 1980; Mannick, 1978; Müller-Wiefel, 1980; Schwartz, 1973; Szilagyi, 1978).

POST-OPERATIVE HAEMORRHAGE

Post-operative haemorrhage (Craver *et al.*, 1973) can be due to coagulation problems, of course, if heparinization is not neutralized or is going to be continued. Usually one does not need any anticoagulants to save an operative result, such haematomas as well do as a rule not make a re-operation necessary unless in case of a great amount of blood loss with expanding oedema; then a reintervention should be done in time. We never found direct post-operative haemorrhage from the anastomotic suture but from loosening of a branch ligation or whenever such a branch was forgotten to be ligated: the valves of the branch orifice will become insufficient and the bleeding begins (Fig. 1). This cause of haemorrhage was found in less than 1% (five out of 802 saphenous bypasses = 0.6%), yet one of them was bleeding from infection of the upper anastomosis. Four of the cases could be managed well by suturing, the one infected had to be ligated and lost his leg by high amputation (Table III).

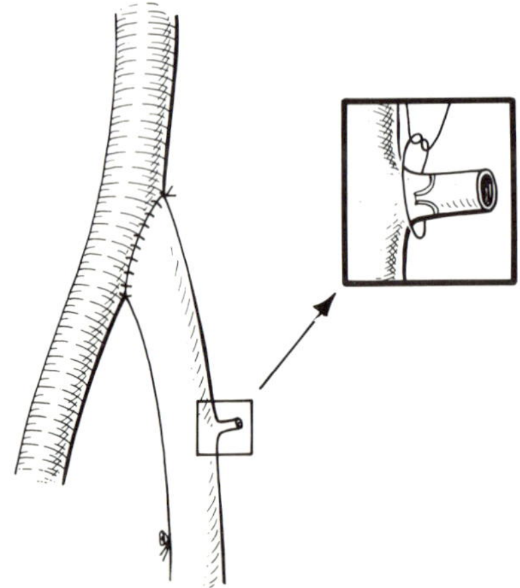

Fig. 1. Loosening of branch ligature.

INFECTION

Fortunately, infection is a rare complication (Stipa *et al.*, 1972, 1977; Szilagyi, 1978). It usually depends, primarily, on distal ulcerative or gangrenous lesions when saphenous vein graft is used for limb salvage. The only

Table III. Early complications: autogenous saphenous bypass.

Femoro-popliteal bypass	*n*	(%)	Treated with success	Amputation	Died
Post-operative haemorrhage	5	0.6	4	1	1
Infection course of graft	11	2.1	8	2	–
Infection anastomosis	6		2	4	1
Occlusion within 30 days	104	13.0	30	53	17
Post-operative mortality other than above					4
Total: 802 operations	126	15.7	44 (5.5%)	60 (7.5%)	23 (2.9%)

explanation we had is injuring of infected lymph vessels, especially in the middle part of the thigh where the saphenous vein has to be exposed for gaining. In this area also blood supply sometimes happens to be affected as well, so that a secondary infection of the following necrosis threatens the underlying graft.

In our 802 femoro-popliteal saphenous bypass procedures we had 17 infections (2.1%). The infected graft in the middle of the thigh — with non-infected anastomoses — could be saved in eight of 11 instances by local management. The vein bypasses remained patent except one. Six anastomotic infections had to be treated by graft ligation and only in two patients we succeeded in saving the leg by extra-anatomic bypass using expanded PTFE. The others (four patients) lost the menaced extremity, two of them died from generalized septicaemia (Table III).

EARLY THROMBOSIS

The most common early complication is sudden intra- or post-operative *thrombotic occlusion* of the inserted graft (Brener *et al.*, 1975; Craver *et al.*, 1973; Gordon *et al.*, 1975; Schwartz, 1973; Stipa *et al.*, 1977). There are three reasons for failure of such a graft. One may be a wrong or desperate indication; since blood inflow (Charlesworth *et al.*, 1975) mostly is sufficient or can be achieved easily, the problem is the outflow or run-off capacity (Fig. 2). Out

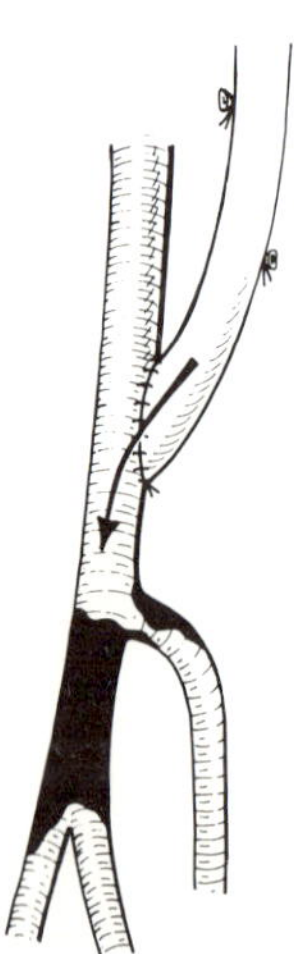

Fig. 2. Run-off impairment from distal arterial stenosis and/or occlusion.

of 104 early thrombotic graft occlusions 46 (44%) were re-operated upon, but only in 30 operations could we achieve a remaining patency, in most instances by prolonging the bypass to a more distal arterial segment; 53 patients (more than 50% of the post-operative thrombotic occlusions) had to suffer a big amputation, and 17 patients died during the post-operative course (Table III). The overall mortality rate concerning autogenous venous bypass in our hands within 30 days after operation is 2.9%.

A second cause of acute post-operative thrombotic graft occlusion could be a certain hypercoagulability — not a good reason because we found clinical blood clotting faster than in other patients, yet a satisfying haemostaseological cause could never be found.

The remaining third cause of early graft failure for thrombotic occlusion certainly is iatrogenic and should be acknowledged as a mistake in surgical technique. In dilating the graft one can find constricting adventitial bands, usually nearby branch ligations, which will work as stenoses one after another, and can easily be cut through (Fig. 3). A twisted transplant means an

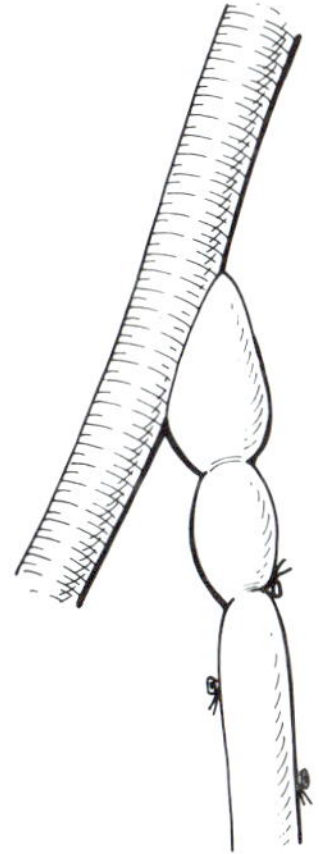

Fig. 3. Narrowing from adventitial bands.

even higher stenosis; some authors developed methods to avoid such distorsion (Gordon *et al.*, 1975; Schwartz, 1973); we think an accurate pulling through of the graft will avoid any torsion (Fig. 4).

The graft itself in certain cases could not be qualified by either being too small in size (Fig. 5) or too large representing a varicose vein with aneurysmatic dilated segments (Fig. 6). The latter actually does not lead to early thrombosis but will be the cause later of peripheral embolism or rupture.

False anastomotic techniques (Stipa *et al.*, 1977; Szilagyi, 1978) (Fig. 7) as well as use of a phlebosclerotic vein (Fig. 8) will certainly cause early graft failure, particularly in the early post-operative period.

If the graft is not long enough (Gordon *et al.*, 1975), one should never extend and stretch it so that the lengthening will fit to bypass the necessary distance (Fig. 9). And sometimes (three times in our 802 cases) it is very difficult to expose the below knee region, especially in second or third re-intervention, so that the younger surgeon sometimes cannot differ between artery and vein and anastomoses the graft to the popliteal vein (Fig.

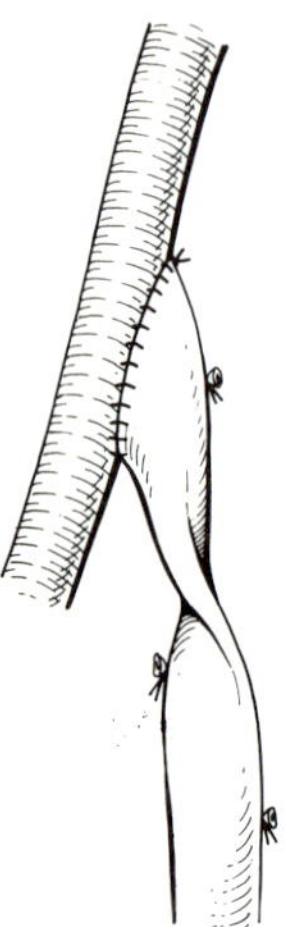

Fig. 4. Twisting of the graft.

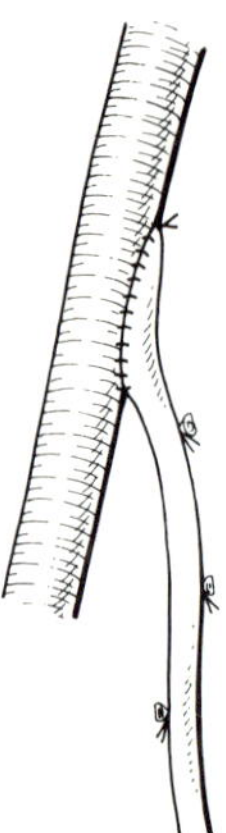

Fig. 5. Small diameter of the graft.

10) — an aggravating mistake which can lead to acute heart failure as well as to loss of the extremity. In our cases this mistake could be revealed during operation by angiography and the correct anastomosis could be accomplished in all three instances afterwards.

COMMENT

Retrospectively it is sometimes impossible to find the exact cause of the graft failure, so that one has to take pains to have a strong indication, a refined surgical technique and a meticulous post-operative care.

In about 40% of our patients we could not find a vein suitable for grafting

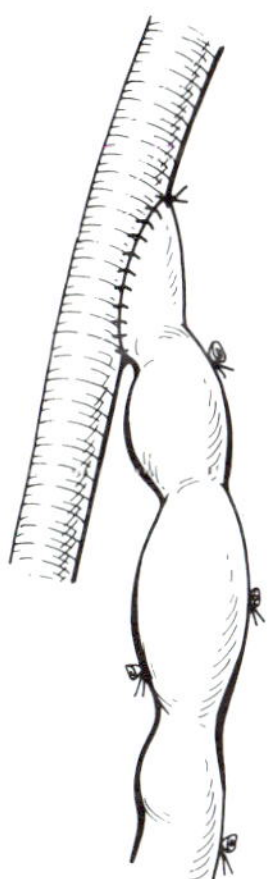

Fig. 6. Aneurysmal graft (from varicosities).

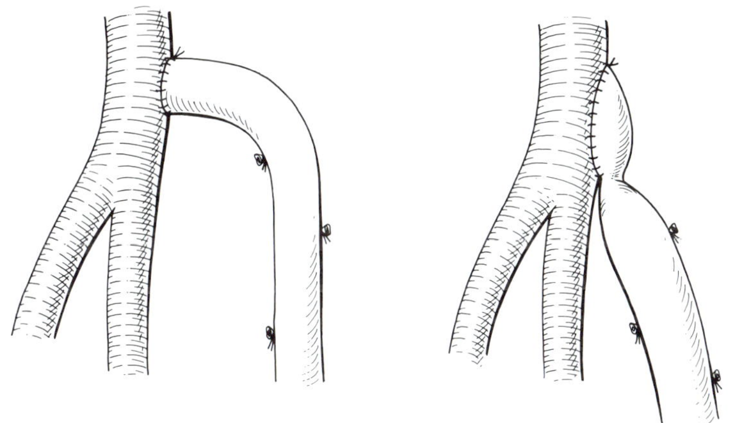

Fig. 7. Not correct technique of anastomosis.

(or not in whole length) so that we tried to find a usable length to at least cross the knee joint in performing a sequential bypass procedure using expanded PTFE for the upper part and the vein separately to cross the joint. The area of the adductorian channel thereby is thrombendarterectomized according to the first describers (DeLaurentis and Friedman, 1972) (Fig. 11). Among 42 of those operations we did not have any early complication yet, so that we incline to favour this kind of combined procedure despite the longer time needed. This refers to occlusive arterial disease only, of course, whereas femoropopliteal aneurysms always can be bypassed by a long saphenous vein.

We did not yet mention other complications such as general disorders (cardiopulmonary system, renal disfunction and others); they are rare whenever a laparotomy can be avoided. Others like the iatrogenic entrapment

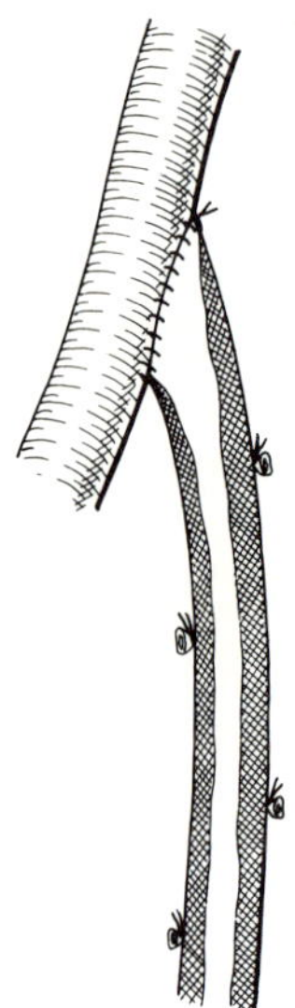

Fig. 8. Diseased vein wall (phlebosclerosis).

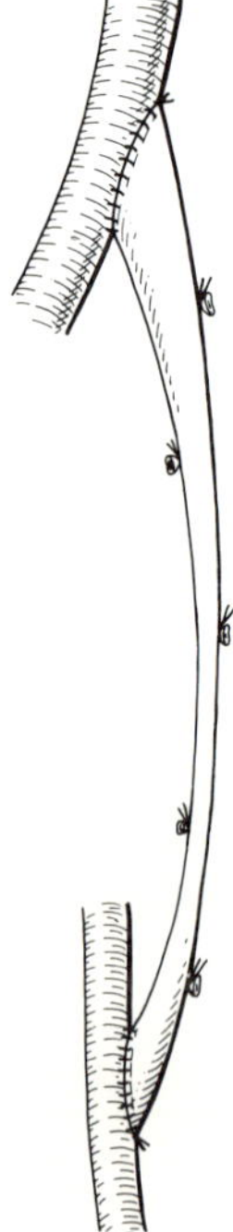

Fig. 9. Stretching of the graft.

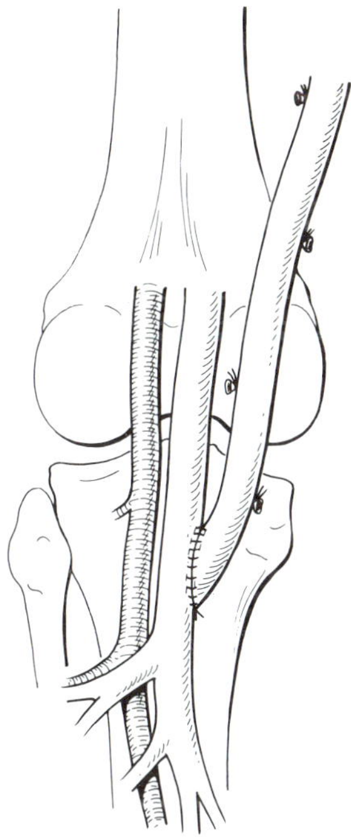

Fig. 10. Distal anastomosis tailored on the popliteal vein (instead of the artery).

syndrome and the post-operative anterior tibial compartment syndrome did not occur in our patients; we also never found an anastomotic pseudo-aneurysm except one rupture of the anastomosis caused by infection.

One other complication to be mentioned is the more or less huge post-operative oedema; this is caused certainly by lymph vessel injury during operation rather than of post-ischaemic origin (Sandman *et al.*, 1976; Schmidt *et al.*, 1978). The oedema usually disappears six–eight weeks after operation unless the occlusive arterial disease is combined with a post-phlebothrombotic syndrome. To avoid those early complications pay attention to the following rules: pre-operatively the indication for surgery is to be planned carefully: in case of limb salvage there is no discussion about doing surgery or not. But it is in the second stage (stage II) with only claudication complaints, where alternative conservative treatment also can achieve lessening or disappearance of the symptoms so that surgery is not needed mostly. Inflow- and outflow-tract deserve attention in planning the operative procedure.

During the operation the condition of the saphenous vein to be gained may be a reason for changing the technique in favour of a sequential bypass. The vein should be carefully dilated and handled. Intra-operative control measurements such as flowmetry (Albrechtsen, 1976; Barner *et al.*, 1968; Bernhard *et al.*, 1971; Cooley and Wukasch, 1979; Flinn *et al.*, 1980; Mannick,

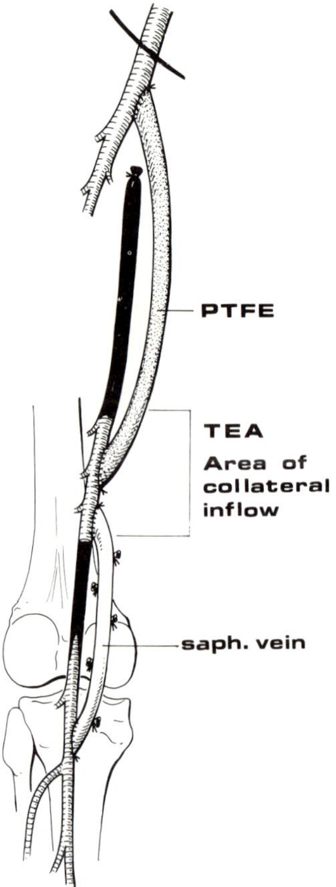

Fig. 11. Composite sequential femoro-popliteal bypass.

1978; Müller-Wiefel, 1980; Szilagyi, 1978) and arteriography (Liddicoat *et al.*, 1975; Pinkerton, 1975; Renwick *et al.*, 1968) can be of great value in detecting and repairing actual faults. Here we think angiography rather than flowmetry should be obligatory. Also we think it is not good to do an additional local thrombo-endarterectomy at the site of the upper and lower anastomosis because we feel that this may also be a cause of a higher post-operative thrombotic occlusion rate than in cases where we could avoid any damage to the anastomotic segment.

In the post-operative period, patients should be mobilized as soon as possible, with some kind of additional rheological treatment and a low-dose heparin prophylaxis or aggregation inhibitors, or both. Vasoactive drugs do not seem to be of any value here. Control of the vascular reconstruction by peripheral pressure measurements and post-operative angiography in case of presumed failure is of course necessary.

REFERENCES

Albrechtsen, D. (1976). Intraoperative hemodynamic findings and their prognostic significance in femoro-popliteal reversed saphenous vein bypass operations. *Scandinavian Journal of Thoracic Cardiovascular Surgery* **10**, 67.

Barner, H. B., Judd, D. R., Kaiser, G. C., Willman, V. L. and Hanlon, C. R. (1968). Blood flow in femoro-popliteal bypass grafts. *Archives of Surgery (Chicago)* **96**, 619.

Bernhard, V. M., Ashmore, C. S., Rodgers, R. E. and Evans, W. E. (1971). Operative blood flow in femoral-popliteal and femoral-tibial grafts for lower extremity ischemia. *Archives of Surgery (Chicago)* **103**, 595.

Brener, B. J., Alpert, J., Brief, D. K. and Parsonnet, V. (1975). Iatrogenic entrapment of femoropopliteal saphenous vein bypass grafts by the gastrocnemius muscle. *Surgery* **78**, 668.

Charlesworth, D., Harris, P. L., Cave, F. D. and Taylor, L. (1975). Undetected aorto-iliac insufficiency: a reason for early failure of saphenous vein bypass grafts for obstruction of the superficial femoral artery. *British Journal of Surgery* **62**, 567.

Cooley, D. A. and Wukasch, D. C. (1979). Femoropopliteal occlusive disease. *In* "Techniques in Vascular Surgery". Saunders, Philadelphia, Pennsylvania.

Craver, J. M., Ottinger, L. W., Darling, R. C., Austen, W. G. and Linton, R. R. (1973). Hemorrhage and thrombosis as early complications of femoropopliteal bypass grafts: causes, treatment and prognostic implications. *Surgery* **74**, 839.

Cronestrand, R., Ekeström, S. and Hambraeus, G. (1968). Pre- and postoperative flow measurements after femoral-popliteal arterial reconstructions. *Scandinavian Journal of Thoracic Cardiovascular Surgery* **2**, 128.

DeLaurentis, D. A. and Friedman, P. (1972). Sequential femoropopliteal bypasses: another approach to the inadequate saphenous vein problem. *Surgery* **71**, 440.

Flinn, W. R., Yao, J. S. T. and Bergan, J. J. (1980). Reoperation for failed femoro-popliteal or femorotibial grafts. *In* "Operative Techniques in Vascular Surgery" (J. J. Bergan and J. S. T. Yao, Eds). Grune & Stratton, New York.

Gordon, A., Williams, J. and Buxton, B. (1975). Optimal length of a saphenous vein segment when used as an arterial substitute. *Cardiovascular Research* **9**, 541.

Gordon, A., Williams, J. and Buxton, B. (1975). Changes in flow and pressure due to rotation of a saphenous vein segment. *Cardiovascular Research* **9**, 539.

Gundry, R. S., Jones, M., Ihihara, T. and Ferrans, V. J. (1980). Intraoperative trauma to human saphenous vein: scanning electron microscopic comparison of preparation techniques. *Annals of Thoracic Surgery* **30**, 40.

Liddicoat, J. E., Bekassy, S. M. and Debakey, M. E. (1975). Intraoperative arteriography during femoropopliteal bypass. *Archives of Surgery (Chicago)* **110**, 839.

Mannick, J. A. (1978). Femoropopliteal and tibial bypass surgery. *In* "Vascular Surgery" (J. S. Najarian and J. P. Delaney, Eds). Thieme, Stuttgart.

Müller-Wiefel, H. (1980). Femoro-popliteal bypass. *In* "Operative Technique in Vascular Surgery". (J. J. Bergan and J. S. T. Yao, Eds). Grune & Stratton, New York.

Pinkerton, J. A. (1975). Operative arteriography. *Archives of Surgery (Chicago)* **110**, 841.

Renwick, S., Royle, J. P. and Martin, P. (1968). Operative angiography after femoro-popliteal arterial reconstruction — its influence on early failure rate. *British Journal of Surgery* **55**, 134.

Sandmann, W., Kremer, K., Kleinschmidt, F. and Günther, D. (1976). Lymphahab-flubstörungen nach Arterien-operationen am Bein. *Chirurg* **47**, 198.

Schmidt, K. R., Welter, H., Pfeifer, K. J. and Becker, H. M. (1978). Lymphographic investigations of oedema of the extremities following reconstructive vascular

surgery in the femoro-popliteal territory. *Fortschrift der Röntgenstrahlentherapie* **128**, 194.
Schwartz, C. F. (1973). Prevention of axial rotation of venous autografts during vascular reconstruction. *Surgery, Gynecology, and Obstetrics* **137**, 97.
Stipa, S., Cavallaro, A., Sciacca, V. and Vincenti, R. (1977). Chirurgia ricostruttiva del tratto femoro-popliteo. *In* "La chirurgia delle arterie periferiche" (Stipa, S., Ed.), p. 233. Piccin, Padova.
Stipa, S., Cavallaro, A., Thau, A. and Palestini, M. (1972). Complicanze e reinterventi nella chirurgia ricostruttiva delle arterie periferiche. *Policlinico, Sezione Chirurgica* **78**, 48.
Szilagyi, D. E. (1978). The greater saphenous vein as an arterial autograft. *In* "Graft materials in Vascular Surgery". (H. Dardik, Ed.). Yearbook Publishers, Chicago, Illinois.

INFECTIONS IN RECONSTRUCTIVE SURGERY: PRINCIPLES OF TREATMENT

J. F. Vollmar and E. U. Voss

Department of Surgery of the University of Ulm, Ulm, West Germany

INTRODUCTION

Wound infection represents the most dangerous complication in vascular surgery. The incidence varies with the experience of the surgical team, the location of reconstruction and the type of graft replacement. A deep wound infection is encountered in 0.6–3.0% of all vascular reconstructions (review by Smith and Szilagyi, 1961; Javid *et al.*, 1962; Szilagyi, 1979; Stirnemann and Nachbur, 1978). A further drastic reduction of the infection rate by the routine use of antibiotics has proved as an unrealistic dream of progress: comparing two own series of 1000 reconstructions using Dacron prostheses without and with antibiotics gave evidence that the infection rate in both groups was quite identical, i.e. 1.1%.

PROPHYLAXIS

Some prophylactic measures most important for preventing deep wound infections are listed in Table I:

(1) Exact disinfection and draping of the operative field. For epilation skin shaving should be avoided, only special creams should be used.

Serono Symposium No. 44, "Peripheral Arterial Diseases: Medical and Surgical Problems", edited by S. Stipa and A. Cavallaro, 1982. Academic Press, London and New York.

Table I. Prophylactic measures against wound infections.

(1) Preparation of the operating field
no skin shaving
(Epilation by special creams)
exact skin disinfection (3 ×)
Plastic drapes (without bullae!)

(2) Surgical tissue dissection
sharp and anatomical
no fingers in the wound!
no damage to lymphatic pathways!

(3) Operating time:
as short as possible
close the groin incision first

(4) Postoperative care:
wound drainages as a routine (Redon-suction-system)
antibiotics only selectively

(2) Exact anatomical tissue dissection using sharp instruments avoiding any damage to surrounding structures such as lympathic collectors and/or lymph nodes. This is especially true for groin incisions.
(3) The operating time should be kept as short as possible (3-S-principle).
(4) Antibiotics not as a routine but selectively in the presence of local or generalized infections.

CLINICAL ASPECTS

The classical signs of inflammation may be expected only in vascular reconstructions in superficial position such as in the groin respectively in the extremities. These signs will be usually missed in deep infections affecting the retroperitoneal space or the thoracic cavity. For these locations the signs of recurrent fever over a period of more than five days post-operatively in combination with positive blood cultures are high suspective. Effusions round the prostheis proved by CT may give additional evidence for the diagnosis (Haaga *et al.*, 1978). The groin is the area most frequently affected by wound infections and disturbances in wound healing (82%; Vollmar, 1980).
In the spontaneous course of deep wound infection several sequelae may be observed (Fig. 1):

(1) Local abscess formation with spontaneous rupture sometimes resulting in a chronic fistula.
(2) Disruption of the suture line with the development of acute haemorrhage or a false aneurysm.
(3) Extensive wound dehiscence with free exposure of the graft.
(4) Septicaemia with positive blood culture.
(5) Secondary graft occlusion.

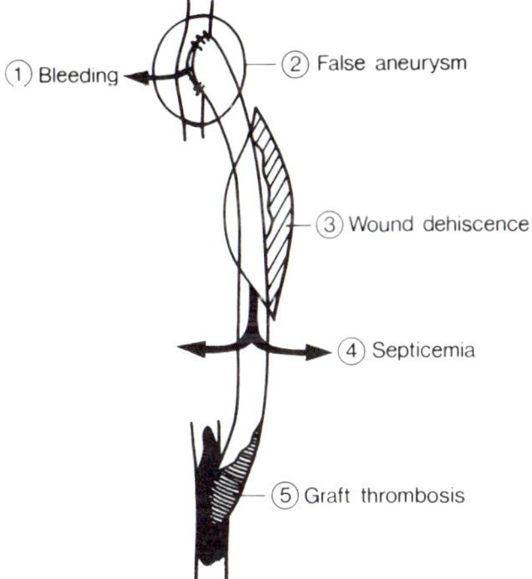

Fig. 1. Sequelae of deep wound infections in vascular surgery.

PROGNOSIS

The overall mortality in deep wound infections following vascular surgery is still between 20% and 37% (Vollmar and Bimler, 1978; Vollmar *et al.*, 1981). By far the worst prognosis have infected aortic grafts with a mortality approaching 75% (Koning *et al.*, 1980). After arterial reconstructions for the extremities the removal of an infected graft leads in 20–40% to secondary amputations (Szilagyi, 1979; Brücke *et al.*, 1975).

PRINCIPLES OF TREATMENT

A conservative therapy with antibiotics in high doses in combination with local anti-inflammatory measures is only defensible during the early phase of subacute infections especially in the retroperitoneal or intrathoracic space. If within a few days local and/or generalized signs of infections persist or increase an active surgical approach is mandatory.

Infected areas in superficial position, e.g. in a groin or in extremities, should be opened early insuring an adequate drainage. Sometimes the graft must be widely exposed in order to have free access and control of the whole infected area. This is specially true for the femoro-popliteal segment. Surgical debridement and the daily application of antiseptic solutions such as Polyvinylpyrrolidone or Rivanol, offer in 10–20% of these patients the chance of preserving the graft (Vollmar *et al.*, 1981). The success of such a local aggressive surgical approach depends on several prerequisities: (a) no signs of general septicaemia, (b) the anastomotic area should not be affected, i.e. no impending complications from the suture line, (c) the wound infection should not be older than four–six weeks after surgery in the presence of a full patent vascular graft. Autologous graft but also double velour Dacron and expanded PTFE prostheses justify such a local open wound treatment because these materials have a remarkably higher resistance to infection than other conventional knitted or woven grafts including all types of biografts (Pasternak *et al.*, 1977; Ehrenfeld *et al.*, 1979; Vollmar *et al.*, 1981).

The external velour layer favours a fast tissue invasion, preventing the spread of infection along the vascular prosthesis frequently seen in normal knitted or woven graft (Fig. 2). On the other hand the degree of neo-intima formation seems to be an important factor counteracting graft infections via the bloodstream (Roon *et al.*, 1977).

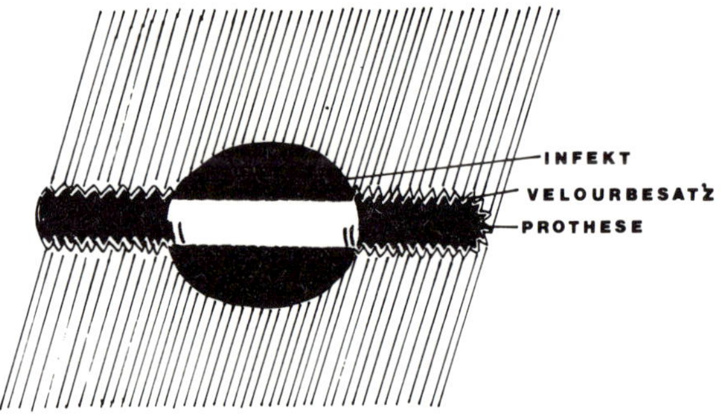

Fig. 2. Early contact between Dacron velour prosthesis and the surrounding tissue prevents spread of infection along the vascular prosthesis.

After clean-up of the wound the acceptance of the pulsating prosthesis by the surrounding granulation tissue is announced by the change of its colour from pale to pink and further on by its progressive fixation in the wound ground. At this stage a secondary wound closure helps a great deal to shorten the healing process either by a turned soft tissue flap (for the groin) or a "buried precedure" (in the extremities). The technique of such a buried operation is demonstrated in Fig. 3. In all four patients with deep wound infections of femoro-popliteal double velour prostheses the buried grafts have healed in with no recurrent infections during a follow-up period of one–three years. There is strong evidence that such a local open wound treatment will fail regularly in late infections, i.e. beyond six–eight weeks after surgery specially when a circular wall of granulation tissue heralds a "sequestration" of the graft. Here the graft should be removed immediately to avoid anastomotic complications or septicaemia (Vollmar *et al.*, 1981). At this stage there is no longer a chance for graft preservation. The removal of the infected graft should be combined when ever possible with a new bypass outside of the infected area preserving the blood supply to the concerned body region. In general, any attempt of a new arterial reconstruction in the infected area includes a high risk of failure and is therefore contraindicated.

A new approach to an *in situ* repair in the infected region opens perhaps the report of Ehrenfeld *et al.* (1979). After removal of the infected aorto-iliac

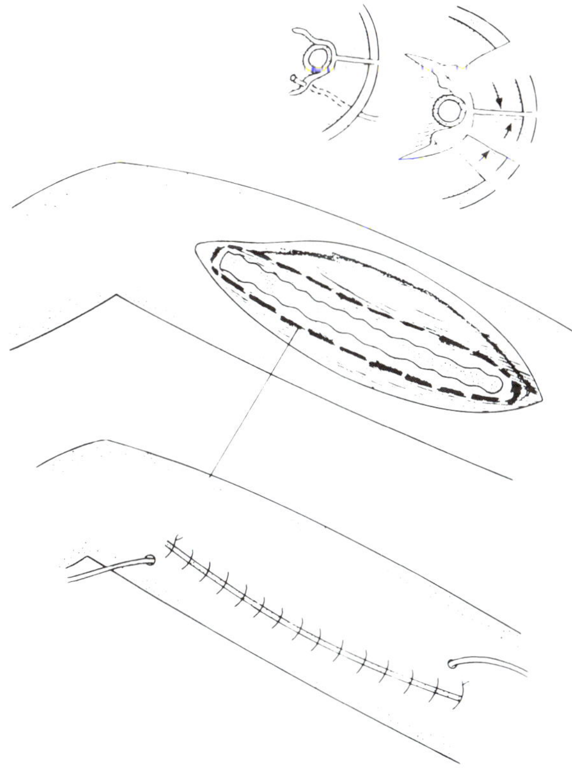

Fig. 3. "Buried procedure" after open treatment of an infected vascular graft (antiseptic solutions). Mobilizing the surrounding soft tissue and covering the graft with complete closure of the wound.

Dacron prostheses the authors used autologous grafts from disobliterated segments of the occluded iliac respectively superficial femoral arteries in combination with venous patches. In 24 patients there was a post-operative mortality of 13% but not recurrent infection. In recent years a variety of operations have been proposed for bypassing the septic focus. Descending thoracic aorta infected vascular prosthesis in this position may be removed with closure of the aortic stumps after a preliminary bypass from the ascending aorta down to the abdominal aorta or as a bifurcated graft to both iliac arteries.

AORTO-ILIAC INFECTIONS

The preferred procedure is an axillo-femoral or axillo-bifemoral bypass with distal anastomoses to an uninfected vascular segment below the inguinal ligament. In unilateral retroperitoneal infection the femoro-femoral bypass is the method of choice. Its long-term results are quite satisfactory with a five-year patency rate of 75%. In contrast most other extra-anatomic reconstructions, e.g. long bypasses from the descending aorta to the inguinal region includes a remarkably higher risk for the patient.

INFECTIONS IN THE GROIN

If the infection is limited to the groin the construction of an obturator bypass is considered as the method of choice (Vollmar, 1980; Vollmar *et al.*, 1981). Its long-term patency is comparable with the femoro-femoral cross-over graft.

FEMORAL-POPLITEAL SEGMENT

If an open local treatment fails or is contraindicated (see above) the attempt of an extra-anatomic atypical bypass using the lateral apsect of the thigh and knee region is justified using if possible an autogeneous vein graft from the opposite leg or an expanded PTFE prosthesis of 6-mm diameter (Fig. 4). The other solution is the attempt of *in situ* repair using a semi-closed thrombo-endarterectomy with autologous venous patches for the upper and distal anastomoses after removal of the infected graft. The outcome of all these procedures are equivocal with respect to limb salvage.

EXTRA-ANATOMIC GRAFT INFECTIONS

In the supraclavicular graft position, i.e. carotid-subclavian Dacron bypass, deep wound infections are rare conditions. In 200 cases there were two infections. One healed spontaneously after open wound treatment, the second graft had to be removed and replaced by an axillo-axillary Dacron prosthesis. This procedure offers a simple and excellent approach for by-passing supraclavicular graft infections.

Infected axillo-femoral Dacron grafts include several solutions of a secondary aseptic bypass. We feel the best approach is the return to the anatomical arterial pathway. When groin infections have happened before we do not hesitate to insert a second graft to the common femoral artery if the wound has healed completely for three months at least (Vollmar and Bimler, 1978). Another alternative is an aorto-iliac thromboendarterectomy avoiding any artificial materials.

GRAFT REACTION VERSUS GRAFT INFECTION

Only a few reports are recently available describing a peculiar clinical picture with recurrent fluid accumulation around Dacron prosthesis (Kaupp *et al.*, 1979). There is no bacterial contamination of the plasma-like fluid. A

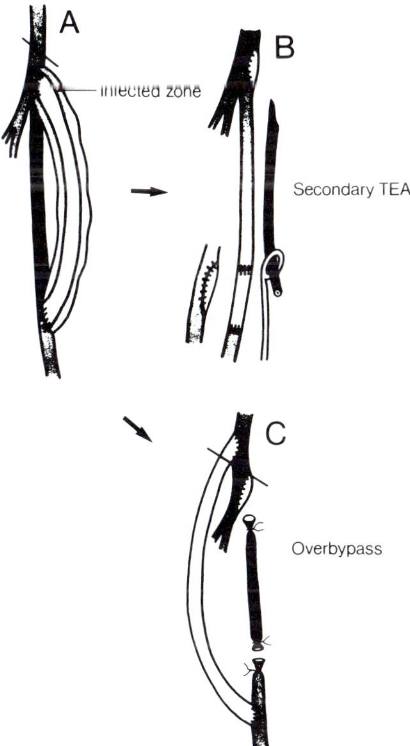

Fig. 4. Secondary reconstructions after infected femoro-popliteal grafts: B, after complete removal of the infected graft restoration of the arterial pathway by semi-closed ring disobliteration of the superficial patch or interposition of a venous graft; C, aseptic "overbypass", using great saphenous vein or expanded PTFE-prosthesis.

pronounced foreign body tissue reaction characterizes the histological picture. The time interval between graft insertion and the first clinical signs varies between months and years (Fig. 5). A through wall healing of the prosthesis is missed. The question is still open if this non-healing phenomenon mainly seen in Dacron velour prostheses in extra-anatomical position is caused by a hypersensitive or allergic reaction on the synthetic material.

Anyway there is only one real chance of definitive healing: taking out the total Dacron prosthesis and insert another synthetic material such as expanded PTFE. As an example, in a 58-year-old man: no less than six vascular repairs were done after a carotid-subclavian Dacron velour bypass complicated by recurrent formation of cysts along the new inserted double velour segments in axillo-axillary position. After removal of all Dacron material and insertion of an expanded PTFE prosthesis a definitive healing was established.

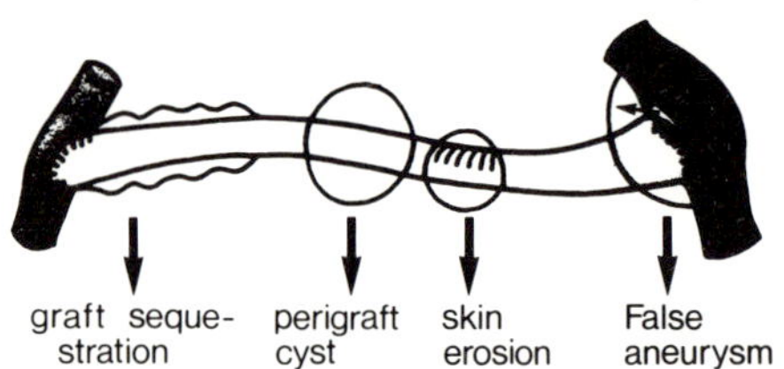

Fig. 5. Aseptic perigraft reaction. Allergic hypersensitivity and foreign body overreaction.

SUMMARY

(1) Deep wound infection is still the most serious complication in vascular surgery threatening limbs, organs or life. The most important prophylactic measures include exact skin preparation and disinfection avoiding any shaving for epilation. Any tissue damage specially to the lymphatic pathways has to be avoided. The routine use of antibiotics is not a realistic approach to eliminate such a disaster.

(2) Late wound infections of vascular grafts (beyond the six–eight weeks after surgery) affords nearly regularly the removal of the infected arterial substitute in combination with the insertion of an aseptic new arterial pathway. An *in situ* repair using autologous arteries and/or veins may be an alternative in selected cases.

(3) Early infections (one–six week post-operationem) of synthetic vascular prostheses (double velour Dacron, expanded PTFE) in superficial position, e.g. in the groin and/or extremities justify the attempt of graft preservation by early opening of the wound and local antiseptic treatment. After wound cleaning a secondary wound closure (buried procedure) may be done with excellent results.

(4) Hypersensitivity against synthetic material with aseptic fluid accumulation around the prosthesis and missing tissue invasion in the porous graft represents a new clinical entity which has to be differentiated from bland late infections. Total exchange of the graft material (e.g. Dacron versus expanded PTFE) is mandatory and promises an uncomplicated outcome.

REFERENCES

Brücke, P., Denck, H., Piza, F. and Wagner, O. (1975). "Lymphgefässchirurgie septische gefässchirurgie dialyse-shunt-probleme", Vol. VII. Jahrestagg. Österr. Ges. Gefässchir., Linz, 5.–9.6 Egermann-Verlag, Wien.

Ehrenfeld, W. K., Wilbur, B. G., Olcott, N. and Stoney, R. J. (1979). Autogenous tissue reconstruction in the management of infected prosthetic grafts. *Surgery* **85**, 82.

Haaga, J. R., Baldwin, G. N., Reich, N. E., Bevene, E., Kramer, A., Weinstein, A., Havrilla, Th. R., Seidelmann, F. E., Namba, A. H. and Parrish, Ch. M. (1978). CT detection of infected synthetic grafts: preliminary report of a new sign. *American Journal of Roentgenology* **131**, 317.

Javid, H., Julian, O. C., Dye, W. S. and Hunter, J. A. (1962). Complications of abdominal aortic grafts. *Archives of Surgery* **85**, 650.
Kaupp, H. A., Matulewicz, T. J., Lattimer, G. L., Kremen, J. E. and Celani, V. J. (1979). Graft infection or graft reaction? *Archives of Surgery (Chicago)* **114**, 1419.
Koning, J., Barwegen, M. G. M. H. and Van Berge Henegouwen, D. P. (1980). Die behandlung von infektionen nach arteriellen gefässrekonstruktionen. *Angiologia* **4**, 269.
Pasternak, B. M., Paruk, F. A. C. A., Kogan, S. and Lewitt, S. (1977). A synthetic vascular conduit (expanded PTFE) for hemodialysis access—a preliminary report. *Vascular Surgery* **11**, 99.
Roon, A. J., Malone, J. M., Moore, W. S., Bean, B. and Campagna, G. (1977). Bacteremic infectability: function of vascular graft material and design. *Journal of Surgical Research* **22**, 489.
Smith, R. F. and Szilagyi, D. E. (1961). Healing complications with plastic arterial implants. *Archives of Surgery (Chicago)* **82**, 14.
Stirnemann, P. and Nachbur, B. (1978). Der tiefe infekt als komplikation einer aorto-iliaco-femoro-poplitealen rekonstruktion im arteriellen system. *Vasa* **7**, 154. 154.
Szilagyi, D. E. (1979). Management of complications after arterial reconstruction. *Surgical Clinics of North America* **59**, 659.
Vollmar, J. (1980). "Reconstructive surgery of the arteries". Thieme, Stuttgart.
Vollmar, J. and Bimler, H. H. (1978). Chirurgische aspekte bei der behandlung infizierter gefässprothesen. *Aktuelle Chirurg* **13**, 225.
Vollmar, J. F., Hepp, W. and Voss, E. U. (1981). Das infizierte gefässtransplantat—entfernung oder erhaltung? *Aktuelle Chirurg* **16** (In press).

SURGICAL TREATMENT OF BUERGER'S DISEASE

S. Shionoya

Department of Surgery, Nagoya University Branch Hospital, Nagoya, Japan

Although the number of patients with obliterating arteriosclerosis is recently increasing in Japan, there are at present about 5000 patients with Buerger's disease who have to undergo surgical or conservative managements, and the surgical treatment of Buerger's disease is one of the most difficult problems in the field of vascular surgery in Japan. From May 1967 to April 1981, 399 patients with Buerger's disease have been treated at the Department of Surgery, Nagoya University Branch Hospital: 388 males and 11 females. Our diagnostic criteria of Buerger's disease are shown in Table I. The clinical diagnosis of Buerger's disease was made when No. 4 or 5 was present in addition to No. 1, 2, 3, 6 and 7.

Table I. Diagnostic criteria of Buerger's disease.

(1)	Smoker
(2)	Onset of symptom before the age of 50 years
(3)	Arterial occlusion below the knee
(4)	Involvement of the upper extremity
(5)	Phlebitis migrans
(6)	Absence of atherogenic risk factors
(7)	Arteriographic findings
(8)	Histological characteristics

Serono Symposium No. 44, "Peripheral Arterial Diseases: Medical and Surgical Problems", edited by S. Stipa and A. Cavallaro, 1982. Academic Press, London and New York.

ARTERIAL RECONSTRUCTION

In 68 of the 399 patients, 79 arterial reconstructions were performed: seven patients underwent operation twice and two patients three times (Table II).

Table II. Summary of 79 arterial reconstructions from May 1967 to April 1981.

		Occlusion	
(I) Symptoms	No. of cases		
Claudication	22 (27.8%)		
Rest pain	11 (14.0%)		
Ulcer or gangrene	46 (58.2%)		
	79 (100.0%)		
(II) Affected limb			
Upper extremity	3		
Lower extremity	76		
	79		
(III) Type of operation		early	late
Bypass	68	26	16
TEA	9	4	4
Replacement	2	0	0
	79	30	20

At the present time, direct arterial surgery is not frequently feasible for the patients with Buerger's disease because of multiple and diffuse occlusions of the arteries distal to the brachial or the popliteal artery. The rate of arterial reconstruction in our series was 17.0%. As the finger or the palm arteries were diffusely occluded and segmental obstructive lesion in the forearm arteries was rarely seen, arterial revascularization of the upper extremity was uncommonly indicated. Therefore, in the majority of cases, arterial reconstruction was indicated for obstructive lesions of the lower extremity, especially for iliac or femoro-popliteal block.

Ischaemic symptoms for which arterial revascularization was indicated were ulcer or gangrene in 58%, claudication in 28% and rest pain in 14%. From onset of symptoms to the time of follow up, 30 April 1981, trophic lesions occurred in 73% of the patients, and the principal symptom for which surgical procedure was indicated was ulcer or gangrene. As the majority of the patients were in the prime of manhood, prompt relief of claudication was important for them from an occupational standpoint. Judging from the highest absent pulse of the patients when they were first seen, it was of interest that about one-third of them showed an iliac or femoro-popliteal block in addition to infra-popliteal lesions at the first examination, and the rate of arterial reconstruction in the patients with iliac or femoro-popliteal occlusion was 43.4%. Because of poor result of TEA, probably due to the presence of a remnant of the inflammatory lesion in the revascularized segment, we preferred bypass grafting to TEA (Shionoya *et al.*, 1976). According to revascularized segment, results of arterial reconstruction were discussed. The status of all the patients was determined as of 30 April 1981.

Aortoiliac Reconstruction (16 Cases) (Table III)

Table III. Results of aortoiliac reconstruction.

(I) Symptoms	No. of cases		
Claudication	4 (25.0%)		
Rest pain	2 (12.5%)		
Ulcer or gangrene	10 (62.5%)		
	16 (100.0%)		
(II) Type of operation		Occlusion	
		early	late
Bypass: Aorto-femoral	4	0	3
Ilio-femoral	6	1	2
Ilio-popliteal	2	0	1
Femoro-femoral	1	1	0
TEA: External iliac	3	2	1
	16	4	7

Except three vein graftings, bypass procedures with Dacron prosthesis were performed and lumbar sympathectomy was carried out at the same time in eight cases. In our series, 27 patients showed an involvement of the aortoiliac segment in addition to obstructive lesions in femoro-popliteal area. The superficial femoral artery was patent in only four limbs of them, and operative indication was mostly decided by run-off in the deep femoral artery. Such a second distal revascularization as femoro-crural bypass was not feasible in general, and in only one case, iliofemoral and femoro-peroneal bypass grafting were performed at the same time (Fig. 1). Therefore, long-term patency of the only proximal revascularized segment was not ready to be achieved.

Although the proximal revascularization alone was inadequate to completely relieve ischaemia in the lower extremity, successful proximal arterial reconstruction was effective for healing of trophic lesions. Two TEA failed immediately and the other ended up in rupture of the false aneurysm one year after operation.

Femoro-popliteal Reconstruction (58 Cases) (Table IV)

Direct arterial surgery was most frequently performed in this area and autogenous vein was used for bypass procedure in all the cases. When the saphenous veins were occluded or of inadequate diameter, the cephalic or the basilic veins were employed. Concomitant lumbar sympathectomy was

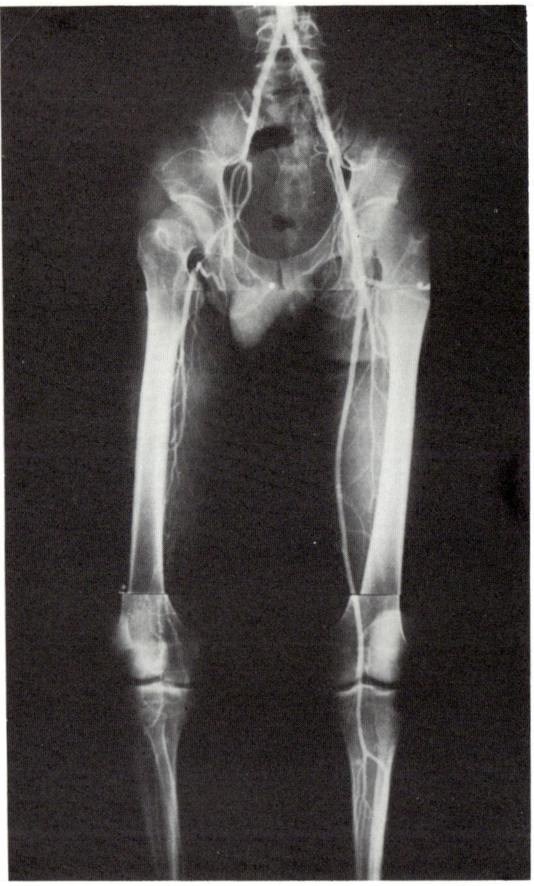

Fig. 1. Arteriogram of a 31-year-old man with Buerger's disease. The right external iliac artery is occluded and only the deep femoral and the peroneal arteries are patent in the right lower extremity. Iliofemoral and femoro-peroneal bypass graftings were performed at the same time.

performed in 29 cases. Poor results of the femoro-popliteal revascularization was due to early failure of bypass grafting, and the main cause of the early occlusion was poor distal run-off. While TEA of the femoral or the popliteal artery failed within one and a half years after operation except one case with profundaplasty, replacement of the femoral artery using autogenous vein functioned well for four years.

Degree of involvement in this group was almost the same as that in the former group, and effects of successful arterial reconstruction on the ischaemia were impressive (Fig. 2.).

Table IV. Results of femoro-popliteal reconstruction.

(I) Symptoms	No. of cases		
Claudication	18 (31.0%)		
Rest pain	6 (10.3%)		
Ulcer or gangrene	34 (58.7%)		
	58 (100.0%)		
(II) Type of operation		Occlusion	
		early	late
Bypass: Femoro-popliteal	12	4	5
Femoro-crural	27	14	3
Popliteo-popliteal	3	1	0
Popliteo-crural	9	3	2
TEA: Femoral	3	1	1
Popliteal	2	0	2
Replacement: Femoral	2	0	0
	58	23	13

Reconstruction of the Forearm or the Crural Artery (5 Cases) (Table V)

Arterial reconstruction was performed to relief ulceration of the finger or rest pain of the hand. Although TEA of the radial artery soon failed, brachio-ulnar bypass with autogenous vein was patent for two months to three years (Fig. 3). Tibiotibial vein bypass in two patients with rest pain or ulcer failed immediately after operation, and thereafter, ulceration of the toe occurred in one case (Fig. 4).

In conclusion, as shown in the cumulative patency rate by life-table method (Fig. 5), the main cause of the poor results was due to early failure and long-term result of revascularization which had escaped from early occlusion was almost satisfactory.

NONINVASIVE DIAGNOSTIC TECHNIQUES

In our hospital, measurement of segmental blood pressure in the extremity has been our routine practice since four years ago and pre-operative assessment of distal run-off has been done with the technique. During the last four years, namely, from May 1977 to April 1981, 39 arterial reconstructions were performed in 36 of 166 patients with Buerger's disease (Table VI). The highest absent pulse of the patients was femoral in 12 (7.3%), popliteal in 58 (34.9%) and ankle in 96 (57.8%), and the rate of arterial reconstruction in the patients with iliac or femoro-popliteal block was 45.7%, because three patients underwent operation twice and four cases had revascularization of the forearm or the crural artery.

Eleven early failures occurred after bypass grafting of which distal anastomosis was below the knee, and the cumulative patency rate by life-table method showed the same pattern as that during the whole term (Fig. 6).

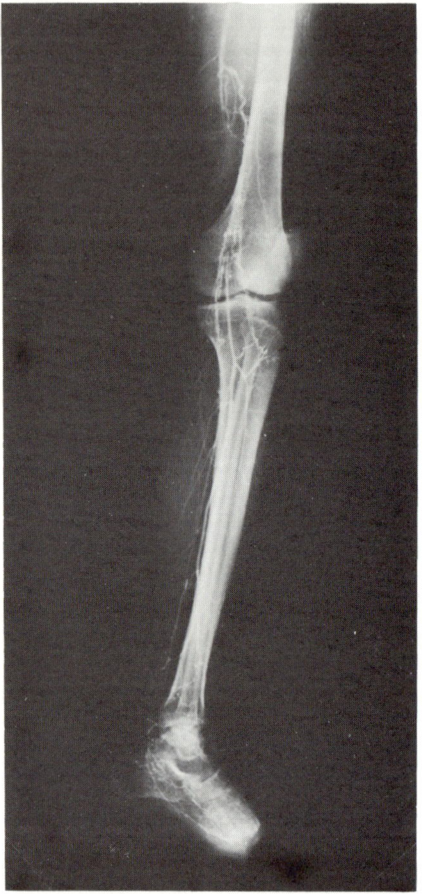

Fig. 2. Arteriogram of a 28-year-old man with Buerger's disease. The left lower superficial femoral and upper popliteal arteries are obstructed. The anterior and posterior tibial arteries are occluded at the mid-tibia level. Intractable ulceration of the stump of the foot which had been amputated near Lisfranc's joint promptly healed after femoro-popliteal bypass grafting.

Post-operative course of the 39 cases showed that ischaemic symptoms were worsened in three of 11 patients with early failure in spite of concomitant lumbar sympathectomy (Table VII).

Judging from the relation of pre-operative ankle or toe blood pressure with follow-up results, pre-operative blood pressure alone did not predict the post-operative course, because arterial reconstruction was successful even in cases with distal low blood pressure before operation (Fig. 7). Post-operative consecutive measurement of the ankle and the toe blood pressure in cases of successful revascularization revealed that the ankle blood pressure

Table V. Results of reconstruction of the arm or the crural artery.

(I) Symptoms	No. of cases		
Rest pain	3		
Ulcer	2		
	5		
(II) Type of operation		Occlusion	
		early	late
Bypass: Brachioulnar	2	0	0
Tibiotibial	2	2	0
TEA: Radial	1	1	0
	5	3	0

immediately reverted to almost normal but the toe blood pressure rose very slightly (Fig. 8). The post-operative incomplete recovery of the toe blood pressure implies multiple and diffuse arterial obstructive lesions in the foot and toes in the patients with Buerger's disease (Shionoya *et al.*, 1980).

In our hospital, by means of a tracer technique with 99mTc-pertechnetate, arterial flow velocity in the foot during reactive hyperaemia has been measured (Shionoya *et al.*, 1981) (Fig. 9). The most characteristic finding in the patients with Buerger's disease was an extraordinary decreased flow velocity in the foot (Fig. 10). When the velocity in the foot was normalized after arterial reconstruction, ulceration healed favourably and the ischaemic limb was salvaged in spite of the incomplete recovery of the distal blood pressure. However, pre-operative measurement of the velocity did not provide valuable data for the correct prediction of arterial revascularization, and pre-operative accurate evaluation of the distal run-off is a topic for further discussion.

SYMPATHECTOMY

As a procedure which produces vasodilatation, sympathectomy has been widely employed for relief of vasospasm in Buerger's disease (Szilagyi *et al.*, 1964). However, it is agreed that no significant alteration occurs in muscle circulation after sympathectomy and sympathetic denervation is not indicated for claudication. Among ischaemic symptoms for which sympathectomy was indicated in our series, the most numerous were trophic lesions (Table VIII). Concomitant lumbar sympathectomy was performed at the same time in 39 arterial reconstructions with the expectation that there might be an increase in arterial flow through the revascularized segment as the result of a reduction in peripheral vascular resistance.

Ulceration healed within one month after operation in about 50% of 53 cases in the last four years but the other half was cured with difficulty within three to five months. Three patients underwent amputation of the extremity (Table IX). Successful outcome of a lumbar sympathectomy depends on

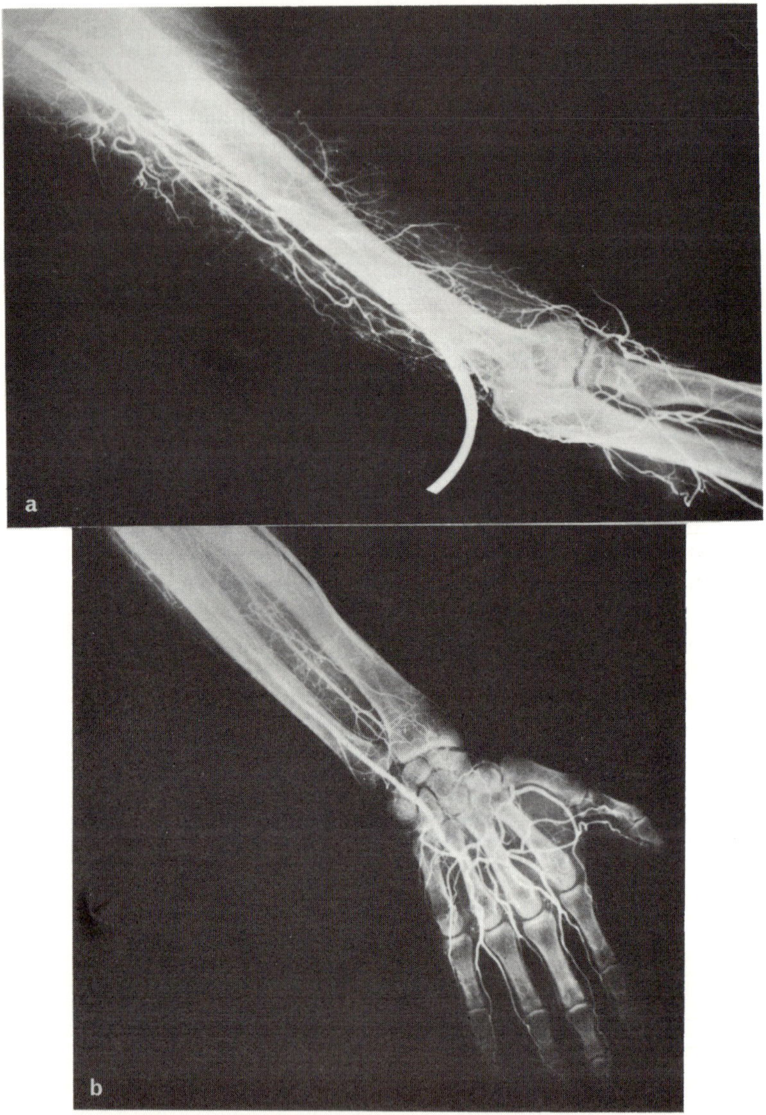

Fig. 3. Arteriogram of a 42-year-old man with Buerger's disease. (a) The brachial artery is occluded above and below the fossa cubitalis. (b) The distal radial and digital arteries are occluded. Brachioulnar bypass was performed.

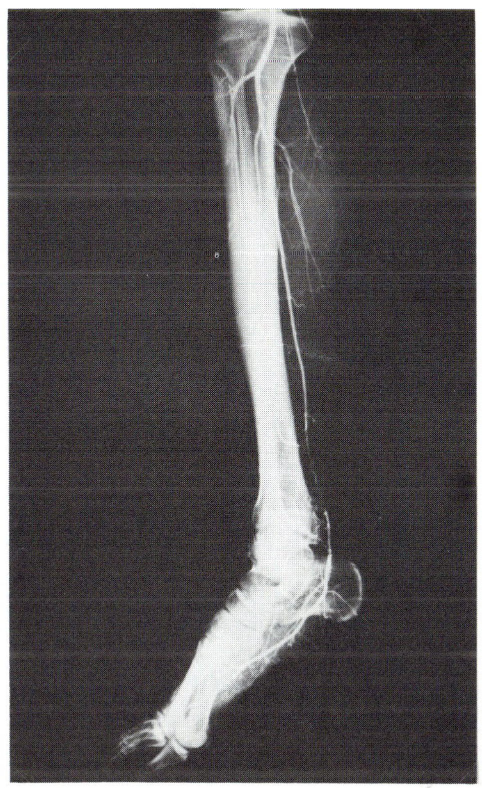

Fig. 4. Arteriogram of a 32-year-old man with Buerger's disease. Tibiotibial bypass was performed for segmental occlusion of the right posterior tibial artery above the ankle.

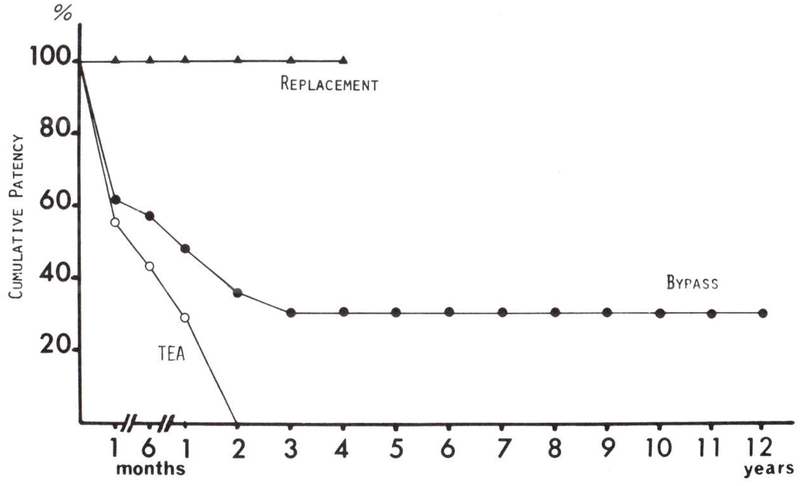

Fig. 5. Cumulative patency rate by life-table method for 79 arterial reconstructions from May 1967 to April 1981. Bypass, 68 cases; TEA, 9 cases; replacement, 2 cases.

Table VI. Summary of 39 arterial reconstructions from May 1977 to April 1981.

(I) Symptoms	No. of cases		
Claudication	9 (23.0%)		
Rest pain	7 (18.0%)		
Ulcer or gangrene	23 (59.0%)		
	39 (100.0%)		
(II) Type of operation		Occlusion	
		early	late
Bypass	36	11	3
TEA	1	0	0
Replacement	2	0	0
	39	11	3

pre-operative evaluation of collateral circulation and vasomotor activity of the extremity. As the ankle blood pressure was unchanged and the toe blood pressure was significantly decreased after lumbar sympathectomy, the distal blood pressure measurement did not predict the outcome of the operation (Fig. 11). On the other hand, of 12 limbs with ulceration, the lesion healed favourably in four limbs which showed normalization of the velocity in the foot after sympathectomy but healing of ulcers was delayed in the other eight limbs without recovery of the velocity. Therefore, the flow velocity correlated with the post-operative clinical course (Fig. 12).

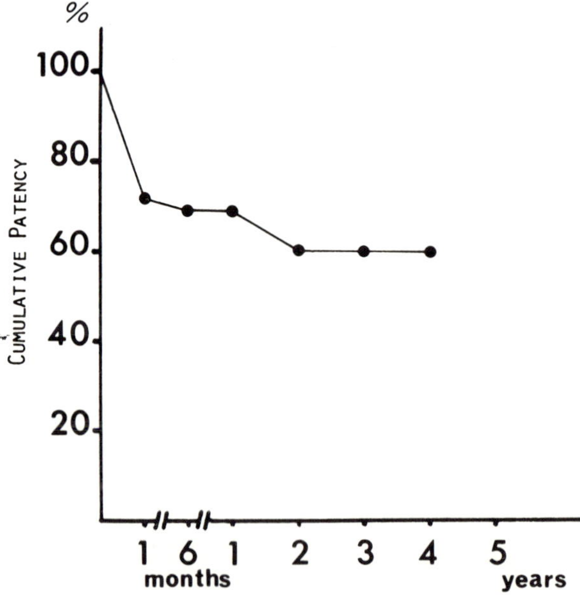

Fig. 6. Cumulative patency rate by life-table method for 39 arterial reconstructions from May 1977 to April 1981.

Table VII. Results of 39 arterial reconstructions according to degree of involvement from May 1977 to April 1981.

Degree of involvement	No. of cases	Better	Same	Worse
Claudication	9 (7)	7	2	0
Rest pain	7 (3)	3	4	0
Ulcer or gangrene	23 (15)	15	5	3
	39 (25) (patent)	25	11	3

CONTINUOUS INTRA-ARTERIAL INFUSION WITH PGE1

Fifty-two patients with intractable trophic lesion for whom neither arterial reconstruction nor sympathectomy was feasible underwent a continuous intra-arterial infusion with PGE1 (Shionoya, 1980), seven cases entered twice and one case four times to the treatment because of recurrence or another trophic lesion. This was done by means of a percutaneous insertion of the catheter with a diameter of 1 mm into the main artery of the affected limb, usually the femoral artery. In the superficial femoral artery, the catheter was detained above the knee and correct insertion of the catheter was always certified by angiography (Fig. 13). After the catheter was connected with the infusion pump, it was fixed on the chest and abdominal wall with adhesive plaster. The solution in the infusion bag consisted of 0.1 ng kg^{-1} min^{-1} of PGE1, 10 mg day^{-1} of heparin and 500 mg day^{-1} of aminobenzyl penicillin. The patient could walk freely in the hospital during the infusion therapy.

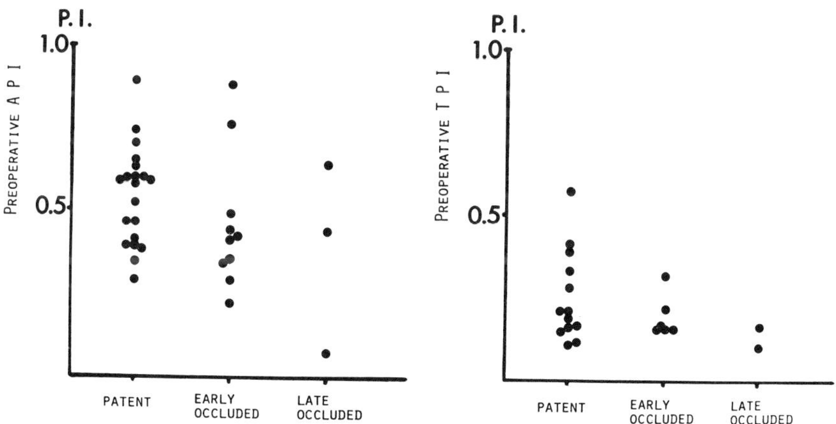

Fig. 7. Correlation of preoperative ankle or toe blood pressure with follow-up results of arterial reconstruction. API, ankle pressure index; TPI, toe pressure index.

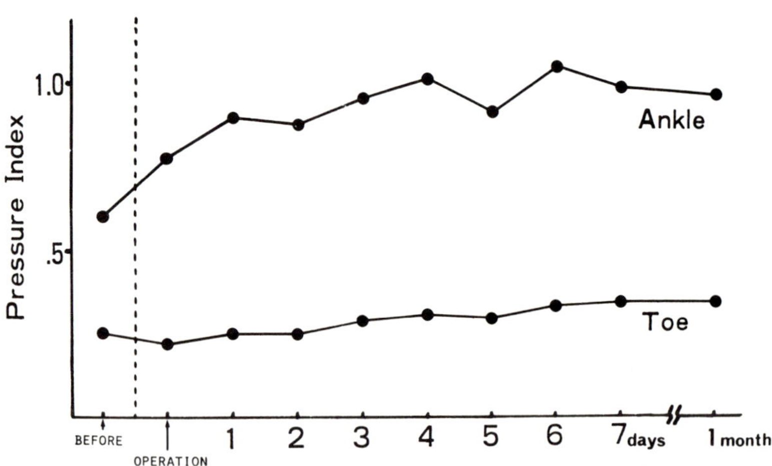

Fig. 8. Comparison of the ankle and toe blood pressures by post-operative consecutive measurement in ten cases with successful arterial revascularization. ●, Mean value of the blood pressure.

The summary of the infusion therapy is shown in Table X. Ten of 15 patients without effect underwent afterwards amputation of the extremity. In all the cases, PGE1 was at first infused at a dose of 0.1 ng kg^{-1} min^{-1} and in 15 cases, swelling or pain was recognized around the knee and the troubles promptly disappeared when the dosage was reduced by half. When the initial dose was ineffective, the dosage was increased to 0.2–0.7 ng kg^{-1} min^{-1} in 25 cases. There was no abnormal variation in the laboratory studies during and after the therapy. However, C-reactive protein test was intensified only during the infusion in 22 cases.

AMPUTATION

In the course of a 14-year follow-up study, 55 patients underwent amputation of the extremity: thigh in five, leg in seven and toe or finger in 43. Four of 45 patients with early or late failure of the arterial reconstruction required amputation: of the leg in two and of the toe in two.

DISCUSSION

The problem that causes the most distress in patients with Buerger's disease is trophic lesion of the extremity and so we should concentrate our attention on limb salvage. Although arterial reconstruction was most effective for healing of ulceration, direct arterial surgery had a very restricted application. Furthermore, it was not easy to avoid early failure due to poor distal run-off,

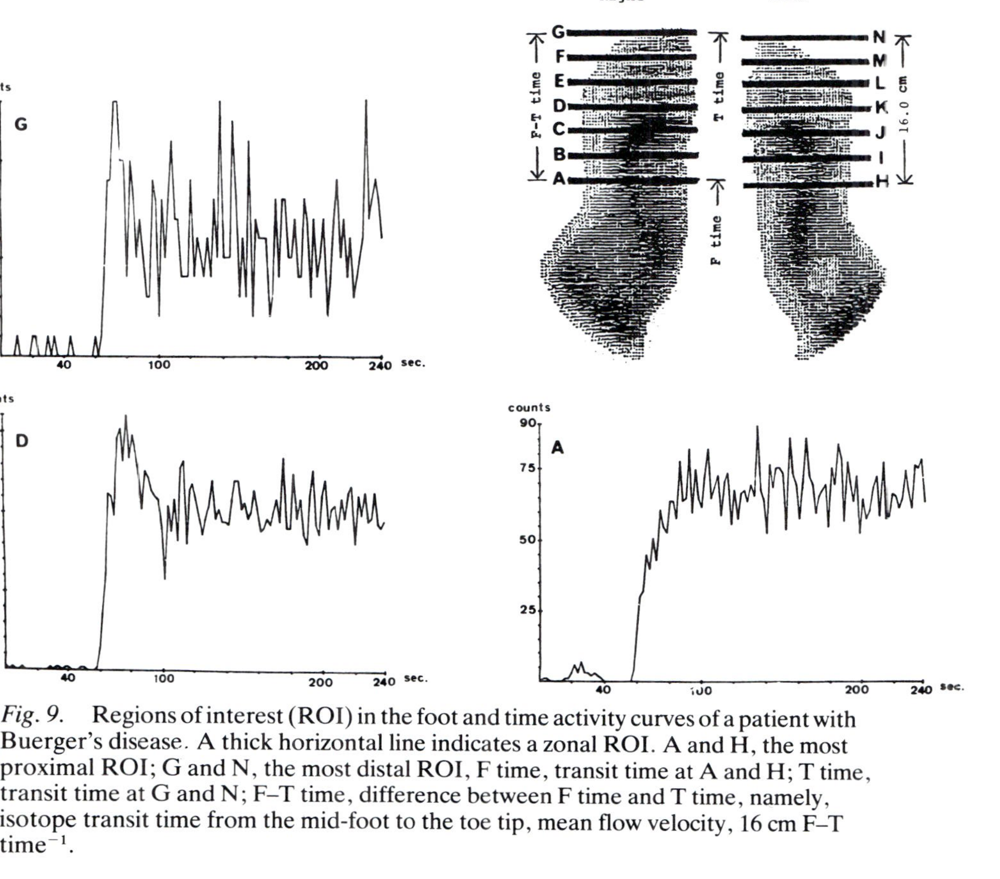

Fig. 9. Regions of interest (ROI) in the foot and time activity curves of a patient with Buerger's disease. A thick horizontal line indicates a zonal ROI. A and H, the most proximal ROI; G and N, the most distal ROI, F time, transit time at A and H; T time, transit time at G and N; F–T time, difference between F time and T time, namely, isotope transit time from the mid-foot to the toe tip, mean flow velocity, 16 cm F–T time^{-1}.

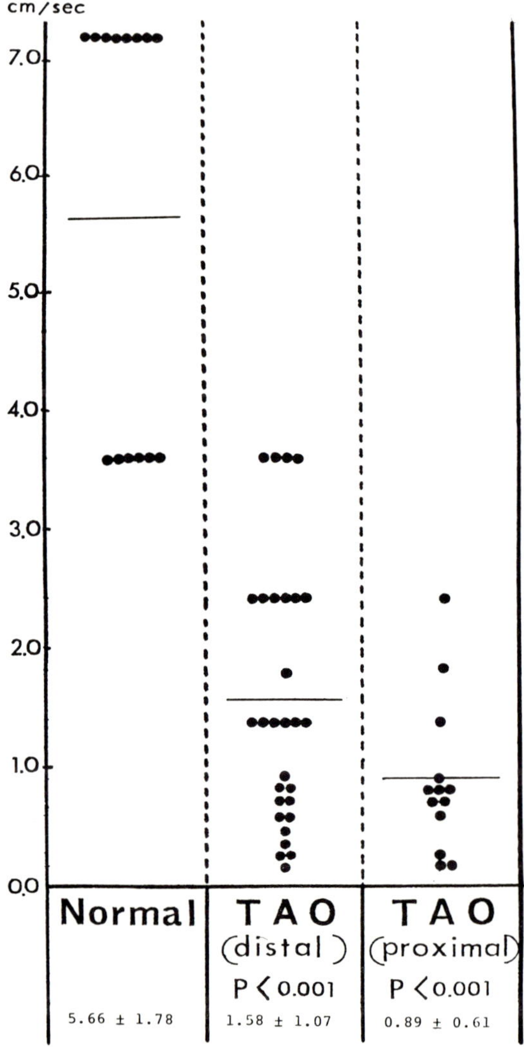

Fig. 10. Flow velocity in the foot in 14 normal limbs and patients with Buerger's disease. Distal TAO: 29 legs of 20 patients with occlusion of the infra-popliteal arteries.
Proximal TAO: 13 legs of 11 patients with occlusion of the arteries proximal to the popliteal artery in addition to obstructive lesions of the infra-popliteal arteries. Lower numerals are mean value and standard deviations in each group.

Table VIII. Summary of 203 sympathectomies from May 1967 to April 1981.

	No. of cases
(I) Symptoms	
Coldness, cyanosis or paresthesia	46 (22.7%)
Rest pain	16 (7.9%)
Ulcer or gangrene	141 (69.4%)
	203 (100.0%)
(II) Site of denervation	
Lumbar	168
Thoracic	35
	203

and pre-operative correct evaluation of the run-off remains to be resolved. A few-month-long patency of the revascularized segment was enough to heal the trophic lesion as a whole, and when late failure occurred after the lesion had healed, ulceration did not recur if the patient completely abstained from smoking.

The patients without indication of arterial reconstruction had to undergo sympathectomy according to involvement, and when sympathectomy failed in healing of ulceration, continuous intra-arterial infusion with PGE1 was the second best treatment.

A good initial result of the treatment of Buerger's disease gave way to recurrence when the patient began to smoke and only the patients who did not abstain from smoking underwent major amputation of the extremity in our series. The arterial occlusion pattern in Buerger's disease was mainly fixed within one to two years after onset of symptoms and thereafter the more proximal extending of the obstructive lesion in the main artery was rarely seen if the patient abandoned smoking (Shionoya *et al.*, 1977). Information elucidating the natural history of Buerger's disease not only has prognostic value but also places in perspective the role of the operation or medical treatment in Buerger's disease (Hill, 1974).

Table IX. Results of 53 sympathectomies for trophic lesions from May 1977 to April 1981.

Site of denervation	No. of cases	Healed within (months) 1	3	5	Extremity amputation
Lumbar	38	16	15 (3)	5 (3)	2 (2)
Thoracic	15	9	3	2	1
		(in association with PGE1 infusion)			

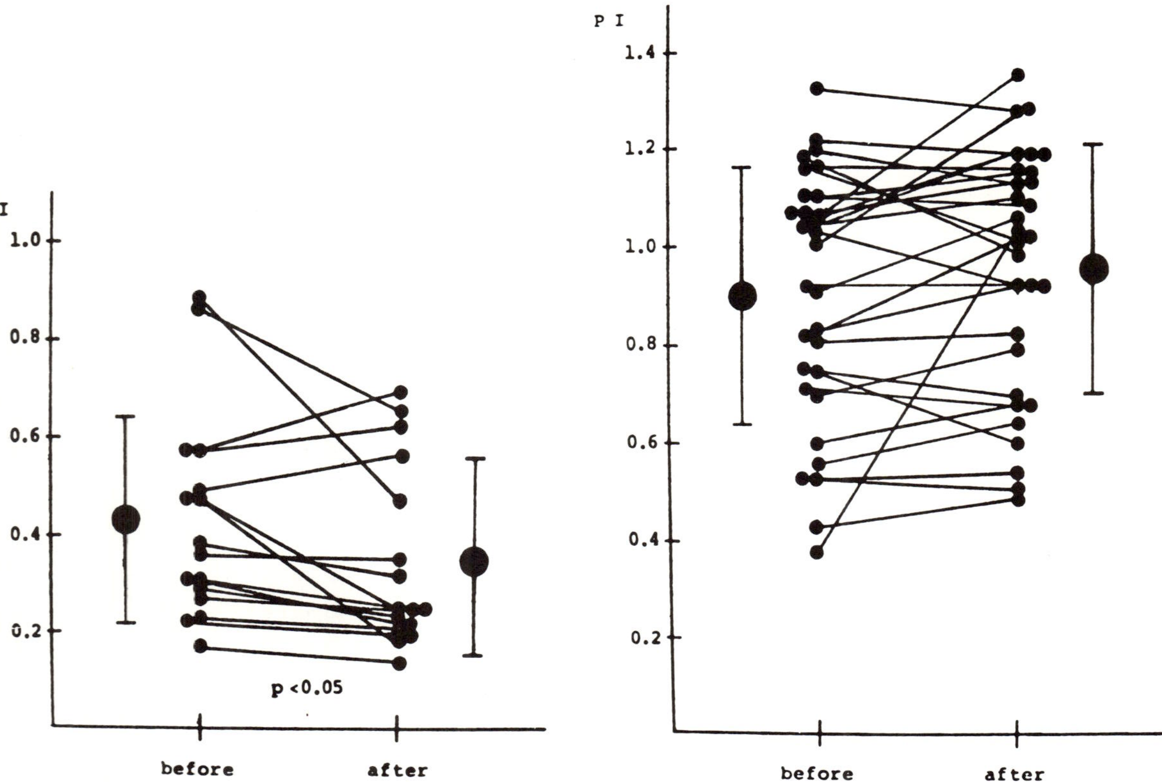

Fig. 11. (a, left) Ankle blood pressure before and after lumbar sympathectomy. (b, right) Toe blood pressure before and after lumbar sympathectomy.

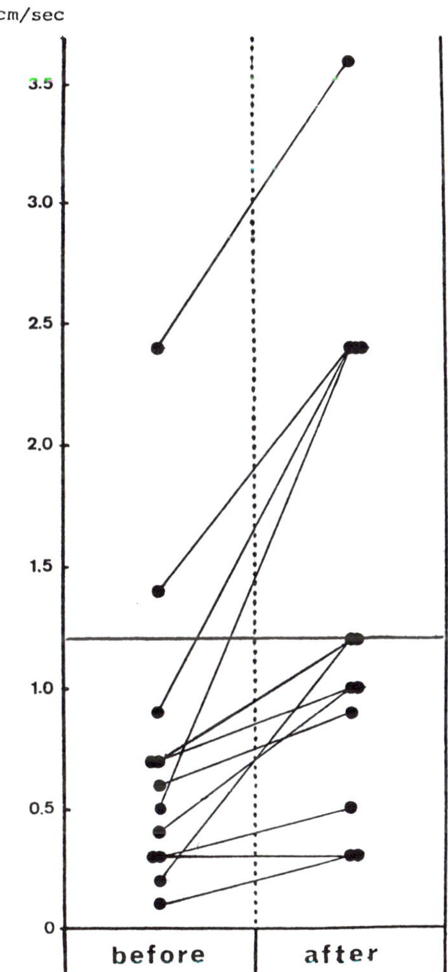

Fig. 12. Flow velocity in the foot of 12 limbs with Buerger's disease before and after lumbar sympathectomy. A solid horizontal line indicates the lower limit of the normal value of the velocity (1.2 cm/s).

SUMMARY

(1) From May 1967 to April 1981, 79 arterial reconstructions were performed in 68 of 399 patients with Buerger's disease and early failure due to poor distal run-off occurred in 30 cases: 74 arterial revascularizations were carried out in 63 of 145 patients with iliac or femoro-popliteal block.

(2) Pre-operative measurement of the distal blood pressure did not predict the result of surgical treatment.

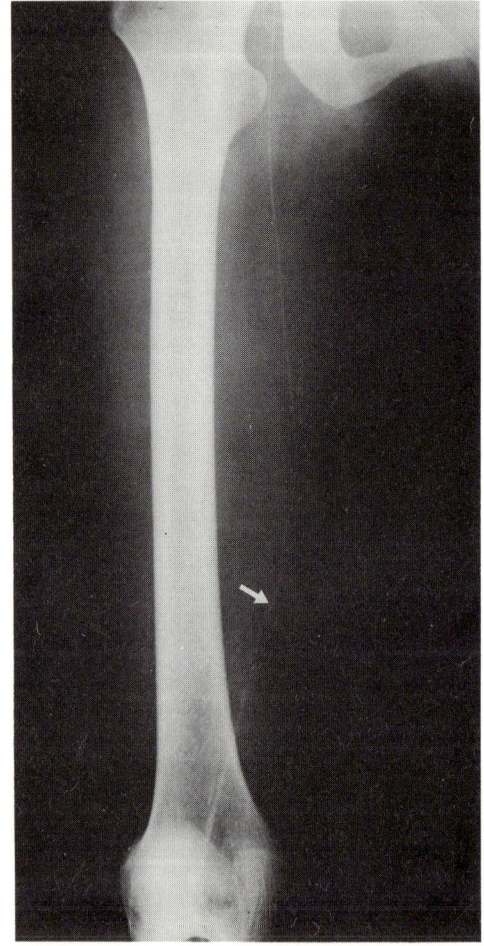

Fig. 13. Right femoral arteriogram through the inserted catheter. Arrow indicates the tip of the catheter.

Table X. Results of continuous intraarterial infusion with PGE1.

Result	No. of cases	Length of infusion (days) Range	Mean
Excellent[a]	22	9–84	34
Good[b]	25	5–140	50
Unchanged[c]	15	1–94	30

[a]Excellent: ulceration healed with the infusion therapy.
[b]Good: ulcers improved but did not completely heal within the infusion period.
[c]Unchanged: lesions were unchanged or worsened during the infusion period.

(3) Arterial reconstruction was most effective for healing of trophic lesions and when sympathectomy failed in healing of ulceration, continuous intra-arterial infusion with PGE1 was the second best treatment.

(4) The most characteristic feature of Buerger's disease was a stagnation of the distal arterial circulation and the flow velocity in the foot was a sensitive predictive index of limb salvage.

(5) Natural history of Buerger's disease was uneventful if the patient completely abstained from smoking.

REFERENCES

Hill. G. L. (1974). A rational basis for management of patients with Buerger syndrome. *British Journal of Surgery* **61**, 476.

Shionoya, S. (1980). Continuous intraarterial infusion-therapy of prostaglandin E1 for ischemic ulceration of the extremity. *In* "Adaptability of Vascular Wall" (Z. Reinis, J. Pokorny, J. Linhart, R. Hild and A. Schirger, Eds), p. 563. Avicenum Czechoslovak Medical Press, Prague and Springer-Verlag Berlin, Heidelberg, New York.

Shionoya, S., Ban, I., Nakata, Y., Matsubara, J., Hirai, M., Miyazaki, H. and Kawai, S. (1976). Vascular reconstruction in Buerger's disease. *British Journal of Surgery* **63**, 841.

Shionoya, S., Matsubara, J. and Kamiya, K. (1977). Fortschreiten des verschluss-prozesses bei thromboangiitis obliterans. *Vasa* **6**, 249.

Shionoya, S., Hirai, M. and Ohta, T. (1980). A prospective study of hemodynamic changes associated with distal arterial bypass in the leg. *Thorac. cardiovasc. Surgeon* **28**, 200.

Shionoya, S., Hirai, M., Kawai, S., Ohta, T. and Seko, T. (1981). Hemodynamic study of ischemic limb by velocity measurement in the foot. *Surgery* (In press).

Szilagyi, D. E., DeRusso, F. J. and Elliott, J. P. Jr. (1964). Thromboangiitis obliterans. Clinico-angiographic correlations. *Archives of Surgery (Chicago)* **88**, 824.

TREATMENT OF BUERGER'S DISEASE

J. van der Stricht

L'Université de Bruxelles, Brussels, Belgium

DEFINITION OF THE DISEASE

Despite an impressive number of works since those of Leo Buerger himself, thrombo-angeitis obliterans (TAO) remains interpreted in several ways. Too often it is diagnosed only because arteriopathy occurs in a young patient. Yet, in this case, the atheromatous disease can also be found, even more and more frequently.

As for us, the absence of calcification of the arterial lesion despite the length of its existence, is one of the fundamental criteria of the diagnosis of TAO, not a frequent ailment (2% of arteriopathies). This leads us to eliminate from the strict outline of the disease all the lesions starting on the main trunks themselves, whatever the age of the patient. Thus, we keep to the following chart to define TAO.

(1) Men and women aged less than 40 at the beginning of the disease.
(2) Cigarette smokers.
(3) Consulting for ischemic trophic troubles or for venous thrombosis, sometimes for foot claudication, most exceptionally for calf claudication.
(4) Showing clinical and arteriographical signs of restriction or obstruction of the distal arteries of the limbs, the upper as well as the lower limbs.
(5) Arterial lesion due to an inflammatory fibrous cicatricial thickening but never to an atheroma.
(6) Showing thus no radiological picture of arterial calcification.

Serono Symposium No. 44, "Peripheral Arterial Diseases: Medical and Surgical Problems", edited by S. Stipa and A. Cavallaro, 1982. Academic Press, London and New York.

SURGICAL THERAPEUTICAL POSSIBILITIES

For the very reason of this definition, direct arterial surgery has only a very limited scope in the treatment of TAO. It is thus on indirect arterial surgery that one should rely. Two forms may be considered: on one hand endocrinal surgery, that is surgery of the adrenal glands; on the other hand sympathic surgery, that is cervico-thoracic and lumbar gangliectomies.

Adrenal Surgery

Adrenal surgery started at the beginning of this century with Von Opel (1921) and later Constantini (1927) who advised medullo-adrenalectomy. Leriche and Stricker practised subtotal adrenalectomies before the Second World War (Leriche and Stricker, 1928). After the Second World War, adrenalectomies became total and bilateral. Let us mention amongst others Ferrand and Elbaz (1958) of Algiers. From 1956 to 1970 we have ourselves operated TAO by medullo-adrenalectomies, subtotal or total bilateral adrenalectomies. These interventions had a real curative purpose. With them was born the hope of correcting the cause of the disease.

From a theoretical point of view these interventions could be justified. Experimenting on dogs in 1960 (van der Stricht and De Schaepdryver) we have proved that total bilateral medullo-adrenalectomy suppressed the reservoir of catecholamines and, at the same time, the sudden and massive discharge of adrenalin in the circulating blood (Fig. 1). But nothing proved that the excess of adrenalin was the cause of TAO. Moreover, if the immediate results of the human intervention were satisfactory from the clinical point of view, the study of future results was negative. We have indeed presented in 1973 (van der Stricht *et al.*) a follow-up of two batches, one grouping isolated sympathectomies, the other the adrenalectomy–sympathectomy association. The result of this study was that after 5, 10 or 15 years, only the "tobacco factor" allowed to show a difference between good and bad results. We have thus given up adrenal intervention.

Sympathetic Surgery

Considering that the consequence of TAO is an ischemia, it appears logical to try to increase, to its maximum, the flow of the arteries that are still permeable by preserving their constriction as a response to sympathic stimulations. Let us note here that a high thoracic sympathectomy of the upper limb, a lumbar sympathectomy of the lower limb suppress the sympathic tonus and the vasoconstriction of the skin of the extremity of the considered limb (Grimonster symposium, 1979). Now it is precisely there, at the extremity of the limb, that the ill consequences of TAO appear. The benefactory effect of sympathectomy and the maleficent effect of TAO show themselves in the same region.

The indication of the sympathectomy is thus logical in case of TAO. Nevertheless, it should be understood that the operation proves itself useful to act on the ischemic consequences of the disease and that it does not act at all

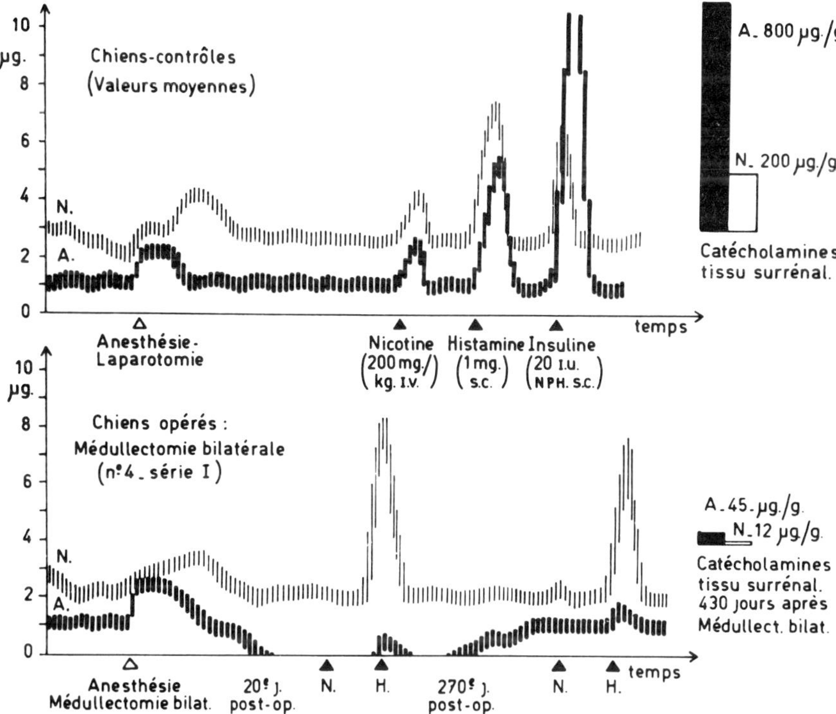

Fig. 1. Output of adrenalin and noradrenalin in intact and medullo-adrenalectomized dog. (Differential fluorimetric estimation.) (van der Stricht and de Schaepdryver, 1960).

on the disease itself. Thus, it should be suggested only in case of trophical trouble or threat of it. Let us make a note that lumbar sympathectomy must be limited to the third and fourth ganglions in order to avoid perturbing ejaculation.

Pre-operative Arterial Balance

Therapeutical results are of course in function of the extension of the vascular injury. To qualify this injury one should first of all establish the morphological circulatory balance by means of an arteriography and the functional balance by means of a vasomotor test. To this purpose we use in our own practice the Pentothal test which we perfected about 20 years ago (van der Stricht, 1962). It consists of practising a cutaneous thermometry before and after the general anesthesia, justified by the angiographic examination.

Before the narcosis, without premedication the patient is, generally, in a state of spontaneous vasoconstriction. The degrees of cutaneous temperature

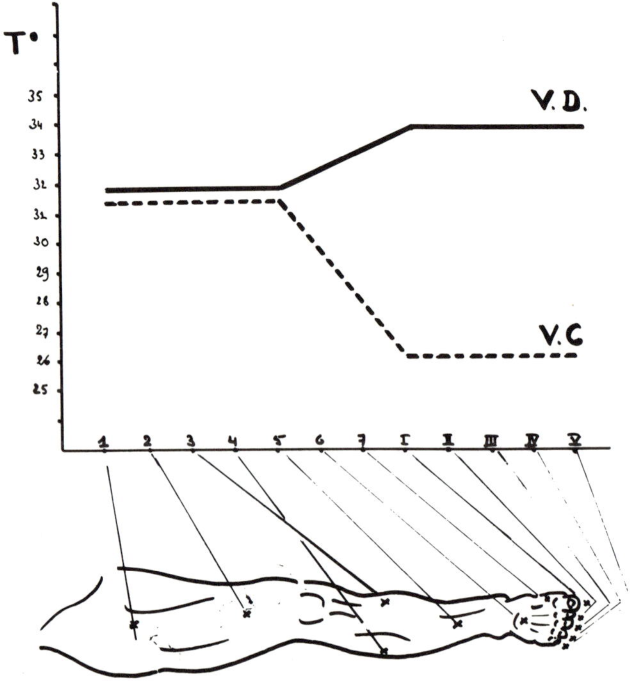

Fig. 2. Normal skin temperature curve in vasoconstriction and in vasodilatation.

measured from the root to the extremity of the four limbs describe a descending curve (Fig. 2). In the case of normal circulation, from 3 to 5 min after the intravenous injection of Pentothal, the shape of the curve reverses. It becomes ascending and shows the state of maximum vasodilatation. In the case of TAO the warming up of the extremities is less strong and more slow according to the importance of the obstructing lesions (Fig. 3).

The Results of Sympathectomy in the Case of TAO

They vary according to:

(1) The vasomotor response to Pentothal.
(2) The limb considered. Lasting as far as the foot is concerned, the result of the operation is limited as time goes on as far as the hand is considered.
(3) Whether smoking is given up or not.

Immediate Results

The Pentothal test is able to predict the immediate result. In case of a satisfactory response to the test, clinical cure follows the sympathectomy. Incomplete response allows to expect an improvement of the trophicity with a

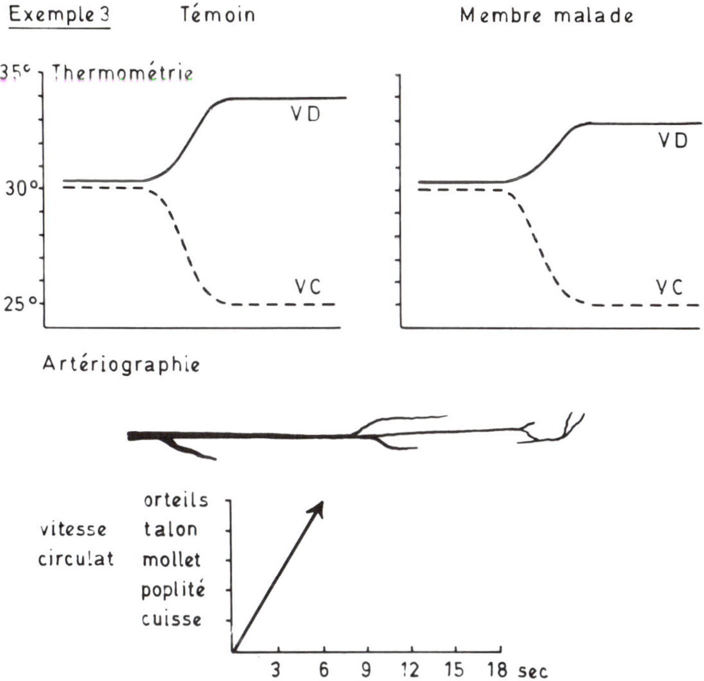

Fig. 3. Normal skin temperature response after pentothal injection on the right. Partial response on the left limb, enough to indicate a lumbar sympathectomy.

limitation of the mutilations but does not leave out the necessity of a partial amputation (one finger, one toe, sometimes part of the foot).

Late Results

They are ruled by the tobacco factor. We shall thus consider separately the results in the long run in case of operated patients who have completely given up cigarette smoking and in case of irreclaimable smokers.

(a) In case smoking has been completely given up.

Upper limb: the effect of sympathectomy fades but the arterial disease is stabilized. The cure remains established.

Lower limb: the effect of sympathectomy persists. Circulation improves as time goes on (Fig. 4).

(b) In case of continuation of tobacco intoxication.

Upper limb: sympathectomy does not protect any longer against a new extension of the disease. Recurrence is to be feared.

Lower limb: the disease progresses but it is compensated, as time goes on, by the development of the collateral net, stimulated by lumbar sympathectomy. However, it is to fear that TAO will win in the long run (Fig. 5).

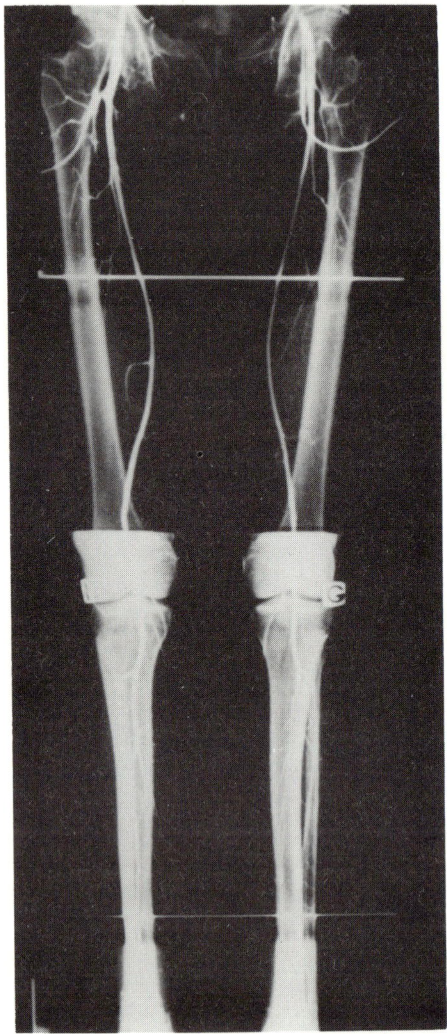

Fig. 4. TAO in a man of 35 years with gangrene. He stopped smoking and had bilateral lumbar sympathectomy. Arteriography was given 18 years later: the disease did not progress and there was no atheroma.

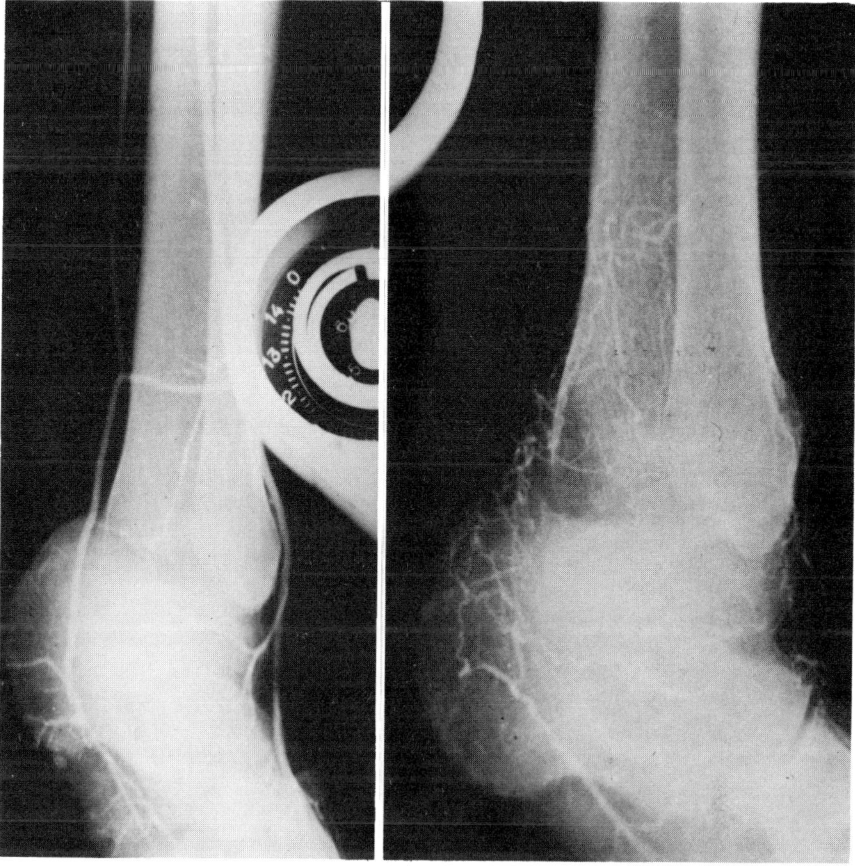

Fig. 5. TAO: despite sympathectomy, considerable extension of the lesions occurred after four years. The patient did not stop cigarette smoking.

CONCLUSIONS

Giving up cigarette smoking stops the development of Buerger's disease and sympathectomies lessen the ischaemic injuries that it produces.

SUMMARY

The Buerger's disease or thrombo-angeitis obliterans (TAO) is an inflammatory arteriopathy affecting the distal arteries of the limbs. Direct arterial surgery is seldom applicable. Surgery of the adrenal glands does not stop the evolution of the disease. Only the sympathectomies are beneficial by opposing the ischemy-producing effect of disease. Nevertheless, lasting good results are observed only in case of complete and definite giving up of tobacco smoking.

REFERENCES

Constantini, H. (1927). A propos d'une surrenalectomie pour gangrène artérielle chez un sujet jeune. Une opération à tenter: La medullosurrénalectomie. *Mémoires de l'Academie de Chirurgie* **53**, 529.

Ferrand, J. and Elbaz, C. (1958). La surrenalectomie bilatérale dans le traitement des artérites malignes. *Ed. Expansion Scientifique Franç.*

Grimonster symposium (1979). 50 years of Lumbar sympathectomy. *Journal of Cardiovascular Surgery* **20**, 279–342.

Leriche, R. and Stricker, P. (1928). Données générales sur les artérites oblitérantes juvéniles. *Bulletin et Mémoires de la Société de Chirurgie* **54**, 201.

van der Stricht, J. (1962). Modificateurs de la vasomotricité au cours de l'artériographie. *Presse Medicale* **70**(24), 1217.

van der Stricht, J. and De Schaepdryver, A. (1960). Essai de justification de la medullosurrenalectomie dans le traitement de l'artérite juvénile. *Bulletin de la Société Internationale de Chirurgie* **2**,193.

van der Stricht, J., Goldstein, M., Flamand, J. P. and Belenger, J. (1973). Evolution and prognosis of thromboangeitis obliterans. *Journal of Cardiovascular Surgery* **14**, 9.

NON-SURGICAL TREATMENT OF BUERGER'S DISEASE

J. A. Dormandy

St James' and St George's Hospitals, London, UK

The first two days of this meeting have concentrated on the problems and successes of surgical treatment of arterial disease. But we all realize that for the large majority of patients with occlusive arterial disease surgical treatment is inappropriate. This is because of the relatively poor results of reconstructive arterial operations, where even in a highly selected group the failure rate below the inguinal ligament is nearly 50% within three years and 25% above the inguinal ligament. In addition there is a significant mortality in the latter group. Therefore, unless the patient's disability is very severe we would not advise surgical treatment. This is particularly true in Buerger's disease, which tends to affect the smaller more distal vessels. It is important that, even as primarily surgeons, we should recognize the scope and limitations of non-surgical treatment and perhaps even play a part in attempting to find improvements in medical therapy. (It is salutory to rememebr that in the past 20 or 30 years we have failed to improve significantly the results of surgical treatment).

Ideal treatment would achieve dissolution of the vascular narrowing and there is now some objective evidence that this indeed can be achieved in atherosclerosis, but only at the cost of the most rigorous dietary discipline, combined often with gastro-intestinal bypass surgery and the massive use of potent lipid manipulating drugs. In the case of Buerger's disease, whose pathology is understood even less than that of atherosclerosis, there is also no specific treatment of the arterial lesion itself.

There is nevertheless a consensus of opinion, with which I do not personally totally agree, that Buerger's disease only affects smokers and certainly

Serono Symposium No. 44, "Peripheral Arterial Diseases: Medical and Surgical Problems", edited by S. Stipa and A. Cavallaro, 1982. Academic Press, London and New York.

stopping smoking is very often of considerable benefit. The mechanism of this is unknown and there is no evidence that the pathological narrowing of the vessels is relieved. This leaves only the possibility, both in Buerger's disease and in atherosclerosis, of compensating for the vascular narrowing by altering the flow properties of the blood travelling through them. An improvement in the flow, or haemorheological, properties may improve blood flow through the unchanged narrow vessels.

Haemorheology may be considered under two headings: macrorheology and microrheology. Chronologically, the macrorheology or blood viscosity was the first to be investigated, and is now recognized to be dependent on three pincipal determinants. Most importantly is the concentration of red cells, that is the haematocrit. From the point of view of bulk blood flow, the "effective" haematocrit or packed cell volume is also dependent on the degree of aggregation of the red cells, and the second determinant of blood viscosity is therefore the plasma, in particular the plasma fibrinogen, which will largely determine red cell aggregation. (The viscosity of plasma itself may also be important particularly in the microcirculation.) Finally, bulk blood viscosity is determined by the deformability of the individual red cells. Red cell deformability is also thought to be the most important influence on microrheology, that is the ability of the red cells to flow through channels much narrower than seven microns.

From the therapeutic point of view, there would therefore seem to be three basic possible approaches to achieving a haemorheological improvement: decreasing the red cell concentration, altering the plasma constituents particularly lowering the fibrinogen concentration and, third, improving the deformability and flow properties of the red cells themselves. These possibilities will be considered in turn.

Lowering the haematocrit in the peri-operative period by haemodilution has now become widely accepted in many countries as being a safe way of saving blood. There is also considerable evidence that down to a haematocrit of about 35% the loss in the oxygen carrying capacity of the blood is more than compensated by the increased flow due to the lowering of the blood viscosity decreasing peripheral resistance and increasing cardiac output. The haemoglobin level immediately before reconstructive arterial surgery has been shown to be correlated with the incidence of rethrombosis, and similar results have also been obtained in relation to healing of distal amputation stumps. In both cases, the higher the pre-operative haemoglobin the greater the risk of failure, thus strengthening the argument in favour of peri-operative haemodilution in patients with small distal vessel disease. The application of haemodilution to the treatment of chronic peripheral ischaemia is more controversial because many of these patients will also have central or cardiac ischaemia which may limit the ability of the heart to increase cardiac output. It has, however, been used successfully to increase cerebral blood flow by workers at Queen's Square in London, whilst both Rieger in Germany and ourselves in London have shown objective improvement in leg blood flow on intermittent claudicants following normovolaemic haemodilution. Although there is an overall increase in oxygen delivery to the ischaemic leg, the optimal degree of haemodilution seems to vary from patient to patient. In clinical practice, it is not possible to pinpoint a particular haematocrit to aim at in all cases. At the moment we repeat the peak leg blood flow measurements after each venesection to detect when further dilution ceases to be beneficial. The optimal haematocrit seems to vary from patient to patient but usually lies between 35% and 45%. In the immediate period following venesection there is theoretically an increased risk of thrombosis due to platelet changes and although we have not seen this complication we now prophylactically administer low doses of Aspirin to these patients for a week. Experience with long-term repeated haemodilution is at the moment insufficient to draw any definite conclusion. It is interesting to remember in this context that regular smoking increases the haematocrit and that this can be reversed if smoking is discontinued.

The second practical haemorheological approach to the non-surgical treatment of peripheral ischaemia is to decrease plasma viscosity and red cell aggregability, and hence whole blood viscosity, by lowering the plasma fibrinogen concentration. This may be particularly helpful in Buerger's disease where the plasma fibrinogen is abnormally high. However, even if its concentration is in the normal range, there is no doubt that the fibrinogen level can be reduced down to 20% of normal with complete safety. This has been shown to be feasible, by us as well as other workers, using subcutaneous injections of Arvin two or three times a week. The consequent fall in whole blood viscosity was accompanied by a parallel improvement in leg blood flow. This is of course theoretically a more attractive way of reducing viscosity than haemodilution because the oxygen-carrying capacity of the blood remains unchanged. Unfortunately, however, Arvin cannot be used long term because it is antigenic and at the moment there is no drug on the market which will lower the plamsa fibrinogen below normal over long periods.

Plasma exchange, or plasmapheresis, has recently been shown to be beneficial in many cases of small vessel ischaemia, particularly in Raynaud's phenomena. This benefit may well be partly due to the lowering of the plasma fibrinogen.

The third haemorheological approach to the treatment of peripheral ischaemia is the improvement of the flow properties of individual red cells, and this can also be achieved by plasma exchange. Perhaps, surprisingly, the improvement in red cell deformability following a course of plasma exchange persists of at least two to three months. The mechanism of this effect is unknown, but we have some evidence that the decreased red cell deformability associated with acute or chronic ischaemia is mediated by a plasma factor which is removed during plasma exchange. The normalization of red cell deformability by plasma exchange has been correlated with clinical improvement. Whilst we do not know whether plasma exchange could be beneficial in patients with normal red cell deformability, there have been several reports of the deleterious effect of smoking on the physical as well as biochemical properties of red cells.

There are now also a number of drugs, like Pentoxyfylline, Flunarazine, Isoxysuprine and Buflomedil, which have been shown to improve red cell deformability *in vitro*, and in some cases *in vivo* as well. Properly conducted clinical trials are now beginning to emerge using these drugs in patients with peripheral ischaemia, including Buerger's disease, to see if the drug induced improvement in the flow properties of the red cell is accompanied by an objective clinical improvement.

In summmary, I will return to the general basic practical problem of the non-surgical management of patients with Buerger's disease, or any other type of peripheral ischaemia. General advice about life-style, in particular giving up smoking, is especially important in Buerger's disease. I believe that supervised regular exercise is also beneficial, although this has never been adequately proved objectively. We then have to consider the use of one of the many drugs for which there may be at least a theoretically valid indication, remembering in this context the very definite placebo effect which can be obtained with any medication. Vasodilators are now generally accepted to have been totally discredited. Anticoagulants may be useful to prevent sudden deterioration due to thrombosis, but the danger of long-term anticoagulation probably outweighs any possible advantage. This is even more true of fibrinolytic therapy. The administration of drugs either acting on the platelets or lipid metabolism is completely irrational unless some abnormality in these measurements can be demonstrated and even then there is little objective evidence that their normalization is clinically beneficial. Steroids are only indicated in an acute and rapidly deteriorating arteritis usually with a high erythrocyte sedimentation rate. The value of prostaglandins has not yet been fully evaluated. We are then left with the haemorheological approaches discussed earlier and it will probably be in this area that really useful drugs will emerge producing significant benefit. Certainly in the near future we are more likely to achieve success by compensating for the vessel narrowing by altering the flow properties of the blood, whether by using drugs, haemodilution or plasma exchange, rather than attempting to reverse the disease process in the vessel walls themselves.

NON-SPECIFIC AORTOARTERITIS (TAKAYASU'S ARTERITIS): ETIOLOGY AND CLINICAL PICTURES

E. Lupi-Herrera

National Institute of Cardiology "Ignacio Chávez", Mexico

Nonspecific aortoarteritis (NSAA) was first described by Savory in 1856. Fifty-two years later Takayasu (1908) noted the ocular changes of the disease in a 21-year-old woman. In discussing this case Onishi and Kagoshima pointed out in two cases with similar ocular manifestations the absence of peripheral arm pulses (Takayasu, 1908). This disease entity has been labeled with many eponyms, which reflect some of its many features, such as pulseless disease, aortic arch syndrome, young female arteritis, idiopathic aortitis, reversed coarctation, occlusive thromboaortopathy, Takayasu's arteritis as well as NSAA (Shimizu and Sano, 1951; Strachnan, 1964).

Clinical and pathological studies have demonstrated that the arteritic process could involve the aortic arch and its branches, the thoracic descending and abdominal aorta and also the pulmonary artery (Nasu, 1962; Lupi *et al.*, 1975).

On the basis of this observation the disease could be subdivided into four types (Modified Ueno classification) (Lupi *et al.*, 1975).

Type I. Shimizu-Sano variety is when the involvement is localized to the aortic arch and its branches (with an incidence of 8%).

Type II. With Kimoto variety the lesions involve the thoracic descending aorta and the abdominal aorta without involvement of the arch (11%).

Serono Symposium No. 44, "Peripheral Arterial Diseases: Medical and Surgical Problems", edited by S. Stipa and A. Cavallaro, 1982. Academic Press, London and New York.

Type III. Inada variety or mixed variety contains features of both (types I and II) with an incidence of 65%.

Type IV. This type which may involve any of the arteries affected in types I, II or III in addition involves the pulmonary artery with an incidence of 45% (Lupi *et al.*, 1977).

In a recent series of 54 cases Ishikawa (1978) proposed a new classification:

Group I. Patients with NSAA with or without involvement of the pulmonary artery, with narrowing or occlusion in some region of the aorta and/or its main branches, but without any of the vascular complications present in group II (see below).

Group II. Patients with NSAA with one of the following complications: (a) retinopathy, (b) secondary hypertension, (c) aortic regurgitation and (d) aortic or arterial aneurysm. If NSAA was mild or moderate it was considered to be in group II-A and group II-B if NSAA was severe.

Group III. Patients with two or more of the complications listed for group II.

ETIOLOGY

More than 100 years after its original description and inspite of a voluminous literature on the subject, a specific cause for NSAA has not been forthcoming.

Attempts have been made to relate it to rheumatic fever, rheumatoid arthritis, collagen vascular disease (such as systemic lupus erythematosus, polymyositis and sclerodermia), parasites (nematodes), ankylosing spondylitis, giant cell arteritis, syphilis, to patterns of inheritance, to an autoimmune etiology and to tuberculosis.

The possible role of tuberculosis in NSAA was pointed out initially by Shimizu and Sano (1948). They considered this possibility on the basis of the presence of Langhans giant cell granulomas morphologically resembling tuberculosis lesions. Many authors have shown the coexistence of pulmonary or extrapulmonary tuberculosis foci in NSAA, especially in juxta arterial and para-aortic lymph nodes (Nasu, 1962; Sen *et al.*, 1963; Lupi, *et al.*, 1973; Takezawa *et al.*, 1966; Sanchez, 1971).

Furthermore, some investigators have reported a strikingly higher incidence of tuberculin skin reactivity to both *Mycobacterium tuberculosis* and atypical mycobacteria in patients with NSAA when compared with the general population, raising the possibility of a relationship with tuberculosis (Lupi *et al.*, 1972a). Other investigators have found that when *M. tuberculosis* is inoculated into the subadventitial layer of the carotid artery of the rabbit changes similar, but not identical to those of NSAA are produced, and also the disease pattern was closer to that of NSAA when the rabbits were previously sensitized (Sen *et al.*, 1972). These pathological, clinical and experimental observations suggest that tuberculosis may play a role in NSAA. However, these may only be related observations. Recently at our institution we searched for humoral antibodies against four different mycobacterial products as well as for immune complexes which react with human C1q in 24 patients suffering NSAA in the chronic inactive phase. No single case showed circulating immune complexes and only three (12%) had antimicobacterial antibodies. The presence of immunopathogenic mechanism in chronic NSAA is not supported by this work (Rojas *et al.*, 1981).

A susceptible genetic background may play a role in the etiology of the disease. The association between HLA B5 and Bw52 described in Japanese patients was confirmed in our Mexican patients, although not as marked as in the Japanese population (Castro *et al.*, 1981). The occurrence of lymphocytotoxic antibodies (LCTA) in human sera has been recognized for many years. Recently an increased frequency of LCTA was noted in sera from patients suffering temporal arteritis. Serum was obtained from 25 patients with chronic NSAA and we found that the frequency of LCTA in NSAA was extremely low and was not different from our normal population, in contrast with the high frequency of LCTA in patients with systemic rheumatic diseases. Our findings, although negative, have an important significance considering the possible natural occurrence of LCTA in human disease, since both mycobacterial and viral infection, where LCTA are present, have been implicated in the pathogenesis of NSAA.

On the other hand the postulated theory by some authors that an autoimmunologic mechanism is in operation is supported by certain findings: high gamma globulins, circulating antiaorta antibodies, the failure to detect any etiologic agent in the lesions of the arterial wall and the systemic arterial nature of the disease (pulmonary and aortic involvement). Overall, the bulk of evidence favors an auto-immune etiology. Although antiaortic antibodies have been detected in patients with this disease, there is no definitive evidence at present that these antibodies are the direct cause of NSAA.

Most of the difficulties in determining the cause of the disease arise because the pathologic observations are usually made in cicatricial or chronic states and only a few during active arteritis. Further experimental work should be encouraged in NSAA in order to find the cause of the disease. It is possible that the arteritis represents the final common pathological expression of a number of different stimuli.

PATHOLOGY

The basic pathological process is that of marked internal proliferation and fibrosis, fibrous scarring and degeneration of the elastic fibers of the media, with round cell infiltration of variable intensity. The adventitia and intima become markedly thickened and vasa vasorum are destroyed. The proliferation process leads to obliterative luminal changes in the aorta and involved arteries. The end result of the marked fibrosis and thickening of the arterial wall is usually a constriction or occlusion and occasionally a saccular aneurysm (Nasu, 1962; Lupi *et al.*, 1972b; Rentería and Contreras, 1978). Calcification in the aortic and arterial walls is a late complication (Lupi *et al.*, 1973).

THE CLINICAL PICTURE

The disease occurs predominantly in females in a ratio of 8.5 to 1, with age of onset between ten and 20 years, although cases beginning in infancy or late middle age have been reported (Lupi *et al.*, 1977; Lupi *et al.*, 1972b).

The Onset

NSAA is characterized in half of the cases by the sudden onset of constitutional symptoms (fever, anorexia, weight loss),joint pain, symptoms and signs of a local circulatory deficit, high blood pressure and elevated erythrocyte sedimentation rate. This clinical picture called first acute clinical inflammatory phase may disappear partly or completely in about three months' time, only to reappear in a chronic phase some months later. However, some patients already have advanced arterial obstruction and evidence of collateral circulation when they first develop symptoms.

These patients as well as those who go through to the so-called initial systemic phase or first acute inflammatory phase present the following clinical picture: diminished or absent pulses in 96%, bruits in 94%, hypertension in 74%, usually with a diastolic blood pressure 140 mmHg (79%), abnormal fundi in 41% and heart failure in 28% (Lupi *et al.*, 1977; Nakao *et al.*, 1967).

It is important to recognize the four types of NSSA for diagnostic and therapeutic reasons (Lupi *et al.*, 1975, 1977). The discriminating clinical features among the four types are the absence of arterial hypertension in patients with type I arteritis. Patients with types I and III manifest those findings that are considered to be most typical of this disease, namely "reversed" coarctation of the aorta with absent or diminished upper body pulses and barely detectable blood pressure in the arms, higher pressures in the lower extremities, syncope and manifestations of ischemia at various affected sites.

Pulmonary artery involvement (type IV) should particularly be suspected when right heart strain is observed in the electrocardiogram or if there are clinical suggestive signs or radiological data of pulmonary arterial hypertension (Lupi *et al.*, 1975). One complication could mark the disease: aortic regurgitation that leads to normal or even wide arterial pulse. In fact, hypertension (an extremely important complication of this disease) may be difficult to recognize because of the diminished pulsations in the arms. Arterial hypertension appears to arise mainly from involvement of the renal arteries (62%) as demonstrated by aortography and necropsy studies, as well as from hemodynamically significant coarctation of the aorta; decreased aortic capacitance and reduced baroreceptor reactivity may be contributory.

The neurologic symptoms result from arterial hypertension or cerebral or spinal cord ischemia (Lupi and Sanchez, 1972). Variations among neurologic symptoms can be explained on the basis of irregular distribution of arterial lesions and of the development of collateral circulation. The neurologic lesions can be permanent and also transient resulting from transient vascular impairment.

Heart failure when present in NSAA is usually seen in very young patients and appears to be a consequence of systemic and pulmonary hypertension and rarely from aortic regurgitation or coronary artery involvement that could lead to direct myocardial damage. It should be stressed that the pathologic findings in the heart are usually non specific related to heart failure and systemic and pulmonary artery hypertension. Symptoms of coronary artery involvement rarely occur in the absence of other manifestations of NSAA, and coronary involvement is itself a rare complication (Lupi *et al.*, 1977; Ishikawa, 1978; Roberts and Wibin, 1966).

MEDICAL TREATMENT

The response to treatment for heart failure and systemic arterial hypertension is usually good. Some authors have obtained remarkable clinical remissions with corticosteroids. However, we feel at present that this therapy needs further evaluation and there are not enough clinical and experimental data to justify the routine use of corticosteroids. The exact role of anticoagulant drugs is at present also uncertain. Medical treatment for tuberculosis is indicated only when active tuberculosis is found and is not justified in all cases until its exact role in NSAA is well established (Lupi *et al.*, 1977; Ishikawa, 1978; Nakao *et al.*, 1967).

SUMMARY

A review of the etiology and clinical pictures of NSAA is presented. Inspite of a voluminous literature on the subject, a specific cause for NSAA has not been forthcoming. The disease predominated in females (8.5:1), with age of onset usually less than 20 years. The most frequent variety of NSAA is type III, in which the supra-aortic trunks and the abdominal aorta are involved. However, it is important to recognize the four types of NSAA for diagnostic and therapeutic reasons. The predominant clinical features are reduction of amplitude of peripheral arterial pulses, vascular bruits, raised blood pressure and heart failure. Treatment for hypertension and heart failure should be employed when indicated. Treatment with corticosteroids, anticoagulant drugs and for tuberculosis is not justified at present in all cases.

REFERENCES

Castro, G., Chávez-Peón, F., Sanchez, T. G. and Reyes, P. (1981). HLA and B antigens in Takayasu's arteritis.

Ishikawa, K. (1978). Natural history and classification of occlusive thromboaortopathy (Takayasu's Disease), *Circulation* **57**, 27.

Lupi, H. E. and Sanchez, T. G. (1972). Arteritis inespecífica y paraplejia intermitente. *Archivos de Instituto de Cardiologia de Mexico* **42**, 131.
Lupi, H. E., Sanchez, T. G. and Castillo, P. V. (1972a). Reactividad cutánea al PPD y a los antígenos de mycobacterias atípicas (Kansasii, avium y fortuitum) en pacientes con arteritis inespecífica. *Archivos de Instituto de Cardiologia de Mexico* **42**, 717.
Lupi, H. E., Contreras, R., Espino, V. J., Sanchez, T. G. and Horwitz, S. (1972b). Arteritis inespecífica en la ninez. Observaciones clínicas y anatomopatológicas. *Archivos de Instituto de Cardiologia de Mexico* **42**, 477.
Lupi, H. E., Horwitz, S. and Sanchez, T. G. (1973). Calcifications in Takayasu's arteritis. *Vascular Surgery* **7**, 259.
Lupi. H. E., Sanchez, T. G., Horwitz, S. and Gutierrez, F. E. (1975). Pulmonary artery involvement in Takayasu's arteritis. *Chest* **67**, 69.
Lupi, H. E., Sanchez, T. G., Marcuschamer, J., Mispireta, J., Horwitz, S. and Espino, V. J. (1977). Takayasu's arteritis, clinical study of 107 cases. *American Heart Journal* **93**, 94.
Nakao, K., Ikeda, M., Kimoto, S., Nhtani, H., Miyahara, M., Ishimi, Z., Hashiba, K., Takeda, Y., Ozawa, T., Matsushita, S. and Kuromochi, M. (1967). Takayasu's arteritis: clinical report of eighty-four cases and immunological studies of seven cases. *Circulation* **35**, 1141.
Nasu, T. (1962). Pathology of pulseless disease: systematic study and critical review of twenty-one autopsy cases reported in Japan. *Angiology* **14**, 225.
Rentería, V. G. and Contreras, M. (1978). Aorto-arteritis inespecifica. Estudio anatomopatológico de 18 casos. *Archivos de Instituto de Cardiologia de Mexico* **48**, 80.
Rojas, E., Sanchez, T. and Reues, P. A. (1981). Estudios inmunológicos en la arteritis de Takayasu. I. Anticuerpos circulantes a productos de micobacterias y complejos inmunes circulantes. *Archivos de Instituto de Cardiologia de Mexico* **51**, 185.
Roberts, W. C. and Wibin, E. A. (1966). Idiopathic panaortitis, supra-aortic arteritis, granulomatous myocarditis and pericarditis. *American Journal of Medicine* **41**, 453.
Sanchez, T. G. (1971). Arteritis inespecífica y enfermedad tuberculosa. Aspectos clínicos. *Archivos de Instituto de Cardiologia de Mexico* **41**, 255.
Savory, W. S. (1856). Case of a young woman in whom the main arteries of both upper extremities and of the left side of the neck were throughout completely obliterated. *Med. Chir. Trans. Lond.* **39**, 205.
Sen, P. K., Kimare, S. G., Engineer, S. D. and Parulkar, G. B. (1963). Middle aortic syndrome. *British Heart Journal* **25**, 610.
Sen. P. K., Kinare, S. G., Kelkar, M. and Nanivad-Kar, S. A. (1972). Non-specific stenosing arteritis of the aorta and its branches. *Mount Sinai Journal of Medicine* **39**, 221.
Shimizu, K. and Sano, K. (1948). Pulseless disease. *Clinical Surgery (Tokyo)* **3**, 337.
Shimizu, K. and Sano, K. (1951). Pulseless disease. *Journal of Neuropathology and Clinical Neurology* **1**, 37.
Strachnan, R. W. (1964). The natural history of Takayasu's arteriopathy. *Quarterly Journal of Medicine* **33**, 57.
Takayasu, M. (1908). Case with unusual changes of the central vessels in the retina. *Acta Societas Ophthalmologicae Japanicae* **12**, 554.
Takezawa, H., Sakakura, M., Kokan, Y. and Hamaguchi, Y. (1966). Report of two cases of Takayasu's disease complicated with tuberculoid like exanthemas. *Japanese Circulation Journal* **30**, 1045.

NON-SPECIFIC AORTOARTERITIS IN INDIA

G. B. Parulkar, M. D. Kelkar, S. G. Kinare, S. R. Panday
and S. Bhattacharya

*Department of Cardiovascular Surgery, KEM Hospital
& Seth GS Medical College, Bombay, India*

NON-SPECIFIC AORTOARTERITIS IN INDIA

Since our earlier reports on management of aortoarteritis we have now had the opportunity of studying 190 such cases. This lesion, which causes acquired narrowing of the thoracic and upper abdominal aorta, has been found to be twice as frequent as cases of congenital coarctation observed by us during the same period. The disease syndrome has rather characteristic clinical and pathological behaviour and poses specific problems regarding the management and both aspects will be briefly discussed in this paper.

Material

Age and sex incidence is shown in Table I. The youngest patient was three years and oldest 45 years. The highest incidence is evident in the age group between 11 and 30 years and the disease is more than three times more frequent in females as compared with males.

The typical patient in our series was a young female in her second or third decade presenting with symptoms of severe hypertension, namely headache, claudication of lower limbs, symptoms of cerebral insufficiency, aches in the arm and, rarely, abdominal angina. Heart failure associated with hypertension and significant cardiomegaly was noted in younger patients. The main symptoms observed have been summarized in Table II.

Serono Symposium No. 44, "Peripheral Arterial Diseases: Medical and Surgical Problems", edited by S. Stipa and A. Cavallaro, 1982. Academic Press, London and New York.

Table I. Aortoarteritis.

Age in years	Male	Female
3–10	7	23
11–20	13	60
21–30	19	54
31–40	6	7
41 and above	1	0
	46	144

The clinical features of aortoarteritis can be easily differentiated from Leriche's syndrome of aortoilliac thrombosis. However, the features summarized in Table III usually help to differentiate the congenital coarctation of aorta from aortoarteritis because in both conditions hypertension in the upper extremity and feeble and delayed or absent femoral pulsations are observed.

Aortogram is the most useful investigation in differentiating the congenital coarctation from aortoarteritis. While in the former the involved segment is usually short and often ring like and single at the classical site, in aortoarteritis the stenotic segment is elongated and may be at multiple sites. Collaterals are well developed in congenital coarctation, whereas poorly formed or absent in aortitis. Moreover, involvement of major arteries such as renal, carotid, subclavian and mesenteric is characteristic of aortoarteritis.

The ascending aorta alone was not involved in any case. Arch alone was not involved in any case. Descending thoracic aorta was involved in 24 cases. Descending thoracic and abdominal aortas was involved in 75 cases. Arch and descending thoracoabdominal portion was involved in 18 cases. Ascending arch and descending portion was involved in two cases and ascending and abdominal aorta in six cases. The lesions in the aorta varied from mere irregularity of the lumen without stenosis, stenosis of aorta, complete obstruction of the aorta or aneurysm formation or combination of stenosis with aneurysm.

The renal artery involvement was present in 115 cases. The carotid arteries were involved in 26 cases, the left subclavian arteries in 70 cases, coeliac axis in 18 cases and superior mesenteric in 15 cases. Inferior mesenteric was involved in three cases. Iliac arteries were involved in 11 cases.

Table II. Aortoarteritis (190).

Hypertension	156
Heart failure	70
Cerebral insufficiency	81
Claudication	55
Abdominal angina	8

Table III.

	Aortoarteritis	Congenital coarctation
Sex	Female	Male
Claudication	Present	Absent
Bruit	Abdominal	Thoracic
Rib notching	Rare	Usual
Aortogram involved segment	Elongated	Short narrow
Branch involvement	Common	Rare

Management

Basically the disease is panaortoarteritis and thus affecting all coats of aorta and the management is determined by the haemodynamic disturbance produced by the lesion and the symptoms resulting from it.

No specific medical treatment is yet known for the condition. Early lesions, very extensive multiple lesions, very poor general condition and refusal for surgery formed the indications for medical treatment, which was given to 84 cases in this series.

The medical treatment consisted of use of antihypertensive drugs. Many of these patients were observed to be resistant to this treatment. Diuretics and digitalis were used to control heart failure. Cerebral vasodilator drugs were used for symptomatic relief of cerebral insufficiency but in general the drugs were ineffective. Antituberculous drugs like streptomycin and isoniazide were advised to those patients in whom there was clinical evidence of tuberculous disease of lymph nodes, lung or bone. While the tuberculous lesions were controlled in these patients, there was no demonstrable improvement in the aortic or arterial lesion but perhaps the disease process arrested. Cortisone was advocated in all patients, who presented with active lesions associated with high ESR and we feel long-term cortisone therapy may help in controlling the progress of the arterial lesion.

Out of 84 patients who received medical treatment, 35 patients expired during observation. Twenty-eight patients are lost to follow up and 21 patients are alive 2–12 years after the treatment was started, only seven of these patients have minimal or no symptoms. In other patients the hypertension has persisted and the disease process seems to have progressed as compared with initial observation.

Surgical treatment was offered to 142 patients but only 106 cases agreed to undergo surgery. In three patients no operative procedure was possible after exploration. All three patients expired during observation. Significant aortic obstruction as demonstrated on aortogram or intraaortic pressure gradient of more than 60 mmHg was considered as indication for surgery. Presence of renal hypertension, symptoms such as cerebral insufficiency and severe claudication and associated localized aneurysm formed the other indications for surgery.

Surgical management posed many problems. The severe uncontrollable hypertension and heart failure posed serious anaesthetic hazard. Nutritional state of many of these patients was poor and danger of wound infection was high. The involved segment of aorta and arteries were densely adherent to the surrounding tissues and their dissection was technically difficult. Many times the lesions were multifocal and extensive and the surgeon after careful clinical assessment of the patient and study of the aortogram had to decide which critical lesions required to be attended to.

Variety of operative procedures were performed in these 106 cases depending on the critical lesion and the decision of the attending surgeon (Table IV).

In ten cases only nephrectomy was performed as revascularization of renal artery was not advisable for the atrophied kidney. The opposite renal artery was normal at the time of first surgery. During follow up three patients have expired, two are lost to follow up and five are alive 3–15 years after follow up and three of them are symptom free.

Thrombointimectomy was attempted in four cases but it failed in all the cases. One of these patients underwent a bypass operation at a later date.

Patch angioplasty was performed in two cases. One patient expired due to severe pesistent hypertension secondary to renal artery stenosis which was not detected at first operation. In general, the patch angioplasty is not recommended as there are dense adhesions in the involved segment which is thick walled and the lesion in the aorta generally involves elongated segment.

The most common type of operation performed for aortic obstruction due to aortitis was aortoaortic bypass. The bypass operation was performed in 38 cases using a synthetic graft. The authors consider this as method of choice. The bypass graft is sutured to the aorta well proximal and distal to the involved aortic segment. This technique has been observed to have several advantages. The difficult dissection in the region of the involved aortic segment is avoided. The bypass graft can be sutured to the healthy aorta well proximal and distal to the diseased aortic segment thus preventing the possibility of late occlusion of the graft due to possible progress of the disease. By selecting a synthetic graft of suitable length and adequate diameter the blood in the obstructed aorta can be bypassed and the haemodynamic effects of aortic obstruction can be relieved.

Table IV. Surgery (106).

No procedure	3
Nephrectomy only	10
Aortoaortic bypass	38
Thrombointimectomy	4
Patch angioplasty	2
Excision of aneurysm	6
Renal revascularization	45
Carotid subclavian revascularization	16
Mesenteric revascularization	1
Reoperations	4
Multiple revascularization	14

Table V. Results of aortoaortic bypass surgery.

	Total	Mortality	Follow up
Thoraco-thoracic	8	0	6
Thoraco-abdominal			
Dorsal	17	3	9
Ventral	11	5	4
Thoraco-iliac	2	1	1
	38	9	20

Out of the 38 cases (Table V) in whom the bypass technique was used, in eight patients the bypass graft was used to relieve localized obstruction to the thoracic aorta only. There was no operative mortality. Two patients lost to follow up. Six patients have been followed up for 8–16 years and at the last follow up the bypass graft was functioning in all. All patients are symptom free. Post-operative aortogram performed in four patients demonstrated the functioning graft. From this experience it is evident that when aortic obstruction is limited to a short thoracic segment alone, the aortoaortic bypass within the chest yields gratifying results. No effort should be made to either do thrombo-intimectomy or patch grafting or excision of the involved aortic segment.

In 30 patients, the aortic obstruction was in the thoracic and abdominal aortic segment or in the high abdominal segment.

In 17 cases the bypass graft was sutured proximally to the descending thoracic aorta just distal to the origin of subclavian artery and distally to the abdominal aorta just proximal to the aortic bifurcation because both these segments of aorta are almost invariably free from any disease. The proximal anastomosis is performed through the fifth left intercostal space and distal anastomosis through the mid-line abdominal incision. The Dacron graft was brought down through the diaphragm and was placed in the retroperitoneal tissue by the side of the abdominal aorta. There were three hospital deaths in this series, one each due to infection, haemorrhage and heart failure. Five patients have been lost to follow up. Nine patients have been followed up for 2–18 years. Eight patients are symptom free and are in minimal medication. One patient who had had concomitant renal revascularization has persistent hypertension and needs continued medical treatment for the same.

In 11 patients, the aortic obstruction was so extensive that the descending thoracic aorta just distal to origin of left subclavian was also involved. In these cases the proximal anastomosis of the bypass graft was carried out intra-pericardially to the ascending aortic segment. The distal end of the bypass graft was anastomosed to the abdominal aorta. The exposure in all these cases was obtained through the mid-line sternum cutting incision and mid-line abdominal incision. The authors, however, feel that the proximal anastomosis to the ascending aorta could be performed through anterior thoracotomy through the right second or third interspace to avoid the morbidity of the long sternum cutting incision. During our earlier experience the bypass graft was brought into the abdomen behind the stomach. There were five hospital deaths, two due to progressive heart failure, two due to gastric erosion and one due to secondary haemorrhage from the proximal anastomotic site. At present the bypass graft is brought from the intrapericardial position into the abdomen through the left dome of diaphragm into the retroperitoneal region and is allowed to lie in the left paracolic gutter and is brought inwards behind the sigmoid colon for anastomosis to the abdominal aorta. The authors are at present investigating other techniques of ascending aorta to abdominal aortic bypass. Two patients in this series are lost to follow up and four patients have been followed up for 7–12 years. Two patients have persistent hypertension due to unrelieved concomitant renal artery obstruction. The other two are doing well.

In two cases in whom the disease had involved even the lower abdominal aorta including aortic bifurcation in addition to involvement of thoracic and high abdominal aortic segment. Both these patients underwent bypass grafting from descending thoracic aorta to both iliac arteries. One patient expired due to post-operative infection. The other patient has been followed up to four years and is doing well.

In addition to the variety of aortoaortic bypass procedure, the authors carried out revascularization procedures for renal arteries (45 cases), carotid artery and/or subclavian artery (16 cases), mesenteric artery (one case). In 14 cases multiple revascularization procedures were performed. Four patients underwent reoperations. In four cases localized aneurysms of aorta and in two cases aneurysms of iliac artery were excised and replaced with graft.

Out of 96 cases who underwent operation other than just nephrectomy 20 patients expired soon after surgery. Eighteen patients are lost to follow up. The remaining 58 are undergoing detailed evaluation at the present time.

It will be interesting to observe that 63 out of 106 patients (Table VI) who underwent surgery are alive, whereas only 21 out of 84 patients who were only treated medically are alive. This observation suggests that properly selected operative procedure would provide palliation by relieving aortic obstruction and critical narrowing of vessels such as renal arteries and carotid arteries.

Table VI. Results and follow up.

	Total	Dead	Lost to follow up	Alive
Medical therapy	84	35	28	21
Surgical therapy				
Nephrectomy	10	3	2	5
Definitive	96	20	18	58
	190	58	48	84

SUMMARY

Aortoarteritis affecting thoraco-abdominal aorta and its main branches can be now identified in India as distinct clinical entity, which can be differentiated from congenital coarctation of aorta and acquired lesions described by Takayasu and Leriche. The authors have studied 190 patients with this lesion during the period 1959–1980. Bypassing the obstructed aorta by suturing a Dacron graft well proximal and distal to the involved aortic segment was found by the authors to be the most rational surgical approach. The operative procedures which included bypass operations and revascularization procedures were planned according to the extent and criticality of the aortic and arterial disease in each case. Follow up for 1–18 years has shown that the surgery provided significant palliation in this curious multifocal disease of the aorta and major branches.

EXPERIENCE WITH 219 OPERATIONS DONE FOR NON-SPECIFIC AORTOARTERITIS

A. V. Pokrovsky

The Bakulev Institute of Cardiovascular Surgery, Moscow, USSR

Non-specific aortoarteritis is a systemic disease of the autoimmunic inflammatory genesis; the main specific feature of which is a stenosing lesion of the aorta and its branches or atypical coarctation. Opinion, that aortitis is a common disease only found in Japan or India is wrong, since it is seen in many countries. Among 287 cases of non-specific aortoarteritis in the residents of the European part of this country 80% of them were Caucasian. The rate of non-specific aortoarteritis ranks second after atherosclerosis as cause of the disease of the aorta and magistral vessels.

The most part of investigators believe that this disease is of autoimmune origin. Our investigations have shown that previous rickettsiosis might be a cause of the development of aortoarteritis. However, it does not mean that rickettsioses are a specific cause of aortitis. Any inflammatory or infectious disease could contribute.

Morphologically, we can distinguish the following stages of disease: acute inflammatory, subacute and sclerotic. It is interesting to note that the sclerotic (fibrotic) stage prevails. The granulomatous inflammatory picture is very rare. We have seen no cases of tuberculosis. These data differ from those seen by others.

We distinguish three variants of vascular lesions: stenotic, which is most commonly seen; aneurysmal, which is rarely seen and deforming, in which the aorta is not stenosed, but its wall is affected and the ostia of arteries are

---

Serono Symposium No. 44, "Peripheral Arterial Diseases: Medical and Surgical Problems", edited by S. Stipa and A. Cavallaro, 1982. Academic Press, London and New York.

narrowed. This disease is more commonly seen in women; 70% of patients are under 30 years and 6% of them are children under ten years.

Many years' experience allows us to distinguish ten clinical syndromes on the basis of which the clinical picture is outlined.

The first syndrome is a general inflammatory reaction consisting of general cardiac and pulmonary syndromes, which are seen in acute period. This syndrome is noted in the anamnesis of 32% of patients.

The second syndrome is a lesion of the aortic arch branches; this syndrome is seen in 74% of patients and is specific for signs of cerebral ischaemia and upper limb ischaemia. Usually, patients have complaints of arm weakness and pain, dizziness, headache, absent arterial pulsations in one of the arms.

The third syndrome is the stenosed descending aorta. It is revealed as two regimens of circulation in the upper and lower part of the body and is seen in 18% of patients. The clinical picture is like the symptoms for coarctation of the aorta and therefore many authors wrongly call them atypical coarctation. Clinical signs are specific for hypertension in the upper part of the organism.

The fourth syndrome is vasorenal hypertension due to renal arterial lesions. For its occurrence it ranks second in aortoarteritis. It is seen in 55% of our patients. It is worth noting that 62% of patients have bilateral renal arterial lesions.

The fifth syndrome is abdominal visceral ischaemia. Clinically it is not often seen (about 9%). Nevertheless, this lesion of the abdominal aortic visceral branches is seen in one-third of patients. Therefore, aortography must be taken in the lateral plane in order to reveal lesions in the ostia of the visceral arteries.

The sixth syndrome is a lesion of the infrarenal aortic part, which can be accompanied with a lesion of the iliac arteries and is seen in the form of lower limb and abdominal visceral ischaemia. It is seen in 18% of patients.

The seventh syndrome is a coronary one seen in 10% of patients. It is specific for cardiac pain and very quickly transient changes on the electrocardiogram. Autopsy material shows frequent arterial lesions.

The eighth syndrome is aortic insufficiency associated with a lesion of the ascending aorta and dilatation of the aortic ring. Here is an echocardiographic picture of aortic insufficiency. Clinically it is seen in rare cases (1.5%). According to the data of Japanese authors aortic insufficiency is more often seen.

The ninth syndrome is pulmonary arterial lesion seen in 5% of patients, though in autopsy material this localization is more often seen. The trunk and main pulmonary branches are involved.

The tenth syndrome is aneurysmal formation seen in 10% of patients.

It is interesting to note, that in most patients there is combination of lesions of several aortic and arterial segments.

The diagnosis of the aortoarteritis is based on auscultation of vessels, definition of arterial pulsation and arterial pressure. Standard clinical examination of patients helps to establish the correct diagnosis in the most part.

An indication for surgical treatment of patients with aortoarteritis is stable hypertension secondary to renal arterial lesion or aortic stenosis, cerebral ischaemia, abdominal visceral ischaemia, limb ischaemia and, rarely, aneurysms. A relative contraindication to operation is cardiac, coronary insufficiency and, rarely, renal failure and acute inflammation. Preliminary treatment can exclude these contraindications. Total aortic calcification and obliteration of the distal part of the artery at the site of reconstruction may be a contraindication.

Taking into consideration multiple character of a lesion in aortoarteritis, it is necessary to eliminate the leading syndrome (cerebral ischaemia or hypertension) first.

In case of the associated lesions of the aortic arch branches and renal arteries we use a hypotensive test to define a sequence of stages. When there is poor cerebral hypotension tolerance reconstruction of the brachiocephalic branches of the aortic arch goes first; if there is good cerebral tolerance, operation for hypertension is done.

Of all types of reconstructions used for aortoarteritis we prefer resection and replacement. In total, we have performed 219 operations, their character is shown in Table I.

Table I. Non-specific aortoarteritis.

Reconstructive operations	184
Nephrectomy	14
Palliation	21
Total	219

Reconstruction of the brachiocephalic branches was performed in 67 patients (Table II). It is worth noting, that common and external carotid and subclavian arteries are often involved. Taking into account character of the arterial lesions endarterectomy at these sites is impossible. Multiple lesions make replacement necessary in many cases (52 operations). It is important that distal anastomosis between prosthesis and innominate or carotid artery is always of end-to-end type. In 29 patients we have used bifurcation prostheses. In the recent years, when it is possible, we use extrathoracic bypass grafting:

Table II. Aortitis: reconstruction of aortic arch branches.

Type of operation	Number
Bifurcation replacement of carotid arteries	17
Bifurcation replacement of carotid and subclavian arteries	12
Replacement of carotid artery	3
Replacement of innominate artery	5
Subclavian–carotid bypass	9
Carotid–subclavian bypass	4
Replacement of subclavian artery	8
Bypass of subclavian artery	9
Total	67

Table III. Aortitis: reconstruction of the thoraco-abdominal aorta.

Type of operation	Number
Resection and replacement descending aorta	9
Resection and replacement of thoraco-abdominal aorta	11 (7)
Thoraco-abdominal replacement	2 (2)
Thoraco-abdominal bypass	4 (3)
One- or two-stage resection of the thoracic and abdominal aorta	4 (2)
Total	30 (14)

carotid–subclavian or subclavian–carotid. In several cases with a lesion of the proximal subclavian artery one can implant it into the carotid artery.

In the stenosis of the descending aorta the operation is performed under moderate hypothermia. Of 30 operations (Table III) there were 26 operations of resection and replacement and only four operations of thoraco-abdominal bypass grafting at the beginning of our experience. Since this process involves

Table IV. Aortitis: operations on renal arteries: reconstruction of one renal artery.

Type of operation	Number
Replacement	14 (8)
Bypass	5 (2)
Transaortic endarterectomy	10 (2)
Replantation	7 (3)
Nephrectomy	13
Total	49 (15)

not only thoracic but also abdominal aorta, in 20 patients we have performed thoracic and abdominal aortic replacement at one time. Only reconstructive operations of the aorta may be insufficient. In particular, vasorenal hypertension might remain. Therefore, 14 patients underwent a replacement of renal or visceral arteries.

In total, 89 operations were performed for correction of vasorenal hypertension (Tables IV and V), among those 48 are one-stage complex reconstructions. In patients with aortoarteritis we perform renal arterial replacement and distal end-to-end anastomosis often. Reconstruction of one renal artery was performed in 49 patients. With experience having been gained, it has become evident that at the sclerotic stage of aortitis it is possible to perform transaortic endarterectomy using an original technique.

We would like to state that using our method of transaortic endarterectomy in 22 patients we managed to perform simultaneous revascularization of both kidneys. In 40 patients one-stage reconstruction of both renal arteries was performed (Table V). Primary nephrectomy was done only in seven patients.

In 51 patients reconstruction of the visceral branches of the abdominal aorta was done (Table VI).

Table V. Aortitis: operation on renal arteries: reconstruction of two renal arteries.

Type of operation	Number
Transaortic endarterectomy	22 (21)
Transaortic endarterectomy and replacement	3 (3)
Replacement	7 (4)
Replantation	1 (1)
Combined reconstruction	5 (4)
Bypass	2
Total	40 (33)

In 1971 we offered a new type of operation on visceral arteries — transaortic one-stage endarterectomy through the thoraco-phreno-lumbotomic approach, during which the aorta is opened along the posterior–lateral surface and endarterectomy is done *en bloc* out of the aorta and visceral branches and out of renal arteries, when necessary. This type of operation was done in 16 patients. Simultaneous endarterectomy was done out of visceral and renal arteries.

If visceral branches are involved, even without symptoms of the abdominal ischaemia, we believe that it is necessary to perform reconstruction simultaneously with correction of the aortic and renal arterial lesions.

In several cases in order to enlarge blood flow to the visceral arteries, which originate from the stenosed aortic segment, we perform a long oblique anastomosis of the graft and aorta in the shape of a patch. When necessary, this patch widens arterial ostium, for example, of the coeliac trunk.

Table VI. Aortitis: visceral arterial reconstruction.

Type of operation	Number
Transaortic endarterectomy	16
Replacement	11
Replantation	6
Bypass	2
Patch of aorta	16
Total	51

Table VII. Aortitis: visceral arterial reconstruction.

Type of operation	Number
Reconstruction of the a. coeliaca	17
Reconstruction of the a. coeliaca and a. mes. sup.	20
Reconstruction of the a. mes. sup.	8
Reconstruction of the a. mes. inf.	4
Reconstruction of the a. mes. sup. and inf.	2
Total	51

Table VII shows which artery is reconstructed. It is worth noting that in 20 patients simultaneous operation is performed on the coeliac trunk and superior mesenteric artery. The surgical technique is more improved for lesions of iliac arteries, infrarenal segments and aortic bifurcation (Table VIII). Thirty-six patients underwent a resection of the abdominal aorta and 25 an additional reconstruction of the renal and visceral arteries. Bypass

Table VIII. Aortitis: abdominal aortic reconstruction.

Type of operation	Number
High abdominal aortic resection	27 (24)
Resection and replacement of the abdominal aortic bifurcation	9 (1)
Total	36 (25)

procedures are not used. In high occlusion of the abdominal aorta we offer to perform operation through thoraco-phreno-lumbotomic approach. Using this approach we can reconstruct visceral arteries, replace the abdominal aortic bifurcation and construct distal anastomoses to femoral arteries. Eight patients underwent a resection of the aortic aneurysm, three thoracic aneurysms and others abdominal aneurysms. Five underwent an additional replacement of the aortic branches (Table IX).

In conclusion, we wish to emphasize several specific features of surgical treatment. In aortoarteritis the affected zone is always larger than aorto-

Table IX. Aortitis: operation for aortic aneurysms.

Type of operation	Number
Resection and replacement thoracic aorta	1
Resection and replacement thoraco-abdominal aorta	1 (1)
Resection and replacement abdominal aorta	5 (4)
Two-stage resection of the thoracic and abdominal aorta	1
Total	8

graphy reveals. Here we prefer resection and replacement. In the presence of hypoplasia of the aorta we apply a method of the oblique anastomosis between the graft and aorta. We support one-stage correction and that is why nearly one-half of patients underwent complex reconstructions of several vessels. At present, post-operative mortality is 3%. In total, 94% of patients leaving hospital were with significant improvement. The results are variable depending on the localization of the process. In case of brachiocephalic reconstruction good results are seen in 57% of patients within ten years.

The best results were obtained in patients with the stenosed thoracic aorta. Regional hypertension disappeared in all patients. After operation done for vasorenal hypertension in 84% of patients there was marked hypotensive effect.

On the whole, significant improvement was noted in 83% of patients with aortoarteritis in the follow-up period, this fact evidences great possibilities for reconstructive vascular surgery in such patients.

HORTON'S DISEASE

L. A. Healey

The Mason Clinic, University of Washington, Seattle, Washington, USA

HORTON'S DISEASE

The best-known manifestation of Horton's disease is temporal arteritis, wherein an elderly patient with severe persistent unilateral headache, possibly an inflamed tender swollen temporal artery and a very rapid erythrocyte sedimentation rate. The diagnosis is established by biopsy of the artery which shows a characteristic histology with inflammation, giant cells, and fragmentation of the internal elastic lamina. The disease responds well to corticosteroid treatment but does carry the risk of blindness.

In his initial report, Horton recognized that this was apparently a "focal localization of some unknown systemic disease". Subsequent experience and investigations have shown that this statement is correct. For example, the temporal artery is a branch of the external carotid whereas the central retinal and ophthalmic arteries, the two vessels which when occluded lead to blindness, are branches of the internal carotid. Autopsy studies have shown that giant cell arteritis, far from being limited to the temporal artery, may involve the aorta, its branches and other large- and medium-sized arteries with an apparent predilection for those of the head and neck. The prospective study of Ostberg (1972) found histologic evidence of giant cell arteritis in 1.7% of 889 post-mortem examinations. When the inflammation is minimal, the lesions are asymptomatic and the disease would not have been recognized except for the systematic search of the vascular tree that Ostberg carried out.

Serono Symposium No. 44, "Peripheral Arterial Diseases: Medical and Surgical Problems", edited by S. Stipa and A. Cavallaro, 1982. Academic Press, London and New York.

More severe inflammation can lead to occlusion of the vessel or damage to the arterial wall and manifest clinically.

The different manifestations of giant cell arteritis may conveniently be divided into general symptoms, manifestations of a systemic disease, and localized syndromes which depend on the particular vessel involved (Healey and Wilske, 1978). Systemic manifestations include the rapid sedimentation rate, anemia, fever, weight loss, anorexia and malaise which can be severe enough to suggest an occult malignant disease, abnormal liver function tests (especially the alkaline phosphatase) and polymyalgia rheumatica. This rheumatic syndrome of pain and pronounced morning stiffness of shoulder and pelvic girdles is a frequent accompaniment of giant cell arteritis and responds dramatically to low doses of corticosteroid.

The localized syndromes include the headache and loss of vision already mentioned. Another visual complaint is transient diplopia which is caused by paralysis of extra-ocular muscles and presumably is due to occlusion of either the artery supplying these muscles or of the vascular supply to the oculomotor, trochlear and abducens nerves.

Jaw claudication, that is pain in the jaw with talking or chewing, stems from ischemia of the masseter muscle due to inflammation of the facial artery. Horton considered it a pathognomonic symptom of temporal arteritis and as such it provides another clue to the diagnosis. Less common manifestations of cranial artery blockage may include scalp gangrene, blanching or even necrosis of the tongue and pain in the ear or throat.

As mentioned, histologic evidence of arteritis can be demonstrated in the aorta and its branches. Severe inflammation can lead to occlusion or damage and manifest clinically as aortic arch syndromes or aneurysm with dissection and rupture. Such cases are seen with varying frequency in all reported series of the disease. For example, of Hamrin's 93 patients, 14 were noted to have an aortic arch syndrome with claudication in arms or legs, paresthesias of the hands or Raynaud's phenomenon. Eight of these patients had angiographic studies demonstrating narrowing and stenosis of branches of the aorta. The same author also reported bruits over carotids, subclavian, axillary, brachial or femoral arteries in 60% of patients in whom careful auscultation was performed. Other investigators have not found the same frequency of bruits as described by Hamrin (1972).

Some estimate of the frequency of aortic arch syndrome can be found in the report by Klein *et al.* (1975) from the Mayo Clinic who reviewed 248 patients with proven giant cell arteritis encountered between 1968 and 1974. They found definite evidence of large artery involvement in 23 (9%) and symptoms indicating possible aortic arch involvement in an additional 11 (5%). Their criteria for the diagnosis included histologic findings at post-mortem examination, changes on aortogram, absent large artery pulse or intermittent claudication and presence of a bruit.

The most common symptoms noted were intermittent claudication in arms or legs, Raynaud's phenomenon, paresthesias, gangrene of toes, abdominal angina or chest pain. Aortic aneurysm or dilatation were also seen and three of the 248 patients with rupture of aortic aneurysm. In most of their patients, treatment with corticosteroid produced improvement in claudication, increase in pulses and disappearance of Raynaud's phenomenon.

As shown in Fig. 1, angiographic studies may be helpful in deciding that aortic arch syndrome is due to giant cell arteritis. The features that suggest the occlusion is due to arteritis rather than atherosclerosis are the following: the changes are localized primarily to upper extremity rather than lower extremity arteries, the irregular plaques of arteriosclerosis are absent, arteries show smooth tapering occlusions which involve long segments and alternate with areas of normal caliber. As with all other presentations of Horton's disease, a very rapid erythrocyte sedimentation rate, often exceeding 100 mm h^{-1} (Westergren) should arouse suspicion of the diagnosis that can then be established by temporal artery biopsy.

The anatomic distribution and histology of the lesions in giant cell arteritis are of interest. Both focus attention on the internal elastic lamina as key tissue. Based on a careful evaluation of 12 cases in all of whom there was adequate post-mortem examination, Wilkinson and Russell (1972) noted that there seemed to be a clear correlation between the susceptibility to giant cell arteritis and the amount of elastic tissue in the media of the individual arteries of the head and neck. This was notably exemplified by severe inflammatory involvement of the vertebral and internal carotid vessels to the point of dural perforation where there is a significant reduction in elastic tissue of vessel walls. This is also true for the ophthalmic and posterior ciliary arteries which

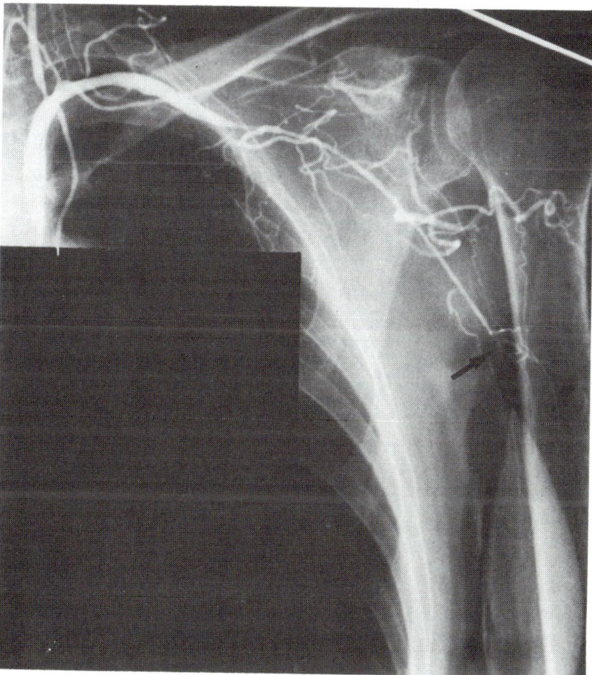

Fig. 1. Angiogram in a 72-year-old woman with giant cell arteritis. Long tapered narrowing of left axillary artery with occlusion near origin of brachial artery (arrow).

are involved by the disease much more often than the central retinal artery which loses its elastic tissue as its penetrates the optic nerve sheath. This theory is attractive in that it would provide an explanation for the relative sparing of intracranial arteries, coronary arteries and the arterioles of kidney and lung. Both clinically and pathologically, these are infrequently involved in Horton's disease in contrast to polyarteritis nodosa.

At histological examination, the inflammation is located on either side of the internal elastic lamina which is markedly fragmented and distorted. The infiltrate consists of histiocytes, lymphocytes, epithelioid cells and the giant cells which have given the lesion one of its traditional names. The lumen is markedly narrowed by thickened edematous intima and at times occluded by clot. Even after the acute inflammation has been treated with corticosteroids and subsides, recognizable changes remain. The lumen is narrowed, intima thickened and striking fragmentation and destruction of internal elastic membrane readily recognized.

Electron microscopic examination reveals that histiocytes and giant cells are in close proximity with fragments of elastic lamina. The ground substance of the elastic tissue is markedly changed from normal, appearing dense and granular, as though it had undergone some unexplained change. While it is not possible to demonstrate phagocytosis of elastic fragments by giant cells, the close proximity of the granulomatous reaction to degenerating elastic tissue suggests that the two might be related. This appearance is consistent with that of a cell-mediated immune response, possibly provoked by elastic tissue that has been altered in some way (Healey and Wilske, 1978). As yet there is no experimental evidence to confirm this hypothesis.

The cause of Horton's disease is unknown but the incidence provides provocative clues. It is a disease of the elderly. Most reported patients are 65 years or older, and it is most unusual for a patient to be seen under the age of 50 years. Second, it is almost exclusively a disease of Caucasians. Documented biopsy-proven cases in blacks or orientals are extremely rare. It seems to occur more often in Northern Europeans and particularly in Scandinavians. It is intriguing that this might explain the experience of Dr Horton and those who followed him at the Mayo Clinic in Rochester, Minnesota as well as our own experience in Seattle, Washington. Both of these states are well known for their large populations of Scandinavian ancestry.

CONCLUSIONS

Horton's disease, also known as temporal arteritis, cranial arteritis, giant cell arteritis or arteritis of the aged, is an inflammatory vasculitis of unknown cause. Available evidence suggests it is an immune response to an unknown stimulus that may primarily affect the internal elastic lamina tissues in genetically susceptible individuals, almost all of whom are elderly Caucasians. The disease has a predilection for the aortic arch and its branches particularly in the head, neck and upper extremities. Such symptoms as fever, anemia, weight loss or polymyalgia rheumatica are indications of the systemic nature of the illness. Localized symptoms such as headache, blindness, diplopia, jaw claudication and aortic arch syndromes depend on the particular artery or arteries involved. If treated early, both systemic and local symptoms respond dramatically to corticosteroids, but the disease can also produce irreversible catastrophic effects such as loss of vision and aortic aneurysm.

REFERENCES

Hamrin, B. (1972). Polymyalgia arteritica. *Acta Medica Scandinavica, Supplementum* **533**, 1.

Healey, L. A. and Wilske, K. R. (1978). "The Systemic Manifestations of Temporal Arteritis." Grune & Stratton, New York.

Klein, R. G., Hunder, G. G., Stanson, A. W. *et al.* (1975). Large artery involvement in giant cell (temporal) arteritis. *Annals of Internal Medicine* **83**, 806.

Ostberg, G. (1972). Morphological changes in the large arteries of polymyalgia arteritica. *Acta Medica Scandinavica, Supplementum* **533**, 135.

Wilkinson, I. M. and Russell, R. W. (1972). Arteries of the head and neck in giant cell arteritis. A pathological study to show the pattern of arterial involvement. *Archives of Neurology (Chicago)* **27**, 378.

POLYARTERITIS NODOSA

R. W. Lightfoot Jr.

Rheumatology Section and Arthritis Center, Medical College of Wisconsin and Veterans Administration Pilot Rheumatology Project, Wood Veterans Administration Medical Center, Milwaukee, Wisconsin, USA

Since its description by Kussmaul and Maier in 1866, polyarteritis nodosa (PAN) has served as a prototypic vasculitis syndrome. The term polyarteritis derives from the characteristic necrotizing inflammation of multiple arteries in multiple areas of the body, the term nodosa from the occasional nodularity that develops in involved arteries. This necrotizing vasculitis can involve small- to medium-sized arteries in virtually any organ system of the body. The approximate incidence of involvement of the various organ systems is shown in Table I as reviewed in Lightfoot (1980). The symptoms exhibited by patients with polyarteritis include (1) those reflecting systemic illness, such as

Table I. Incidence of organ system involvement in PAN[a].

Systemic	75%	G. I. symptoms	62–77%
Kidney	75%	Liver	40–70%
Proteinuria	60%	Nervous system	80%
Hematuria	40%	CNS	35%
Hypertension	60%	PNS	54%
Myocardium	70%	Skeletal muscle	54%
Lung	54%	Skin	5–15%

[a]From Lightfoot (1980).

Serono Symposium No. 44, "Peripheral Arterial Diseases: Medical and Surgical Problems", edited by S. Stipa and A. Cavallaro, 1982. Academic Press, London and New York.

fever, weight loss, night sweats and anorexia, which are often absent and (2) symptoms resulting from impairment of function in the specific organ systems involved, e.g. myocardial failure from coronary vessel involvement, renal failure and hypertension when the renal vasculature is involved, digital gangrene when the peripheral arterial system is involved (Table II). The organ dysfunction seen is a result either of vascular occlusion secondary to the necrotizing process or of hemorrhage from the aneurysmata that can form in involved vessels.

Table II. Clinical syndromes caused by vasculitis involving vessels to specific organs.

Clinical picture	Vessel involvement
Myocardial infarct or failure	Coronary arteritis
Pulmonary infarct or infiltrate	Pulmonary arteritis
Azotemia/hypertension	Renal arteritis
Peripheral mononeuritis	Vasa nervorum
Abdominal angina	Mesenteric arteritis
Intestinal infarction	Mesenteric arteritis
Gastro-intestinal hemorrhage	Mesenteric arteritis
Stroke	Cerebral arteritis
Digital/extremity ulcers or gangrene	Peripheral vasculitis

Involvement of the heart, kidney, lung or peripheral nervous system rarely presents to the vascular surgeon, such patients more often being referred to the general internist or rheumatologist. Patients are more likely to be seen by vascular surgeons when they are mistakenly thought to have the much more common arteriosclerotic occlusive syndromes, such as abdominal angina, mesenteric infarction, Raynaud's phenomenon, digital or extremity ulceration or gangrene or transient ischemic attacks.

PATHOLOGY AND PATHOGENESIS

In PAN the classic acute lesion reveals (Fig. 1) necrosis with fibrinoid change, polymorphonuclear leukocyte infiltration and interruption of the internal elastic lamina. Later, a mononuclear cell infiltrate may also be seen. Giant cells are not present. Weakening of the muscular wall may result in formation of small aneurysms. With healing, aneurysms may disappear and fibrotic nodularity may occur.

The resemblance of the arterial lesions seen in PAN to those found in classical serum sickness was noted earlier in this century (Rich, 1946–1947). However, identification of the reactants that might cause idiopathic vasculitis did not occur until 1970 when Gocke *et al*. reported hepatitis B antigen (HBAg) in patients with PAN. Others have since reported the presence of

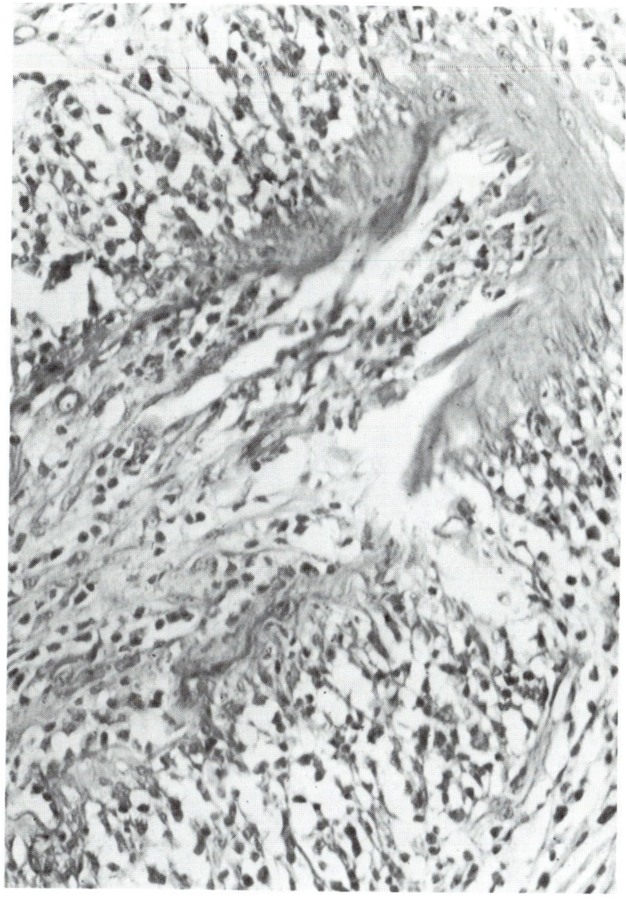

Fig. 1. Spectrum of vasculitis syndromes and size of vessels involved.

HBAg or antibody in 36–69% of PAN patients (Sergent *et al.*, 1976). In 1974, Sergent and Christian (1974) reported PAN in seven patients occurring two weeks to seven months after acute serous otitis media. Another "vasculitic" disease representing a response to a specific infectious agent is subacute bacterial endocarditis, in which hypocomplementemia, rheumatoid factor, mixed cryoglobulinemia, immune deposit nephritis and vascular deposits occur. Whereas a number of investigators have reported the deposition of IgG and complement in vessel walls of patients with a variety of vasculitides (Miescher *et al.*, 1965; Sams *et al.*, 1975), in most instances the causative agent remains unknown and hypocomplementemia is the exception.

SIGNS AND SYMPTOMS

The symptoms of polyarteritis nodosa can be mimicked precisely by a variety of vasculitis syndromes listed in Table III, although in most of those which involve smaller or larger vessels than in PAN, the spectrum of symptoms reflects dysfunction of those vessels.

In evaluating the patient with peripheral or visceral vascular insufficiency syndromes, the clinician must consider a number of nonvasculitic conditions (Table IV) that can mimic either vasculitis or the more common atherosclerotic occlusive syndromes because some of the conditions listed can be permanently relieved by innocuous therapies. Thus, in anyone with peripheral, mesenteric or cerebral vascular occlusion bacterial endocarditis or atrial myxoma should be considered in the differential diagnosis. Conversely, in rare patients a syndrome classical for small vessel vasculitis can be mimicked by cholesterol embolization from an ulcerated atheromatous plaque.

Specific symptoms that may be seen by the vascular surgeon include classical Raynaud's (Fig. 2), nail-bed infarcts (Fig. 3), livedo reticularis and

Table III.

Classification of Vasculitis Syndromes and Spectrum of Vessels Involved

Clinical Syndromes	Vessels involved
Takayasu's arteritis	Large (aorta, cranial arteries)
Temporal arteritis	
Polyarteritis nodosa	
Idiopathic	
Hb antigen positive	Medium-sized muscular arteries
Infantile form	
Associated with i.v. drug abuse	
Wegener's granulomatosis	
Allergic granulomatosis (Churg-Strauss)	
Vasculitis associated with rheumatic diseases	
Rheumatoid arthritis	Small muscular arteries
SLE	
Dermatomyositis	
Mixed connective tissue disease	
Leukocytoclastic vasculitis	
Henoch-Schoenlein purpura	Venules arterioles
Essential mixed cryoglobulinemia	
Sjögren's	
Other	

Table IV. Syndromes mimicking vasculitis.

Atrial myxoma
Hypertensive arteritis
Bacterial endocarditis
Cholesterol "vasculitis"
Thoracic outlet syndromes
Ergot poisoning

telangiectasia, which can result during healing of an involved vessel. Even in the absence of systemic symptoms or evidence of renal, cardiac or other visceral involvement an evaluation for possible vasculitis is in order in anyone in whom a more classical vascular abnormality cannot be demonstrated.

DIAGNOSTIC EVALUATION

The studies utilized in diagnosing a patient with vasculitis include (1) serological studies, (2) angiographic studies, (3) biopsy of involved vessels. Whereas the most specific way of demonstrating unequivocally the presence of vasculitis is histologic examination of the involved vessels, many patients will exhibit serologic abnormalities that strongly suggest the presence of a vasculitis syndrome. Many patients develop vasculitis secondary to a more common primary underlying illness (e.g. SLE, rheumatoid arthritis, bacterial endocarditis, scleroderma). It is reasonable to conduct a panel of serological

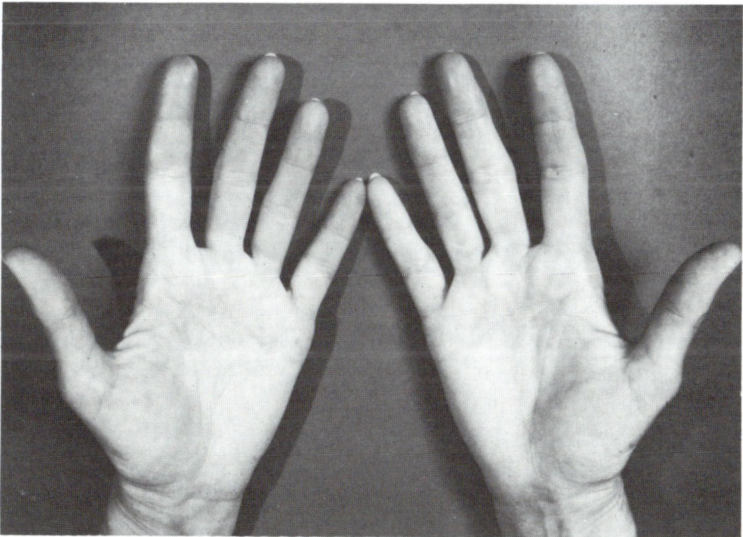

Fig. 2. Nail bed infarctions, suggesting embolic or vasculitic disease.

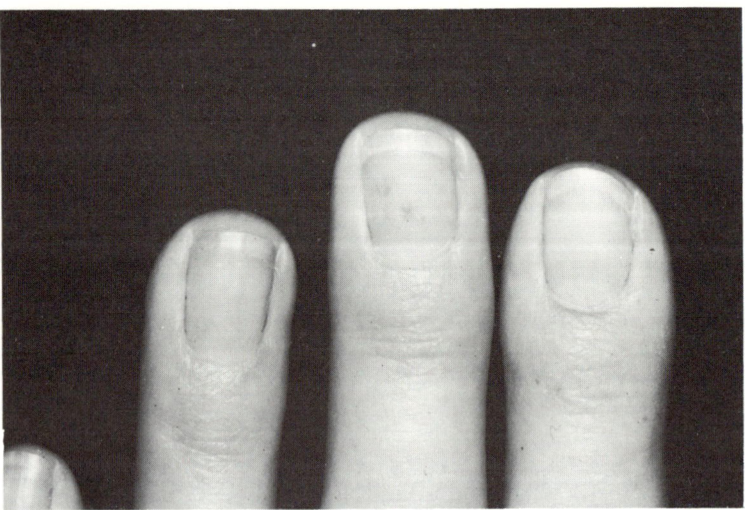

Fig. 3. Necrotizing arteritis in the biopsy of a patient with periarteritis nodosa.

studies looking for evidence of these primary syndromes. Thus, an antinuclear antibody might be suggestive of rheumatoid arthritis, lupus erythematosus or scleroderma. Cryoglobulinemia and hypocomplementemia suggest possible underlying SLE or a primary cryoglobulinemia syndrome. The presence of rheumatoid factor suggests the possibility of bacterial endocarditis or one of the connective tissue disorders. Blood cultures would be essential in ruling out bacterial endocarditis. Liver function tests and studies for HBAg and antibody might suggest that form of PAN. Finally, about one-third of patients with idiopathic polyarteritis may have rheumatoid factor or a positive antinuclear antibody. Any patient undergoing this differential diagnostic survey should also have echocardiography performed to look for atrial myxomata.

The *sine qua non* for polyarteritis is the demonstration of the classical necrotizing arterial lesion in histologic specimens. Generally, the area biopsied should be that most easily and safely accessed. This will most often be skin and muscle. If skin/muscle histology is normal and laboratory evaluation suggests renal or hepatic abnormalities, needle biopsy of these organs may yield a histologic diagnosis. In some instances, abnormalities of pulmonary roentgenograms have led to diagnostic open biopsies in that organ. It is not reasonable to risk percutaneous or open biopsy of these viscera in patients exhibiting no laboratory or X-ray manifestations of abnormalities therein.

If biopsy of those organ systems exhibiting abnormalities does not yield a diagnosis, angiographic studies should be considered. Large vessel angiography may suggest the possibility of embolic disease from proximal atherosclerosis, whereas distal arteriography may suggest the abrupt tapering seen in scleroderma and the other connective tissue diseases causing peripheral arteritis. Similarly, the diagnosis may be made upon the observation of aneurysms in hepatic, renal or mesenteric systems during visceral angiography. Whereas Doppler studies may help localize the area of attenuated flow, they do not give specifically diagnostic information in the vast majority of instances.

TREATMENT

In those connective tissue disorders associated with serological abnormalities such as hypocomplementemia, positive antinuclear antibodies and cryoglobulins, treatment with corticosteroids may not only improve vasculitis but ameliorate the serological abnormalities accompanying it. In classical PAN, where serological abnormalities are usually absent, there is much less compelling evidence that steroids alter the clinical course. This is largely because most of the reported cases existed in the pre-steroid era and were generally critically ill. In more recent years anecdotal experience has suggested that steroid therapy can mitigate a progressive course (Sergent *et al.*, 1976). Similarly, patients unresponsive to steroid therapy have been tried on immunosuppressive medications with anecdotal reports of success. Clearly, surgery to bypass local obstruction in a large artery (e.g. popliteal) would be contraindicated if that patient had multiple other areas in large or small arteries involved with PAN. In the case of mesenteric or renal infarction, surgery to remove the necrotic tissue may be life-saving. Similarly, in the occasional instance in which a vasculitic aneurysm ruptures, it may be advisable to interrupt flow into the area using ligation or angiographically placed embolization to accomplish this.

PAN is a chronic and often fatal disease that can progressively involve multiple organ systems over a period of time. Thus, the primary aim should be to diagnose the arteritis and to initiate systemic treatment using surgery only to manage emergent local complications as they occur.

REFERENCES

Gocke, J., Hus, K., Morgan, C., Bombardieri, S., Lockshin, M. and Christian, C. L. (1970). "Association between polyarteritis and Australia antigen". *Lancet* **2**, 1149.

Kussmaul, A. and Maier, R. (1966). "Über eine bisher nicht beschriebene eigenthümliche Arterienerkrankung (panarteritis nodosa), die mit Morbus Brightii und rapid fortschreitender allgemeiner Muskellähmung einhergeht". *Deutsche Archiv fur Klinische Medizin* **1**, 484.

Lightfoot, R. W. Jr. (1980). The vasculitis syndromes. *In* "Arthritis and Allied Conditions" (D. J. McCarty, Ed.), p. 723. Lea & Febiger, Philadelphia, Pennsylvania.

Miescher, P. A., Paronetto, F. and Koffler, D. (1965). *In* "Immunopathology, IV International Symposium" (P. Graber and P. Miescher, Eds), p. 446. Grune & Stratton, New York.

Rich, A. R. (1946–47). *Harvey Lectures* **42**, 106.

Sams, M. W. Jr., Claman, H. N., Kohler, P. F. *et al.* (1975). "Human necrotizing vasculitis: immunoglobulins and complement in vessel walls of cutaneous lesion and normal skin" *Journal of Investigative Dermatology* **64**, 441.

Sergent, J. S. and Christian, C. L. (1974). "Necrotizing vasculitis after acute serous otitis media". *Annals of Internal Medicine* **81**, 195.

Sergent, J. S., Lockshin, M. D., Christian, C. L. *et al.* (1976). "Vasculitis with hepatitis B antigenemia: long-term observation in nine patients". *Medicine (Baltimore)* **55**, 1.

RICKETTSIAL ARTERITIS? A CRITICAL APPRAISAL OF DIAGNOSTICS

E. A. Edlinger

Unité de Diagnostic Virologique et Rickettsiales, Institut Pasteur de Paris, Paris, France

The hypothesis of neurovascular sequelae was heavily discussed during the 1960s (Review, 1963). But, recently, some authors persist on the rickettsial aetiology of some chronical vascular diseases (Bartolo and Rulli, 1980) and of multiple sclerosis (Szekeres *et al.*, 1980). A paper published in 1979 considers as sequelae of rickettsial and "pararickettsial" infections the following diseases: Buerger's disease, Raynaud's disease, coronaritis, myocardial infarct, multiple sclerosis, Parkinson's disease, epilepsy, thalamic syndrome and, even, schizophrenia (Le Gac, 1979).

Evidently, so many sequelae would induce some scepticism and, as a matter of fact, most authors admit to only some sequelae like Buerger's disease and various other arteritis. However, as we will later show the principal basis of the sequelae hypothesis is the same for vascular and neural harms. Yet, at first, I wish to recall some notions about rickettsias and rickettsial diseases. The most important species of the genus *Rickettsia* are:

(1) *Rickettsia prowazeki*, the agent of epidemic typhus transmitted by body lice.

(2) *Rickettsia typhi (mooseri)*, responsible for murin typhus, the vector is the rat flea.

(3) *Rickettsia conori* and *R. rickettsii*, the source of spotted fever, ticks are the hosts and the vectors.

Serono Symposium No. 44, "Peripheral Arterial Diseases: Medical and Surgical Problems", edited by S. Stipa and A. Cavallaro, 1982. Academic Press, London and New York.

(*Scrub-Typhus*, present in South-East Asia, due to *Rickettsia tsutsugamushi*, transmitted by chiggers, is not considered as an origin of sequelae.)

Rickettsiae are bacterias with an appropriate metabolism that can be arrested by antibiotics, but multiplication can only start within eucaryotic cells. *Rickettsia prowazeki* and *R. typhi*, near antigenic relatives, present only a DNA homology of 70%. Among *R. rickettsii* and *R. typhi* (or *R. prowazeki*) the DNA homology is not more than 35–40% (Myers and Wisseman, 1980). In human organisms, endothelial cells of small vessels, arterioles and capillaries are the favourite targets; it is known that endothelial cells of great vessels are not the same cell type as microvascular endothelium (Weibel and Palade, 1964). Hence, the fundamental lesion in typhus and spotted fever is a microvascularitis, localized principally in the skin (which produces exanthema) and the brain (which results in typhus), but it can spread to the kidney, lung and myocard with the corresponding tissues injuries: glomerulonephritis, pneumonia and myocarditis. Small-vessel damage leads to increased capillary permeability, thrombocytopenia and, the less common, coagulopathy which happens in cases of Rocky Mountain spotted fever. Most fatalities occur during the second week of illness, corresponding to the time of most severe microvascular damage. Deaths are usually due to shock, brain and/or pneumonia oedema or myocardial or renal impairment. Later, vascular healing is followed by reabsorption of interstitial fluid and a marked diuresis. But whatever is the gravity of the illness, the convalescent does not show any vascular sequelae. The degree of gravity is very variable; it is known that, especially among children, clinically inapparent infections can occur.

Only epidemic typhus, but not the other rickettsial diseases, can rise again, as the mostly mild Brill-Zinsser disease.

Q fever whose agent is *Coxiella burneti*, transmitted by aerosol of dejections of infected cattle is also considered as a rickettsial disease. *Coxiella burneti* shares with the rickettsias the obligatory intracellular parasitism but its characters are very different; infection is frequently inapparent; the target cells are interstitial cells of the lung and the usual clinical manifestation is a typical pneumonia. There is no vascularitis. In rare cases *C. burneti* can affect the cardiac valvule, which leads to a mostly fatal endocarditis.

Diagnostic of typhus and spotted fever is easy if epidemiological data are also taken on account (presence of body lice, contact with rats, tick bite).

Laboratory diagnostics use two procedures: isolation of the agent, which is rather difficult and seldom successful, and serology.

To appraise the results of serology several factors must be considered. Specific antibodies (immunoglobulins) are only the immunological scar of a former infection and are not *per se* the sign of an affection. An acute disease is proved by the presence of specific IgMs or by the increase of antibody titre between early and convalescent serum. The tests used must be reliable; they should be specific and sensitive. Yet, a high specifity is at the cost of sensitivity and vice versa. A compromise must be searched for, but first specifity must be required. The hypothesis of the rickettsial aetiology of arteriopathies is founded on the positive results of a single serological test: the microagglutination on slide according to Giroud and Giroud (1944). This test is executed with a kit of antigens called *R. prowazeki, R. mooseri* and *R. burneti* and Neo-rickettsia Q. 18 (a strain of *Chlamydia psittaci*). The above mentioned authors obtain by this test numerous positive results in cases of arteriopathies and neurological syndromes.

However, these positive results put many questions, for example:

(1) How a person who was always living in a country without epidemic typhus can carry anti *R. prowazeki* antibodies? Some people try to explain that by inapparent forms of typhus; but how can they admit that such a serious disease is only inapparent and in a country without proliferation of vectors, body lice?

(2) How admit a spotted fever without tick bite? According to Giroud *et al.* (1966) "The antigen of *R. prowazeki* has undergone a modification to *R. conori* during its intrahuman latency."

A transformation of one species to another, very little relative, as we have shown, needs some hundred simultaneous mutations. Why in Central Africa, in spite of a high frequency of rickettsial diseases, arteritis of legs, phlebitis and coronaritis are exceptional, according to Charmot (Review, 1963). Why in the United States, rickettsial diseases are only known as acute diseases (Fuller see Review, 1963). Finally, all depend on reliability of the test of slide micro-agglutination. Compared with other serological tests, the former gives much more positive results (but sometimes also negative results in clinically unquestionable rickettsial diseases).

Le Gac (1979) attempts an explanation: antigens used in other tests, like in complement fixation reaction (CFR) or immunofluorescence (IF) are too much purified. However, the positive results obtained by Hungarian authors (Szekeres *et al.*, 1980) in cases of multiple sclerosis were obtained by the Girouds' test with antigens purified by Fiset (personal communication). (The Girouds' test is not to be confounded with the micro-agglutination according to Fiset *et al.* (1969). This latter test gives results that are comparable with the results of CF and IF tests.)

We have examined 560 sera from patients with chronic neurological and cardiovascular diseases, considered to be "sequelae of inapparent rickettsial infections", all of which gave us negative results by CF and IF tests with the antigens *C. burneti*, *R. typhi* and *R. conori* (Edlinger, 1979). But the sera of patients with acute boutonneuse fever gave with two methods (CF and IF) positive results with good agreement; however, the IF test appears preferable as the use of specific anti-IgG and anti-IgM sera make it possible to differentiate between recent and past infections. Similar results with epidemic typhus sera were obtained by Ormsbee *et al.* (1977). Furthermore, these methods have shown that in great majority of cases rickettsial antibodies disappear two or three years after infection.

To sum up, rickettsial genetic, cytopathology and clinical decrement of rickettsial diseases and epidemiological data are not in favour of neurovascular sequelae. The eventual persistence of specific antibodies is the trace of an anterior immunization but not the sign of a disease. However, mostly a false positive result obtained by the test of micro-agglutination on slide makes believe in the persistence of antibodies for decades. The hypothesis of a rickettsial aetiology of chronical arteriopathies is only founded on a serological test where the sensitivity is greater than the specifity.

REFERENCES

Bartolo, M. and Rulli, F. (1980). La rickettsiosis en patologia vascular. *Angiologia* **32**, 171.

Edlinger, E. (1979). Serological diagnosis of mediterranean spotted fever. *Annales de Microbiologie (Paris)* **130A**, 203.

Fiset, P., Ormsbee, R. A., Silbermann, R., Peacock, M. and Spielmann, S. M. (1969). A microagglutination technique for detection and measurement of rickettsial antibodies. *Acta Virologica (English Edition)* **13**, 60.

Giroud, P. and Giroud, M. L. (1944). Agglutination des rickettsies. Test de séro-protection et réaction d'hypersensibilité cutanée. *Bulletin de la Societé de Pathologie Exotique* **37**, 84.

Giroud, P., Capponi, M. and Rageau, J. (1966). Le typhus épidémique peut-il se conserver en dehors du pou et de l'homme son véritable réservoir? *Bulletin de l'Organisation Mondiale de la Santé* **35**, 119.

Le Gac, P. (1979). Rickettsie e pararickettsie. Loro micro-agglutinazione: tecnica, risultati, importanza della riattivazione. *Annali dell'Istituto Superiore di Sanità* **15**, 745.

Myers, W. F. and Wisseman, Ch. L. Jr. (1980). The taxonomic relationship of *Rickettsia canada* to the typhus and spotted fever groups of the genus *Rickettsia*. *In* "Conference on Rickettsiae and Rickettsial diseases", p. 1. RML Hamilton, Montana, September 1980.

Ormsbee, R., Peacock, M., Philip, R., Casper, E., Ploerde, J., Gabre-Kidan, T. and Wright, L. (1977). Serological diagnosis of epidemic typhus fever. *American Journal of Epidemiology* **105**, 261.

Review (1963). Réunion d'information sur les rickettsioses et leurs complications vasculaires. *Bulletin de la Societé de Pathologie Exotique* **56**, 565.

Szekeres, J., Palffy, Gy. and Paradi, J. (1980). Rickettsia specific antibodies in multiple sclerosis. *Lancet* **2**, 1089.

Weibel, E. R. and Palade, G. E. (1964). New cytoplasmic components in arterial endothelia. *Journal of Cell Biology* **23**, 101.

RICKETTSIAL ARTERITIS: CLINICAL PICTURE

A. Sciacca

Istituto Patologia Medica VI, Università di Roma, Rome, Italy

It is well accepted that rickettsiae, like many other viruses, have a remarkable angiotropism. The observation of the vessels' involvement, particularly for typhus fever and for Rocky Mountain Spotted Fever, was made far before identification of the aetiological agents (*Rickettsia prowazeki*, *R. rickettsiae*) involved. *Rickettsia mooseri*, *R. conori*, *R. tiphy* and, particularly, *Coxiella burnetii*, may be responsible for arterial diseases. Such an event has been observed by many authors using serological techniques and, sometimes, through isolation of the agent. More recently, new agents, namely Neorickettsie (X14, X18, Q18, V13), have been recognized as a possible cause of arterial involvement. It is interesting to point out that not only can the arterial districts be injured, but also the venous (phlebites, thrombophlebites) and cardiac areas (endocarditis, myocarditis, pericarditis). All such localizations can appear alone or variously associated.

Many other areas, however, can suffer rickettsial infections, for instance, the nervous system (meningitis, meningo-encephalitis, pyramidal syndromes, multiple sclerosis, epilepsy, radiocoloneuropathy), the eyes (uvcitis, keratoconjunctivitis, chorioretinitis), the liver (hepatitis), the serous membranes (serositis, poliserositis), the urogenital apparatus (urethritis, oophoritis) and the dermis. There even seems to exist a rickettsial pathology during pregnancy. All these localizations can be due to a vascular pathogenesis, perhaps through arteriolar involvement. Thus, the clinical features of rickettsial arteriopathy can evolve separately or in conjunction with others in the clinical picture.

Serono Symposium No. 44, "Peripheral Arterial Diseases: Medical and Surgical Problems", edited by S. Stipa and A. Cavallaro, 1982. Academic Press, London and New York.

Review of the medical literature of the last 30 years shows a number of papers concerning rickettsial and neo-rickettsial cardio-angiopathies with the most different syndromes due to the districtual localizations and to the feature of the onset of the course. Semilologically it must be stressed that the variety of symptoms depends on the localizations, single, multiple or associated.

The onset can be:

(1) contemporaneous to the general features of the rickettsial diseases, more or less transitory,
(2) protopathic or apparently protopathic, or
(3) as a sequela, sometimes appearing after some years after the infection, sometimes neglected. This can be explained by the fact that rickettsiae often assume a latent behaviour in the organism. The course of the disease can vary, spacing among transitory, acute, subacute and chronic aspects.

Owing to the multiplicity of localizations, the way of onset, the variety of the course and the possible associations, it is very difficult to define the aspects of the syndrome on a specific or paradigmatic scheme. Under the circumstances, we feel that facing a clinical picture characterized by non-bacterial arteritis or polyarteritis localized in any district *per se* or following a not well-defined infection, the rickettsial or neorickettsial aetiology always should be taken into account. The evidence for such a suspicion can be obtained through the epidemiological, anamnestical and laboratory findings.

Giroud and co-workers have recognized a rickettsial aetiology in many cases of vasculitis of the limbs, of the heart and of the brain, particularly in patients coming from countries where such diseases are endemic. Giroud and Le Gac (1960) observed the presence of rickettsial and neorickettsial antibodies (*R. mooseri, conori, burnetti, Neorickettsia* Q14, V14, T13) in 13 cases of myocardial infarction. Delanoe (1963) obtained significant serological results for rickettsial antibodies in 11 out of 53 cases of angiopathies. In the younger patients the average positive results increased from 20.7% to 41%. These authors stress the possibility of a role played by rickettsiae in the pathogenesis of arteriosclerosis.

Nuzzolo, Zardi and others (Nuzzolo *et al.*, 1966, 1980), reviewed 230 cases of arterial syndromes, observed from 1962 to 1980, including localization to the limbs and the heart (coronary arteries and endocardium), single or associated. In 53 cases (23%) a rickettsial aetiology was suggested by complement fixation and micro-agglutination tests mostly for *C. burnetii*.

Sometimes the morbid pictures, because of their extension, severity and course, are similar to the ones observed in Buerger's disease. The Rickettsiae infections, however, respond favourably to therapy with tetracyclines. In order to maintain a sharp distinction from Buerger's disease we define such pictures as Buerger-like. It is important to stress that many authors consider Buerger's disease as a rickettsial infection. Such an hypothesis was made by Goodman in 1916; subsequently (1937) the author obtained a series of epidemiological and clinical data supported by specific skin tests and he came to the conclusion that the infection can be asymptomatic or oligosymptomatic in the early phase; the latency interval between the acute stage and thromboangioitis can be delayed.

Angelescu *et al.*, since 1930, in Rumania, postulated that typhus infection could be responsible for chronic thromboangioitis. Troisier and Horwitz (1933) stated that juvenile thromboangioitis and typhus fever have the same connexions existing between the progressive paralysis and syphilis and between Parkinson's disease and epidemic encephalitis.

Giroud and co-workers in the 1950s supported such an hypothesis and, in 1959, Michon and his colleagues observed out of 27 cases of rickettsial infections, 13 cases with simil-Buerger features. Bernard *et al.* (1962) in ten out of 20 cases of juvenile arteritis observed the presence of rickettsial antibodies. Delanoe (1963) discussed, on the basis of his research, the prevailing role of the rickettsiae in Buerger's thromboangioitis. Many other authors, mainly from Eastern Europe (Surdan, 1968; Mandache *et al.*, 1977), have stressed this concept on the basis of serological data. Similar results were obtained by Bartolo *et al.* in Italy in 1980.

However, we agree with the criticism of Scaffidi and Cucchiara (1971) and Mansueto (1975). These authors suggest care in labelling as rickettsial any kind of angioitis, taking just anamnestic data and the low positivities of serological tests as insufficient. In this connexion we recall what Adorisio, Vulcano and Zardi stated in 1977 — that only the isolation of the agent, the demonstration through immunofluorescent techniques and a significant seroconversion, may demonstrate the proper aetiology. We should like to add that a discriminating evaluation of Buerger's disease should be obtained with the aid of angiographic and histopathological methods. The pathological picture obviously differs in relation to the severity and the extension of the arterial damage, starting from simple ischaemia and ending with necrosis. It is also important to consider the involvement of single or multiple vascular districts. Anyhow we would limit our description to the lesions of the arterial wall characterizing the various stages.

The elective localization of rickettsiae is represented by endothelium. Princoff and Shaw (1933) were able to demonstrate rickettsiae in the endothelial cells of interstitial and subendocardial capillary vessels, staining myocardial slices with Giemsa. More recently, Walker, Paletta and Cain (1980), in several cases of Rocky Mountain Spotted Fever myocarditis, have confirmed this particular affinity using a specific immunofluorescent technique. These authors have found the presence of rickettsiae in the endothelium of capillary vessels, arteriolae and veinulae. The interstitial mononucleated cell infiltration with oedema mainly surrounds the site of vascular involvement. Rickettsiae can be observed also in the endothelium and in the walls of the main coronary vessels. The endocardial localizations are rare and the myocardial one is completely absent. According to these authors the pathway of the rickettsial myocarditis should follow this scheme:

(1) haematogenic diffusion of the rickettsiae to the endothelium of the myocardial vessels,
(2) lesions of the infected endothelial cells,
(3) increase of the vascular permeability with oedema and, rarely, focal thrombosis and ischaemic necrosis, and
(4) inflammatory reaction with leucocyte interstitial infiltration. The myocardial fibres seem to be uninvolved.

The absence of rickettsiae in the myocardial fibres is a good differential diagnostic criterion from other types of myocarditis as Chagas, toxoplasmosis and coxackiosis; in these diseases the myocardial fibres are always parasitized and damaged.

A case published by Nuzzolo *et al.* (1966) in the course of research performed in our department was identified as polyarteritis due to *Coxiella burnetii.* In fact, the complement fixation tests gave high titres with the Q fever antigen (I/4096 and I/8192). In addition the agent was isolated and tipped after serial passages in guinea-pigs and embryonated hens' eggs. The patient was a man aged 33. The arterial involvement had begun four years before, associated at first with endocarditis of the mitral valve and, later on, of the aortic valve. The arteritic process involved, progressively, both inferior and superior limbs with evident local ischaemic phenomena and intermittent claudication. There were also relapsing episodes of fever of different intensity, increased ESR and mild neutrophilic leucocytosis. Cardial function was progressively impaired until fatal heart failure occurred. Arterial biopsy was performed during the first observation and four years later many samples of arteries were obtained on autopsy. It was likewise possible to carry out a complete evaluation of the histopathological lesions, both in various vascular districts and in various stages of the disease: acute, subacute and chronic. The biopsy of posterior tibial artery of the left leg was performed after an angiography during the first ischaemic episode. There was a conspicuous infiltration of mononucleated cells in the adventitia also involving the external layers of the media. The vasa vasorum were infiltrated and congested. The media was not associated with oedema and the degeneration of the muscular fibres was slight. The internal elastic lamina was undamaged and the intima was thickened with thrombosis of the lumen. Biopsy on the left humeral artery was performed four years later, seven days before the exitus, and the findings were surprisingly similar to those found in the former biopsy. In both arteries the phlogosis was at an acute stage and this confirmed that rickettsiae may develop, at any time — even long after infection — an acute arteritis in various and unpredictable sites. In other arterial districts, such as the right humeral, femoral, popliteal and tibial arteries, the infiltration was less important, localized in the adventitia and in the contiguous layers of the media, spread or limited in small foci. Thickening and sclerosis of the intima and thrombosis were common observations.

REFERENCES

Adorisio, F., Vulcano, G. and Zardi, O. (1977). Le rickettsiosi sono problema di attualità. *Arch. Casa Sollievo Sofferenza* **11**, 291.

Angelescu, C., Georgescu, G. and Burolanu, G. V. (1930). Exanthematous typhus as an etiologic factor in chronic arteritis obliterans. *Spitalul* **50**, 401.

Bartolo, M., Rulli, F. and Raffi, S. (1980). Buerger's disease: is it a rickettsiosis? *Angiology* **31**, 660.

Bernard, J. G., Ougier, J., Duboureau, L. H. and Benzenou, A. (1962). Aspects cliniques et étiologiques des artérites juveniles. *Archives des Maladies du Cœur et des Vaisseaux* **55**, 926.

Delanoe, G. (1963). Sur le rôle des rickettsioses atypiques ou méconnues dans la pathologie vasculaire. *Archives de Maladies du Cœur et des Vaisseaux* **56**, 205.

Giroud, P. and Le Gac, P. (1960). L'infarctus du myocarde peut étre une complication des rickettsioses, des néo-rickettsioses ou des affections du group psittacose. *Medecine et Hygiène* **18**, 277.

Goodman, C. (1937). Thrombo-angioitis obliterans and typhus. Evidence of etiologic relationship. *Archives of Surgery (Chicago)* **8**, 1126.

Mandache, F., Prodescu, V., Costantinescu, S., Kover, G. H., Abranescu, N., Popa, F., Cantaragiu, S. and Popescu, G. (1977). Medullosclerosis, controlateral adrenalectomy and splanchnicosympathectomy in severe essential arterial hypertension and thromboangiitis. Part II. *Revue Roumaine de Medecine et Endocrinologie* **15**, 161.

Mansueto, S. (1975). Sulla eziologia rickettsiosica delle arteriopatie obliteranti croniche. *Minerva Cardioangiologica* **10**, 599.

Michon, P., Giroud, P., Mathieu, L., Bernard, J. G., Larcan, A. and Huriet, C. (1959). Rickettsioses et affections cardio-vasculaires. A propos de 27 observations. *Bulletins et Mémoires de la Société Médicale des Hôpitaux de Paris* **75**, 3.

Nuzzolo, L., Pierangeli, L., Ravetta, M. and Vellucci, A. (1966). Arterite da *Coxiella burnetii. Gazzetta Internazionale di Medicina e Chirurgia* **72**, 24 bis, 1.

Nuzzolo, L., Zardi, O., Carmenini, G. and Di Giacomo, V. (1980). Le arteriti da rickettsie: aggiornamento della letteratura ed osservazioni personali. Rendiconto della Società Italiana di Medicina Interna, Atti 80° Congresso, p. 132.

Princoff, M. C. and Shaw, C. C. (1933). The Eastern type of Rocky Mountain spotted fever. Report of a case with demonstration of rickettsiae. *Medical Clinics of North America* **16**, 1097.

Scaffidi, L. and Cucchiara, E. (1971). Coronarite primitiva da *Rickettsia burnetii. Giornale di Malattie Infettive e Parassitarie* **23**, 964.

Surdan, C. T. (1968). Le contribution roumaine à l'étude des infections latentes provoquées chez l'homme par les rickettsies et les prerickettsies. *Bulletin de la Societé de Pathologie Exotique* **61**, 737.

Troisier, I. and Horowitz, A. (1933). Maladie de Buerger et typhus exanthématique. *Bulletins et Mémoires de la Société Médicale des Hôpitaux de Paris* **49**, 151.

Walker, D. H., Paletta, C. E. and Cain, B. G. (1980). Pathogenesis of Myocarditis in Rocky Mountain Spotted Fever. *Archives of Pathology* **104**, 171.

THE ROLE OF RECONSTRUCTIVE ARTERIAL SURGERY IN THE TREATMENT OF CHRONIC RICKETTSIAL ARTERITIS: A PERSONAL EXPERIENCE

A. Cavallaro[1], V. Sciacca[1], M. Garofalo[1], A. Sterpetti[1], S. Cisternino[1] and A. De Giorgis[2]

IV Cattedra di Patologia Chirurgica dell'Università di Roma[1] *and VI Cattedra di Patologia Medica dell'Università di Roma*[2], *Rome, Italy*

The possibility of chronic arterial lesions from rickettsiae has been discussed for many years (Delanoe, 1963; Nuzzolo *et al.*, 1966; Mansueto, 1976; Rigaud *et al.*, 1977), after the hypothesis by Goodman (1937); this kind of pathology should rely on the angiotropism of the micro-organism and on its capability of persisting alive for a long time inside the human body, even in lack of an initial acute event.

According to Giroud (1976), contamination by rickettsiae may be very frequent in most countries: cardiovascular damage could affect predisposed individuals, bearers of congenital or acquired cardiovascular lesions or presenting with lowered general organic resistance.

A close co-operation with medical colleagues particularly interested in the study of arteritides (Sciacca *et al.*, 1981) has enabled us to select, amongst a lot of vascular cases, a group of patients in which the diagnosis of chronic rickettsial arteritis was strongly suspected.

Serono Symposium No. 44, "Peripheral Arterial Diseases: Medical and Surgical Problems", edited by S. Stipa and A. Cavallaro, 1982. Academic Press, London and New York.

CLINICAL MATERIAL

From 1974, initially as a scanty procedure and thereafter with increasing frequency, antirickettsia antibodies were serologically assayed, according to Babudieri and Zardi (1952), in patients affected by chronic peripheral vascular disease.

Initially, the test was performed in patients possibly affected by non-degenerative arteriopathy on the basis of:

(1) Young age.
(2) Absence of lipid metabolism inbalance.
(3) Angiographic pattern of arterial lesions.

Later on, the serological assay was performed almost routinely in all peripheral vascular patients. The present report deals with the first 104 patients, examined from late 1974 up to June 1980. The same patients formed the basis for a report to the XII World Congress of Angiology (Athens, 7–12 September 1980).

A significantly positive result was obtained in 14 patients (13.5%): to Rickettsia Burnetii in 11, Rickettsia Q 18 in 2, Rickettsia Conori in 1.

All patients but one (patient 6 of Table I, who was born and lived many years in Egypt) had always lived in Italy.

Upper limb involvement was present in three female patients (aged 31, 31 and 43 years) complaining of arm claudication (one) or arm ischaemia (two) and showing at angiography stenosing or occlusive lesions of the subclavian and/or axillary arteries.

The patient complaining of claudication has been under medical treatment three years: for the first two years, in spite of relapsing episodes of fever, her circulatory impairment remained rather stable and acceptable (Fig. 1); serology against Rickettsia Burnetii was positive: 1:160 in July 1978; 1:20 in September 1979, and was negative in June 1980; quite recently (May, 1981) there was a worsening of upper limbs circulation coinciding with a prolonged episode of fever; the patient is actually being evaluated by repeated serology assays and angiography is programmed.

The other two patients, complaining of arm ischaemia, were submitted to axillary-to-contralateral brachial bypass with autologous vein. One refused any subsequent medical therapy and is actually doing very well after 81 months (a slight and till now not significant steel phenomenon is evident in the donor arm); two years ago, she delivered a healthy baby. The second one was affected by a subocclusive critical impairment of the bypass with marked flow imbalance and reappearance of symptoms, one year after the operation (Fig. 2); this critical condition completely subsided under an aggressive therapy with antibiotics cortisone and anticoagulants; the patient has since followed cycles of wide spectrum antibiotic therapy and her upper limb is actually in satisfactory trophic and functional conditions after a follow-up period of 78 months.

Also one male patient, aged 60, complained of arm claudication with typical subclavian steel syndrome; he was submitted to axillary–axillary bypass with autologous vein and did not follow thereafter any antibiotic

Table I. Summary of clinical data for patients with lower limb arteries involvement.

Patient	Operative indication	Operation	Follow-up period (months)	Result	
				Anatomical	Functional
1	Rest pain	Fem. to post. tibial bypass (vein)	76	Thr. 30 months	Good
2	Rest pain	Fem. to post. tibial bypass (vein)	61	Good	Good
3	Rest pain	Fem. to post. tibial bypass (vein)	26[a]	Good	Good
4	Gangrene	Fem. to ant. tibial bypass (vein)	43	Thr. 3 months	Fair
5	Gangrene	Fem. to ant. tibial bypass (vein)	37[b]	Good	Good
6	Heavy claudication	TEA common il.	12[c]	Good	Good
7	Gangrene	Fem. pop. bypass (PTFE)	27	Good	Fair
8	Heavy claudication	Dacron aorto-bifem. graft	34	Good	Good
9	Gangrene	Dacron aorto-bifem. graft	26	Good	Good
10	Heavy claudication	Dacron axillo-femoral graft	26	Thr. 3 months	Status quo

[a]Died, myocardial infarction. [b]Transmetatarsal amputation of big toe. [c]Died, lung cancer.

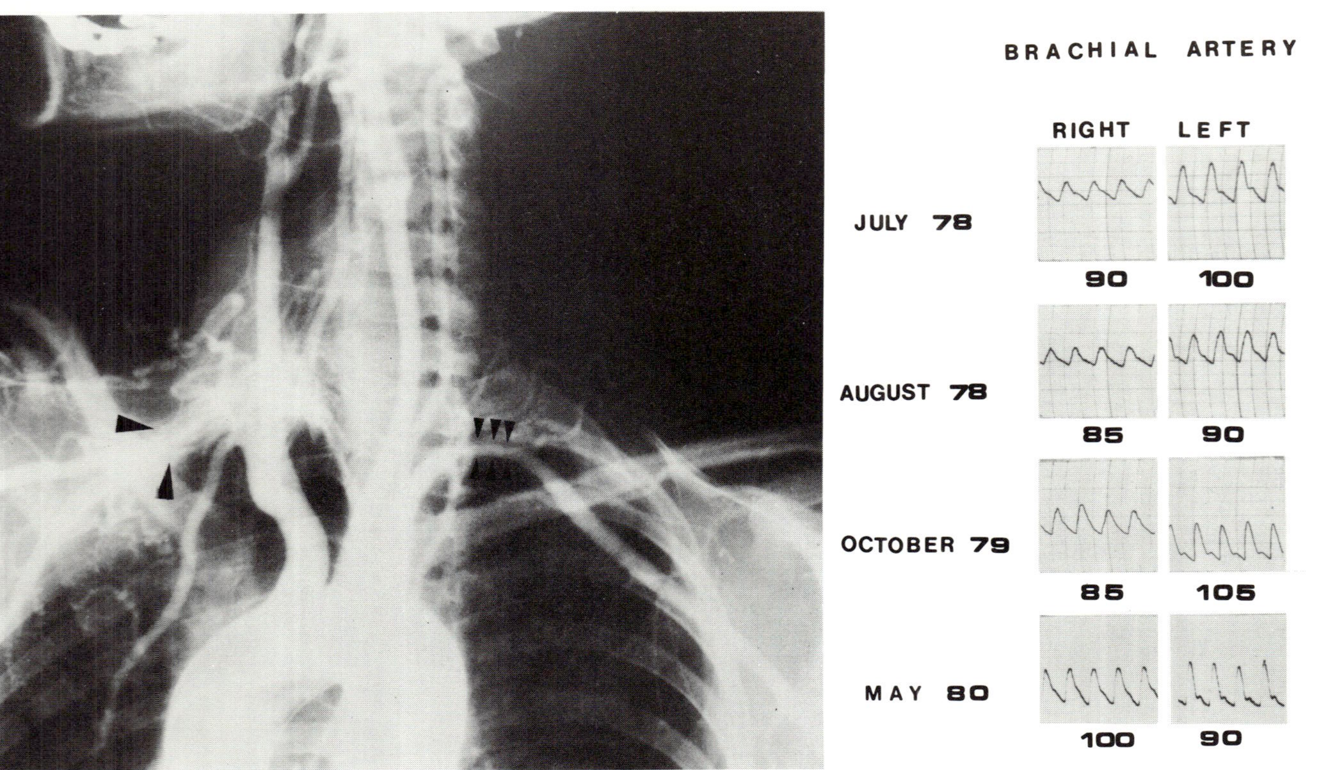

Fig. 1. Left: aortic arch, angiography showing involvement of subclavian arteries (July 1977). Right: CW Doppler recordings on brachial arteries (numbers refer to systolic arterial pressure).

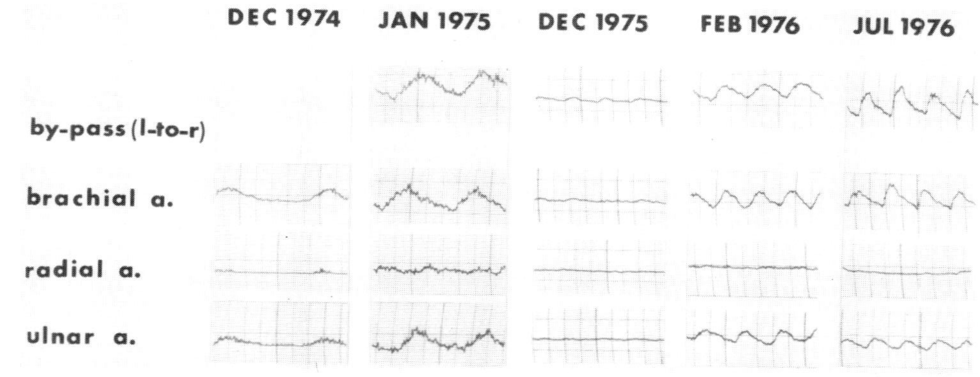

Fig. 2. CW Doppler recordings: critical low flow state one year after the operation (see text).

therapy: the graft eventually thrombosed after two months and he refused a second operation, remaining in the pre-operative status.

In ten male patients (aged 32–71, mean 55) lower limb involvement was present with heavy claudication in three, rest pain in three, gangrene in four. They were submitted to reconstructive surgery according to the site of predominant lesions, as listed in Table I together with the respective follow-up and results. Only few of them accepted to be submitted to regular antibiotic therapy, and these seemed to offer the best results, sometimes with a surprising behaviour of both arterial lesions and grafts (Figs 3 and 4).

COMMENT

Surgery can play a significant role in the treatment of chronic arterial lesions attributable to rickettsiae: mainly as a means of rescue from particularly critical hepisodes of circulation impairment. Obviously, one is brought to believe that the medical therapy remains the fundamental one, even if this is a debatable assertion at least from our limited experience, may be on account of a degenerative pathology coexistent with the inflammatory one.

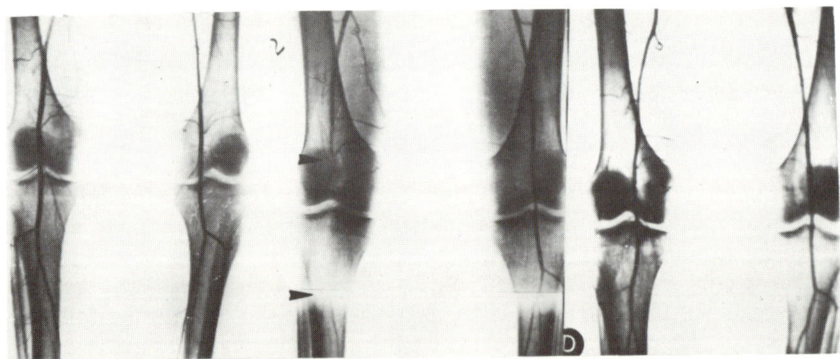

Fig. 3. (patient 1 of Table I) Left: angiography performed in May 1972, when the patient complained of left leg claudication; left lumbar sympathectomy was performed with definite improvement. Middle: angiography on December 1974, when the patient was affected by rest pain of right foot and leg; full resolution of symptoms followed the construction of a femoral-to-posterior tibial bypass. Right: after failure of the bypass with persistence of peripheral pulses and without reappearance of symptoms, angiography (July 1977) showed the recanalization of the popliteal artery. The patient never followed anticoagulant therapy; is following regular cycles of wide spectrum antibiotics since July 1977, when the hypothesis of rickettsial arteritis was expressed. Serology for Rickettsia Q 18: July 1977, 1:80; November 1977, 1:80; December 1977, 1:80; April 1978, 1:640; November 1978, 1:20; January 1979, 1:20; May 1980, 1:20; November 1980, 1:20; April 1981, 1:20. The patient was entirely free from symptoms in May 1981.

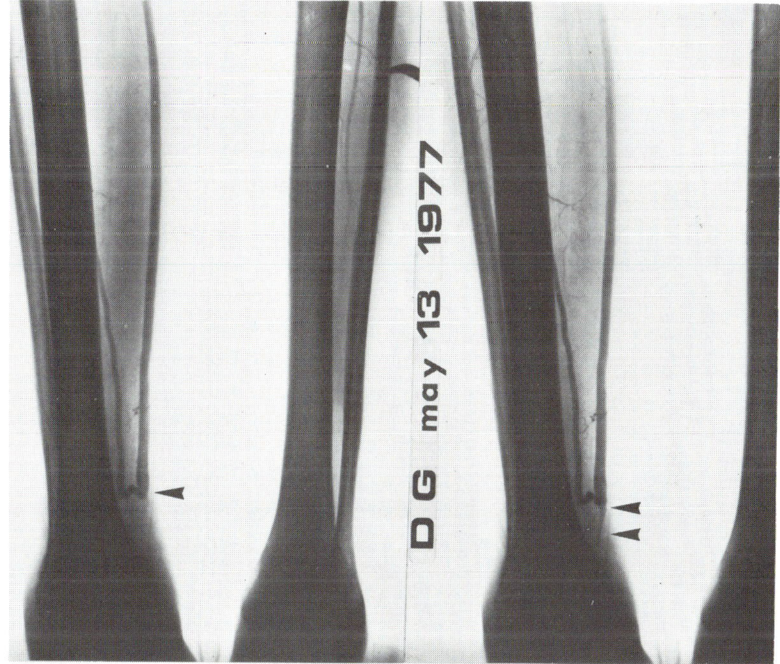

Fig. 4. Control angiography in patient 2 of Table I. Bypass patent from 12 months, in spite of impaired forward outflow at distal anastomosis. Bypass still patent and patient free from symptoms in May 1981.

We must also keep present in our mind that rickettsiosis is not an absolutely stated aetiological factor in our patients, lacking the culture of micro-organism and the tissue immunofluorescence studies: in fact, the arterial specimens when available were studied only by conventional microscopy, always resulting a diagnosis of aspecific arteritis without the degenerative changes typical of atherosclerosis but for the aortic specimens (patients 8 and 9 of Table I) which showed extensive atherosclerotic involvement.

REFERENCES

Babudieri, B. and Zardi, O. (1952). Ricerche diagnostiche della febbre Q. *Giornale di Malattie Infettive e Parassitarie* **4**, 190.

Delanoë, G. (1963). Sur le rôle des Rickettsioses atypiques ou méconnues dans la pathologie vasculaire. *Sémaine des Hôpitaux* **39**, 1430.

Giroud, P. (1976). Les lésions cardio-vasculaires des Rickettsioses et des Chlamydioses (néorickettsioses). *Angéiologie* **28**, 175.

Goodman, C. (1937). Thrombo-angeitis obliterans and typhus. Evidence of etiology relationship. *Archives of Surgery (Chicago)* **6**, 1127.

Mansueto, S. (1976). Les artérites rickettsiennes. *Angéiologie* **28**, 167.

Nuzzolo, L., Pierangeli, L., Ravetta, M. and Vellucci, A. (1966). Arterite da *Coxiella burnetii. Gazzetta Internazionale di Medicina e Chirurgia* **71**, 24 bis, I.

Rigaud, J. L., Sirol, J., Barabe, P., Delprat, J., Maistre, B., Segonne, J. and André, L. J. (1977). Artérite rickettsienne due à *Coxiella burnetii. Archives des Maladies du Cœur et des Vaisseaux* **70**, 185.

Sciacca, A., Di Giacomo, V. and Carmenini, G. (1981). "Les Arteriopatie ad Impronta Flogistica". (L. Pozzi, Ed.). Rome.

DIABETES AND MACROANGIOPATHY

A. Strano, S. Novo, G. Davì, G. Avellone and A. Pinto

Institute of Clinical Medicine and Medical Therapy of University of Palermo, Palermo, Sicily

Clinical, epidemiological and pathological investigations demonstrate that the degree of atherosclerosis and the consequent morbidity and mortality are increased in diabetics (Jarret, 1977; Jarret and Keen, 1975) and that the mean life expectancy of diabetic patients is about one-third lower than that of non diabetic patients (Crofford, 1975).

Diabetics are susceptible to diseases of both the large muscular arteries (particularly those supplying the myocardium, the brain and the lower limbs) and the capillaries, of which those in the retina and the glomerulas are the more important under a clinical aspect.

The disease of the large vessels is atherosclerosis which, in diabetes, differs neither in distribution nor in morphology from atherosclerosis in non-diabetics (Strandness *et al.*, 1964). In the Framingham study (Garcia *et al.*, 1974), subjects with diabetes mellitus (men and women) had a stronger tendency to develop cerebral, coronary and peripheral vascular diseases than non-diabetics and the incidence of intermittens claudication was particularly high in the diabetics. The mortality rate from cardiovascular diseases in diabetics was about three times higher than in the whole population.

Also in the Tecumseh study, atherosclerotic complications were more frequent in diabetics than in non-diabetic patients (Ostrander *et al.*, 1965). And in the Bedford study the frequency of cardiovascular diseases was higher in the diabetic group, intermediate in the borderline group and lower in the subjects with normal blood sugar levels (Keen and Jarret, 1973).

Serono Symposium No. 44, "Peripheral Arterial Diseases: Medical and Surgical Problems", edited by S. Stipa and A. Cavallaro, 1982. Academic Press, London and New York.

In the AMAT study (Rini *et al.*, 1980) the presence of coronary heart disease at first examination was 23.9% in the whole population examined and 47% in patients with diabetes mellitus.

In the Comungas study (Rini *et al.*, 1980) the presence of coronary heart disease (CHD) at first examination was 26.28% in all the subjects and 53.5% in patients with diabetes mellitus. Therefore, in the AMAT study the incidence of CHD per year per 1000 was 8% in non-diabetics and 24% in diabetics, with a risk increase of about three times.

In the epidemiological study which we have carried out at Trabia (Fig. 1), on behalf of the Research Group ATS RF2 of the Italian National Research Council (1981), in a randomized population sample, the prevalence of arterial vascular diseases of the lower limbs was 4.66% in the whole population, 4.30% in non-diabetics and 7.27% in diabetic patients. An exception to the association of diabetes and CHD occurs in the American Pima Indians, which have a low prevalence of CHD despite a very high prevalence of diabetes (Ingelfinger *et al.*, 1976). Thus the majority of the epidemiological studies confirms the association between diabetes and cardiovascular diseases.

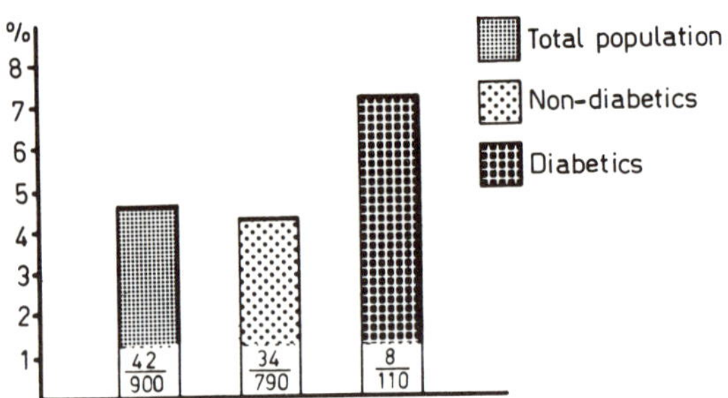

Fig. 1. Prevalence of atherosclerotic vascular disease of the lower limbs at first examination in diabetics and in total population sample in Trabia study (on behalf of the Research Group ATS-RF2 of the Italian Research Council).

On the other hand, clinical investigations have demonstrated that, in patients with ischaemic heart disease (Wahlberg and Thomasson, 1968), there is frequently an abnormal oral or intravenous glucose tolerance test; therefore, hyperglycaemia has very often been found in patients with angiographically demonstrated peripheral (Kingsbury, 1966; Sloan *et al.*, 1970) or coronary heart (Heinle *et al.*, 1969; Falsetti *et al.*, 1970) disease.

Although various clinical studies do demonstrate that diabetics have a higher prevalence of vascular diseases consequent to an extensive atherosclerosis (Epstein, 1967), it is not clear, from retrospective clinical studies, if the relationship between diabetes and atherosclerotic vascular disease is dependent from the other risk factors commonly found in diabetes, such as hyperlipidaemia, hypertension and obesity, or independent and consequent to hyperglycaemia or other metabolic disorders present in diabetes, such as insulinism, or in part consequent to a thrombophilic state often present in diabetes.

HYPERGLYCAEMIA

Experimental findings and epidemiological studies suggest that hyperglycaemia is not an independent risk factor for atherosclerosis in diabetes.

In experimental diabetes induced by pancreasectomy or by alloxan administration, hyperglycaemia is not atherogenic (Woolf, 1971)

Hyperglycaemic alloxanized rabbits fed high cholesterol diet developed fewer vascular lesions than control animals fed the same diet, despite similar serum cholesterol levels in the two groups (Duff and McMillan, 1949; McGill and Holman, 1949). The alloxanized diabetic rabbits treated with insulin developed vascular atherosclerotic lesions like the control animals (Duff *et al.*, 1954).

Epstein has recently synthesized the results of some epidemiological studies in which the relationship between hyperglycaemia and atherosclerotic vascular complications of diabetes mellitus has been analysed (Epstein, 1976). In several epidemiological studies a positive correlation has been found between hyperglycaemia during OGTT (Tecumseh, Epstein, 1967; London, Fuller *et al.*, 1976; Israel, Epstein, 1976; Medalie, 1979) and CHO risk or between glucose tolerance index and CHD (Framingham, U.S. Public Health Service, 1971) or between positive history for diabetes and CHD (Göteborg, Elmfeldt *et al.*, 1976).

This correlation was independent from other risk factors (Epstein, 1976). In the Bedford (Keen and Jarret, 1973) and Honolulu (Gordon *et al.*, 1974) studies positive correlation between hyperglycaemia and vascular atherosclerotic complications of diabetes depended on the other risk factors.

In the Chicago (Stamler, 1975) and Finland (Epstein, 1976) studies a definite correlation could not be demonstrated.

In the Puerto Rico (Gordon *et al.*, 1974) and Basel (Epstein, 1976) studies no correlation was found between hyperglycaemia and atherosclerotic complications of diabetes.

Recently, Stamler and co-workers, on the basis of the epidemiological studies carried out in Chicago, brought forth the hypothesis that hyperglycaemia is not an independent risk factor for cardiovascular diseases (Stalmer *et al.*, 1979).

It has been hypothesized that hyperglycaemia could be an injury favouring the beginning of atheromatosis as is clear from experimental evidence. In fact, the polyol pathway does not depend on the presence of insulin, and the rate of sorbitol formation increases with rising glucose concentrations (Gabbay, 1973).

Extracts of rabbit aorta, incubated in high-medium glucose concentrations, showed an increased concentration of sorbitol and a rise in water content and a depressed oxygen uptake (Morrison *et al.*, 1972). This may alter the metabolism of the arterial wall and possibly contribute to the production of arterial lesions. Therefore, the role of polyol pathway in the pathogenesis of atherosclerosis in diabetes is not yet clear and requires other experimental data.

Hyperglycaemia determines also high plasmatic concentrations of glycosilated haemoglobin (Wise and Yeates, 1978) and the glycosilated haemoglobin concentrations are a better indicator of metabolic control of diabetes.

Glycosilated haemoglobin should have a high affinity for oxygen and thus reduce the tissutal oxygen uptake.

The tissutal hypoxia should determine a thickening of basal membrane and should be an injury for arterial wall according to Ross and Glomset (1976).

HYPERINSULINISM

Various experimental and clinical–epidemiological findings support the hypothesis that there is a relation between hyperinsulinism and vascular atherosclerotic complications of diabetes mellitus.

In fact there is recent evidence that the incidence of atherosclerosis in diabetes increased after the beginning of insulin therapy. This increase does not seem to be consequent to an augment of the mean life of diabetic patients (Fedele *et al.*, 1980).

It has been found, in experimental research, that insulin administration inhibits spontaneous regression of atheromatosis in chicks fed a hypercholesterolaemic diet, whereas this regression normally takes place when the birds are brought back to normal diet (Stamler *et al.*, 1980).

Insulin stimulates lipidic synthesis in the vascular wall (Stout, 1968) and, if administered daily to chicks, determines a lipidic infiltration in the arterial wall (Stout, 1970).

Insulin inhibits lipolysis in human arteries and consequently determines a greater deposition of lipids in the arterial wall (Mahler, 1971).

Insulin stimulates also a dose-dependent concentration proliferation of cultured arterial smooth muscle cells (Stout *et al.*, 1975).

When insulin and saline were infused respectively into the right and left femoral arteries of alloxan-diabetic dogs, the insulin-treated artery developed intimal and medial proliferation and contained more cholesterol and fatty acids than the control artery (Cruz *et al.*, 1961).

Recently Epstein (1976) examined the papers concerning the problem of insulin like a possible pathogenetic factor for atherosclerotic complications of diabetes.

This author examines the findings from 19 studies in which insulin had been dosed after an oral glucose tolerance test in population samples, in patients with subclinical or latent diabetes, in children of diabetic patients and in twins born of diabetic parents. In seven studies insulin secretion was increased and the insulin/blood glucose ratio augmented (Chiles and Tzagournis, 1970; Danowski *et al.*, 1969; Florey *et al.*, 1972; Jackson *et al.*, 1972; Reaven *et al.*, 1971; Seltzer *et al.*, 1967). In other seven studies insulin secretion and insulin/blood glucose ratio were normal (Grodsky *et al.*, 1965; Serrado-Rios *et al.*, 1970; Siperstein *et al.*, 1973) or diminished (Cerasi *et al.*, 1973; Colwell and Lein, 1967; Pyke *et al.*, 1970). In other five studies, increased or variable values of insulinaemia were demonstrated (Fajans *et al.*, 1974; Johansen, 1972; Ostrander *et al.*, 1973; Ricketts *et al.*, 1966; Welborn *et al.*, 1969).

The hypothesis that high insulin levels predispose diabetic patients to atherosclerotic complications is confirmed by several data on insulin secretion in patients with atherosclerosis, both in basal conditions (Christiansen and

Decher, 1968; Boden, 1971; Enger and Ritland, 1973; Schenk *et al.*, 1974; Sorge *et al.*, 1976) and after oral glucose tolerance test (Sloan *et al.*, 1970; Ostrander *et al.*, 1973; Peters and Hales, 1965; Nikkila *et al.*, 1965, Tzagournis *et al.*, 1967; Kasyap *et al.*, 1970, Malherbe *et al.*, 1971; Gertler *et al.*, 1972; Berchtold *et al.*, 1972).

We have studied the behaviour of insulin and blood glucose in basal conditions and after OGTT (Notarbartolo *et al.*, in press) in diabetics with macroangiopathy in comparison with diabetics with microangiopathy and control subjects without diabetes and atherosclerosis.

The insulin area after OGTT was significantly higher in diabetics with macroangiopathy than in those with microangiopathy and in control subjects. Vice versa, the blood glucose levels were higher in diabetics with micro-angiopathy than in those with macroangiopathy and in control subjects.

The patients with insulinism and macroangiopathy showed also evident abnormalities of lipidic metabolism characterized by a significant increase in total cholesterol, triglycerides, VLDL-cholesterol, VLDL-triglycerides, LDL-cholesterol, apo-B and a reduction in the levels of HDL-cholesterol, HDL-C/LDL-C ratio and LDL-C/apo-B ratio.

Our findings agree with various clinico-epidemiological data which confirm the pathogenetic role of hyperinsulinism in the genesis of macrovascular complications of diabetes.

LIPIDIC METABOLISM ABNORMALITIES

Several retrospective studies demonstrate a clear, but moderate, hyper-lipidaemia in diabetes (Avogaro *et al.*, 1972; Patrassi and Crepaldi, 1971; Wahl *et al.*, 1974).

In the Framingham study there was no significant difference in triglycer-ides, cholesterol and HDL-CT levels between diabetic and non-diabetic men; vice versa, there was a significant difference in triglycerides and HDL-CT between diabetic and non-diabetic women (Garcia *et al.*, 1974).

In the Trabia study, total cholesterol levels > 240 mg dl^{-1} were found in 36% of the diabetics and in 13.8% of the normal subjects, whereas trigly-ceridaemia was > 170 mg dl^{-1} in 33.80% of the diabetics and in 14.34% of the non-diabetics (Fig. 2).

In contrast with the epidemiological findings in Trabia (The Research Group ATS RF2 of the Italian National Research Council, 1981), well controlled diabetics in our wards did not show significant differences in triglycerides, total cholesterol and glycosilated haemoglobin in comparison with control subjects (Fig. 3), but HDL-cholesterol and HDL-CT/TC were significantly lower in diabetics compared to controls.

The lowest HDL-cholesterol levels were present in diabetics on glyben-clamide plus phenformin, whereas diabetics on insulin had intermediate levels (Fig. 4). The groups of diabetic patients with macro-angiopathy showed significantly higher HDL-C levels than diabetics without angiopathy (Davì *et a.*, in press) (Fig. 5).

Thus the increase of plasmatic lipids in diabetics is not a constant finding

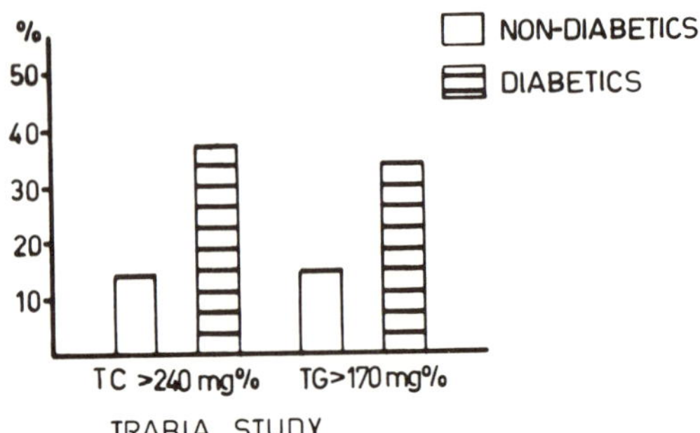

Fig. 2. Percentage of subjects with total cholesterol > 240 mg dl^{-1} and with triglycerides > 170 mg dl^{-1} in diabetics and in non-diabetics in Trabia study.

but, in the presence of a bad metabolic control, plasmatic triglycerides are likely to increase (Nikkila and Hormila, 1978).

Hypertriglyceridaemia in diabetic patients can be consequent to:

(1) An increased liver synthesis of VLDL determined by hyperinsulinism in overweight diabetics (Reaven *et al.*, 1967).

(2) A reduced plasmatic clearance of triglycerides and VLDL for deficit

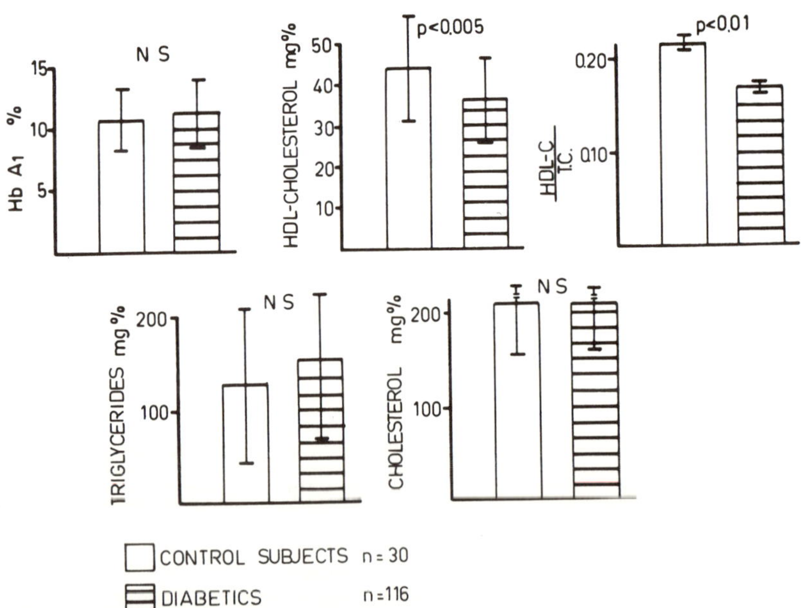

Fig. 3. Behaviour of HbA_1, triglycerides, total cholesterol, HDL-C and HDL-C/TC ratio in well controlled diabetics in our wards in comparison to control subjects. Only HDL-C levels are significantly lower in diabetics.

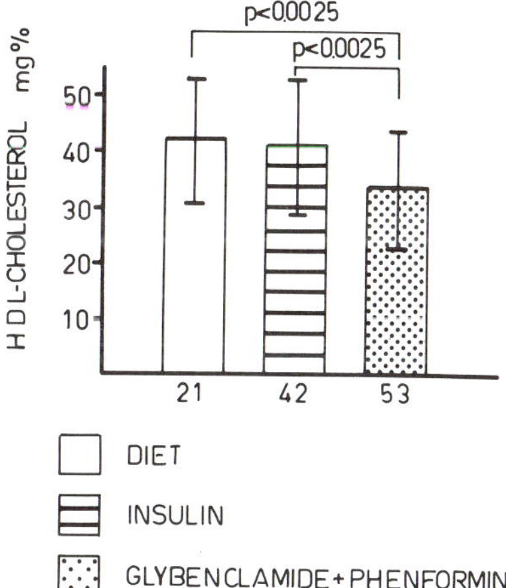

Fig. 4. HDL-cholesterol levels in well-controlled diabetics in our wards on diet, insulin and glybenclamide + phenformin. Diabetics on phenformin have the lowest levels of HDL-C.

of insulin dependent lipoprotein-lipase (Bagdade *et al.*, 1968; Lewis *et al.*, 1972).

(3) An activation of tissutal lipolysis with overafflux of FFA to the liver and oversynthesis of VLDL and triglycerides (Crepaldi *et al.*, 1978). This abnormality normally coexists with a deficit of clearance in insulin-dependent diabetics.

Thus, hypertriglyceridaemia is often present in diabetics both with decreased or increased insulin secretion, because insulin is able, on the one

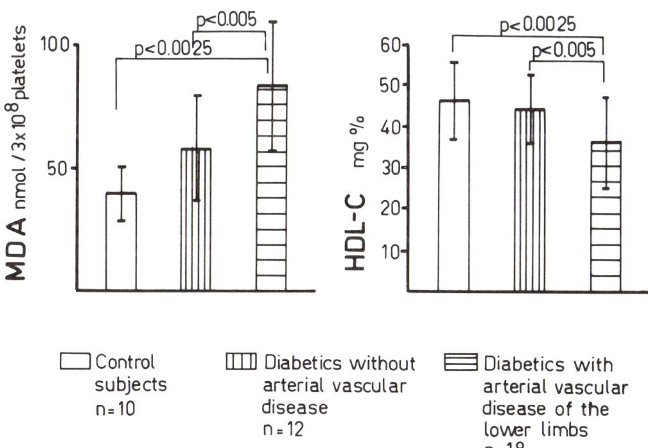

Fig. 5. Diabetics with atherosclerotic vascular disease of the lower limbs in our wards have higher levels of MDA and lower levels of HDL-C in comparison to diabetics without arterial vascular disease and to control subjects.

hand, to stimulate the liver synthesis of VLDL but, on the other hand, is necessary to remove VLDL from plasma. Hypertriglyceridaemia, perhaps, can be an intermediary between diabetes and atherosclerotic vascular complications of this disease (Carlson and Bottiger, 1972; Nikkila *et al.*, 1971).

OBESITY

Mature onset diabetes often goes together with obesity.

In the Framingham study an overweight of 35% was positively correlated with a more frequent incidence of CHD and atherosclerotic brain infarction (Gordon and Kannel, 1973).

Obesity as a pathogenetic intermediary between diabetes and atherosclerosis is still under discussion. This relation is still uncertain; but overweight could stimulate atherosclerotic complications through a more frequent incidence of hypertension as demonstrated in the Framingham (Gordon and Kannel, 1973) and Israel (Medalie, 1979) studies. Furthermore, overweight can act through the presence of hyperinsulinism (Bagdade *et al.*, 1968) and hypertriglyceridaemia (Pelkonen *et al.*, 1977).

In fact it is likely that at least part of the hypertriglyceridaemia associated with obesity is due to high insulin levels promoting triglyceride production, and the high basal insulin levels of obesity will also promote triglyceride synthesis in obese diabetics (Stout, 1979; Bagdade *et al.*, 1967).

Thus obesity could be another aspect of the problem that we have already examined.

HYPERTENSION

In diabetic patients there is a correlation between hyperglycaemia and hypertension (Jarret, 1977) and the same can be said for diabetic children (Florey *et al.*, 1976). Hypertension is found more often in women with diabetes than in diabetic men (Edeiken, 1945) and this rate increases in elderly diabetics (White, 1956).

Among the Du Pont workers hypertension, for each class of age, was more frequent in diabetics than in non-diabetics and in hypertensive diabetics the incidence of CHD was twice as high (Pell and D'Alonzo, 1967). In spite of this, in the Framingham study hypertension was not (Garcia *et al.*, 1974) an independent risk factor for cardiovascular diseases in diabetics.

In the Trabia study (The Research Group ATS RF2 of the Italian National Research Council, 1981) the percentage of hypertensive patients was 15.42% in normal subjects and 38.02% in diabetics (Fig. 6).

Therefore, Ostrander *et al.* (1965) deem that hypertension is not an intermediary between diabetes and atherosclerosis, although Nikkila *et al.* (1971) found a positive correlation between insulin levels after OGTT and arterial hypertension in men aged 31–49 years.

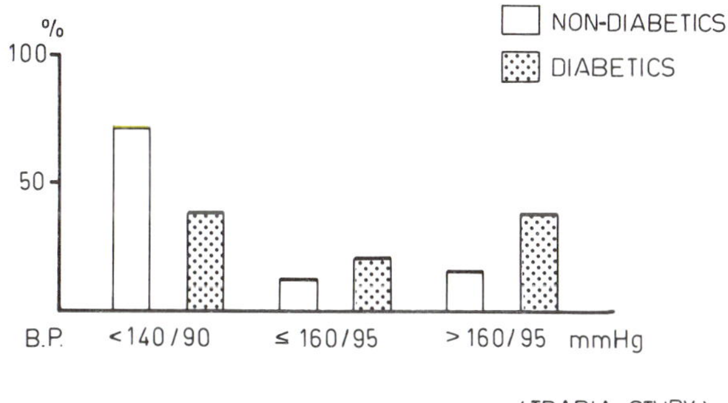

Fig. 6. The prevalence of high blood pressure (> 160/95 mmHg) at first examination was more frequent in diabetics in comparison to non diabetics in Trabia study.

THROMBOPHILIC STATE

Several investigations indicate that in diabetic patients there is an early involvement of the haemostatic system (Neri Serneri, 1980). This involvement could be consequent to a generalized condition of endothelial injury consequent to a state of hypoxia or dismetabolism present in diabetes. If an endothelial lesion exists in early diabetes, this can easily explain the alterations of platelet function, clotting and fibrinolysis present in diabetes mellitus.

Platelets of diabetic patients show a more evident sensibility to aggregating agents (ADP, collagen, epinephrine) (Fig. 7) (Bensoussan *et al.*, 1975; Heath *et al.*, 1971; Sagel *et al.*, 1975). Furthermore, a decrease of platelet half-life has been demonstrated using ^{75}Se (seleniomethionine) labelled platelets (Ferguson *et al.*, 1975) and an enhanced platelet turnover is shown by a reduction of platelet regeneration time according to Stuart *et al.* (1975) (Figs 8 and 9). A consequence of accelerated platelet turnover is an increase in circulating megathrombocytes, younger and functionally more active cells than platelets (Karpatkin, 1972). A possible interpretation of this phenomenon is the existence, in diabetes, of an increased peripheral platelet consumption due to formation of intravascular aggregates (Colwell *et al.*, 1977) with consequent accelerated thrombocytopoiesis (Garg *et al.*, 1972).

The presence of an enhanced platelet function in diabetes mellitus is confirmed by a more evident release of beta thromboglobulin (Fig. 10) (Burrows *et al.*, 1978) and PF4 (Bern, 1978) and by an increased number of circulating platelet aggregates (Neri Serneri, 1980).

The increased platelet aggregation occurs very early in the natural history of the disease because an increased number of platelet aggregates can be observed also in pre-clinical diseases (Neri Serneri, 1980). Platelet hyperaggregability is probably related to the changes of glucose metabolism which are demonstrated even in pre-clinical diabetes, and in part due to an increased activity of the endoperoxide–thromboxane forming metabolic pathway.

In fact, patients with diabetes mellitus, especially if complicated by macro-

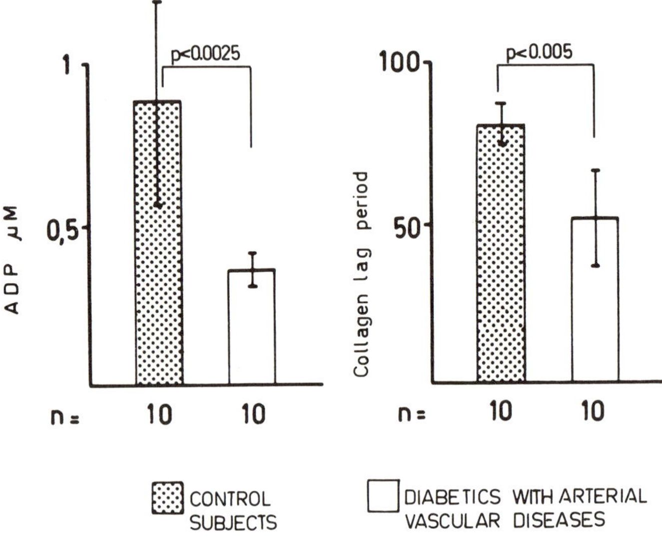

Fig. 7. The threshold dose for irreversible platelet aggregation induction and the collagen lag period are significantly lower in diabetics with atherosclerotic vascular disease of the lower limbs in comparison to control subjects.

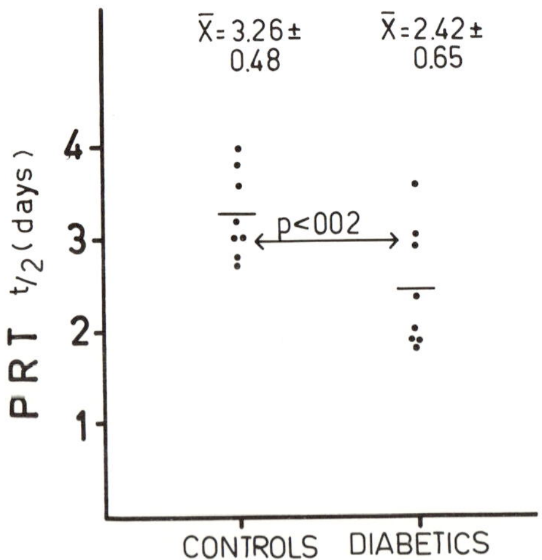

Fig. 8. Platelet regeneration time is significantly shorter in diabetics than in control subjects.

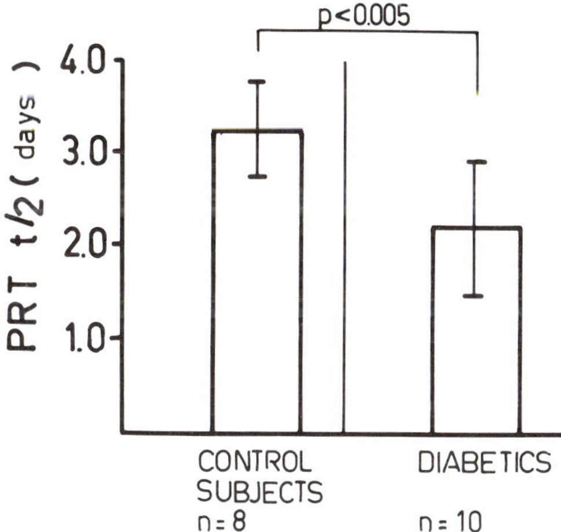

Fig. 9. Platelet regeneration time is significantly shorter in diabetics with CHD than in controls.

angiopathy, show an increased formation of malondialdehyde when platelets are stimulated by thrombin (Neri Serneri, 1980) and an enhanced level of circulation TxB2.

Recently we have demonstrated that in diabetes mellitus there is an increased production of thromboxane and a raised release of beta thromboglobulin and PF4 (Fig. 10) with a decreased platelet sensitivity to prostacyclin with small levels of HDL-CT. These findings seem to indicate that an alteration of platelet function occurs in diabetic patients (Davì *et al.*, in press).

HDL-cholesterol reduced levels together with an increased platelet thromboxane production, suggest that the formation of arachidonic acid metabolites is increased, perhaps in relation to the different phospholipid/cholesterol ratio in platelet membrane.

In patients with clinical diabetes and in those with vascular atherosclerotic complications, the enhanced platelet formation is due, in addition to the enhanced malondialdehyde biosynthetic pathway, to a platelet aggregating plasmatic activity (Kwaan *et al.*, 1972).

In experimental diabetes there is also a decreased synthesis of release of PGI_2 (Harrison *et al.*, 1978), a substance which inhibits adhesion and aggregation of platelets to the endothelium (Vane, 1976).

The decreased production of PGI_2 and the increased levels of TxB2 indicate the existence, in diabetes, of an altered balance between the two metabolic pathways derived from arachidonic acid.

It has also recently been shown that platelets of diabetics have a low sensibility to the anti-aggregating effect of PGI_2 (Betteridge *et al.*, 1980).

Furthermore, there is, in diabetes, an enhanced coagulation activity demonstrated by increased levels of fibrinopeptide A especially in patients with latent diabetes, with clinical diabetes and with complicated diabetes, but not in pre-diabetics (Neri Serneri, 1980).

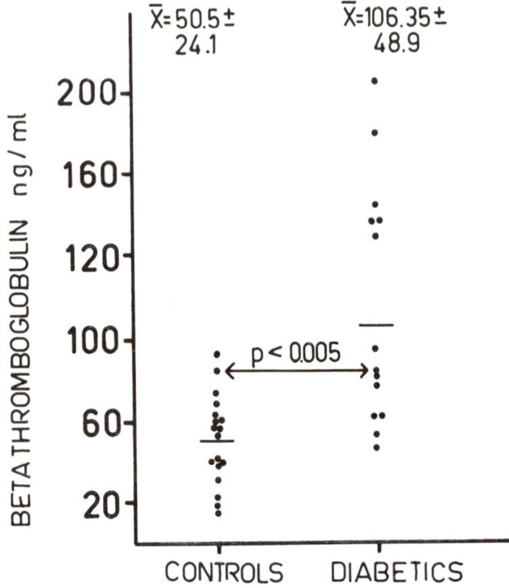

Fig. 10. Plasmatic levels of beta thromboglobulin are significantly higher in diabetics in comparison to control subjects.

Disorders of the whole activity of factor VIII have been shown in (Bensoussan *et al.*, 1975; Neri Serneri, 1980) clinical and complicated diabetes, whereas in latent diabetes there is an increase of vW:F VIII R and AG:F VIII R (Neri Serneri, 1980).

The pathogenetic significance of these findings is uncertain. Perhaps, increased levels of vWF could be consequent to an enhanced release of this factor by damaged endothelial cells (Coller *et al.*, 1978; Gensini *et al.*, 1979).

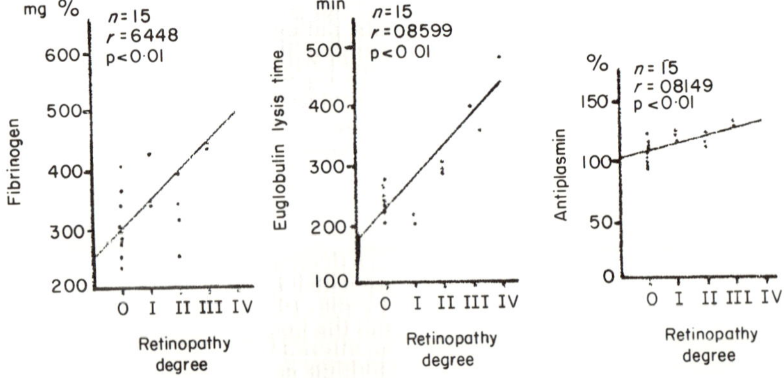

Fig. 11. In diabetic patients with microangiopathy there is a significant correlation between the retinopathy degree and the fibrinogen and antiplasmin levels and the euglobulin lysis time.

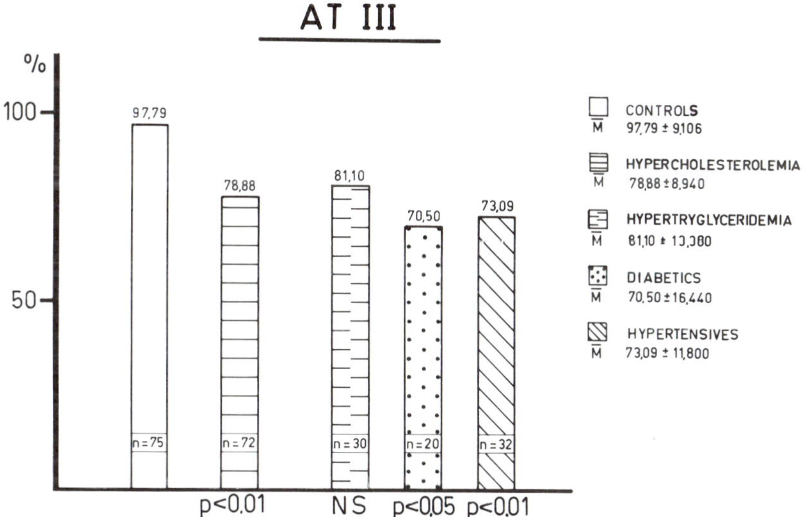

Fig. 12. Diabetics in our wards show antithrombin III lower levels in comparison to control subjects.

Furthermore, there are, in diabetes, increased concentrations of fibrinogen (Fig. 11) (Strano *et al.*, 1980), decreased levels of biological activity of AT III (Fig. 12) and a depression of blood fibrinolytic activity (Fig. 13) especially in diabetes associated with obesity or hyperlipoproteinaemia (Novo *et al.*, 1978) and an increase of antiplasmin activity (Strano *et al.*, 1980) (Fig. 14).

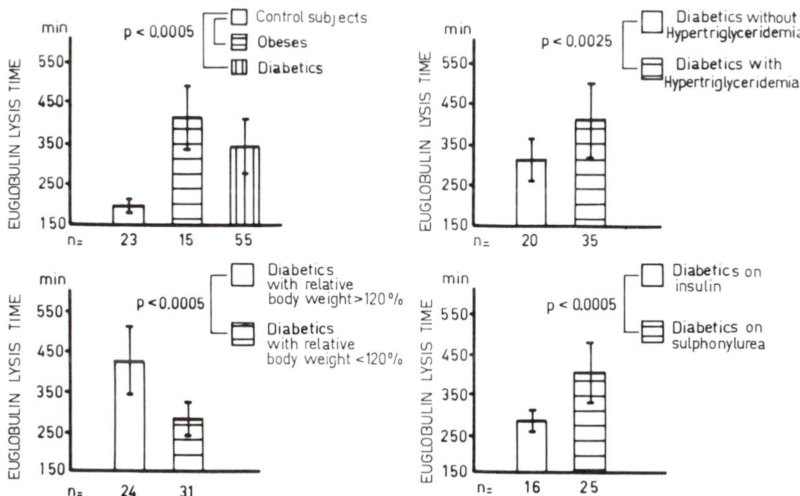

Fig. 13. Euglobulin lysis time is significantly higher and fibrinolysis depressed in diabetics, especially if hypertriglyceridemia or overweight is associated; therefore, diabetics on sulphonylurea show a more depressed fibrinolysis.

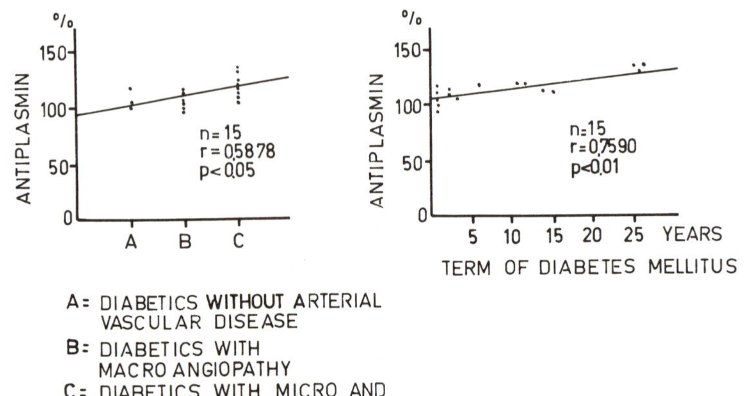

Fig. 14. Antiplasmin activity is significantly correlated with the term of diabetes mellitus.

CONCLUSIONS

Clinically, epidemiological and pathological studies confirm that diabetes goes together with an enhanced frequency of vascular complications in cerebral, coronary and peripheral districts.

Hyperglycaemia in itself does not seem to be an important risk factor for vascular complications of diabetes, whereas recent studies point to insulinism as a possible promoting factor for macroangiopathy in diabetes (Stout, 1979).

Insulinism, in fact, is often present in mature diabetes which is associated with obesity; but on the other hand, even in insulin-dependent diabetics, and therefore insulin-treated, there are often abnormal circulating levels of insulin (Stout, 1979). And hyperinsulinism can favour atherosclerosis both directly (Stout, 1979) and through the determination of lipidic metabolism alterations as we have found in our macroangiopathic diabetic patients (Notarbartolo *et al.*, in press).

Moreover, almost all the risk factors for atherosclerosis are present in diabetics in higher percentage than in non-diabetics. And though none of these factors is in itself an independent risk factor for the appearance of macrovascular complications in diabetes it is, nevertheless, possible that the sum of these risk factors may increase the possibility of developing a diabetic macroangiopathy.

Of importance is the frequent finding, in diabetic patients, of a thrombo philic syndrome with an enhanced platelet function. Such alterations of the haemostatic balance could accelerate the onset of progression of athero-sclerotic lesions and predispose to thrombotic complications. Furthermore, we must underline that platelet function alterations appear very early in diabetes and seem thus determined to diabetes itself.

It is likely that each factor analysed plays a role in the pathogenesis of diabetic macroangiopathy.

Further studies should take into account all these factors and, through a multivariate analysis, should determine the extent to which each factor increases the probability of a macroangiopathy in diabetes.

REFERENCES

Avogaro, P., Capri, C., Cazzolato, G. and Paris, M. (1972). Alterazioni lipidemiche nel diabete mellito. *Acta Diabetologica Latina* **9**, 540.

Bagdade, J. D., Bierman, E. L., Porte, D. R. (1967). The significance of basal insulin levels in evaluation of the insulin response to glucose in diabetic and nondiabetic subjects. *Journal of Clinical Investigation* **46**, 1549.

Bagdade, J. D., Porte, D. J. and Bierman, E. L. (1968). Acute insulin withdrawal and regulation of plasma triglyceride removal in diabetic subjects. *Diabetes* **17**, 127.

Bensoussan, D., Levy-Toledano, S., Passa, Caen, J. and Canivet, J. (1975). Platelet hyperaggregation and increased plasma levels of von Willebrand factor in diabetics with retinopathy. *Diabetologia* **12**, 307.

Berchtold, P., Bjorntorp, P., Gustavson, A., Lindholm, B. and Tibblin, G. (1972). Glucose tolerance, plasma insulin and lipid in relation to adipose tissue cellularity in men after myocardial infarction. *Acta Medica Scandinavica* **191**, 35.

Bern, M. M. (1978). Platelet function in diabetes mellitus. *Diabetes* **27**, 342.

Betteridge, D. J., El Tahir, K. E. H., Reckless, J. P. D. and Williams, K. I. (1980). A study of the sensitivity of platelets from patients with diabetes mellitus to inhibition of ADP-induced aggregation by prostacyclin. *Clinical Science* **59**, 24.

Boden, G. (1971). Hormonal and metabolic disturbances during acute and subacute myocardial infarction in man. *Diabetologia* **7**, 240.

Burrows, A. W., Chavin, S. J. and Hockaday, T. D. R. (1978). Plasma thrombo-globulin concentrations in diabetes mellitus. *Lancet* **1**, 235.

Carlson, L. A. and Bottiger, L. E. (1972). Ischaemic heart disease in relation to fasting values of plasma triglycerides and cholesterol. *Lancet* **1**, 865.

Cerasi, E., Efendic, S. and Luft, R. (1973). Dose-response relation between plasma insulin and blood glucose levels during oral glucose loads in prediabetic and diabetic subjects. *Lancet* **1**, 794

Chiles, R. and Tzagournis, M. (1970). Excessive serum insulin response to oral glucose in obesity and mild diabetes. Study in 501 patients. *Diabetes* **19**, 458.

Christiansen, I. and Decher, T. (1968). Glucose tolerance, plasma lipids and serum insulin in patients with ischemic heart disease. *Acta Medica Scandinavica* **184**, 283.

Coller, B. S., Frank, R. N., Milton, R. C. and Gramnick, H. R. (1978). Plasma co-factor of platelet function: correlation with diabetic retinopathy and haemo-globin A. *Annals of Internal Medicine* **88**, 311.

Colwell, J. A. and Lein, A. (1967) Diminished insulin response to hyperglycemia in prediabetes and diabetes. *Diabetes* **16**, 560.

Colwell, J. A., Sagel, J., Crook, L., Chambers, A. and Laimins, M. (1977). Correla-tion of platelet aggregation, plasma factor activity and megathrombocytes in dia-betic subjects with and without vascular disease. *Metabolism* **26**, 279.

Crepaldi, G., Tiengo, A., Segato, T. and Molinari, M. (1978). Hyperlipidaemia and Diabetes. *In* "Selected Topics in Diabetes", p. 141. Cordani, Milan.

Crofford D. (1975). "Report of the National Commission on Diabetes". Dhew. Pus. No. (NIH), 76. Government Printing Office, Washington D.C.

Cruz, A. B., Amatuzio, D. S., Grande, F. and Hay, L. J. (1961). Effect of intrarterial insulin on tissue cholesterol and fatty acids in alloxandiabetic dogs. *Circulation Research* **9**, 39.

Danowski, T. S., Lombardo, Y. B., Mendelsohn, L. V., Corredor, D. G., Morgan, C. R. and Sabeh, G. (1969). Insulin patterns prior to and after onset of diabetes. *Metabolism* **18**, 731.

Davì, G., Rini, G. B., Averna, M. R., Novo, S., Di Fede, G., Pinto, A., Notarbartolo, A. and Strano, A. (1981). Correlation between platelet function and apo/lipoproteins changes in complicated diabetes mellitus. *In* "3rd European Symposium on Metabolism". Padua, May 28–30 (In press).

Davì, G., Novo, S., Riolo, F., Mendola, G., Avellone, G., Muzzo, P. and Russotto, M. (1982). Formazione di malondialdeide piastrinica in pazienti con diabete mellito. *Il Progresso Medico.*

Duff, G. L. and McMillan, G. C. (1949). The effect of alloxan diabetes on experimental atherosclerosis in the rabbit. I. The inhibition of experimental atherosclerosis in alloxan diabetes. II. The effect of alloxan diabetes on the regression of experimental cholesterol atherosclerosis. *Journal of Experimental Medicine* **89**, 611.

Duff, G. L., Brechin, J. H. and Kinkelstein, W. E. (1954). The effect of alloxan diabetes on experimental cholesterol atherosclerosis in the rabbit. *Journal of Experimental Medicine* **100**, 371.

Edeiken, J. (1945). Diabetes mellitus as observed in 100 cases for 10 or more years: cardiac studies. *American Journal of the Medical Sciences* **209**, 8.

Elmfeldt, D., Wilhelmsen, L., Wedel, H., Vedin, A., Wilhelmsson, C. and Tiblin, G. (1976). Primary risk factors in patients with myocardial infarction. *American Heart Journal* **91**, 412.

Enger, S. C. and Ritland, S. (1973). Glucose tolerance, insulin release and lipoprotein pattern in patients with myocardial infarction. *Acta Medica Scandinavica* **194**, 97.

Epstein, F. H. (1967a). Hyperglycemia. A risk factor in coronary heart disease. *Circulation* **36**, 609.

Epstein, F. H. (1967b). Some uses of prospective observations in the Tecumseh Community Health Study. *Proceedings of the Royal Society of Medicine* **60**, 55.

Epstein, F. H. (1976). Diabete e arteriosclerosi: aspetti epidemiologici. *Giornale dell'Arteriosclerosi* **14**, 107.

Fajans, S. S., Taylor, C. I., Floyd, J. C. and Conn, J. W. (1974). Some aspects of the natural history of diabetes mellitus. *In* "Diabetes" (W. J. Malaisse and J. Pirat, Eds), p. 329. Excerta Medica, Amsterdam.

Falsetti, H. L., Schnatz, J. D., Greene, D. G. and Bunnell, I. L. (1970). Serum lipids and glucose tolerance in angiographically proved coronary artery disease. *Chest* **58**, 111.

Fedele, D., Baggio, G. and Crepaldi, G. (1980a). Diabete e rischio aterogeno. *Giornale dell'Arteriosclerosi* **18**, 89.

Fedele, D., Fellin, R., Lapolla, A., Baggio, G., Baiocchi, M. R., Frigato, T. and Tiengo, A. (1980b). Lipidi plasmatici e controllo metabolico nella malattia diabetica. *In* "Emoglobina Glicosilata e Diabete Mellito" (G. Erle, Ed.), p. 121. Vicenza, 1980.

Ferguson, J. C., Mackay, N., Philip, J. A. D. and Sumner, D. J. (1975). Determination of platelet and fibrinogen half life with 75 Se(seleniomethionine): studies in normal and diabetic patients. *Clinical Science and Molecular Medicine* **49**, 115.

Florey, C. V., Milner, R. D. G. and Miall, W. E. (1972). Insulin excess as the initial lesion in diabetes. *Lancet* **2**, 227.

Florey, C. V., Uppal, S. and Lowy, C. (1976). Relation between blood pressure, weight and plasma sugar and serum insulin levels in schoolchildren aged 9–12 years in Westland, Holland. *British Medical Journal* **1**, 1368.

Fuller, J. H., McCartney, P. and Colwell, L. M. (1976). Blood sugar as a predictor for coronary heart disease. *Diabetologica* **2**, 343.

Gabbay, K. H. (1973). The sorbitol pathway and the complications of diabetes. *New England Journal of Medicine* **288**, 831.
Garcia, M. J., McNamara, P. M., Gordon, T. and Mannel, W. B. (1974). Morbidity and mortality in diabetics in the Framingham population. Sixteen year follow-up study. *Diabetes* **23**, 105.
Garg, S. K., Lackner, H. and Karpatkin, S. (1972). The increased percentage of megathrombocytes in various clinical disorders. *Annals of Internal Medicine* **77**, 361.
Gensini, G. F., Abbate, T., Favilla, S. and Neri Serneri, G. G. (1979). Changes of platelet function and blood clotting in diabetes mellitus. *Thrombosis et Diathesis Haemorrhagica* **42**, 983.
Gertler, M. M., Leetma, H. E., Saluste, E., Rosenberger, J. L. and Guthier, R. G. (1972). Ischemic heart disease: insulin, carbohydrate and lipid interrelationships. *Circulation* **46**, 103.
Gordon, T. and Kannel, W. B. (1973). The effects of overweight on cardiovascular disease. *Geriatrics* **28**, 80.
Gordon, T., Garcia-Palmieri, M. R., Kagan, A., Kannel, W. B. and Schiffman, J. (1974). Differences in coronary heart disease in Framingham, Honolulu and Puerto Rico. *Journal of Chronic Diseases* **27**, 329.
Grodsky, G. M., Karam, J. H., Pavlatos, F. C. and Forsham, P. H. (1965). Serum insulin response to a glucose load in prediabetic subjects. *Lancet* **1**, 290.
Harrison, H. E., Reece, H. A. and Johnson, M. (1978). Effects of insulin treatment on prostacyclin in experimental diabetes. *Life Sciences* **23**, 351.
Heath, H., Bridgen, W. D., Canever, J. V., Pollock, J., Hunter, P. R., Kelsey, J. and Bloom, A. (1971). Platelet adhesiveness and aggregation in relation to diabetic retinopathy. *Diabetologia* **7**, 308.
Heinle, R. A., Levy, R. I., Frederickson, D. S. and Gorlin, R. (1969). Lipid and carbohydrate abnormalities in patients with angiographically documented coronary artery disease. *American Journal of Cardiology* **24**, 178.
Ingelfinger, J. A., Bennet, P. H., Liebow, I. M. and Miller, M. (1976). Coronary heart disease in the Pima Indians. Electrocardiographic findings and post-mortem evidence of myocardial infarction in a population with a high prevalence of diabetes mellitus. *Diabetes* **25**, 561.
Jackson, W. P. U., Von Mieghem, W. and Keller, P. (1972). Insulin excess as the initial lesion in diabetes. *Lancet* **1**, 1040.
Jarret, R. J. (1977). Diabetes and the heart atherosclerosis. *Clinics in Endocrinology and Metabolism* **6**, 389.
Jarret, R. J. and Keen, H. (1975). Diabetes and atherosclerosis. *In* "Complications of Diabetes" (H. Keen and R. J. Jarret, Eds), p. 179. Arnold, London.
Johansen, K. (1972). Normal initial plasma insulin response in mild diabetes. *Metabolism* **21**, 1177.
Karpatkin, S. (1972). Biochemical and clinical aspects of megathrombocytes. *Annals of New York Academy of Sciences* **201**, 262.
Kasyap, M. L., Magill, F., Rosas, L. and Hoffmann, M. M. (1970). Insulin and non esterified fatty acid metabolism in asymptomatic diabetes and atherosclerotic subjects. *Canadian Medical Association Journal* **102**, 1165.
Keen, H. (1971). Factor influencing the prognosis of atherosclerosis in the diabetic. *Acta Diabetologica Latina* **8**, Suppl. 1, 444.
Keen, H. and Jarret, R. J. (1973). Macroangiopathy — its presence in asymptomatic diabetes. *Archives of Metabolic Disorders* **2**, Suppl., 3.
Kingsbury, K. J. (1966). The relationship between glucose tolerance and atherosclerotic vascular disease. *Lancet* **2**, 1374.
Kwaan, H. C., Colwell, J. A. and Suwanwela, N. (1972). Disseminated intravascular

coagulation in diabetes mellitus with reference to the role of increased platelet aggregation. *Diabetes* **21**, 108.
Lewis, B., Mancini, M., Mattoch, M., Chait, A. and Russel Fraser, T. (1972). Plasma triglyceride and fatty acid metabolism in diabetes mellitus. *European Journal of Clinical Investigation* **2**, 445.
McGill, H. C. and Holman, R. L. (1949). The influence of alloxan diabetes on cholesterol atherosclerosis in the rabbit. *Proceedings of the Society of Experimental Biology and Medicine* **72**, 72.
Mahler, R. (1971). The effect of diabetes and insulin on biochemical reaction of the arterial wall. *Acta Diabetologica Latina* **8**, Suppl. 1, 68.
Malherbe, C., De Gasparo, M., Berthet, P., De Hertogh, R. and Hoet, J. J. (1971). The pattern of plasma insulin response to glucose in patients with previous myocardial infarction. The respective effects of age and disease. *European Journal of Clinical Investigation* **1**, 265.
Medalie, J. H. (1979). Risk factors other than hyperglycemia in diabetic macrovascular disease. *Diabetes Care* **2**, 77.
Morrison, A. D., Clements, R. S. and Winegrad, A. I. (1972). Effects of elevated glucose concentrations on the metabolism of the aortic wall. *Journal of Clinical Investigation* **51**, 3114.
Neri Serneri, G. G. (1980). La sindrome trombofilica della malattia diabetica. Bendiconti della Società Italiana di Medicina Interna, Atta 80° Congresso, p. 552.
Nikkila, E. A. and Hormila, P. (1978). Serum lipids and lipoproteins in insulin treated diabetes. *Diabetes* **27**, 1078.
Nikkila, E. A., Pyorala, K. and Taskinen, M. R. (1971). Role of insulinemia in arterial disease. *Acta Diabetologica Latina* **8**, Suppl. 1, 56.
Nikkila, E. A., Miettinen, T. A., Vesenne, M. R. and Pelkonen, R. (1965). Plasma insulin in coronary heart disease. *Lancet* **2**, 508.
Notarbartolo. A., Rini, G. B., Averna, M. R., Montalto, G., Di Fede, G., Fiore, M., Lodato, G. and Novo, S. Lipoprotein, apoprotein and insulin behaviour in not treated diabetic patients. *Acta Diabetologica Latina* (In press).
Novo, S., Avellone, G., Pinto, A. and Davi, G. (1978). Blood fibrinolysis in atherosclerosis and in high risk metabolic disorders. *In* "Proceedings of European Symposium on Coagulation, Fibrinolysis, Platelet Aggregation and Atherosclerosis", p. 249, CEPI, Rome.
Ostrander, L. D., Francis, T., Hayner, N. S., Kjelsberg, M. O. and Epstein, F. H. (1965). The relationship of cardio-vascular disease with hyperglycemia. *Annals of Internal Medicine* **62**, 1170.
Ostrander, L. D., Block, W. C., Lamphiear, D. E. and Epstein, F. H. (1973). Altered carbohydrate and lipid metabolism and coronary heart disease among men in Tecumseh, Michigan. *In* "Second Symposium on Early Diabetes" (R. A. Camerini Davalos, Ed.), Academic Press, London and New York.
Patrassi, G. and Crepaldi, G. (1971). Le iperlipoproteinemie. Rendiconti della Società Italiana di Medicina Interna, Atti 72° Congresso.
Pelkonen, R., Nikkila, E. A., Koskinen, S., Penttinen, K. and Sarina, S. (1977). Association of serum lipid and obesity with cardiovascular mortality. *British Medical Journal* **2**, 1185.
Pell, S. and D'Alonzo, C. A. (1967). Some aspects of hypertension in diabetes mellitus. *Journal of the American Medical Association* **202**, 10.
Peters, N. and Hales, C. N. (1965). Plasma insulin concentrations after myocardial infarction. *Lancet* **1**, 1144.
Pyke, D. A., Cassar, J., Todd, J. and Taylor, K. W. (1970). Glucose tolerance and serum insulin in identical twins of diabetics. *British Medical Journal* **4**, 649.

Reaven, G. M., Lerner, R. L., Stern, M. P. and Farquhar, J. W. (1967). Role of insulin in endogenous hypertriglyceridemia. *Journal of Clinical Investigation* **46**, 1756.

Reaven, G. M., Shen, S. W., Silvers, A. and Farquhar, J. W. (1971). Is there a delay in the plasma insulin response of patients with chemical diabetes mellitus? *Diabetes* **20**, 416.

Ricketts, H. T., Cherry, R. A. and Kirsteins, L. (1966). Biochemical studies of prediabetes. *Diabetes* **15**, 880.

Rini, G. B., Averna, M. R., Di Fede, G., Montalto, G., Fiore, M. and Notarbartolo, A. (1980). Prevalenza ed incidenza di cardiopatie in diabetici di due popolazioni lavorative di Palermo: osservazioni preliminari. *In* "VIII Congresso Nazionale della Società Italiana di Diabetologia". Napoli, 4–7 Maggio 1980.

Ross, R. and Glomset, J. A. (1976). The pathogenesis of atherosclerosis. *New England Journal of Medicine* **295**, 369, 420.

Sagel, J., Colwell, J. A., Crook, L. and Laimins, M. (1975). Increased platelet aggregation in early diabetes mellitus. *Annals of Internal Medicine* **82**, 733.

Schenk, K. E., Quabbe, H. J., Bittner, H., Sasse, H. and Schroder, R. (1974). Insulin-sekretion und coronare Herzerkrankung. *Klinische Wochenschrift* **52**, 1053.

Seltzer, H. S., Allen, E. W., Herron, A. L. Jr. and Brennan, M. T. (1967). Insulin secretion in response to glycemic stimulus: relation of delayed initial release to carbohydrate intolerance in mild diabetes mellitus. *Journal of Clinical Investigation* **46**, 323.

Serrado-Rios, M., Ramos, F., Rodriguez-Minon, J. C. and Vivanco, F. (1970). Studies in prediabetes. Insulin response to oral glucose, intravenous tolbutamide and rapid intravenous glucose infusion in genetic prediabetes. *Diabetologia* **6**, 392.

Siperstein, M. D., Unger, R. H. and Madison, L. L. (1973). Studies of muscle capillary basement membranes in normal subjects, diabetic and prediabetic patients. *Journal of Clinical Investigation* **47**.

Sloan, J. M., Mackay, J. S. and Sheridan, B. (1970). Glucose tolerance and insulin response in atherosclerosis. *British Medical Journal* **4**, 586.

Sorge, F., Schwartzkopf, W. and Neuhaus, G. A. (1976). Insulin response to oral glucose in patients with a previous myocardial infarction and in patients with peripheral vascular disease. *Diabetes* **25**, 586.

Stalmer, R., Stamler, J., Dyer, A., Cooper, R., Collette, P., Berkson, D. M., Lindberg, H. A., Stevens, E., Schoenberger, J. A., Shekelle, R. B., Paul, O., Lepper, M., Garside, D., Tokich, T. and Hoeksema, R. (1979). Asymptomatic hyperglycemia and cardiovascular diseases in the Chicago Epidemiological Studies. *Diabetes Care* **2**, 142.

Stamler, J. (1975). Diet-related risk factors for human atherosclerosis: hyperlipidemia, hypertension, hyperglycemia — current status. *In* "Diet and Atherosclerosis" (C. Sirtori, G. Ricci and S. Gorini, Eds), p. 125. Plenum, New York and London.

Stamler, J., Pick, R. and Katz, L. M. (1980). Effects of insulin in the induction and regression of atherosclerosis in the chick. *Circulation Research* **8**, 572.

Stout, R. W. (1968). Insulin-stimulated lipogenesis in arterial tissue in relation to diabetes and atheroma. *Lancet* **2**, 702.

Stout, R. W. (1970). Development of vascular lesions in insulin-treated animals fed a normal diet. *British Medical Journal* **3**, 685.

Stout, R. W. (1979). Diabetes and atherosclerosis: the role of insulin. *Diabetologia* **16**, 141.

Stout. R. W., Bierman, E. L. and Ross, L. (1975). The effect of insulin on the proliferation of cultured primate arterial smooth muscle cells. *Circulation Research* **36**, 319.

Strandness, D. W., Priest, R. W. and Gibbons, G. E. (1964). Compared clinical and pathological study of diabetic and non diabetic peripheral arterial disease. *Diabetes* **13**, 336.

Strano, A., Novo, S., Davi, G. and Avellone, G. (1980). La sindrome trombofilica della malattia diabetica: studio della fibrinolisi. Rendiconti della Società Italiana di Medicina Interna, Atti 80° Congresso, p. 558.

Stuart, M. J., Murphy, S. and Oski, F. A. (1975). A simple non radioisotope technic for determination of platelet life-span. *New England Journal of Medicine* **292**, 1310.

The Research Group ATS RF2 of the Italian National Research Council (1981). Distribution of some risk factors for atherosclerosis in nine Italian population samples. *American Journal of Epidemiology* **113**, 338.

Tzagournis, M., Seidensticker, J. F. and Hamin, G. I. (1967). Serum insulin, carbohydrate and lipid abnormalities in patients with premature coronary heart disease. *Annals of Internal Medicine* **67**, 42.

U.S. Public Health Service (1971). The Framingham Study: an epidemiological investigation of cardiovascular disease (Section 27): coronary heart disease, atherothrombotic brain infarction, intermittent claudication — a multivariate analysis of some factors related to their incidence — Framingham Study, 16 years follow-up. United States Government Printing Office, Washington D.C., May 1971.

Vane, J. R. (1976). An enzyme isolated from arteries transforms prostaglandin endoperoxides to an unstable substance that inhibit platelet aggregation. *Nature (London)* **263**, 663.

Wahl, P., Hasslicher, Ch. and Vollmar, J. (1974). Diabetes und hyperlipoproteinemien. *Deutsche Medizinisches Wochenschrift* **99**, 2158.

Wahlberg, F. and Thomasson, B. (1968). Glucose tolerance in ischaemic cardiovascular disease. *In* "Carbohydrate Metabolism and its Disorders" (F. Dickens, P. J. Radle and W. J. Whelen, Eds), p. 185, Academic Press, London and New York.

Welborn, T. A., Stenhouse, N. S., Johnstone, C. G. (1969). Factors determining serum insulin response in a population sample. Preliminary Communication. *Diabetologia* **5**, 263.

White, P. (1956). Natural course and prognosis of juvenile diabetes. *Diabetes* **5**, 445.

Wise, P. H. and Yeates, R. A. (1978). Effects of therapy on plasma — high density lipoprotein cholesterol concentration in diabetes mellitus. *Lancet* **2**, 66.

Woolf, N. (1971). Diabetes and atherosclerosis. *Acta Diabetologica Latina* **8**, Suppl. 1, 14.

DIABETES AND LOWER LIMB ARTERIAL DISEASE: THE MEDICAL STANDPOINT

P. J. Guillausseau[1], E. Dupuy[2], C. Guillausseau[3], L. Drouet[2], A. M. Wild[2], A. Basdevant[3], H. D. Nahum[1], E. Kaloustian[1], A. Warnet[1] and J. Lubetzki[1]

Department of Internal Medicine and Diabetology[1], Department of Haematology, Hôpital Lariboisière[2] and Department of Internal Medicine and Nutrition, Hotel Dieu[3], Paris, France

Vascular disease related to diabetes mellitus represents today the most important cause underlying the morbidity and mortality in the diabetic population. Diabetes mellitus leads to microangiopathy — with high incidence of blindness and renal failure in long-term patients — and to macroangiopathy — namely, atherosclerosis.

The Framingham study (Kannel and McGee, 1979) indicates a twofold increase of cardiovascular disease in men and a threefold increase in women when compared with non-diabetics. The lower limb arterial disease accounts for high mortality. In a series of 1.555 autopsies of diabetics, Bell (1952) found about 50% of vascular death, with gangrene in 25.8% of these cases. In a personal study, lower limb arteriopathy accounts for 11% of all causes of death (Lubetzki and Chebat, 1970). Clinical studies offer similar results: in a series of 2.050 diabetic patients, we demonstrated lower limb macroangiopathy in 8.8% of them (Lubetzki and Chebat, 1970).

The pathological lesions are quite different from those of non-diabetics: more distal with tibial and popliteal involvement and often with multisegmental extension. The incidence of gangrene, often bilateral, is also higher, as much as fortyfold (Bell, 1952). Atherosclerosis in diabetics occurs at an earlier age, its evolution is more rapid and severe. All kinds of this hetero-

Serono Symposium No. 44, "Peripheral Arterial Diseases: Medical and Surgical Problems", edited by S. Stipa and A. Cavallaro, 1982. Academic Press, London and New York.

geneous disease are involved — insulin and non-insulin requiring patients or even patients with impaired glucose tolerance.

Before considering medical treatment, we think it is helpful to review the main aspects of the pathogenesis of the large vessel disease in diabetes mellitus.

The deleterious role of hyperglycaemia is now well established in the progression of the retinal and glomerular angiopathy and of the neuropathy (Pirart, 1977). However its place is less obvious so far as macroangiopathy (coronary disease or lower limb arteriopathy) is concerned (Pirari, 1977). These findings must be brought together with those of the Whitehall study (Fuller *et al.*, 1980) which demonstrates a high incidence of macroangiopathy in the intolerant glucose group (IGT) (defined as 2-h post-glucose blood sugar between 7.8 and 11 mM), whereas higher values, well above 11 mM, are needed for the occurrence of retinal damages. These apparently conflicting observations are probably connected by peripheral hyperinsulinism (Stout, 1979), encountered as well in IGT (delayed insulin secretion with exaggerated late response) as in insulin-treated diabetics. In this last occurrence, insulin administration route is an unphysiological one, as high peripheral insulin levels are required to achieve effective portal insulin concentrations.

The cellular basis implicated to pathogenesis of atherosclerosis have been extensively reviewed (Ganda, 1980). The first event in the development of the fibrous plaque, according to Ross and Glomset (1976) is the disruption of the endothelial barrier, with desquamation of the cells and increased permeability. In diabetic vessels, this endothelial injury may be related to numerous factors, among them hypertension, increased shear stress, hyperlipidemia and osmotic changes related to hyperglycaemic state. The key event is the following step: the medial smooth muscle cells then proliferate and migrate through the internal elastic lamina. Many factors are known to stimulate smooth cell proliferation, including insulin (Stout, 1979), the platelet derived growth factor of PDSF (Ross *et al.*, 1974) and growth hormone (Ledet, 1976), the impairment of which is well demonstrated in diabetics in poor control. This step is followed by deposition of cholesterol and interstitial material (collagen, elastic fibres and proteoglycans). This phenomenon is favoured by the frequent lipoprotein abnormalities encountered in diabetic population. An increase of low density lipoproteins (LDL) or very low density lipoproteins (VLDL) or both is often seen in diabetics (Beach *et al.*, 1979; Saudek and Eder, 1979; Reckless *et al.*, 1978), so much more as metabolic control is poor (Nikkila and Hormila, 1978). On the other hand, high density lipoproteins (HDL) have a protective role against cholesterol deposition (Witzum and Schonfeld, 1979). HDL and HDL-cholesterol low values represent vascular risk factors as shown by the Framingham study (Gorton *et al.*, 1977). Conflicting results have been published in diabetes (Beach *et al.*, 1979; Reckless *et al.*, 1978; Nikkila and Hormila, 1978; Elkeles *et al.*, 1978). A fair control seems to increase HDL-cholesterol levels (Lopez-Virella *et al.*, 1977) but this fact needs to be confirmed. Damaged parietal wall permits the formation of microthrombi (which may flow away in the bloodstream and cause microembolism in the peripheral vascular bed) or macro-thrombi responsible of acute ischaemia or gangrene.

Many studies deal with haemostasis and diabetes (Bensoussan *et al.*, 1976; Colwell *et al.*, 1976; Bern, 1978; Dupuy *et al.*, 1979), factor VIII (Lufkin *et al.*, 1979), platelets–vessel walls interactions and fibrinolysis (Almer and Pandolfi, 1976). The place of the antagonist components of the prostaglandin system — prostacyclin and thromboxan A_2 seems to be an important one (Moncada and Vane, 1979). However clinico-haematological correlations are searched in only a few studies (Badawi *et al.*, 1970), and the attention is mainly focused upon retinopathy. The usual lack of non-diabetic controls bearing the same vascular lesions must be stressed. Comparison between diabetic patients with lower limb arteriopathy and non-diabetics with similar vascular lesions is presented here.

SUBJECTS AND METHODS

We studied 27 diabetics with lower limb vascular disease (24 insulin-treated and three with oral treatment), 11 non-diabetic patients with the same kind of lesions. One-hundred-and-sixty-three normal controls were also studied for platelet aggregation tests and 15 normal subjects for factor VIII studies. Clinical features are summarized in Tables I and II.

Platelet aggregation was studied according to the method of Born as previously described (Dupuy *et al.*, 1979). Aggregation was induced by ADP (final concentration 0.6 and 1.2 μM) and collagen (final concentration 8 μg ml^{-1}). The following parameters were studied: maximal aggregation intensity with ADP (0.6 and 1.2 μM) and collagen, velocity with ADP (0.6 and 1.2 μM) and disaggregation pattern with the low ADP concentration. Factor VIII_{AHF}

Table I. Clinical data of the subjects studied.

	Diabetics with lower limb arteriopathy	Controls	Non-diabetics with lower limb arteriopathy
n	27	163	11
Age (mean ± SD) (years)	58.5 ± 13.5	46.3 ± 8.9	54.7 ± 12.1
Age range	28–83	25–63	33–71

Table II. Diabetic patients: subgroups.

	Grade I–III	Grade IV (gangrene)
n	18	9
Age (mean ± SD)	53.9 ± 13.1	67.9 ± 8

was determined by the one-stage assay using deficient factor VIII substrate (Precibio Laboratories), factor $VIII_{RA\text{-}VWF}$ according to the Laurell method (antisera anti-factor VIII provided by Behring Laboratories).

Statistical analysis was performed with chi-square test (with Yates correction if appropriate), unpaired Student t-test and Wilcoxon test.

RESULTS

In diabetics (Fig. 1), with low dose ADP, velocity is higher than in normal controls but does not differ from non-diabetics with arteriopathy. Maximal intensity is higher compared with both groups, and disaggregation abnormalities (Fig. 2) are more frequent in diabetics than in the two other groups. Disaggregation is also impaired in non-diabetics with arteriopathy compared with the controls. With high dose ADP (1.2 μM) (Fig. 3), we find similar velocity values in the three groups, but diabetics exhibit higher aggregation maximal intensity. With collagen (Fig. 4), the aggregation pattern is the same in the three groups.

Factor $VIII_{RA\text{-}VWF}$ (Fig. 5) is normal in diabetics and in non-diabetics with lower limb arterial disease. Factor VIII_{AHF} levels are higher in the only diabetic group.

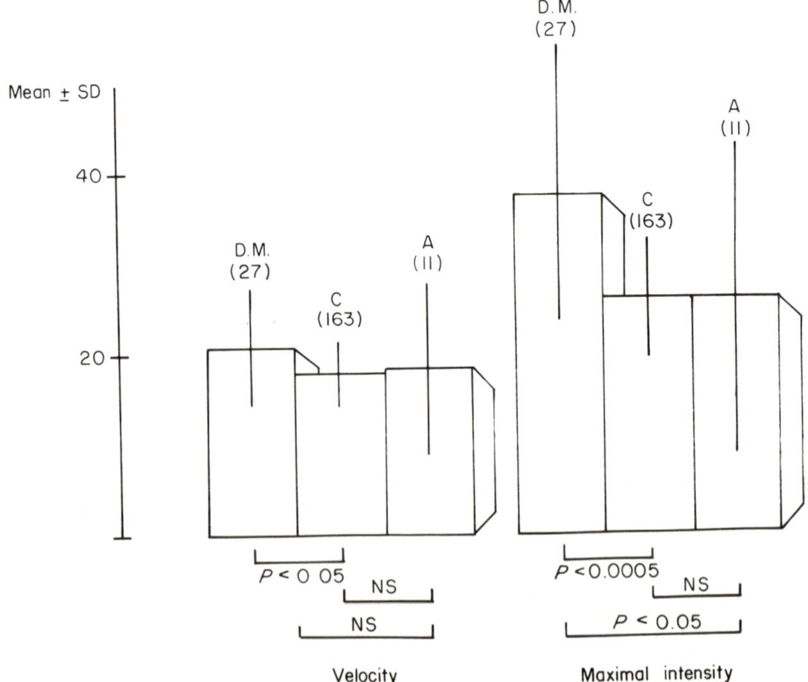

Fig. 1. Platelet aggregation ADP 0.6 μM.

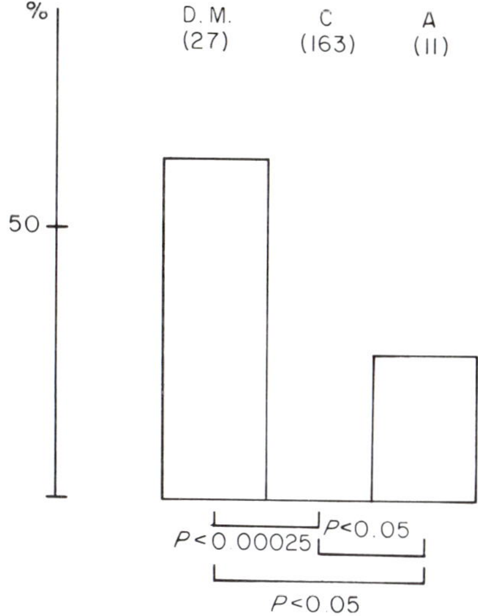

Fig. 2. Platelet aggregation ADP 0.6 μM; absence of disaggregation.

When diabetics are divided into two sub-groups, according to the severity of the vascular lesions (Table II), the less complicated patients (grade I–III) have the most striking aggregation abnormalities (Fig. 6) but no difference is found as far as factor $VIII_{RA\text{-}VWF}$ is concerned (Fig. 7).

No difference is found in the presence (18 cases) or the absence (nine cases) of hyperlipoproteinemia (type IIa and IIb), nor of hypertension.

DISCUSSION

This study demonstrates platelet hyperaggregation with ADP in diabetics when compared with control subjects and non-diabetics bearing the same vascular lesions. It is of interest to notice that the most obvious abnormalities are seen in the group without gangrene. This finding may suggest a preventive role for anti-aggregating agents. As we have seen platelets play also an important role in atherosclerosis (Ross *et al.*, 1974). Further studies are still in progress in our group: determination of *in vivo* platelet activity with beta thromboglobulin assay in plasma and in platelets, thromboxan B2 generation during thrombin aggregation. It is not possible at the present time to study plasma prostacyclin, as non-detectable levels are found with appropriate methods in normal subjects. This was clearly shown by Fernand Dray in the last meeting of the Mediterranean League against Thrombo-embolic Disease (Monte Carlo, October 23–25, 1980).

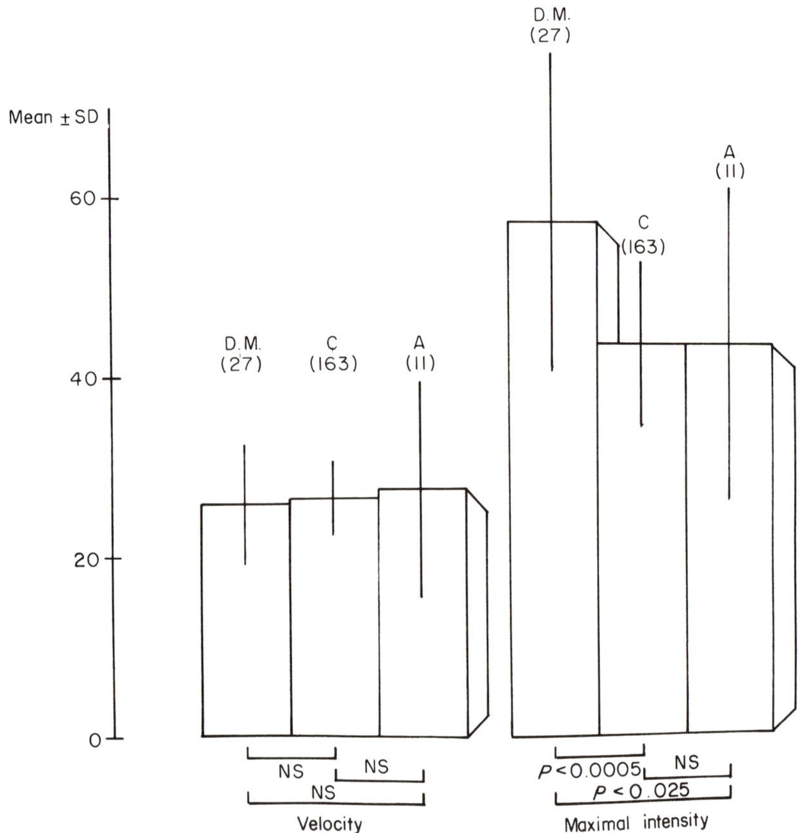

Fig. 3. Platelet aggregation ADP 1.2 μM.

MEDICAL TREATMENT

We have reviewed the pathogenetic basis of the atherosclerosis in diabetes mellitus in order to emphasize the important role of the prophylaxis. In fact, when angiographic studies are performed, arterial lesions are much too often beyond surgical treatment. However, surgical reconstructive procedures should be done in every case when possible.

Optimal glycaemic control must be achieved with insulin (two or three daily injections) or oral hypoglycaemic drugs. Self-monitoring now offers in insulin-requiring diabetes the greatest interest in this field. Body weight normalization, adequate diet and physical exercise are indispensable in all cases. Continuous subcutaneous insulin infusion with portable pump which realizes normal glycaemic profiles is of interest in acute complications (as toe infection) or during post-operative period in order to obtain a rapid healing.

But as we have seen, present administration routes of insulin do not prevent

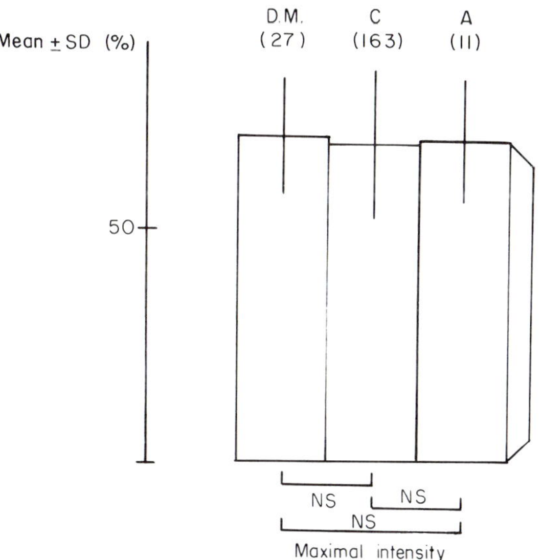

Fig. 4. Platelet aggregation: collagen.

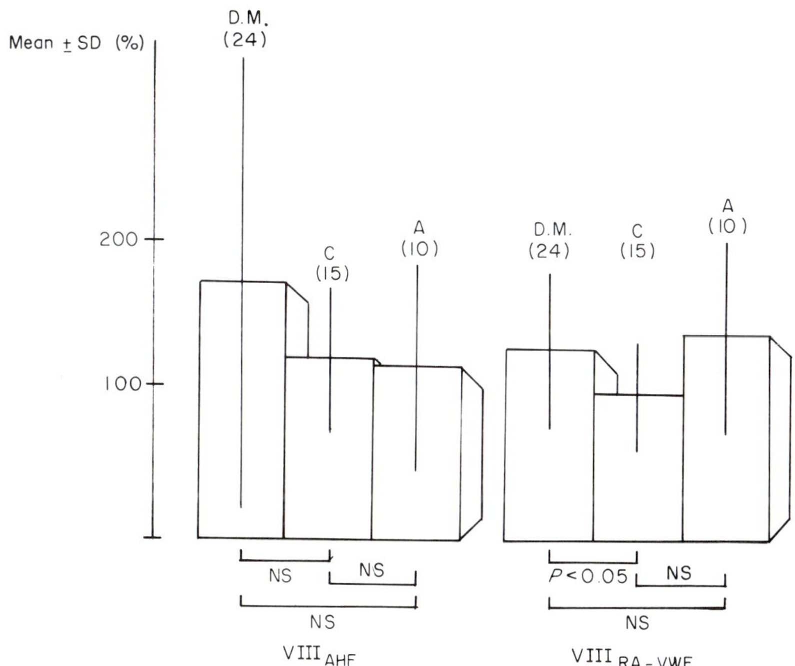

Fig. 5. Factor VIII.

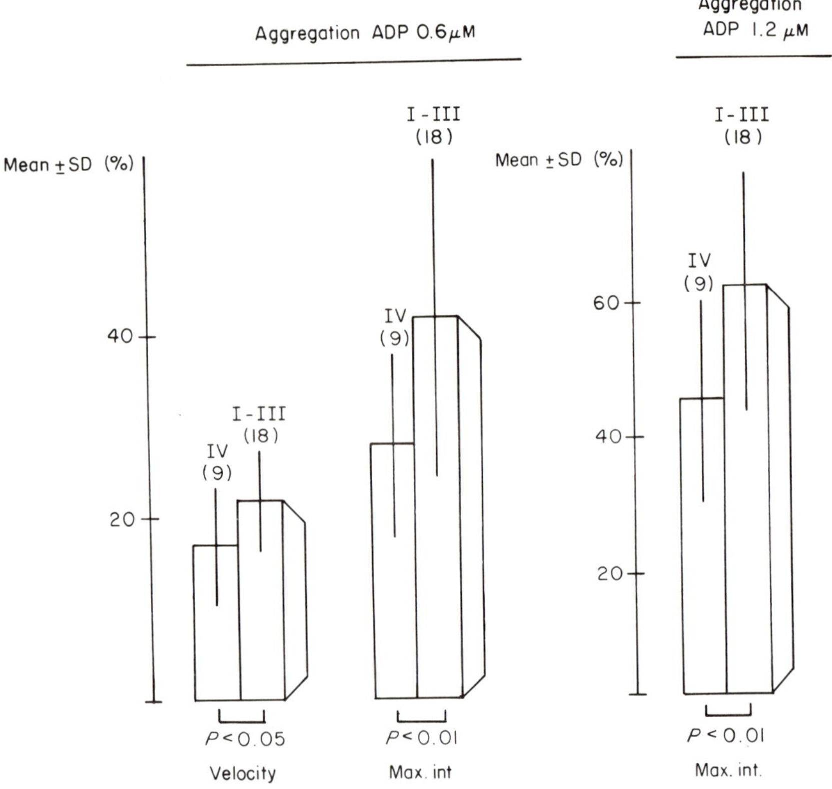

Fig. 6. Aggregation in diabetics according to the severity of the arteriopathy.

macroangiopathy, and new methods are needed in the future, as implantable delivery system with intra-portal insulin infusion or intra-portal islets graft.

Smoking must be forbidden as soon as diabetes is discovered.

Hypertension must be detected early in the careful management and treated. However two cautions should be stressed: avoid a severe blood pressure drop, which causes haemodynamic failure beyond stenotic lesions, and beta blocking agents when arterial disease is present, since these drugs could unmask alpha tonus and thus cause peripheral vasoconstriction.

There is no evidence in the literature of the efficacy of vasoactive drugs. Several authors favour the daily consumption of small quantities of brandy or whisky as vasodilators.

Search and treatment of lipoproteinemia when not controlled by metabolic control is an important point. There is in non-diabetics much evidence that correction of lipid disorders is a benefic preventive action. Polyunsaturated fat diet, clofibrate derivatives or cholestyramine should be used in these cases.

Acute complications such as acute leg ischaemia needs heparin therapy.

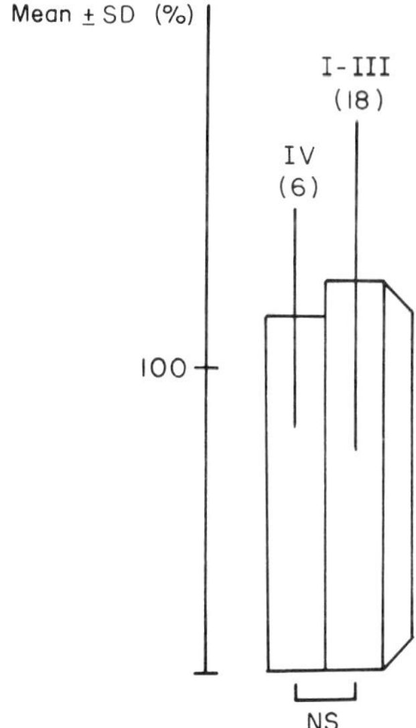

Fig. 7. Factor $VIII_{RA\text{-}VWF}$.

Long-term oral anticoagulant treatment should be reserved for the only patients with prosthetic vascular material.

Distal gangrene is often related to foot or toe infections. Prevention of these accidents is important in the educational programmes of diabetics. When such infection occurs, antibiotic treatment and heparin must be administered very early in order to avoid distal ischaemia secondary to oedema and lymphangitis.

Antiplatelet therapy is more attractive, including Aspirin, the association of Aspirin with dipyridamole, ticlopidine or gliclazide an hypoglycaemic sulfonylurea which corrects haemostasis disorders in diabetics (Ponari *et al.*, 1979).

Conflicting results have been reported in preventive use of anti-aggregating agents in non-diabetics. But we have shown that these patients have less platelet hyperactivity than diabetic subjects. Several prospective studies are in progress in diabetics with Aspirin dipyridamole in the United States (Emanuele *et al.*, 1981) and in France (DAMAD) or with ticlopidine (TIMAD).

Prostacyclin analogues might be helpful in the future (Editorial, 1981).

CONCLUSIONS

Prophylaxis of lower limb arteriopathy and generally of macroangiopathy in diabetics should play an important role in the treatment: adequate diet, physical exercise, reduction of risk factors (hypertension, hyperlipoproteinemia, haemostasis abnormalities).

New physiological means for optimal metabolic control are still needed. These actions may be of benefit in putting off the time of vascular complications.

Earlier clinical and plethysmographic detection in careful follow-up studies may permit angiographic studies and more reconstructive attempts at a time when the peripheral vascular bed is still suitable.

REFERENCES

Almer, L. O. and Pandolfi, M. (1976). Fibrinolysis and diabetic retinopathy. *Diabetes* **25** Suppl. 2, 807.

Badawi, H., El-Sawy, M., Mikhail, M., Nomeir, A. M. and Tewfik, S. (1970). Platelets, coagulation and fibrinolysis in diabetic and non-diabetic patients with quiescent coronary heart disease. *Angiology* **21**, 511.

Beach, K. W., Brunzell, J. D., Conquest, L. L. and Strandness, D. E. (1979). The correlation of arteriosclerosis obliterans with lipoproteins in insulin-dependent and non-insulin-dependent patients. *Diabetes* **28**, 836.

Bell, E. T. (1952). A post-mortem study of vascular disease in diabetes. *Archives of Pathology* **53**, 444.

Bensoussan, D., Levy-Toledano, S. and Passa, P. (1976). Anomalies de l'hemostase primaire au cours de la microangiopathie diabetique. *Nouvelle Presse Medicale* **5**, 2383.

Bern, M. M. (1978). Platelet functions in diabetes mellitus. *Diabetes* **27**, 342.

Colwell, J. A., Halushka, P. V., Sarji, K., Levine, J., Sagel, J. and Nair, R. M. G. (1976). Altered platelet function in diabetes mellitus. *Diabetes* **25**, Suppl. 2, 826.

Dupuy, E., Guillausseau, P. J., Gaudeul, P., Kartalis, G., Wild, A. M., Pastureau, A., Soria, C., Malbec, D., Duprey, J., Lubetzki, J. and Caen, J. (1979). Fonctions plaquettaires des diabétiques ayant une angiopathie. *Nouvelle Presse Medicale* **8**, 3123.

Editorial (1981). Prostacyclin in therapeutics. *Lancet* **1**, 643.

Elkeles, R. S., Wu, J. and Hambley, J. (1978). Haemoglobin A1, blood glucose and high-density lipo-protein cholesterol in insulin requiring diabetics. *Lancet* **2**, 547.

Emanuele, M. A., Buchanan, B. J. and Abraira, C. (1981). Elevated leg systolic pressures and arterial calcifications in diabetic occlusive vascular disease. *Diabetes Care* **4**, 289.

Fuller, J. H., Shipley, M. J., Rose, G., Jarrett, R. J. and Keen, H. (1980). Coronary-heart disease risk and impaired glucose tolerance. The Whitehall Study. *Lancet* **1**, 1373.

Ganda, O. M. P. (1980). Pathogenesis of macrovascular disease in the human diabetic. *Diabetes* **29**, 931.

Gorton, T., Castelli, W. P., Hjortland, M. C., Kannel, W. B. and Dawber, T. R. (1977). HDL as a protective factor against coronary heart disease. The Framingham Study. *American Journal of Medicine* **62**, 707.

Kannel, W. B. and McGee, D. L. (1979). Diabetes and cardiovascular Risk Factors: the Framingham Study. *Circulation* **59**, 8.

Ledet, T. (1976). GH stimulating the growth of arterial medial cells *in vitro*. Absence of effect of insulin. *Diabetes* **25**, 1011.

Lopez-Virella, M. F. L., Stone, P. and Colwell, J. A. (1977). Serum HDL in diabetic patients. *Diabetologia* **13**, 285.

Lubetzki, J. and Chebat, H. (1970). Incidence de l'Atherosclerose chez le diabetique. *Journées Annuelles de Diabétologie de l'Hôtel Dieu*, 259.
Lufkin, E. G., Fass, D. N., O'Fallon, W. M. and Bowie, E. J. W. (1979). Increased von Willebrand factor in diabetes mellitus. *Metabolism* **28**, 63.
Moncada, S. and Vane J. R. (1979). Arachidonic acid metabolites and the interaction between platelets and blood-vessel walls. *New England Journal of Medicine* **300**, 1142.
Nikkila, E. A. and Hormila, P. (1978). Serum lipids and lipoproteins in insulin-treated diabetes. *Diabetes* **27**, 1078.
Pirart, J. (1977). Diabètes et complications dégénératives. Présentation d'une étude prospective portant sur 4 400 cas observés entre 1947 et 1973. *Diabètes et Métabolisme (Paris)* **3**, 97 (1st part); 173 (2nd part) and 245 (third part).
Ponari, O., Civardi, E., Megha, S., Pini, M., Portioli, D. and Dettori, A. G. (1979). Anti-platelet effects of long term treatment with gliclazide in diabetic patient. *Thrombosis Research* **16**, 191.
Reckless, J. P. D., Betteridge, D. J., Wu, P., Bayne, B. and Galton, D. J. (1978). High-density and low density lipoproteins and prevalence of vascular disease in diabetes mellitus. *British Medical Journal* **1**, 883.
Ross, R. and Glomset, J. A. (1976). The pathogenesis of atherosclerosis. *New England Journal of Medicine* **295**, 369 (1st part) and 420 (2nd part).
Ross, R., Glomset, J., Kariya, R. and Harker, L. A. (1974). A Platelet-dependent serum Factor that stimulates the proliferation of arterial smooth muscle cells *in vitro*. *Proceedings of the National Academy of Sciences, United States of America* **71**, 1207.
Saudek, C. E. and Eder, H. A. (1979). Lipid metabolism in diabetes mellitus. *American Journal of Medicine* **66**, 843.
Stout, R. W. (1979). Diabetes and atherosclerosis — the role of insulin. *Diabetologia* **16**, 141.
Witzum, J. and Schonfeld, G. (1979). High density lipoproteins. *Diabetes* **28**, 326.

LOWER LIMB ARTERIOPATHY IN DIABETICS: SURGICAL STANDPOINT

R. Soyer

Department of Cardiac Surgery, Hôpital Charles Nicolle, Rouen, France

Lower limb arteriopathy in diabetics is characterized anatomically by three types of lesion.

(1) Proximal arterial lesions similar to those found in non-diabetics.
(2) Distal lesions affecting the arteriolo-capillary system, which are peculiar to this disease.
(3) Angioneuropathy.

These lesions can be isolated or associated with each other. Clinically, they will take on individual characteristics by their frequence and by the precocity of distal cutaneous lesions. Diabetes is effectively an aggravating factor whose high mortality rate is represented by vascular lesions (67%), coronary disease being the most significant (Janneau *et al.*, 1980; Kahn *et al.*, 1974), whereas acute metabolic complications represent only 1% mortality (Strandness, 1970). The causal relationship between metabolic problems and arterial lesions, particularly arteriolo-capillary lesions, has been postulated, but is contended, opinions differing between this concept and the possibility that there is no relationship between specific lesions and diabetes (Les Arteriopathies Diabetiques, 1975; Kahn *et al.*, 1974; Strandness, 1970; Tournigand *et al.*, 1974) (Table I).

The surgical problem is therefore the management of proximal lesions, but also of distal lesions in a patient who is always of advanced physiological age.

Serono Symposium No. 44, "Peripheral Arterial Diseases: Medical and Surgical Problems", edited by S. Stipa and A. Cavallaro, 1982. Academic Press, London and New York.

Table I. Arteriopathy of the lower limbs in diabetics.

1,800 operated cases	(%)
Coronary artery disease	30
Hypertension	30
Cerebro-vascular disease	15–20
Renal vascular disease	5–10
Associated diseases (>2)	30–40
Acute metabolic complication	1

The purpose of our study is to consider arterial lesions of the aorta down to distal arteries, and particularly reconstructive arterial surgery. Angioneuropathic lesions are not considered. We must insist on the fact that close and permanent collaboration between physician and surgeon is absolutely necessary.

The clinical symptoms of arterial occlusion or stenosis are well known (Les Arteriopathies Diabetiques, 1975; Tingaud *et al.*, 1973; Guilmet *et al.*, 1968). Arteriopathy in diabetics however, which reaches the same proportion in males and females, is generally more severe: it is complicated in 70–75% of cases by early distal cutaneous lesions, manifested clinically at first by small plaques of distal cutaneous necrosis. These lesions may remain localized distally, in which case prognosis is relatively good, or they may develop to gangrene. The main risk here is infection, the most extreme form being the diabetic phlegmon. In 1,800 cases, studied from the literature (Les Arteriopathies Diabetiques, 1975; Cecile, 1974; Fontaine *et al.*, 1971; Janneau and Cormier, 1980; Tingaud *et al.*, 1973, 1974), diabetic arteriopathy is characterized by the rapidity of its evolution (55–67% grade IV); 65–70% of these cases appear at this stage without any warning; only 30–35% are in stage II but even here, evolution is usually less than five years (Table II).

Table II. Arteriopathy of the lower limbs in diabetics.

1,800 operated cases — clinical findings		(%)
Trophic disturbances		70–80
Distal cutaneous necrosis		15–30
Gangrene		40
Diabetic phlegm		5–10
No trophic lesions		20–30
Evolution		
	Grade II	20–30
Four–five years		
	Grade IV	55–67

Surgically, it is necessary to know that there is no connexion between clinical gangrene and the importance of proximal and distal arterial lesions, and that arteriography is always essential. Unfortunately, in most cases reconstructive arterial surgery will be impossible, and can be attempted in only one case out of five. Arteriography, showing up proximal lesions but also the quality of the distal network, indicates whether or not reconstructive arterial surgery will be performed.

The predominance of distal arterial lesions in diabetics is a recognized fact (Les Arteriopathies Diabetiques, 1975; Tingaud *et al.*, 1973; Strandness, 1970; Tchobrousky *et al.*, 1974) (Table III). The arteriographic patterns are:

(1) The importance of vascular surcharge with many stenoses; it is often surprising to find such vessels still permeable.
(2) Iliac arteries are not affected.
(3) Femoro-popliteal axis is always stenosed but rarely thrombosed.
(4) The predominance of lesions at the level of the terminal part of the femoro-popliteal artery and of the leg arteries.
(5) Thrombosis is more frequent at this level. On rare occasions, one or two leg arteries are found to be injected.
(6) Another characteristic pattern, considered important by many authors (Cecile, 1974; Courbier *et al.*, 1976; Levy *et al.*, 1975; Van Der Stricht, 1969) is the damage to the deep femoral artery, which often presents a thrombosis of its distal part.
(7) The presence of important calcifications.

As well as these characteristic arterial aspects, we must also look for arterial lesions at the level of the aorta, iliac and femoral arteries, as these obviously increase distal disturbances by reducing the distal flow, immediately affecting arteriole capillaries. On the other hand, arteriole capillary lesions are much more difficult to appreciate from arteriography. The Doppler effect in diabetic arteriopathy enables us to show diminution of the distal flow and especially rigidity of the artery wall, and to estimate the degree of lesions of the proximal trunks. Unfortunately, the picture is not always so clear. In a very small number of patients, there will be no visible difference between diabetic and non-diabetic lesions and centrifugal evolution reaching arterial trunks. In most cases, however, diabetic lesions will rapidly extend to distal arteries without attaining the proximal trunks.

Table III. Arteriopathy of the lower limbs in diabetics.

1,800 operated cases — arteriographic findings	(%)
Disease of proximal trunks	12–20
Disease of femoral bifurcation deep femoral artery	60
Disease of distal network femoro-popliteal bifurcation	70–80

Three possibilities are open to the surgeon.

Reconstructive arterial surgery including thromboendarterectomy with angioplasty or not, prosthesis and distal bypass.

The indications and the results are the same at aortic and ilio-femoral levels whether the patient is diabetic or not. Unfortunately surgery is rarely advisable (Table IV).

Table IV. Arteriopathy of the lower limbs in diabetics.

1,800 operated cases — surgical technics	(%)
Reconstructive surgery	12–22
Thromboendarectomy	
Prosthesis	
Distal bypass (6%)	
Venous autograft	
Gore-tex + venous autograft	
Venous homograft	
Lumbar sympathectomy	45–57
Immediate amputation	15–30

At the level of femoral bifurcation in cases where there is a stenosis at the orifice of the deep femoral artery, often associated with a stenosis or a thrombosis at the orifice of the superficial femoral artery, it will be possible to carry out an endarterectomy of the common femoral artery prolonged into the deep femoral artery with a venous patch enlargement. This simple surgical technic is without risk and can be performed when distal network is relatively sound. For this reason, it will rarely be possible but may sometimes be associated with distal reconstructive surgery, which must also be carried out in presence of a sound distal network. As arteriography, and particularly peri-operative arteriography, remains the only means of assessment, it is difficult to appreciate its functional value. Distal anastomosis must always be performed on the distal part of the femoro-popliteal artery, when this is permeable, and when the distal network includes at least one or two sound leg arteries, otherwise it must be peformed on a leg artery. A thromboendarterectomy is, in fact, impossible at this level on calcified lesions. The femoro-popliteal bypass will be performed with a venous autograft which has been described widely in the literature (Cecile, 1974; Cormier, 1979; Garrett *et al.*, 1968; Kessler, 1971; Tchobrousky *et al.*,1974; Tingaud *et al.*, 1974). In some patients, venous autograft cannot be used; it can be replaced by the use of gore-tex + venous autograft or, which is perhaps better, a venous homograft (Les Arteriopathies Diabetiques, 1975; Levy *et al.*, 1975). The use of prosthesis is exclusively reserved for cases where there is no infection, unfortunately rare in diabetic arteriopathy. Proximal anastomosis is usually carried out just below the orifice of the superficial femoral artery by end-to-end anastomosis, associated or not with an endarterectomy. Distal anastomosis must always be performed from end to side, so as to divert the flow into branches above it.

LUMBAR SYMPATHECTOMY

Its effects have been widely analysed (Les Arteriopathies Diabetiques, 1975; Tournigand *et al.*, 1974; Van Der Stricht, 1970). It creates a state of vasodilatation which is permanent and irreversible. This vasodilatation is characterized at rest by a preferential distribution of blood to the skin and to subcutaneous cellular tissue of the lower extremity, foot and toes. It has a beneficial effect on the collateral compensatory circulation, induced by suppression of the peripheral resistance, thus increasing the pressure gradient. The importance of the permeability of the deep femoral artery is mentioned in several publications (Levy *et al.*, 1975; Tingaud *et al.*, 1973; Van Der Stricht, 1969, 1970). However, a certain percentage of failures (15–30% for grade II, more than 50% for grades III and IV) lead us to consider that lumbar sympathectomy does not always improve the blood flow to the distal arteries. We feel that angiography should be associated first with a certain number of circulatory dynamic tests which would show the reactivity of the vasomotor system: phlethysmography, isotopes (Les Arteriopathies Diabetiques, 1975), test with pentothal (Van Der Stricht *et al.*, 1974), hyperaemia test (Courbier *et al.*, 1976; Rettori *et al.*, 1979). Furthermore, lumbar sympathectomy is effective where there is an adequate vascular network, few or no lesions at aorto-iliac level, and good permeability of the deep femoral artery, which is not always the case in diabetic arteriopathy. When reactive hyperaemia is negative, lumbar sympathectomy can be tried only if there is no other alternative, either medical or surgical. Surgical treatment will often be either lumbar sympathectomy or immediate amputation or both, duc to the failure of medical treatment, the extent of the lesions, and the impossibility of carrying out reconstructive arterial surgery.

Lumbar sympathectomy reduces time of healing and protects the limb while reducing the risk of recurrence.

AMPUTATION

Amputation at leg or thigh level will be necessary in 15–30% of cases (Les Arteriopathies Diabetiques, 1975; Janneau *et al.*, 1980; Langeron and Mulliez, 1975). Distal excision, if necessary atypical, in 70–85% of cases leads to healing with preservation of weight bearing.

INDICATIONS

The indications for surgery must be carefully analysed. They depend on the human and clinical context, age, arteriographic findings and results of vascular dynamic tests, particularly after the age of 70.

Study of the 1,800 operated cases from the literature is difficult because information is not always given, and the criteria of assessment are not always comparable. We can, however, retain some points (Table V).

Table V. Arteriopathy of the lower limbs in diabetics.

1,800 operated cases — indications — results	Good results (%)	Amptuation (%)	Mortality (%)
No trophic lesions			
Immediate amputation 10–22%			3
Lumbar sympathectomy 45–55%	55–65	4	2–5
Reconstructive surgery 2–10%	72–84	3	2
Trophic disturbances			
Immediate amputation 15%			7
Lumbar sympathectomy 55%	35	15	4–7
Reconstructive surgery 10–22%	58	25	11

(1) Absence of trophic disturbances is rare. Only 2–10% (Les Arteriopathies Diabetiques, 1975; Fontaine *et al.*, 1971, Haimovici, 1967; Rettori *et al.*, 1979) of patients present proximal arterial lesions and may be treated by reconstructive procedure and, at the same time, lumbar sympathectomy. The result is the same in diabetics and non-diabetics (72–84% satisfactory results). In the remaining patients, lumbar sympathectomy may be performed where possible, but with a certain risk (2–5% mortality). This justifies a full analysis of the situation, and explains why some surgeons decide on immediate amputation after results of vascular dynamic tests. Lumbar sypathectomy gives 55–65% good immediate results but some failures in patients at grade II and IV.

(2) Trophic disturbances are found in the majority of patients. Here too, reconstructive surgery is rarely advisable at aortic and iliac level and the results are the same in diabetics and non-diabetics. Procedure at the femoral bifurcation is also an exception, the results depending on the quality of the distal network. It has the advantage of being simple and without risk. It can, in any case, be associated with reconstructive surgery of the femoro-popliteal bifurcation or leg arteries, which has been seen to have growing indications during the past few years. A careful analysis of the arteriographic findings permits a better assessment of the distal network. Bypass, with a venous autograft is the best procedure. It must be noted, however, that a venous autograft bypass on an unsound distal network can bring about the healing of a gangrene, but that a post-operative thrombosis will always result in amputation at thigh level; whereas a limited excision would have been possible in the first place. Lumbar sympathectomy can be associated with reconstructive surgery or, where the latter is impossible, to a limited excision. It obviates the necessity for major amputation and shortens healing time, but is totally inadvisable in angioneuropathy.

AMPUTATION

There is a high percentage of amputations in all the series (ranging from 27.7 to 30.4%). Unfortunately 12–15% of these must be performed immediately. In 22–28% of cases, amputation is the result of failure of conservative surgery. Limited excision is often possible (Les Arteriopathies Diabetiques, 1975; Fontaine *et al.*, 1971; Janneau and Cormier, 1980; Kunlin *et al.*, 1967; Van Der Stricht, 1969). The study of these series enables us to find a relationship between percentage of amputation and type of arterial lesions. In proximal lesions or in arteriopathy with no major trunk lesions, amputation was not necessary, whereas the percentage of amputations was very high in femoro-popliteal and leg artery diseases, though limited amputation was often possible in these cases.

CONCLUSION

Arteriopathy in diabetics is very serious because the lesions are often deeper and more widespread than in other patients and are highly susceptible to infection. The indications for surgery must be very carefully considered.

Few of the patients had lesions permitting reconstructive surgery which is thus only rarely indicated, though some authors are reconsidering distal reconstructive surgery.

In some patients with ischaemia disturbances, healing may be obtained after an appropriate surgical procedure (reconstructive surgery and/or lumbar sympathectomy), or by isolated excision. Unfortunately, in many cases, the only possible procedure remains amputation.

SUMMARY

The authors analyse the characteristics of arteriopathy in diabetics and undertake a full study of the angiographic findings in this disease.

Surgical procedures are described, particularly reconstructive arterial surgery; the major difficulty is consideration of the criteria of assessment of the distal network.

Lumbar sympathectomy, alone or associated with vascular reconstructive surgery, markedly increases the chances and shortens the time of healing in patients with ischaemic trophic lesions. The indications must be very carefully considered, especially in patients of over 70 years of age.

REFERENCES

Cecile, J. P. (1974). "L'artériographie du Pied. Journées Angéiologiques de Langue Française", p. 446. Paris, 13–15 mars 1974. Expansion scientifique, 1974.

Cormier, J. M. (1979). Chirurgie des artères distales des membres inférieurs. *In* "Actualités de Chirurgie Cardiovasculaire de l'Hôpital Broussais", p. 157. Masson, Paris.

Courbier, R., Jansseran, J. M., Reggi, M., Buril, T., Forlot, P. and Ifrgane, A. (1976). Résultats objectifs de la sympathectomie lombaire. Etude statistique fondée sur les épreuves fonctionnelles vasculaires. *Nouvelle Presse Medicale* **5**, 633.
Fontaine, J. L., Rezek, C. and Fontaine, R. (1971). Bilan de 289 lésions vasculaires dites diabétiques observées et traitées à la clinique chirurgicale de Strasbourg. *Journal de Chirurgie* **101**, 505.
Garrett, H. E., Kotch, P. I., Green, M. T., Dietrich, E. B. and De Bakey, M. E. (1968). Distal tibial artery by-pass with autogenous vein grafts. *Surgery* **63**, 90.
Guilmet, D., Brunet, A., Broc, A., Soyer, R., Gandjbakhch, I. and Dubost, Ch. (1968). Dérivation fémero-tibiale distale. Presse Médicale **76**, 589.
Haimovici, H. (1967). Patterns of arteriosclerosic lesions of the lower extremity. *Archives of Surgery (Chicago)* **918**, 95.
Janneau, D. and Cormier, J. M. (1980). La place de la sympathectomie lombaire dans le traitement des artérites diabétiques. *Journal des Maladies Vasculaire* **5**, 211.
Janneau, D., Lagneau, P. and Cormier, J. M. (1980). Les artériopathies diabétiques. Indications chirurgicales à propos d'une série de 416 cas. *Journal des Maladies Vasculaire* **5**, 115.
Kahn, O., Wagner, W. and Bessman, A. N. (1974). Mortality of diabetic patients treated surgically for lower limb infections and for gangrene. *Diabetes* **33**, 287.
Kessler, I. I. (1971). Mortality experience of diabetic patients. A twenty six years follow-up study. *American Journal of Medicine* **51**, 715.
Kunlin, J. *et al.* (1967). Vein grafts in arteritis obliterations of the popliteal artery or tibio-peroneal tract (technique and results). *Journal of Cardiovascular Surgery* **8**, 408.
Langeron, P. and Mulliez, Ph. (1975). "Les Divers Types d'Artériopathies du Diabète. Incidences Chirurgicales. Journées Angéiologiques de Langue Française", p. 137. Paris, mars 1975. Expansion scientifique, 1975.
Les Arteriopathies Diabetiques (1975). "Rapport au 9e Congrès du Collège Français de Pathologie Vasculaire Journées Angéiologiques de Langue Française", p. 13. Paris, mars 1975. Expansion scientifique, 1975.
Levy, J. B., Rettori, R. and Olivier, C. (1975). Indications et résultats du traitement chirurgical de l'artériographie diabétique. A propos de 196 cas. *Journal de Chirurgie* **111**, 547.
Quancard, X., Plagnol, Ph., Masson, B., Mamere, L., Janvier, G. and Tingaud, R. (1976). Problèmes posés par la chirurgie de restauration des artérites diabétiques. *Annales de Chirurgie* **30**, 147.
Rettori, R., Levy, J. B. and Olivier, C. (1975). "Indications et Résultats du Traitement Chirurgical de l'Artériopathie Diabétique. A Propos de 196 cas. Journées Angéiologiques de Langue Française", p. 117. Paris—mars 1975. Expansion scientifique, 1975.
Rettori, R., Levy, J. B. and Olivier, Cl. (1979). Place de la sympathectomie dans l'artériopathie diabétique. *Journal des Maladies Vasculaire* **4**, 277.
Strandness, D. E. (1970). Exercise testing in the evaluation of patient undergoing direct arterial surgery. *Journal of Cardiovascular Surgery* **11**, 192.
Tchobrousky, C., Assan, R., Tutin, M., Hautecouverture, M. and Slama, G. (1974). Comment faire progresser, la thérapeutique anti-diabétique. *Nouvelle Presse Medicale* **3**, 1379.
Tingaud, R. *et al.* (1973). Considérations sur l'artérite des membres chez le diabétique. *Bordeaux Medical* **6**, 105.
Tingaud, R., Masse, C., Boissieras, P., Baste, J. C. and Plagnol, Ph. (1974). Diabetic arteriopathies. *Journal of Cardiovascular Surgery* **15**, 54.
Tournigand, P., Dureau, A., Quilichini, F., Mercier, C. and Lena, A. (1974). Les artériopathies diabétiques: considérations cliniques et thérapeutiques; à propos de

155 malades. *Revue Française d'Endocrinologie* **11**, 395.

Van Der Stricht, J. (1969). De l'indication des sympathectomies à la lumière de l'épreuve radiothermométrique au Pentothal. *Revue de Médicine* **9**, 533.

Van Der Stricht, J. (1970). Indications chirurgicales en fonction du type d'artérite. *Angéiologie* **22**, 103.

Van Der Stricht, J., Ledant, P. and Vanhove, J. (1974). Diabetic arteriopathy. Nosologic entity. *Journal of Cardiovascular Surgery* **15**, 62.

ADVANCES IN THE MANAGEMENT OF FOOT PROBLEMS IN PATIENTS WITH DIABETES

G. M. Williams, R. T. Rolley and H. A. Pitt

Division of Transplantation and Vascular Surgery Service, The Johns Hopkins University School of Medicine, Baltimore, Maryland, USA.

Among the numerous complications of diabetes, foot problems are responsible for more days spent in the hospital (Pratt, 1975). Four pathophysiological processes contribute to this: (1) premature arteriosclerosis obliterans; (2) microangiopathy; (3) reduced resistance to infection and (4) peripheral neuropathy. In reviewing progress in the management of foot complications, each of these pathophysiological processes will be examined from the point of view of prevention and/or management.

PREMATURE ARTERIOSCLEROSIS OBLITERANS

Typical atherosclerosis is more common in diabetic than nondiabetic individuals and is thought to be the result of deranged lipid metabolism. Prevention of the atherosclerotic process is difficult because the physician can guide but not control his patient's diabetic management.

While typical aortic, iliac and femoral occlusive disease is present in the diabetic individual, there is a general consensus that the popliteal and tibial vessels are occluded more frequently than in the non-diabetic. At The Johns Hopkins Hospital we have found a particular propensity for the atherosclerotic process to involve the distal popliteal artery in black diabetic patients. The

Serono Symposium No. 44, "Peripheral Arterial Diseases: Medical and Surgical Problems", edited by S. Stipa and A. Cavallaro, 1982. Academic Press, London and New York.

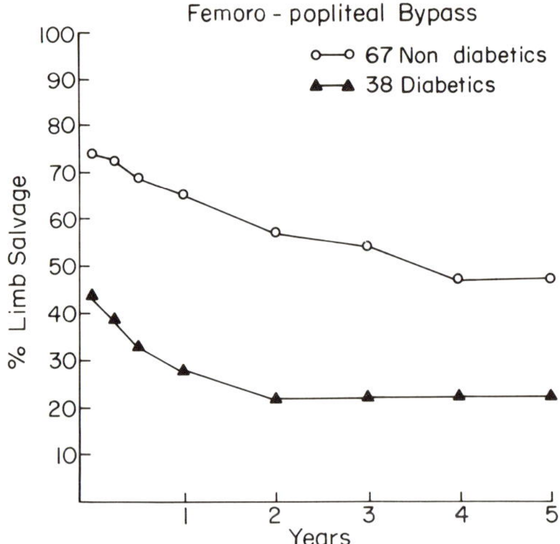

Fig. 1. Comparison of limb salvage rates in diabetic and nondiabetic patients.

frequently reported finding that diabetics fair worse following saphenous vein grafting for femoro-popliteal disease was confirmed in a recent study from our services shown in Fig. 1. When the results were analysed further, we found that the white diabetic undergoing femoral–popliteal bypass had results equivalent to the white nondiabetic patient. However, our results in black patients were very poor with only 9% of the patients undergoing saphenous vein femoro-popliteal bypass maintaining a viable limb one year later. However, when the saphenous vein graft was placed in a tibial or peroneal artery in the black diabetic, limb salvage rates were equivalent to the white nondiabetic having the more traditional procedure (Fig. 2). These data have led us to establish a policy of performing saphenous vein bypass grafts to any and all open arterial systems below the knee in diabetic patients threatened with loss of a foot.

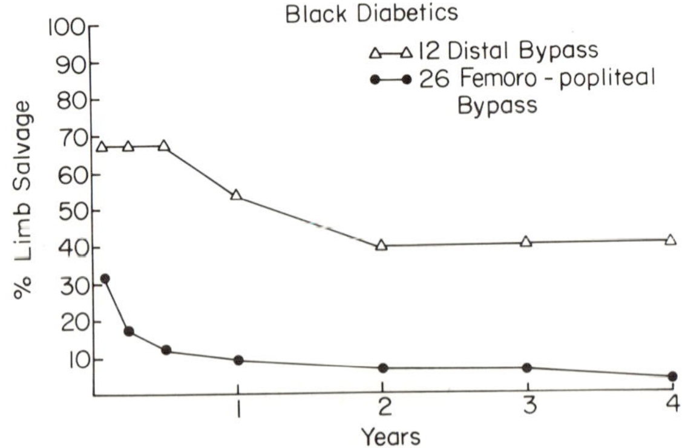

Fig. 2. Comparison of limb salvage rates achieved by femoral-popliteal and femoral tibial bypass grafts in the black diabetic patient.

MICROANGIOPATHY

This disease process distinguishes diabetics from other patients with vascular disease. It is responsible for the morbidity of blindness and for the mortality of nephropathy. It is possible that microangiopathy is responsible for degeneration of peripheral nerves and for the loss of articular sensation so common in the diabetic.

Microangiopathy is demonstrated by a particular localization of radioactive microspheres when they are injected intra-arterially at the time of arteriography. In patients with major vessel obstruction, the distribution of blood flow in the extremity is still largely to muscles. In the diabetic, the distribution is fairly distinctive with muscles receiving about the same degree of blood as joints.

While the microangiopathy undoubtedly contributes to the progression of ulceration and gangrene, particularly in the young diabetic, it is unwise for the physician to assume that this is the only major factor. We agree with Wagner (1978) that the principal problem is one of the larger vessel disease. He has demonstrated that if the ischemic index which is the ratio of pressure determined in the part in jeopardy to that present in the arm is greater than 0.45, 93% of diabetic patients will heal ulcers or gangrene with local amputations. Thus, modern surgery stresses the importance of bypass grafting to raise the perfusion pressure at the ankle as a prerequisite for healing.

INFECTION

Various types of defects in the immune response and in host resistance have been ascribed to diabetics (Hardwerger *et al.*, 1980). From the clinical point of view, it has been well established that the diabetic with an infection requires very aggressive medical and surgical therapy. Uncontrolled diabetes leads to defective immune responses which lead to infection which leads to greater difficulty in controlling diabetes. Prompt and wide drainage combined with meticulous control of blood sugar, frequent and conservative debridement and the appropriate use of antibiotics will generally result in cure if the ischemic index exceeds 0.7.

Evidence for this statement is obtained from a study of 53 patients admitted to The Johns Hopkins Hospital because of a foot infection. The presence or absence of diabetes was not associated with salvage of the foot. Rather, our inability to increase perfusion pressure and our failure to include full antibiotic coverage for the patient's organisms were the principal determinants of successful therapy. Of the 29 patients losing their limb, 86% had diminished perfusion pressure and 52% had incomplete antibiotic coverage (Table I).

NEUROPATHY

Loss of sensory nerves leads to lack of perception of painful stimuli and traumatic ulceration due to ill-fitting shoes, burns and ingrown toenails. It is

Table I. Factors influencing the salvage of limbs in patients with foot infections.

	Number of patients	
Factors	Major amputation (29)	Good outcome (24)
Decreased perfusion[a]	25–86%	6–25%
Diabetes mellitus	18–62%	13–54%
Mixed infection	11–38%	5–21%
Incomplete antibiotics[a]	15–52%	6–25%

[a]Significant at 0.05 level.

likely that combined defects in sensory nerves to joints and in motor nerves to the intrinsic muscles of the foot are responsible for the hammer-toe deformities. This deformity results in plantar deflection of the metatarsal heads, the formation of callus and eventual breakdown of the joint and skin. Controversy exists of how best to deal with these "neurotrophic ulcers". Many surgeons advocate resection of the metatarsal head resulting in a pseudoarthrosis and a straighter phalanx. On the other hand, the author has not seen a convincing demonstration of a serious plantar space infection originating from a "neurotrophic plantar ulcer". It is likely that this type of ulcer begins inside the joint as a sterile inflammatory process. The joint itself breaks down and is extruded through the callus. Sufficient sterile inflammation results from this process so that the communication through the skin is already walled off from surrounding tissues by firm fibrous tissue. Many of these lesions will heal if the patient is provided with properly fitting shoes or a metatarsal arch bar. Silvadene cream has proved to be a very effective antibacterial for long-term use in such patients. The best policy is to be either aggressive and excise the open lesion and joint or to be conservative. Local debridement breaks down the fibrous barrier and opens the way for serious infection.

CONCLUSIONS

In our experience, an aggressive approach in three areas offers the patient with diabetes an increased probability of surviving with intact lower extremities. While the ultimate solution to early atherosclerosis awaits correction of the fundamental metabolic abnormalities in diabetes, much can be accomplished by traditional or even heroic efforts to bypass occlusive lesions. If one can establish normal perfusion pressures in major arteries of the ankle and foot, the probability of healing a gangrenous digit or a serious infection is excellent.

However, healing will not occur without appropriate surgical drainage and debridement. With respect to the former, it must be extensive. The surgeon cannot control a plantar space infection even with appropriate antibiotics unless the drainage is wide and complete. The principles of drainage of the various spaces within the foot have been well described and our recent experience only validates the principles previously espoused.

There exists a mystique that diabetic foot infections are more serious and tend to have more peculiar bacteria than infections in nondiabetic patients. This is really not the case, provided that drainage and revascularization can be achieved. However, since most foot infections contain mixed flora, it is mandatory to provide coverage against Gram-positive bacteria, Gram-negative bacteria and anaerobic bacteria. We currently advocate the combination of a penicillin derivative, an aminoglycoside and either clindamycin or chloramphenicol.

The young surgeon is frequently discouraged by the appearance of the infected diabetic foot after one or two weeks of therapy. The final lesson learned by surgeons experienced in the care of the diabetic foot is that much patience is required. When granulations appear in some area of the wound, particularly at proximal areas, one can be confident that eventual healing will occur with daily care consisting of conservative debridement. Contrary to what has been written about the acceptance of split-thickness skin on the plantar surface of the foot, we have had excellent results, provided the patient is fitted with proper shoes once healing has occurred. Thus, five ingredients are necessary for the proper care of the diabetic with ischemia, gangrene or ulceration: (1) revascularization of major arteries; (2) drainage and debridement; (3) control of blood sugar; (4) broad antibiotic coverage and (5) persistence.

REFERENCES

Hardwerger, B. S., Fernandes, G. and Brown, D. M. (1980). Immune and autoimmune aspects of diabetes mellitus. *Human Pathology* **11**, 338.

Pratt, R. C. (1975). Gangrene and infection in the diabetic. *Medical Clinics of North America* **49**, 987.

Wagner, F. W. (1978). The diabetic foot and amputations of the foot. *In* "DeVries' Surgery of the Foot" (Roger A. Mann, Ed.). C. V. Mosby, St. Louis, Missouri.

During the Symposium the following communications were presented.

G. Zannini, G. C. Bracale, E. Contieri, P. Rocco and B. Amato
"Treatment and results of abdominal aortic aneurysms surgery"

C. Spartera, E. Pastore, A. Zaccaria, M. Ventura and G. R. Pistolese
"Considerations on the causes of mortality in ruptured abdominal aortic aneurysms"

G. Marinelli, A. Pierangeli, P. Panisi and B. Turinetto
"Our experience on infra-renal aneurysms of abdominal aorta"

R. De Nunno, F. Prestipino and A. Bertolini
"Ruptured aneurysms of the abdominal aorta"

M. Guastamacchia, G. Cianfanelli, B. Borreani, E. Zepponi and L. Brizio
"Ruptured aneurysms"

P. Bigazzi, A. Tacconi, F. D'Angelo, M. Maggi, F. Zucco, B. Puglisi and B. Mattassi
"Four cases of abdominal aortic aneurysms ruptured in caval vein. Therapeutical behaviour and results"

A. Pouché, S. M. Giulini, A. Lazzarini and G. Tiberio
"Luetic aneurysms of infrarenal abdominal aorta"

S. Lo Scudo, G. Rabitti, B. Ragusa, G. Gentili and G. Chidichimo
"Dissecting aneurysms of the aorta"

F. Giordanengo, P. Mingazzini, S. Miani and E. De Carlis
"Femoral anastomotic false aneurysm (ethiologic and therapeutic patterns)"

A. Agresti, F. Lo Schiavo and F. Freda
"Indications and limits of axillary-femoral by-pass in lower limb chronic ischaemia"

G. P. De Riu and E. Ballotta
"Routine use of by-pass distal anasthomosis on patch enlarged arteriotomy in tibial and leg small arteries reconstruction"

P. Cavaliere, G. Orsi, S. Camera, A. Schirru, D. Panero and C. Ferrari
"Retrospective appraisal of long-term results in over 200 surgical treatments of arterial diseases"

A. Tacconi, F. Miele, F. D'Angelo, R. Mattassi and P. Bisetti
"Modified bovine carotid artery as heterologous arterial graft"

B. Gozzetti, E. Gizzi, P. Marini, R. Massa and F. Benedetti Valentini, Jr.
"Homologous vein grafting for arterial reconstructions in the lower limbs"

G. Motta, G. B. Ratto, E. Spinelli and M. Leonardi
"Clinical experience in vascular reconstructions with processed human umbilical vein (Meadox-Dardik biograft)"

P. M. Mikus, G. Arpesella, L. Forlani, V. De Rosa, P. Bacchini, L. Tabacchi, R. Brioli, A. Zanoni, M. Cassani and A. Pierangeli
"The preservation of the homologous saphenous vein: is it possible an alternative solution to the glutaraldeheyde in theory?"

A. Argenteri, A. Bagliani and R. Moia
"Surgical experience in Buerger's disease"

S. Miani, R. Piglionica, M. Cugnasca and P. Pelli
"Present knowledge and current views on Buerger's disease"

G. Carmenini, V. Di Giacomo, F. Meloni, F. Di Maio and A. Sciacca
"Diagnostic criteria for Buerger's disease"

V. Di Giacomo, F. Meloni, G. Carmenini, D. Leonori and C. Kamaris
"Giant cell arteritis: is the term to maintain?"

F. Ippolito and A. Di Carlo
"Telethermography with cryostimulation in the study of microangiopathies"

A. Tribulato, A. Lombardo, A. Spitaleri, S. Musumeci, N. Sozzi and A. Giovinetto
"Behaviour of some hemorreological and hemocoagulative parameters in Raynaud's syndrome"

G. M. Andreozzi, S. Signorelli, V. Magnano, D. Tornetta and F. Sorrentino
"Pharmacological simpathectomy in the therapy of the POAD (preliminary results)"

S. Mansueto
"Rickettsial arteritis: our experience"

C. Allegra, G. Pollari, A. Criscuolo and V. Tonelli
"Preclinical diabetes revealed by rheography and capillaroscopy"

A. Bagliani, R. Moia and M. Salvini
"Surgical therapy of diabetic lower limb arteriopathy"

F. Giordanengo, P. Mingazzini, D. Gai and L. Franch
"Impotence in the diabetic patient (diagnostic research)"

A. Agresti, C. D'Antonio and P. Petronella
"Diabetic foot: conservative surgical treatment"

M. Cagetti, S. Scattone, R. Staico and G. Garau
"Diabetes and chronic ischemia of the lower extremities. Therapeutic indications and surgical treatment"

And the following posters were exposed.

A. Agresti, A. Fontanarosa, P. Petronella and F. Lo Schiavo
"Complications in axillo-femoral by-pass"

G. F. Azzena, R. Alvisi, A. Guberti, P. Mondini, N. G. Cavallesco and S. Pollice
"The back pressure of the profunda femoris as haemodynamic value of distal run-off"

B. Borreani, G. Cianfanelli, M. Guastamacchia, L. Brizio and E. Zepponi
"Our experience on infrarenal aortic aneurysm surgical treatment"

L. Brizio, G. Cianfanelli, B. Borreani, M. Guastamacchia and E. Zepponi
"Our experience with the treatment of real and false aneurysms of peripheral arteries"

F. Castaldo, V. Trombetta and A. Cavallaro
"Traumatic aneurysms of thoracic aorta"

P. Cavaliere, G. Orsi, S. Camera, A. Schirru, D. Panero and C. Ferrari
"Arteriosclerotic multiple-aneurysms disease. A case report"

S. de Franciscis, C. Coviello and L. Scaramuzzino
"The doppler in the diagnosis of acute arterial thrombosis"

V. Di Giacomo, A. Cavallaro, F. Meloni, G. Carmenini, M. Garofalo and A. Sterpetti
"Subclavian steal syndrome in a case of Takayasu's arteritis with multiple vascular localizations and with late clinical beginning"

V. Di Giacomo, F. Meloni, A. Cavallaro, V. Sciacca, D. Leonori and G. Carmenini
"Syphilitic aetiology of some aneurysms of abdominal aorta"

M. Garofalo, A. Sterpetti, L. Di Marzo, A. Mingoli and A. Cavallaro
"The diabetic foot"

G. Gozzetti, F. Spigonardo, G. Belcaro and L. Bonomo
"Diagnosis of aortic aneurysms by CT scanning"

A. Agresti, C. D'Antonio, F. Lo Schiavo, V. Argenzio and F. Freda
"Microsurgery in the surgical treatment of diabetic foot"

S. Miani, F. Giordanengo, P. Mingazzini and A. Odero
"Leakages of abdominal anastomosis after arterial reconstruction"

G. Motta, G. B. Ratto, E. Spinelli, C. Lunghi, M. Tomellini, R. Agati, G. Poloniato and A. Sacco
"Morphological findings of Meadox-Dardik biograft inner surface: an experimental study by light and SEM"

F. Pancrazio, R. Adovasio and P. Pietri
"Evaluation of a laminar airflow system in the prevention of synthetic vascular grafts infections"

A. Petrassi, A. Scarpelli, P. Formisani, A. Lannello and L. Aiello
"Local area treatment with urokinase of obstructive arterial disease of limbs"

C. Pratesi, A. Alessi Innocenti, V. Lazzeri and G. Credi
"About visceral aneurysms: report of a case of post-traumatic celiac tripod aneurysm"

P. Rubba, A. Iannuzzi, B. Amato and G. C. Bracale
"Increase in calf arterial flow at rest after by-pass surgery"

L. Scaramuzzino, C. Coviello and S. de Franciscis
"The doppler in the femoral-popliteal by-pass"

A. Sterpetti, M. Garofalo, S. Cisternino and A. Cavallaro
"PTFE prostheses in leg arteries reconstruction"

The papers are published by Editor L. Pozzi (Rome) in a special issue of the Journal Policlinico sez. *Chirurgica* **88**, 1981.

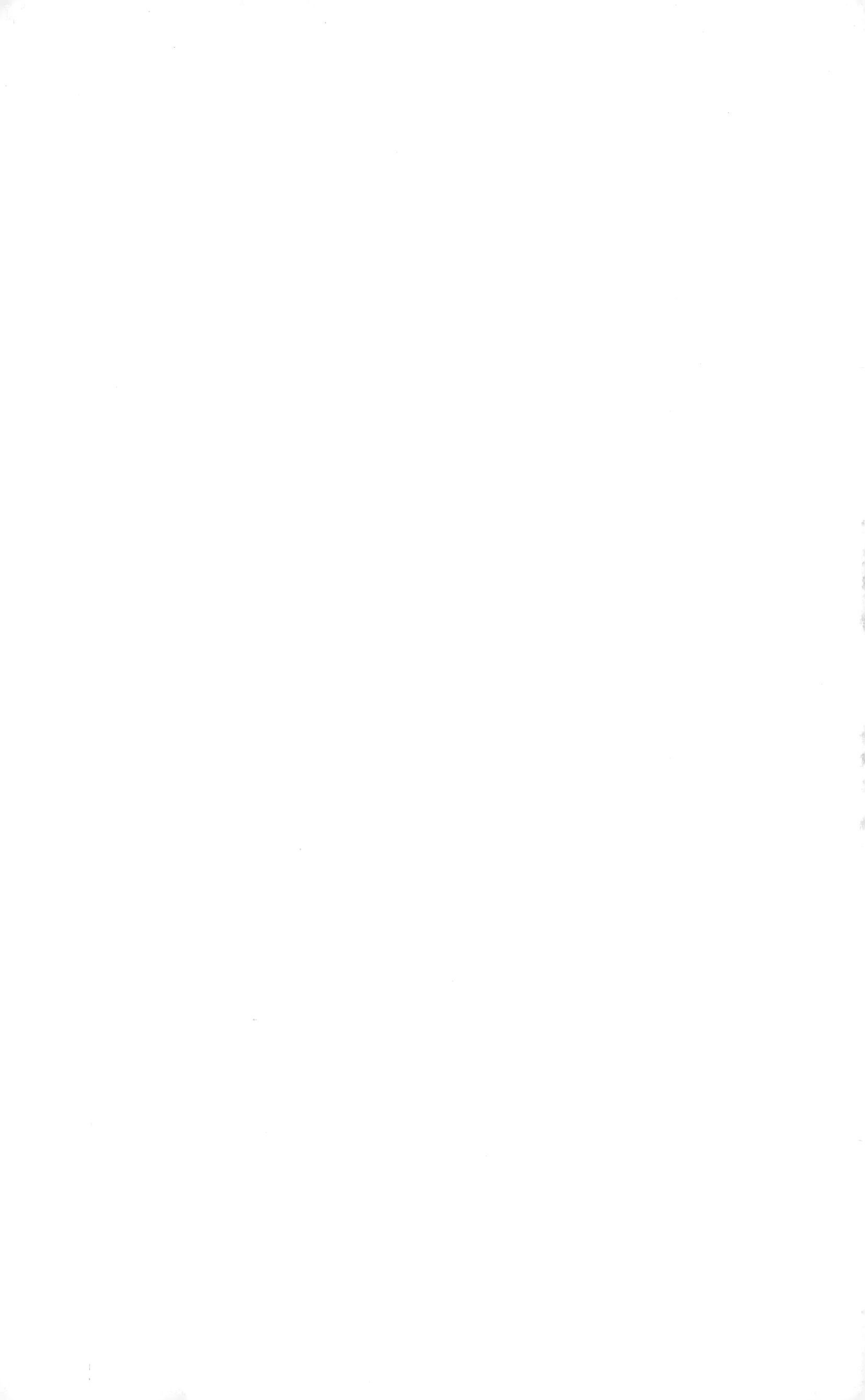